# HEAL THE HURT CHILD

# HEAL
# THE
# HURT
# CHILD

*An Approach through Educational*
*Therapy With Special Reference to*
*the Extremely Deprived Negro Child*

BY HERTHA RIESE, M.D.

FOREWORD BY
NATHAN W. ACKERMAN

**THE UNIVERSITY OF CHICAGO PRESS**

CHICAGO & LONDON

Library of Congress Catalog Card Number: 62–19623
The University of Chicago Press, Chicago and London
The University of Toronto Press, Toronto 5, Canada

© 1962 by The University of Chicago. All rights reserved
Published 1962. Third Impression 1967
Printed in the United States of America
Designed by Adrian Wilson

# FOREWORD

In child guidance today there is surely no scarcity of new publications; if anything, the trend is the other way, toward a plethora of books and articles that spreads over the entire landscape. But this book is a different one; it is, in fact, unique. So far as I know, it is the first offering of a comprehensive program to heal the hurts of the rejects of our society, the deprived children of destitute Negro families. It describes a method of "educational therapy" developed by the author over a period of twenty years at the Educational Therapy Center in Richmond, Virginia.

Twenty-five years ago, Lawson G. Lowrey said to a group of us working in child guidance: "There are many books on the psychopathology of children, but there is not a single definitive work on child psychotherapy." Clearly, this is no longer the case today. The literature is a growing one. The journals are filled to the brim with such writings, and there are now respectable tomes devoted to the problems of child psychotherapy. Despite this spate of published material, we are nonetheless faced with a strange contradiction. Lowrey's challenge of a quarter a century ago was an astute one. Its essence is pertinent to the situation today almost as it was then. In some deeper sense, despite the merit of recent contributions, we do not even now have a definitive work on the methods of child psychotherapy. We cannot assert a valid claim to the achievement of an integrated system of child psychotherapy, nor can we yet be proud of the results of the treatment of disturbed children. They are none too good.

Both in theory and in practice, the secret of a truly effective child psychotherapy still eludes us. It is like the game of hide-and-seek. We are getting warmer, we come ever closer to the place where the treasure is hidden, but we have not yet discovered it. The findings of this present study on educational therapy of the extremely deprived child, noteworthy in their own right, affirm this conclusion.

The author of this work, Dr. Hertha Riese, writes as a sensitive artist paints a canvas. She has that rare combination of the competent scientist and the gifted artist. With the flow of her sensitive pen, she vividly depicts the hunger, the aloneness, pain, fright, and anger of the deprived Negro child. She does not visualize the hurt child alone and apart; rather, she draws a picture of the misery of the child within the panorama of the miseries of the whole way of life of the destitute Negro family. The child is the end product of a culture of poverty and degradation. The destitute Negro family of the South does not live; it exists. "Life is not lived; it is undergone." The distress and disablement of the disadvantaged Negro subculture is a festering sore on the back of the parent society. It is the disorganized, depressed, "dirty" fringe of the larger community.

The hurt child is the product of this oppressed way of life, a hand-me-down of sickness and disorder of three or four generations in the destitute Negro community. Sixty per cent of these families are one-parent families, by death, desertion, divorce, separation or by reason of no marriage. Illegitimacy is not merely frequent; it is almost the rule. Families of six or seven children with changing fathers is a frequent pattern. In the larger community, the father is a nonentity. He is valued not as a person but only for his service as "handyman": no work, no status. Within his own home he is denigrated for non-support. All too often, out of sheer despair, he deserts. The mothers escape into drink and sex. By the standards of the white community, these women are promiscuous. By the standards of their own subculture, they are merely seeking surcease from an agonizing loneliness. By the conventions of the white community, these mothers seem to neglect their children and yet, paradoxically, they are frequently warm and devoted.

The child in such a family is emotionally stultified; he is oppressed, depressed, isolated, and withdrawn. He is in despair; his hope is crushed; he is frightened, suspicious, and angry. He is out of touch with his world. In episodic bursts, he makes contact by means of an aggressive assault on his surroundings. He cannot communicate except through an inner language, the primitive language of the emotions and of the body. He is retarded in learning. He is frozen emotionally and socially. He is flighty, shallow, evasive. He lives only in the present. He bashes his head against a world which seems not to care about him. In every sense, this is a condition of arrested emotional development.

Interestingly enough, the author chooses not to throw into sharp relief the obvious, the difference in skin color. She does not "find the Negro-ness of the child," as such. It is there, but of itself it seems to fade into dim consciousness. Instead, she emphasizes in the most poignant way, the signs of aloneness, fright, and the desperate lashing out of a severely deprived child. Clearly, the implications of this point of view extend far beyond the confines of the Negro subculture, as important as this is in itself.

Several conclusions, based on the author's twenty-year study, stand out sharply. Contrary to the traditional position of child guidance, the extremely deprived child is in no sense "untreatable." To pin these children with the label "untreatable" is, at the very least, a misconception. Beyond that, it is an instance of discrimination of a subtle kind, which nonetheless has devastating consequences. Scientifically, it is simply not so that such children are untreatable. It is grossly misleading to expect a Negro child, reared in an extraordinarily disordered and depriving environment, to fit into a pattern of child-guidance procedure, predetermined to meet the needs of children of intact and economically capable families. What else can one anticipate, except that the lost Negro child must reject a stereotyped guidance program as being utterly unsuited to his special needs. To characterize such children as untreatable is a crude and unfair indictment. It is one dramatic example of deluded professional thinking and inappropriate professional practice. When a standard treatment technique is applied in a stereotyped manner and is given priority over the unique quality of a human problem, the value of psychological specificity is completely lost. The treatment procedure must inevitably miscarry in such circumstances. As in every branch of the healing profession, a correct understanding of the specific nature of the human problem is the primary responsibility; after that comes the development of an appropriate method of treatment. Within this framework, diagnosis is primary, therapy is secondary. In child guidance, our obligation is surely to fit the therapeutic method to the needs of the child, rather than to force the child to submit to a preordained procedure.

The findings of this program at the Educational Therapy Center demonstrate not only that these children are treatable, but rather much more. They can be salvaged socially as well as psychiatrically. In times past, a high percentage of such children, unresponsive to traditional child guidance practices, were committed to a training school. Admission to a training school is a euphemistic phrase which means "serving time" in a reform institution. As the author shows, in many instances this extreme measure can be prevented. However, prevention of such commitment can be accomplished only under special conditions. An effective program requires total care for the total child within his total life situation. This is more than therapy. It is no less a task than changing a whole way of life. It means protection, support, education, and, finally, psychotherapy. It demands continuous concern with the needs of survival, the patterns of social training and sustained support for the creative unfolding of these children. It necessitates a comprehensive program for the psychosocial support of the entire family unit, as well as for the child. In its basic orientation, total care of this kind merges the goals of social support, education, therapy, and prevention.

The case for such a program is amply documented in this volume. Within a special segment of the human community, the author illustrates the profound interconnection of social disorder and mental disorder. The two categories of failing adaptation are not the same, but the overlapping of one with the other is profound. A condition of persistent social disorganization leads ultimately to mental disorganization. The psychiatric deviations of these children are the end result of a perpetuated pattern of social disorder in these families. The children are the victims of a "culture of poverty."

The lesson learned in the prodigious labor of rescuing the starved and hurt Negro child has a far wider application. It points sharply to the deficiencies of theory and practice in the whole field of child guidance. The principles demonstrated in this study are pertinent to the emotional problems of the deprived child in every segment of society, white or dark, rich or poor. When a helpless child is maimed, hurt, or caused to suffer, all of society feels distressed. Unconsciously, every member of the community takes his share of guilt and blame. In our heart of hearts and in secret silence, each of us feels we have a part in causing this suffering. We are secretly ashamed that our community makes scapegoats of these children. They are the tragic victims of our competitively driven social pattern. The hurt of the parents is visited upon the children. A generation back, the parents were the hurt children. It goes on and on.

But what do we do about it? Each of us carries a private guilt. The more guilty we feel, the less we are prone to assume a realistic responsibility. We turn our face away from the pain of it. Each of us feels defensively the urge to deny and project the guilt and blame.

When an innocent child is afflicted with mental suffering, whom shall we accuse and punish—the child himself, his mother, his family, or society at large? Curiously enough, we find in this study that the child turns all the blame on himself. Society either turns its face away, or points an accusing finger at the mother. The mother may turn about to attack the father. The father may assume the blame or turn against the mother and the child and desert. This is passing the buck on a truly grand scale.

In a strange way, we professionals, being a part of this culture, get caught in the same vicious cycle. We unconsciously participate in a process of emotional scapegoating of a segment of the human community and in a tendency to set one part of the family against another. If, instead, we faced the pain and shame squarely and assumed a realistic responsibility for this human distress, we would be less tempted, unwittingly, to comply with and fortify this unrational trend toward scapegoating of helpless people.

The conflict, fear, pain, and disablement of the deprived Negro child cannot be his struggle alone. It can only be the struggle of the child joined to those people with whom he shares a way of life and who care enough to ally with him in the battle for life and health. The psychiatry of children cannot grow by itself. It can only move ahead as we develop along a parallel path an effective psychiatry for the family and for the whole community. As I have said elsewhere, in the years ahead, we shall be talking less of child psychiatry and rather more of family psychiatry. We must modify our perspectives. We must recognize that our traditional conception of a child as individual is both incomplete and inaccurate. The child is part of the family and the family is part of the child. The processes of individuation of child personality emerge within the broader matrix of the twin processes of emotional joining and separation in family bonds. The deviant components of child development can then be better understood within the larger frame of total development; the sick parts can be seen in relation to the preserved healthy parts of growth, both in the child and in his family. We need now to shift here from the more or less exclusive emphasis on the study and treatment of the single patient to the study and treatment of clusters of persons who share identity, emotions, and a whole way of life. Only in this way can we merge the goals of therapy and prevention. We need, therefore, a new set of mental health practices which approaches child and family as an indivisable unity.

Dr. Riese's work is an admirable start in this direction and should point the way for others who work with less dramatic aspects of the emotional disturbances of children.

NATHAN W. ACKERMAN, M.D.

# PREFACE

One of the vital problems facing any society that calls itself democratic and humanitarian is the relationship between the individual and that society. How much conformity can the latter impose on the individual in order to sustain the complex web of human relations and how much freedom must the individual preserve for his own well-being and for the development of his full potentialities? What happens when an injurious imbalance sets in, when society overwhelms the individual? These are the questions which the social and behavioral sciences are attempting to answer. The purpose of this book is to point up these problems and to indicate one method of their solution, or, at least, alleviation, in one special area: the emotionally disturbed, the neglected, or hostile children and, particularly, such Negro children of the South.

It must be clarified at this point that I do not want this to be considered a study exclusively of the deprived Negro child—it is, strictly speaking, a study of the child in socioeconomic destitution. Furthermore, in my many years of work with the Negro child, I have not found "the Negro" in him. What I found was a greater despondency than in the white child, a deeper muteness when in a state of depression, also a deeper hopelessness that talking will not help. Because of greater hopelessness generally, the adolescent Negro boy may resort to expressions of violent despair. But all such more marked negative attitudes are not caused by any "Negro-ness" in these young people—it is generated by particularly damaging pressures and deprivations imposed on them as Negroes.

This book stems from the experience of eighteen years of work with such children in the Educational Therapy Center in Richmond, Virginia. It intends to transmit this experience as plastically as possible without becoming a textbook. It may hopefully serve as an indication of what the method used in this setting can accomplish; professionals, as well as intelligent and concerned laymen, may find it helpful to retrace with us our steps and convince themselves of the possibilities of progress with children who have largely been abandoned and considered beyond help.

We shall focus a searchlight on the conditions under which these children try to grow up and how they feel, or, in other terms, we shall look into their lives as the workshop within which their emotional disturbance was forged and explain their treatment as well as suggest general preventive measures.

This book may be regarded as a basis for exchanging experience rather than as a scientific treatise. It is meant for a wide public and not only for professionals concerned with the complex work with emotionally disturbed children. As an individual the reader is not unaffected by the problem, and, as a citizen who feels some responsibility for the welfare of his country, he seeks enlightenment. Therefore, an attempt is made to speak to all potential readers simultaneously. The professional idiom is avoided as far as possible and desirable. Histories, testimonies, recordings or interpretations are stated in such a manner that the professional reader will understand the technical implications. But I also had a reason intrinsic to the therapeutical attitude, which deterred me from spelling out diagnoses and from using classificatory terms.

As a matter of regular procedure, the Educational Therapy Center, now a clinic of the Department of Mental Hygiene and Hospitals, has to include in its monthly reports the diagnosis reached in every referral. While we do not lose sight of the diagnosis and while the child is likely to keep us cognizant of it, we do not allow the diagnosis to "stigmatize" the child and thus to deprive him of the full impact he may have on us as a living and struggling youngster. He is in communication with us by his total behavior. His behavior reflects his environment, his relationships and interactions. It is into the child's moving and changing life that we have to penetrate and in so doing try to exercise a salutary influence. The diagnosis may be discouraging, the revealed background forbidding. But we have found that even the most withered and twisted life can still unfold itself when appropriately tended to. Therefore, we have not allowed our efforts to relax under the pressure of a clinically unfavorable diagnosis. With the proper efforts even the diagnosis may change.

Avoiding technical terminology, we have perhaps indulged in a type of writing more appropriate to intuitive rather than to discursive thinking, particularly in trying to convey an immediate insight into the children's experience. Often language imbued with imagery is more expressive of the child's thoughts, feelings, and reactions. Scientific language cannot be but a somewhat cold approximation. The child uses discourse in thought and speech as a rule only for communication with the adult world. But should we not try to reflect the child's own experience in the most authentic terms?

An attempt to help these children necessarily entails a modification of criteria, including those of treatability and methods. It also entails the willingness to endure emotionally as well as economically the violent and unpalatable manifestations of exasperation and suffering, as well as the criticism, and at times even scorn, of a community that reacts rejectingly, to the hurt children's persistent undoing.

The first faltering steps leading up to the founding of the Educational Therapy Center, and its subsequent painstaking growth, have involved the interest and dedication of a number of concerned and civic-minded individuals, without whose interest and dedication it never would have come into existence and continued to develop. The Center began its work in 1943 as a private foundation. At the beginning I was its only worker. I conceived the idea for such a project when I assisted as a volunteer at the Juvenile and Domestic Relations Court, in Richmond, Virginia. Soon I was fortunate enough to find a small group of interested citizens who, under the inspiring leadership of Mrs. Kitty Dennis, carried the Center administratively and financially, until Dr. Joseph E. Barrett, the commissioner of the Department of Mental Hygiene and Hospitals, invited us to affiliate with his department, under the Mental Health Act of 1947. The affiliation took place in 1948. Commissioner Barrett's staunch support throughout his years of service was a constant source of uplifting encouragement.

The story of the Center's growth, its connections with other agencies, and the various and varying sources of financial support will be told elsewhere in this book. However, it is here that we want to state, with deepest gratitude and conviction, that the arduous up-hill struggle against prejudice and partial original unacceptance would not have been successful without an unusually inspired, determined, and devoted staff, some of whose members have been employed by the Center ever since its affiliation with the Department of Mental Hygiene and Hospitals. In this connection, Miss Ethel Banks deserves special mention: on our staff since 1948, she has, since 1955, fulfilled with tact and wisdom the task of supervising the teachers and co-ordinating the therapeutic and educational work. She has also voluntarily helped with the preparation of the manuscript of this book, aided by Mrs. Georgianna Hawley, to whom gratitude is also extended. The Center is likewise immeasurably indebted to Dr. H. Barrington Bowser, who has donated his services as pediatrician throughout its existence, as well as to Dr. M. M. Gordon, who has been volunteering his services in otolaryngeology and opthalmology, to Dr. George Arrington, our consultant opthalmologist, and Dr. Walther Riese, our consultant neurologist.

The Center owes a great debt to the city officials, who generally supported us consistently—especially to Mr. R. A. Hobson, welfare director, and Judge John Montgomery, formerly of the Juvenile Court, who emphatically and successfully appealed to the City Council in 1953 that it assume a long-overdue responsibility for our urgently needed services. We appreciate the moral support of Mr. Willett, superintendent of public schools and his staff, a support which is implied in the financing of three of our six teachers. Thanks are due to Dr. Barnett, state supervisor of special education, who consents to the sharing of the expenses by the State Board of Education.

Two of our volunteer workers deserve highly to be credited, Mrs. Marie Smith with her outstanding services as a psychologist for the past ten years and for the invaluable assistance in securing approval of our qualification for the National Lunch and Free Milk Program, and Mrs. Lord for fine public relations work and assistance in follow-up study.

In the early difficult days, Dr. Fred McDaniel, then assistant to Commissioner Barrett, provided unforgetful moral and practical support. Great appreciation is also due to the new Commissioner of the Department of Mental Hygiene and Hospitals, Dr. Hiram Davis, and to Dr. J. Funkhouser, Director of Clinics and Research, as well as to Dr. Cyril Mill, chief psychologist, Miss E. Brantly, chief psychiatric social worker, and Miss Edan Lantz, statistician.

We are also very grateful to Mrs. Edythe Allen, our chief psychiatric social worker, for her stimulating suggestions in reference to social work and for referring Dr. Kalif to us, who gave his time and help with the bibliography, a task which I found would make an impossible demand on my limited time. Mrs. Allen is also an instructor at the School of Social Work at the Richmond Professional Institute of the College of William and Mary. Dr. Kalif is head of its School of Social Work. The bibliography was accomplished and brought to its final state by Mr. Jim Lewis with the help of Mr. Bill Woodruff and Mr. Seymour Wolf. Their conscientious and intelligent achievement brought me great relief.

We also want to express here our appreciation of the valued help of Mrs. Phyllis O'Kelly, past chairman of the board of our Center.

We partially owed our early existence to the understanding and generosity of Mr. William Ayres, chief city librarian of Richmond, who, together with Mrs. Belle Boyd Hightower, head of a branch library, gave the Center its very first "domicile," in 1943, in the stack rooms of Mrs. Hightower's branch. We also owe thanks to Mrs. Alma Brown, present board president, through whose assistance the Urban League gave us the Community House as our quarters on Marshall Street.

A number of friends have helped me with the reading of, commenting on, and organizing a growing manuscript written after a day's work and usually into the early hours of dawn. Thanks are owed to Dr. George Arrington, Dr. Joseph Bunzel, Dr. Ivan Freed, Mrs. Sheila Melville, psychiatric social worker, Mrs. Caroline Weatherby, and especially to Dr. Judd Hubert, my son-in-law, whose warm encouragement has often given me the heart to continue.

Particular mention and thanks are owed to Mrs. Miriam Morton, who saw the entire manuscript through its final stages. She succeeded, despite a heavy load of other work, in giving it the final order and polish, using intelligence, devotion, and a sensitive touch. She has done a great deal to improve the manuscript without interfering with the intentions, style, and design.

Special thanks are also due to Miss Roberta Goodwin, whose work in preparing the Index was invaluable, and to Mrs. Yvonne Lindsey, who typed the bibliography.

We cannot forego remembering Frieda Fromm-Reichmann, the regretted friend of a lifetime. The impact of her interest in the Educational Therapy Center and in this book will always remain.

All the aforementioned are only a few of the most outstanding of those who, in an unlimited variety of ways, made the Educational Therapy Center and its work possible. Although we are not mentioning everyone by name, we are, nonetheless, remembering everyone and their help with heartfelt gratitude. All of these enlightened and empathetic people readily understood that disturbed and grossly neglected children deserve help; that not by their own choice have they been denied equal opportunities with their fellows. Although they have become indifferent or antagonistic to the avowed wishes of the community, they are a part of the community and molded largely by it, and thus they are ours.

Dr. Hertha Riese

Richmond, Virginia

# CONTENTS

# INTRODUCTION

*Justification for a New Therapeutic Approach*

The method of educational therapy is devised to assist those children who have not been the concern of the child guidance clinics so far because they meet none of the basic requirements that make a child amenable to treatment by their methods. It is the child in conflict who still relates and communicates—and thus reaches out for help—who is the object of therapeutic assistance in the conventional child guidance clinic. The children with whom the Educational Therapy Center concerns itself, particularly, show only a minimal tendency to relate or to communicate. Also, the children's parents are not readily capable of contributing to their improvement by adequate and sustained cooperation.

Usually institutional care will otherwise be resorted to, and the children would be committed to welfare agencies. The need for treatment, whether in the community or in institutions, is due to the almost total neglect of earliest as well as all subsequent developmental necessities. Any method suited to redeem these children's condition, therefore, cannot begin with requirements which the child is too undeveloped or too misshapen to meet. The disregard by the adult of the child's actual capacity increases his sense of isolation. Communication as well as cooperation are further discouraged as the child senses that his vital needs are not understood and remain unanswered. At best, he will submit and bide his time under coercion and fear. As soon as the support by the structured milieu ceases, the child will act out pent-up frustration impulsively. The sense of isolation and distrust have become intensified through confinement and with it the resentful need to go on provoking motives for a chronic indulgence in hostility.

Our method offers the opportunity for a change in the fundamentally disturbed relationship with the mother and the family. The fact that the treatment occurs within the community, causes the distorted interaction *with* the community to change likewise. As long as the child is disturbed, the relationship with the community, naturally, is reciprocally disturbed; mutual rejection leads to a vicious circle where each opponent nurtures a need for "madness,"[1] and retaliation. Both the child and the community incur damage, but in the final analysis the child falls prey to the untiring hunt that his disturbed parents began and which society has continued until the bitter end. Only when the child is no longer overwhelmed by neglect, rejection, and ambivalence toward him and the values the adult pretends to stand for can he stop interpreting the whole world in a hurt and sensitized way. Only when rejection of him is discontinued can he slowly be pacified and learn to accept the friendlier world of which he becomes a part. Strengthened by support, he can begin to feel and assume responsibility. Impressed by the fond attention of his fellows who no longer submit him to wholesale condemnation, he will overcome his hostile and undiscerning approach to others and himself; and due to his increasing discrimination, he will be prepared to face an inner conflict which is the condition of his recovery. Educational therapy opens the gates to include those who angrily folded up within themselves or defensively attacked their surroundings. But it has first to promote a state of maturation and differentiation where conflict will be sensed and dealt with.

Our approach takes account of the fact that, negativistic as the children are, they still long for gratification in all areas of development when help is offered without danger of hurt or loss of face. Acceptance of the children as they are saves them from the fear that they will be made to change, which they sense as amputation and dislocation, if not as a threat to existence itself. Existence can be maintained only behind the narrow entrenchment into which the hurt child has withdrawn. To cause him as much as to move, therefore, may be viewed as a dangerous dislocation, a ruse for "disarmament" in the face of the enemy. If, however, conditions can be offered so that the children feel safe, so that they can retain their however frail integral selves and be tended to with tact, insight, and regard, they will develop and will actually change. Change will now be accepted. It will be associated with an increasing sense of well-being, with an awareness that one's identity can be maintained and completed rather than mutilated.

However, when thus stricken by anxiety and on the defensive, these children become a real or only potential menace to their environment; they usually are interned in Industrial or Training Schools, not yet equipped to deal with their deep-seated emotional problems by psychiatric means. Only an infinitesimal portion of the children sent to these schools desire commitment as an opportunity for improvement. Many of those who want to go either seek license to be "bad" or feel in need of punishment in order to gratify irateness directed against themselves, or else to have new motives for anger and aggression against others. They also want to "get it over with" considering punishment the accepted right of retaliation by "the other gang" which is society. When children are in need of atonement, it is usually based on the conviction that punishment is necessary.[2] It never occurs to these children to justify their shortcomings and excuse their behavior by their underprivileged condition, much as it might be resented or depress them. In particular, suffering is never thrown into the balance as an atonement already incurred.

Because of the child's coarse, undifferentiated state, his need of punishment also is amorphous and the forthcoming answer will be unspecific and unacceptable. At its worst it may intensify the child's pathological relationship to parental or sibling figures. Punishment and pain will not become what many a child direly hoped for, a ransom for failure and a road to peace. To be opportunities for growth and maturation, punishment and pain must become profound inner experiences for the fruitful and generous elaboration of which a young person necessarily needs assistance. A child in search of the industrial school usually is ignorant of the fact that he has inner conflicts which deserve to be clarified, or else he avoids and escapes clarification.

For children such as we attempt to portray in this book, commitment to penal institutions does not represent a proper solution when the therapeutic approach is neglected or applied half-heartedly. A sizable number of these children can be kept in the community even in those instances where the home cannot be redeemed.[3] Appropriate foster homes are found during treatment by the method used in the Educational Therapy Center. (*The establishment of small therapeutic homes connected with a child guidance clinic or an educational therapy center should be the next step in a nationwide mental health program.*) When the number of children placed in the penal institutions or industrial schools can be reduced to those cases which need the protection of a structured world, the states might be in a position to transform these institutions into really therapeutic units which keep the children until they are well. As long as the industrial schools have the connotation of penal institutions with an educational program, the duration of any child's stay in the institution will have to be limited in view of two main considerations: one, that the duration of punishment cannot be excessive; the other that the training program is exhaustible at least with the means at hand and in reference to the learning potentials of the children.

It is an untold tragedy that after "serving their time," as the children call it, they are placed back in their traumatic homes where an emotional or mental survival is humanly impossible. Help offered to the parents in the absence of their children is usually of short duration and does not touch the problems sufficiently, in particular not the pathological interaction between them and their children. Most of the children, although treated with devotion in those institutions, have not been exposed to psychotherapy. Their overt attitude but not their deep-seated condition is improved. Those who have been subjected to psychotherapy usually are dismissed from these institutions without sufficient regard to the therapeutic situation, because agency policies have precedence.

They are hurriedly released because of overcrowding, and soon will have to be returned, increasing the density of the industrial school population. Repeatedly the children will be shifted back and forth. Each time untreated or in a state or turmoil resulting from a most untimely break of treatment, these children are exposed to a family milieu that would test any human resistance beyond endurance. To expose children to their traumatic home situation when they have fought a difficult uphill battle toward emotional well-being is as cruel as it is unwise. To the child it is a lesson in the vanity of trusting any adult or in the futility of investing love. The child has good reasons to be convinced that either the grown people have no genuine interest in him or they are powerless to help him. As a result, the child's capacity to brace himself against the effects of an unnerving milieu will be weakened.

While verbal encouragement is given to hold on to the results of the training and education received in the institution, the child is exposed to those diametrically opposed influences in his home to which he is particularly sensitive. Thus, at the community level, an exact replica of the mother-child or parent-child interaction is accomplished, where the mother, under the impact of her own impulses, deviously incites him to commit acts that she censures when they are carried out. In the re-exposure to his traumatic milieu, the child is almost bound to see an incitement to act out despite verbal advice to the contrary. What is verbally requested is materially impossible. The child's co-operation again is enrolled in the community interaction as it used to be with the mother. He is made to desire or to succumb to what actually will incur new censure.

Any modern concept of a child's growth, however, includes the environment as a factor and takes account of stimulating or impeding influences, correcting faulty environmental stimulations or remedying the absence of desirable ones. Unless interfered with, pathological needs and interaction will be mutually nurtured, leading to increasing deterioration of the family interrelationship and of each individual's personality development.

Necessarily, the approach has to be twofold: the child's material surroundings have to be altered concretely, as well as the human relationships psychodynamically. In the traditional child guidance clinics this is not generally undertaken, with the result that families such as the ones we have in mind with extreme concrete needs have remained unaided. They are considered untreatable and indeed frequently are. But with an approach modified to suit their needs, a number of most resistant cases can be assisted to the point that treatment can be carried out successfully. Many social agencies pursue serious efforts toward improvement of the material as well as the emotional surroundings of the children they are concerned with. But it must be considered a rare instance where home circumstances can be changed sufficiently after the child's departure to warrant his return. Usually an extreme effort has preceded the children's placement outside the home. Moreover, these parents' weariness and poverty are such that they drop the children into the lap of their guardian and do not have a tendency to brace themselves for the child's return. The parents' insight into their own contribution to the child's behavior is partially, or more frequently totally absent. Life is so difficult that a denial of reality is a necessary defense. When, however, the parents crave pathological interaction with their children, they are motivated exclusively by this need, and will not only avoid assistance but will interfere with the assistance and progress achieved by the child.

Children who are treated successfully usually have achieved a real conversion which has cost them a heavy price in humility, courage to decide for and proceed on a new, unfamiliar course of action, and both the courage and humility to accept one's own home conditions realistically. But a child returned to extremely adverse conditions cannot be expected to fight or otherwise master them before he is of age or independent. To attempt it, he has to overreach himself, the task at hand actually and invariably exceeding even a grown person's resources.

The second aspect of the two-way approach to a child's emotional problem resulting from highly adverse environmental circumstances such as we have in mind, is that it has to be concrete as well as psychodynamic. Only private therapeutic institutions have found it possible to answer the concrete needs of the children, simultaneous with therapy proper.

But these almost exclusively private institutions offer psychotherapy only to the well-to-do. The underprivileged child is left out by both clinics and institutions.

The method outlined in this book does not imply the rejection of theory or practice previously conceived. We approach the task we set ourselves with reverence for the great theoreticians who preceded us and with due respect for our contemporaries. Our actions were not uninspired by the experience of those who were and are trying their hands in helping emotionally disturbed children or those who break out of the ranks. *But being highly motivated to help in an area of great concern where the child psychiatrist considered himself disarmed, we brought inevitable newness into a combined psychotherapeutical and educational approach to the problem of the child who has been the abandoned victim of our discouragement.*

Our plan of approach is the combination of psychiatric treatment of the child and his therapeutic education in a day-care program; it is the combination of a symbolic therapeutic relationship with the necessary concrete approach and the offering of an animated milieu of such a kind that the child could transfer to it qualities which answer practically all of his needs.

We had to be flexible and unorthodox as the only way to help the many underprivileged children who needed psychiatric help, that is treatment that had sufficient depth to give hopes for the child's recovery. We had to explore new horizons in cases where prognosis seemed very poor. We took the risk of failure. This was the price we had to pay for the discovery of new therapeutic zones. However, we never lost sight of the basic consideration that treatment cannot be attempted at the risk of exposing the patient to damage of any kind. To do nothing seemed a cruel abandonment of the helpless child based on a pessimistic and a self-centered attitude of the community of men and its professional exponents.

We had to break rules established for the treatment of children who came from a different background, where neglect was not total, where exposure had not promoted strength and toughness in the struggle for survival. We ventured to treat children in the "open ward," as, in a sense, we may consider our clinic, at a time when it was considered dangerous and counter-indicated. But contrary to what many would expect, we widened considerably the range within which the child patient can benefit by such an approach.

We had, above all, to break the rules of optimal ratio of therapeutic personnel to child patient. Nevertheless we were able by therapeutic means to pacify and domesticate the aggressive child to the point that he became a challenge rather than a menace to the timid and withdrawn child with whom he shared the offerings of the clinic.

We have been encouraged by the awareness that in a number of instances our day-care approach has been accepted elsewhere: The Jewish Board of Guardians instituted a day-care program in 1958. The Memorial Guidance Clinic in Richmond started a day-care program, on a part-time basis, in the fall of 1961. At the same time the Fairfax County Child Guidance Clinic in Falls Church, Virginia, started an Educational Therapy Service, and the Children's Service Center, Charlottesville, Virginia, is bracing itself for a similar endeavor. All of these institutions have been either aware of or influenced by our experiences. That the general trend is moving in our direction becomes apparent in the recent, published and unpublished, literature.

Although we have found our approach suitable for minority groups, *it has a more general validity*. All of the clinics just mentioned cater to the general public but will use day-care for the non-neurotic, emotionally disturbed patient who is non-amenable to the usual approach of *treatment by appointment* as in the classic child guidance clinic.

One of the immeasurably great advantages of day-care educational therapy is that it results in a prolonged daily contact of the child with therapeutically minded supportive adults—about thirty-five hours of weekly concentrated therapeutic attention instead of one hour.

We have been rewarded by the amazing discovery that a dependent therapeutic relationship can nevertheless be established with an autistic child seen at the rate of one weekly session. The attitude of the parents toward their children generally improves while they, as well as their children, could be offered so little.

To explain our results, attempted almost shamefully but with a mixture of fascination for the intellectual challenge and an empathy for the children's state of reduced humanity, we can refer only to Thomas Mann's concept of the density and fertility of time: "Very little can be very much," he asserts in his praise of transitoriness: "Time is sanctified by its creative use."

# I

## The Educational Therapy Center

### A Description of its History, Resources,
### Children Treated, Procedures, and Staff

*History and Resources*

Its present home, which the Educational Therapy Center has occupied since December, 1955, is located in the historic Church Hill section of Richmond, Virginia. It is just two blocks from St. John's
Church, where the Second Virginia Convention met and where, in
1775, Patrick Henry made his impassioned plea for liberty. The building that houses the Center is itself of such historic interest that it
would probably have been restored had it happened to be in nearby
Williamsburg. Indeed, a structure directly across the street from it has
been beautifully reclaimed. However, this part of Richmond, despite
its several historic landmarks and its many buildings that display the
sturdiness and sensitive proportions typical of the best eighteenth-
century American architecture, is now a squalid slum, sheltering a
congested Negro population.

It would seem desirable to treat and re-educate victims of our urban
culture in a milieu close to the soil and things that sprout, a place
where a child can rest with his back on the meadow, his hands delving
in the grass and his glance reaching the blue atmosphere through the
moving foliage of a cathedral of lofty trees. But we made the uplifting
experience that our young patients respond to the appeal of the
therapeutic milieu and to the rewards of human relations. They rise
above the undesirable solicitations of the slums that surround us so
closely.

The condition of most of the families living in this area is traceable
to their tragic socioethnic and socioeconomic past. Society's indifference to their destiny traverses history from before the days of Patrick
Henry to the present. There is a sad but significant incongruity in the

fact that even Patrick Henry, that eloquent champion of liberty, was not averse to Negro slavery, for, as he said, he, too, was "drawn along by ye general Inconvenience" of living without slaves.[1] The general inconvenience of living near desperately deprived descendants of slaves is, regrettably, evoking only a very limited concern among the descendants of former masters. Fortunately, there are also citizens who have realized the vital needs and basic worthiness of these people, and of their children, whose deprivation is often total—economic, emotional, educational, and social; they have devoted their efforts to the establishment and the development of social services, one of which is the Educational Therapy Center.

In 1942, I held several meetings with Negro citizens in the community to form an agency for the severely disturbed children in the area and in surrounding counties. A number of prominent white citizens were also interested. Mrs. Overton Dennis, who was then on the Board of the Memorial Guidance Clinic, had several conferences with me and with Dr. Harvey De Jarnette Coghill, outstanding local child psychiatrist. It was soon decided that a clinic for such children be established and that it should combine its services with a day-care program—a new approach to the problem of extremely neglected and disturbed children, whose clamors, in the shape of hostile aggression, represented grave dangers to them and to the community. This new approach was conceived mainly by the author. Thus the Educational Therapy Center came into being, in 1943, as a private foundation.

At that time, Dr. Hugh Henry, first commissioner of the department of Mental Hygiene and Hospitals, stated in a conference with Mrs. Dennis, that if the Center proved "effective and needed" after a three-year period of operation, he would approve it as a state clinic. He also supplied the consultation service for the organization of the Center.

To get the Center started $600 was raised by private white donors, $183 by private Negro donors, $815 by local churches. It was first called the Family Counseling Center and began with twelve Negro children. The staff at first consisted of one member, its director throughout the existence of the Center. I was assisted occasionally by volunteers at that time. The first annual budget was a mere $1200.

The stack room of the City Library, Bowser Branch, was made

available as the Center's first home. The children had to be kept quiet so as not to disturb the users of the Reading Room below, and the staff had to resort to near-magic to keep a dozen and more boisterous and emotionally keyed-up youngsters from making a noise. Nevertheless we made progress—the number of children who came or were referred to us for help grew constantly, the budget grew with much less momentum, and the stack room remained our quarters for five years.

At that time referrals came only from the public schools. The referring principals had to be personally responsible for releasing the children to us on school time. At that stage they could not be officially enrolled. Credit is given to Mrs. Ethel Thompson Overby. She was the first and for some time the only one who had the vision, conviction and courage to take personal responsibility for the referrals.

In 1948, the use of a part of the Community House of the Urban League, at 2 West Marshall Street, was obtained, and the Clinic was affiliated with the Mental Hygiene Department under the Hill-Burton Act. State and federal funds were matched by funds raised by a chartered board of citizens. At the same time the Center's originally suggested name Educational Therapy Center was restored and it came under the auspices of the Virginia State Department of Mental Hygiene and Hospitals; it continues to be under these auspices.

The Center being financed under the Mental Health Act, derives one-third of its budget from the United States Department of Health, Education, and Welfare, one-third from the Virginia Department of Mental Hygiene and Hospitals, and one-third from the City of Richmond; additional funds (for house maintenance, etc.) must be raised by the Citizens Board. Our current yearly budget of $63,000 provides for the salaries of eight professional workers (two of them part-time), including the psychiatrist-director, and three of the six teachers. The other three teachers are financed by the Richmond City Public School funds for nine out of twelve months; our own budget provides for the remaining two and one-half months of their salary. The yearly budget also includes salaries of three non-professional workers, as well as all other expenses, excluding the house, whose maintenance is the responsibility of the Citizens Board, and the free-lunch program, which is provided under the National Lunch and Special Milk Program.

To return to our housing history, the entire Community House gradually became and remained the Center's quarters for the ensuing seven years. Those premises, in turn, became too small for the ever increasing number of children and even a too slowly increasing staff. A house was finally bought, on North Nineteenth Street, by the Board of Citizens. This is still the location of the Center, but it, too, has become and been most inadequate for a number of years. The three-story building, with its basement, front and back yards, offers a space of 1,880 square feet for the fifty children in day-care, the staff members, and a varying but large number of children in individual treatment, as well as parents, grandparents, guardians, and foster parents, who visit the Center for a number of reasons.

Our space is already so limited that only too often one of the larger therapeutic offices has to be used by several therapists alternately. Obviously this is not good for the patient who should be able to associate his therapist with one stable and familiar location. We are also in want of two classrooms.

## The Center's Child Population

During the first nine months of the calendar year of 1961, the Center carried an active case load of 107 children. There were 40 children in day-care, 67 in treatment, excluding day-care. During the same period, 24 additional cases were evaluated but not, or not yet, taken into treatment. Of these children all those in day-care were Negroes; of the children not in day-care 90 per cent were Negroes and 10 per cent white. The laws of Virginia used to restrict the institutional contact of the races. Since the need of Negro children has been so much greater, we have limited our day-care services to Negro children. The day-care program is now also limited to boys because we cannot adequately treat girls in the inadequate space and with the limited facilities available to us. Non-day-care treatment is available to boys and girls. Of the children treated in individual therapy outside the day-care program, during this nine-month period, 47 were boys and 37 were girls, not counting diagnostic services. In the course of these nine months 23 cases were dismissed; 6 are in intake at this writing.

Eligible for treatment are children of school age—the age range for intake in day-care is 6 to 14 years; at times a younger child may be included. Children may terminate treatment at the age of 17. This wide age range is conducive to creating a home and family atmosphere in the day-care milieu. The children start as rivals and end up helping each other, the older ones strongly identifying with father figures. Children of borderline mentality, as well as those who do not communicate readily or verbalize their problems, are accepted for day-care or individual treatment. We do not refuse children who are victims of extreme parental neglect and parental as well as community rejection. We would consider such a refusal as penalizing a child for having been penalized by fate.

Not eligible are larger, aggressive boys, who would cause constant disquietude to the smaller and weaker ones, whether the latter are provocative and acting out or sensitive and tending to withdraw. Children who are not toilet trained are not accepted into the day-care program.

When the home environment is constantly destructive to the child's emotional health, or resists any endeavor at rehabilitation, the child is placed in a foster home, through the offices of a public or private agency and, usually, with parental co-operation and consent. If this occurs, intense work with parents, foster parents, and social agencies is necessary. We continue working with the parents to help them with their hostile dependency on the child, their collaboration with foster home placement, and for the achievement of a changed outlook on life and parenthood when the child is ready to return home. Of the 40 children in our day-care program during the first nine months of 1961, 13 were already in foster homes or placed there following our recommendation, 24 remained in parental homes, 2 lived with grandparents, 2 with other relatives.

## Procedures

### DEFINITION OF "EDUCATIONAL THERAPY"

Succinctly, educational therapy can be said to represent a "global" approach to the needs of children who have responded to early and constant neglect or rejection by aggressive hostility or by withdrawal of a hostile or sensitive nature. Such manifestations reflect an underdevelopment in every phase of maturation: sensorimotor, mental, social, and emotional—usually of serious proportions. It is readily conceivable that a child inadequately equipped to meet the challenges of ordinary life tends to regress further when he encounters increased distress, whether real or imagined.

Two closely interacting services are in operation at the Educational Therapy Center five times a week, from 8:30 A.M. to 5 P.M. One is that of the Clinic proper and the other is the day-care milieu, an enlarged family setting and a minor world. The availability of these two services helps the children to succeed without further loss of love and self-esteem. Through individual and group therapy, the Center offers opportunity for a revision of first object relationships; through daily living in the day-care group the Center becomes a testing ground for relationships with substitute siblings as represented by the other children. Teaching and activities provide sources of necessary experiences, which, in the past, were totally missed because of material and emotional deprivation and because of an emotional scarring, withdrawal, and lack of mental development.

Academic schooling at the child's specific level is offered in a permissive atmosphere, either in small groups or individually. Learning a craft or trade at the Center is an important source of education and presents a first approach to learning. Frequent outings provide education as well as experience in acceptable ways of enjoyment.

## Referral

Referrals come to the Educational Therapy Center, through official channels, from the public schools, the juvenile court, county and city welfare agencies, county schools, parents, physicians, other child guidance and medical clinics, and from private agencies and schools. Sometimes children themselves apply for admission or suggest it to their educators, when they have had contact with another child who has been helped by the Center.

Motivations for applications from children are many. The permissiveness of the Center seems to be its major appeal because the children sense that, in the Center, they will be accepted, acceptable, and more adequate, and will have a chance for fulfilling the potentialities in themselves that they dimly sense they have, thereby finding their place and their role in life. In the Center the mother figure and the the other children substitute for a much-needed real mother and the street group. Children may also be attracted by the recreational activities such as the craft class, or they may wish to have an education and catch up with their own age group, or they may seek to fulfil superior ambitions. They may want treatment for some neurotic manifestation such as stuttering. Sometimes they are sexually attracted to some child in the Center. Each of these requests is seriously followed up by contact with the parents or guardians and with the children's schools.

## Our Functions in Reference to Mental Hospitals and Industrial Schools

Since we have been interested specifically—though not exclusively —in the child who has become a public concern or liability, we have been, in the majority of cases, at least in this area of the state, the only possible solution to these children's problems. Previous to our existence no therapeutic approach was available to extremely deprived children with serious emotional disturbances. Their condition did not yet make it advisable or possible to place them in institutions, but they were headed inevitably for an asocial or antisocial adaptation. These children could not find a place in school; they could not find psychiatric treatment.

Until a few years ago, many such children, who now can be kept in the community, had to be committed to the industrial schools. Their actual condition, at times an early psychotic state, was not always fully recognized and would not be treated. The atmosphere of a mental hospital would have been even less appropriate for their recovery. Electric shock, moreover, was earlier an impending menace. The rate of readmissions of children dismissed from the industrial schools was extremely high.

The state welfare is now assisted by a small but efficient mobile clinic, which operates under the auspices of the Department of Mental Hygiene and Hospitals. It is our pride to have practically no commitments to make to the state welfare; on the contrary, many children returning to the community from the industrial schools are referred to us by the Mobile Clinic. In certain instances the children's stay in the industrial school can be shortened because of our availability to those of them who return to the community in need of further psychotherapy. We also assume responsibility for after care of the children returning from the Mental Hospitals.

A very small percentage of the children referred to us have had to be committed to the state hospitals. However, we have been able to reduce greatly the absolute as well as the relative number of these commitments.

In the fiscal year 1958–1959 we committed 9 out of 147 children treated or diagnosed that year.

In the fiscal year 1959–1960 we committed 7 out of 156 children treated or diagnosed that year.

In the fiscal year 1960–1961 we committed out of 163 children treated or diagnosed one adolescent returnee from the industrial school, newly referred to us, simply because he had no home and could not find one. The mother promoted his acting out and his exclusion. His response to the Clinic had been impressive and his institutionalization seemed truly tragic.

While the children are in the institutions we endeavor to improve the general and emotional climate to which they will be returned. In particular, an attempt is made to wean the mother from her destructive dependency on the child, or her ruling his existence and committing him to his or her needs. No child in sufficient contact with reality was committed anywhere without previous discussion with him of the reasons for commitment and without obtaining his consent based on confidence, and even insight into the inevitability of the decision and the benefit to be derived from the step to be taken. In the majority of cases the children contributed to the decision arrived at in treatment at the Educational Therapy Center, hoping to liberate themselves from the bondage of their emotional illness. They co-operated with the hospital to the extent that this could be expected.

## THE INTAKE

The emergency of the children's problems and the strained family relationships that, at the time of referral, have culminated in the straining of the community in terms of antisocial behavior are good reasons for avoiding a waiting list.

There is wisdom in accepting one's limitations and in delaying the intake of new children when the staff is already overburdened by obligations, but this wisdom is inevitably practiced at the expense of a very sick child in desperate need of assistance. Our Clinic usually has no alternate choice. The referring agencies are otherwise compelled to resort to less specific solutions or to refer the children to institutions that would prefer not to be involved with such cases because they are not equipped to meet their needs.

Unfortunately the patient's emergency is lost sight of too frequently. Agencies and their workers are prone to feel the need of defending their physical health and professional integrity by taking the attitude that the victim's unrelieved peril is a case of absolute necessity for which the agency has however to, at least temporarily, refuse responsibility. Such an attitude is practical in laying the responsibility at the doorstep of the community upon whom it is incumbent to finance adequate services. It is sometimes felt that the neglect of obvious needs will inevitably advertise these needs most effectively. But when it concerns the outcast or outlawed child, whom it is easier to impeach for his blatant shortcomings than to relieve from the emergencies he reveals, which simultaneously highlights the community's own involvement with them, nothing or very little might be gained. Also, in the case of our potential patients, deferment of intake might soon result in so serious a condition that the Clinic services would no longer be useful. Moreover, the hostile involvement of patient and community may intensify to such an extent that the community's insistence on angry punishment can no longer be controlled and understanding cannot even be expected.

Officers of an agency are often subject to interference by the public in their immediate sympathy with the patient. The unsparingly dedicated worker might, as a result of his dedication encourage the community to burden him with an impossibly heavy load of responsibilities. In order to avoid this, the worker has to consent to an even greater loss, that is to sacrifice the immediately needed service of fellowship, the solemn duty of the physician. The dilemma between professional integrity which is expressed by unsparing dedication and/or the decision to restrict it in order to maintain the proper standard of craftsmanship and the gains to be obtained through intensified rather than repeated experience and insight is a truly great dilemma. The patient himself may be more sensitive and thus more responsive to the intangibles of an immediate and unconditioned empathy with him than to a craftsmanship that may prove a lesser safeguard to him than the worker's ornament and pride.

In this undeniably painful dilemma, we have attempted, through the years, to be imaginative in order to reconcile the justified concerns and inevitable limitations of the staff, with the goal of avoiding deferment of children's intake. In addition to the general reasons for making help available when it is needed, we have to keep in mind that deferment of help is sensed by the child and his parents as a new rejection or exclusion from privileges and a hurt which can motivate rationalizations for further failure; in short, it is distinctly antitherapeutic.

*In view of these considerations, an intake study is initiated within days of the request for it.* Cases distinctly unsuitable for our approach can immediately be eliminated without loss to the child. A well-considered substitute solution is presented at all times, and no child is left entirely without assistance. When none of the therapists are free to take on more cases at the moment, those children whom we believe to be our own concern are placed on our "inside waiting list," that is, in the day-care group. Thus, help is offered immediately. The child is made to belong somewhere and to feel wanted. Though undecided whether to yield to the lure of acceptance or refuse it, he can already begin to work through his ambivalence in the understanding presence of his therapeutically minded teachers and to benefit by group interaction. Therefore, an initial success usually is achieved and the majority of the children artlessly reveal that, despite their antagonistic behavior in the group, they respond to acceptance to the point that at least they attend the Clinic and rapidly forget to act out in the street.

The child soon notices that he has no psychotherapist and may feel slighted. One of the functions of the day-care group, for the new ones, is to make psychotherapy appear to them as a sought-for privilege. To avoid the danger that the new child will feel left out, we point out to him, in the initial interview that it is genuine interest in him which prompted us to accept him despite the shortage of personnel and that it is not lack of interest that may cause the delay in assigning him to a therapist. We may have difficulties in being convincing with the sullen, hostile, pre-adolescent or early adolescent who will look for motivation of hostile expression everywhere and with the younger boys who need to be attracted by individual maternal acceptance. They tend to accept the female teachers as an answer to their dependency needs. But either the young boy who displays or the growing boy who conceals his need of dependency through his cockiness can be assisted by the teacher's staff until treatment is available. Some children will be gratified by the teacher to whom they are assigned; others will seek and find individual attention elsewhere, or join an adolescent discussion group with the teacher supervisor.

## SOCIAL WORK WITH PARENTS

The *social work* staff feels the greatest burden in adjusting to the heavy demands for service, particularly with additional treatment of the new parent whose child may be only in day-care for a while or already in one of the therapeutic groups. If the parents are not taken into the Clinic family at this time, their suspicions and resistance become more pronounced and they may be willing to turn over their responsibilities for the child's welfare entirely to the Clinic. Thus, once more, they deny immediate parental care to the child. Or they may act out hostility aggressively toward the Clinic and interfere with the treatment plan or procedure for their child or children.

A tentative solution to this problem is the formation of an intake group made up of five or six new parents who have been through the usual intake procedure and whose families have been accepted for treatment. This group gives these new parents an opportunity to find answers for their questions about the Clinic, to express their suspicion, their fears, and their resentment concerning the treatment.

At this time the general exposition of the total family tragedy occurs and concrete help is given in clearing the scene where treatment will be staged. At the same time peripheral problems concerning siblings, relatives and friends which, significantly, are coming to the fore, immediately tend to give the worker a first directive for understanding of parental attitudes. In helping the parent in a subjectively marginal and, therefore, a less sensitive area of their concerns, the way may be paved for a dawning awareness of their own contribution to their difficulty. But depending on the degree of anxiety, the need to discuss immediate problems will arise sooner or later. A relief is derived from being heard and understood. Readiness of the parent for treatment can be assessed and his transfer to an individual therapist, when available, or to a place in an ongoing therapeutic group, can be arranged. No special number of sessions are prescribed in advance, but they relate to the needs of the group and the availability of staff.

Parents whose child is mentally retarded or those who have an autistic child need special assistance in expressing their feelings about their limited and isolated youngsters and how to motivate, support, and improve them in regard to day-to-day living. Parents of emotionally disturbed children who are acting out aggressively are assigned to special groups. Their own behavior may vary greatly. They may be withdrawn, inhibited, rigid, or outgoing with varying degrees of warmth. More mothers than fathers respond to the encouragement to join the group. The fathers tend to take less responsibility for their children and consider the management of problems the function of the mother.

However, do what we may, we cannot absolve the community as a whole from assuming increased responsibility. Unless the public, convinced by its enlightened and courageous citizens or representatives, shares responsibilities with those who want to reform their ways and with those who attempt to help them, successful work, rather than being an asset, may paradoxically become a liability because of the pressure of increased demands. The story of success tends necessarily to increase intakes as well as parental co-operation. To the public it seems that the more help is offered, the more sickness is brought into the open. For the workers it becomes increasingly difficult to cope with the new intake and with the correspondingly accrued obligations to pursue psychiatric social work or treatment with the new as well as unfinished treatments. Not only can tangible therapeutical results be obtained more rapidly with the child when the parent assumes the responsibility to change, but what is also gained is a higher quality and greater depth of recuperation in both parent and child.

Lately emphasis has been laid on the fact that group therapy is not merely a means of solving the problem of the great demand for help, in numbers, but rather one specifically indicated in some instances.[2] We cannot overlook, however, that whenever group therapy is indicated and proves to be a necessary and sufficient therapeutic approach, it also solves a problem of numbers. When, for instance, we have a group of six patients in a one-and-a-half-hour session, granting a whole hour for the more complex note-taking of group dynamics and interaction, and its evaluation in reference to each patient's individual problem, it means that we have used two and a half hours for six patients instead of nine hours, at the rate of one hour for each treatment and one-half hour for required note-taking. But assuming that the session lasts only fifty minutes and only ten minutes are used for note-taking, we still have six hours versus two and a half hours of time investment to consider, or a precious gain of three and a half hours which might represent another group treatment and a fifty-minute hour with note-taking. In other words, this makes it possible to help an additional seven patients that day. We realize that no time is thus gained in staff and supervisory sessions since discussions will concern not only the group dynamics but each individual's family dynamics and personal relationships as well.

Group work with parents has, on the whole, developed more slowly than group work with children. The obstacles are obviously connected with the economic distress under which a great number of these mothers of destitute families labor. Many of them have to work and cannot absent themselves from their jobs to attend group therapy sessions. These difficulties are connected further with these families' sense of isolation in the community and their sensitivity to the experience of rejection, or of acceptance only in those areas where instrumental use can be made of their services. Above all, a profound distrust of each other has to be conquered and the inclination to be self-rejecting, often projected on an agency that, in their mind, depreciates itself by being available to their social group, failures that they feel they are.

The families have to be convinced against a high wall of resistance that the Clinic services are worth being used and that they are offered after due deliberation and with consideration not because these services are not acceptable elsewhere or because its workers are not aware of whom they are trying to serve. It goes without saying that rejection of help may be total because of resentment and holding society as a whole responsible for the state of misery and suffering in which these families exist. Even when a great deal of preparatory work has been done, some of these impediments may persist, in addition to the resistance that developed during the treatment or due to a tendency to react by withdrawal or by losing interest and the incentive for struggling. Important concrete hindrances stand in the way and new ones are likely to come up when we deal with impoverished large-size families where many health problems may interfere with the mother's attendance, to mention but one of the myriad of obstacles. It seems, for instance, almost impossible to bring together a group of women who may have great difficulties in saving sufficient carfare to come and go, or to have a few hours of leisure in daytime, which includes the time to prepare for a neat appearance. To some of these women making a good appearance is a condition *sine qua non* for feeling sufficiently at ease and for sharing with others a faith in the possibility of change under forbidding circumstances, and in the responsibility for the child's condition and for his improvement.

These parents are so preoccupied with economic problems and with physical care for their large families, that consideration for the children's emotional welfare emerges as a new idea or as a way of thinking that has not been part of their daily life. Initial concern for the children's feelings is resisted and these parents use the group as a sounding board to describe and berate the children's overt behavior. Such attitudes are accepted in the group, but parents are slowly guided and encouraged to think out what their children may be trying to express by their behavior. As they begin to examine behavior in terms of experience disclosed by their children, they are almost compelled to think of their own past behavior in terms of their own childhood. For obvious reasons the parents with less resistance and hostility tend to release these factors and are first to bring them into the group discussion. In this way they stimulate self-examination in the more repressed and withdrawn parent. Before these parents can detect solutions for their present family problems, they have to find some way of understanding the past. Their rigid, patterned, automatized reactions, as well as their sensitized behavior in meaningful and difficult experiences, are an outgrowth of responses to early inappropriate stimuli. Their own locked sibling relationships, resulting from the inadequacies of their childhood experiences, can be recognized, conditioning or failing to condition their relationship with the contemporary generation. The bearing it has on their socioeconomic and family adjustment can also be seen. Though these parents vary in their ability to relate, share, and comprehend, even the most withdrawn parents show that they are gaining insight from the proceedings of this particular milieu. The gain is derived not only from the acceptance by the leader, but the knowledge shared and conquered by mutual interaction. This interaction actually is the first positive experience in a mature unfolding and dealing with sibling dissensions and a search for solutions or the capacity to live with problems unsolved or resolved by mutual concession.

At first the symbolic support by the parent figure in the person of the leader is needed to give the patients the reassurance that they are adequate to the test of mature interaction. The most anxious and dependent ones may ask for an individual session in their need of encouragement for facing the test in the group of their "contemporaries." The interaction between parents therefore implies that, unconsciously, problems are tested and worked through for the elaboration of which the patients lend and use each other. The gaining in self-awareness consequently can be transferred to the patient's present family life, with the benefit of deepening emotional experience and understanding. The fact that the term "contemporaries" has no chronological implication emphasizes the symbolic character of the reported relationship. The parents may be of varying ages and the leader might be a young person.

We can see in the parents' discussion group a first outline of a resolution of a competitive and combative interaction between contemporaries, real and symbolic siblings, neighbors or co-workers, an interaction so characteristic of many of our patients. In the group, which is a symbolic family with an impartial parental figure, competition for superiority becomes unnecessary and vain. It liberates the group members for an impartial search for themselves and their problems. A fundamentally new attitude is made possible in reference to the children with whom they will now compete less and less, and in reference to whom they will not have to assert themselves by predominance. Benefiting by the example of the group leader, they will learn to evaluate problems and situations, to guide and convince with greater calm and, when it is wise, to yield.

In spite of overwhelming difficulties encountered in social work, at the time of this writing 75 per cent of the parents of our children who come for therapy, benefit from the parent groups or are being helped by individual psychiatric social work; formerly only 25 to 33 per cent could be reached. This improvement is due to our own gain in experience with the total complex of reality factors as well as the defenses involving our patients with the surrounding culture. Moreover, a lack in the number of workers used to limit our casework, which is a necessity in overcoming these families' inhibitions in relating, as well as in aiming at intangible values. Their sensitivity has to be surmounted through visits to their homes. Persistent attention and acceptance gradually conquer their sense of inadequacy and rejection and pave the way for insight into the benefits of treatment, including, particularly, the fundamental value of parental co-operation.

About three-fifths of our day-care children live in their own homes. Except for extreme cases where we take the initiative in having the children committed to foster home care, we are able to carry through, due to the merits of the day-care program, the children's treatment and simultaneously to preserve the natural family. In those cases where the children are living in foster homes at time of referral, we contribute, in many instances, to their usually successful restoration to their natural families. Psychiatric social work also is carried on while children have to make a more or less prolonged stay in mental hospitals or industrial schools.

## COMMUNICATION WITH AGENCIES

Our communications to the agencies or institutions have been always as complete and elaborate as has been necessary to convey our insight into the children's behavior and the family dynamics. We take the stand that, if anyone deserves the privilege of helping a patient, he also deserves to be trusted with the available tools necessary for the patient's treatment.

Our children and their parents at worst "don't care," but they more usually are confident that our revelations are made with the object of assisting them. They hope that through these reports a continuity of endeavor is being established when the child has to be referred to a mental hospital. They hope that the treatment in the hand of another autonomous therapist does not have to begin from scratch and that the territory conquered will not have to be given up again. The new therapist thus does not start as as a complete stranger and does not appear as such when the existence of a community with the old therapist, with whom the child had a relevant relationship, is felt. In other cases the new therapist may be helped to advance safely if warned of the already explored, vulnerable areas.

Wrong decisions can be prevented in court by a profound understanding of the child's behavior and the forces that menace him from without and within, rendered in a full written report. Contrary to a prevailing belief, we have found that busy judges or the therapeutic personnel of institutions do not feel imposed upon by the obligation to give time for the study of a portrait of a child or his family when it might benefit them. Our reports are generally appreciated and often make friends for us among our professional contacts.

## The Staff

We began, nineteen years ago, with a staff of one—the psychiatrist-director, who was assisted occasionally by a limited number of volunteers. Our present staff consists of the same psychiatrist-director, three psychologists, one part-time volunteer psychologist, four psychiatric social workers, two of whom are on part-time, four male teachers, two female teachers, two clerical workers, and a part-time janitor.

One of the two women teachers is the supervisor and co-ordinator between the Clinic team and the educational staff; the other woman teacher instructs in crafts and home economics, and manages the important lunch program, discussed elsewhere in this book. Of the four full-time male teachers, two are special academic teachers, one is a teacher in recreation and crafts, and the fourth is a specialist in shop work as well as agriculture and biology. The workshop program includes the maintenance of the house, the agriculture the tending of the garden.

The Center also benefits greatly from the services of a pediatrician, an ophthalmologist, a laryngologist, and a neurologist—all given without remuneration.

In addition to the usual supervisory sessions and staff meetings of the psychiatrist-director with the psychologists and the psychiatric social workers, the entire professional staff meets for weekly discussions of the children's problems and the therapeutic approach to them, and for the discussion of current observations and problems arising in the day-care group. The professional workers' observations of the children and their particular behavior in the day-care group give rise, in turn, to additional individual conferences between those involved directly in therapeutic work and the teachers or their supervisor. These sessions are not scheduled but are held as need arise, in reference to acute problems, mutul information, therapy, work with the family, the child's guardians or interested agencies. In-service-training and individual supervisory sessions are also held with the educational staff; the teachers' supervisor is in charge of these.

Our teaching staff has been very stable—two of the members have served the Center since 1948, others have been with us for extended periods of as long as six years. The stability of the staff is of invaluable importance to children whose treatment is necessarily extended and who need to have, for once in their lives, the experience of the continuity of mutual commitments. Only when such reliability has been tested by time, can the child take it for granted. Encouraged by the experience, the child may then venture out for exploits of courage and curiosity, rise to imaginativeness, and, with less fear of rejection and frustration, trust love and the rewards of the generosity of giving.

On the other hand, the children's reality adjustment will be put to the test when, by force of circumstances, changes occur. However, we consider them most undesirable. Changes cannot always be properly timed and the character of a symbolic home suffers as a result of unfortunate and unplanned timing. Men and women whom we once knew as troubled children like to return in mind or in reality to a "familiar" (with the connotation of "family") place and let us know that they are "making it." Too many changes cause a sense of strangeness. A stabilized community symbol is an asset.

The total endeavor of the psychiatric workers and the teaching staff affords each child in our day-care program 35 hours of therapeutic attention weekly instead of the usual one hour. The duration of treatment has been from eighteen months to four years.

# THE CHILD: HIS BACKGROUND
## AND HIS SYMPTOMS

# II

*The Hurt Child and His Relationship to the World*

## A Behaviorally Oriented Description of the Children

The great majority of the children in our day-care program at the Educational Therapy Center come from the low socioeconomic groups. Because of their isolated status in society, many of them have been largely inaccessible for observation and treatment before coming to us. A valid evaluation of their actual limitations in being able to absorb academic knowledge and of their ability to benefit from new experience presents a considerable challenge to the therapist and educator.

These children's potential and their development have been inhibited by an appalling absence of positive stimulation—sensory, motor, mental, or emotional. At the same time they have been exposed to terrifying experiences and distorting influences. When, later on, they encounter people whose standards are impressively higher than their own, a sense of paralyzing inadequacy hampers their benefiting from belated opportunity and frustrates hope of matching these ideal figures. The flow of a beneficial source which otherwise would have been inspiring seems repugnant.

Not having learned to know in communicable terms what their feelings are, these children cannot help their mystified observers to understand why they do not react positively to good example and mental stimulation. Lacking contact with and understanding of these children, their would-be educators and benefactors become overtly and covertly annoyed and increasingly rejecting. The "grapes" of opportunity will move out of the children's reach with increasing momentum, and for comfort the weary child will declare them totally unpalatable.

The child may bend every sinew in order to keep the threatening world from impinging its hostility on him. He may literally even shut his eyes; his head may sink deep into his shoulders as though continuously ducking the expected blow from an invisible but present assailant. When approached, the child may shrink or cringe and become more and more detached and unresponsive.

In their need to shield their identities from the threatening world these children may pretend that they have forgotten their own names. At times these pretenses may be more than symbolic and may have a basis in reality. Many of them come from such chaotic and confusing family relationships that often they have no clear idea of their own identity.[1] By retreating into anonymity they try to becloud their precarious position in a hostile world. Cyril, who was born out of wedlock, envied his siblings' status, all of whom were legitimate children by his mother, although by different fathers; he would pronounce all paternal names in such a way that they sounded quite alike, including his own father's name.

On the other hand, these deeply ungratified children may remain in a constant search for an object to which they lack identifying clues. Not knowing what they want and unable to recognize what could gratify them, they are condemned to go on hopelessly seeking, touching and testing everything, resentfully destroying the unrewarding material objects grasped. In their perpetual and aimless agitation they ignore word and sentence structure, they talk incessantly and irrelevantly. In this state of chronic and increasing deprivation, the child bypasses opportunities, becomes argumentative, aggressive, destructive, and unmanageable. His threshold for stimulation is so low that even his very clothing seems to disturb him. This irritability may also be partly attributed to malnutrition, inadequate sleep, and other physical factors, but psychological tensions intensify the strain, and motivations for outbursts are continually available. Tragically, the child is not without an awareness that he compares unfavorably with more fortunate people. This awareness increases his suffering and insecurity, as well as his incapacity to collect his thoughts.

When such children have improved, refusal to face certain aspects of learning may reveal that a sense of inadequacy has not been overcome. Now identification with their ideal figures is fraught with the danger that discrepancies between the child and his ideal will be discouraging to him. Intolerance against his own weaknesses may result. A boy who had made a pathetic effort to learn to read, suddenly exploded with sardonic laughter when one of his classmates showed the same inadequacy. He could no longer endure the pitiful and ridiculous deficiency he despised so intensely in himself.

The children feel out of place, wrong, and undesirable—always and everywhere. They identify with the rejection sensed in the family and outside. When they feel better, they talk about this induced self-rejection and finally do much joking about being "dumb" " 'flicted" (afflicted) and "crazy," which shows that they are accepting their rejected condition while hopefully tending to overcome it.

## The Problem of Relating

The hope of relating is based on the joy of being accepted and on the dawning perception of the beauties of existence. But the children's resentment and retaliatory tendencies are initial obstructions. Acceptance of treatment, however, just as any other human co-operative endeavor, presupposes the laying down of arms. Though suspicion may be diminishing, the children may still be driven to overt warfare from fear of assaults or from an "ambush."

As the child becomes accessible to treatment, he accepts, for the first time, the burden of more conscious frustration and inadequacy derived from new identifications and the responsibilities they impose. At the very instant when joy appears on the horizon of incipient love, a period of self-denial begins: "I felt like killing that guy," said a boy, "but then I thought of you [the therapist] and walked away. But I don't know if I can do that all the time." However, suffering no longer has a totally negative content. It has become the necessary corollary to a more complete world. This is the main step toward recovery.

The children long for contact and support, but, at the same time they fear the potential enemy in the other person. This ambivalent attitude is the carry-over of the mother-child relationship, or their relationship to all and their entire world. This ambivalence leads to a tendency to provoke what is feared, as though fear and suspense were harder to endure than the actual hurt which is anticipated. The attitude is usually generalized and the ingenuity of these children in varying the means of provoking the very trouble they fear is impressive. It actually is their way of life—the only means by which they can feel they are living. The need to culminate the fear in concrete trouble becomes so intense that actual occurrences cannot satisfy it any more, and the aggression is imagined, nurtured by fear.[2]

Challenge and competition are more than the child can endure. Anything for which anybody reaches out seems worth trying to catch first. To miss it is distressing regardless of its actual worth or usefulness. The object secured may prove to be disappointing in importance and the more so the more the child is lacking in a capacity for enjoyment. The object may be used the next minute as a missile against the very one who just failed to obtain it. He is the one who, in the aggressor's mind, fooled him into giving in to a false lure and a deceptive promise. The dependency on the act is sensed and resented. The competitor thus calls to mind the enticing and disillusioning mother. He recalls her immediately as a person as well as the symbol of the disappointing object caught—the false lure and deception have become ubiquitous.

Devoid of the security derived from early maternal solicitude and gratification, these children are keenly competitive. They are anxious to be the first ones everywhere, for fear that otherwise nothing will be left for them of whatever it is. They have to exclude the other fellow from the only attainable spot worth conquering. They lack resourcefulness as well as the hope to imagine that there may be other and new horizons spread out before them. Incapable of recognizing that the goal for which they strive is at all times evasive, they surrender themselves to an irresistible drive to attain it. Their world is shrunken into the present instant, inhospitable, and precarious. They have no resources for sharing and for the alleviation of suffering, which is derived from sharing in partnership. The child sees in everyone phantoms of a depriving world, a world to be totally absorbed, or torn down, for the sake of survival.

Destructive interference does not imply simply destruction of material things by the child. An early symptom may be the demand for, and absorption of, all possible attention, vigilance and guidance, as well as a tendency to disrupt the material and therapeutic organization. Their concentrated attack may come from two directions: the upsetting of other children and the distracting of staff members and interfering with their achievement of actual objectives. In the course of treatment, the all-pervading hostility will be reduced to specific trigger areas. From the natural milieu the problems are carried to the therapeutic milieu, where they can be dealt with in the group and by the group, as well as in individual therapy. The child feels understood and protected and becomes dependent on the psychotherapist. When finally belief in unconditional acceptance is born, the privilege to share may be discovered with ecstatic joy.

Thus the bridge is built stage by stage from the isolated individual to the community and to all of mankind.

When the children learn to share, competition becomes positive and constructive. They produce and try to please. Though anxiety is not fully conquered, they voice admiration for other children's work and try to do as well. No longer will the drawings of the other children "just happen" to fall to the ground or be soiled or torn "accidentally." No longer will the objects of clay made by other children be used for raw material. The formerly hostile child now collects the drawings and places them in a folder, because all the children have become a dedicated unit. They have risen from the bondage of isolation and are using the Clinic as an avenue to liberation.

In the microcosm of the world of the Clinic may be observed the first steps taken towards a co-operative community. When the children actually desire to accomplish their daily achievements, no matter how modest they may appear, they are on the road to the goal of becoming part of a united and positively motivated group, where competition becomes an unselfish striving for perfection.

## The Problem of Learning

As long as a child is beset with so many needs and obsessions, whether he is able to learn or not, he thinks of school as just another device of the grown group to prevent his pursuit of satisfactory ways of discovering the world—of the kind of world he is willing to accept. The gift of knowledge offered by our modern schools in as pleasurable a way as possible, cannot be accepted because of the threatening involvement with it and with the people who represent it. The child fears the responsibility associated with it, "the change of mind," as he may call it. Moreover, he has built up prejudices against "gifts" because they rarely, if ever, have been truly satisfying. They create burdensome and disappointing dependency. The "gift" of food may have been "seasoned" with adverse emotional tensions at all phases of his existence and by animosity of everyone against everyone in his home; the child usually can remember food given by the wrong person, in inadequate amounts, improper quality and uninspiring monotony, at a time when he was exhausted from waiting and in need of sleep rather than nourishment.[3] Competition, when there are too many vying for too little, may have represented another exhausting element. The longed for, the avidly required gratification was thus turned into its opposite. Whatever anticipation the child may have fostered was frustrated. Such chronic experiences, which usually have been undergone since infancy, prior to a stage that can be remembered, explain why such children have become afraid of the gifts offered by the adult, why they have such a short frustration span and cannot wait for gratification. Whatever gratification school learning may have to offer is delayed. It presupposes too many investments from a child who has no funds.

To children who are sensitized by an unending series of disconcerting experiences, with gratification delayed or denied, the future is a most uncertain thing and is usually discounted. At times it is more than skepticism that affects the child. He represses his frustrating, as well as his humiliating, experiences, and thus, he reduces[4] his imagery and the usefulness of his concepts; he atrophies his capacity for anticipation. The food of knowledge, like all food, is poisoned. They tell you so.

## A Child's Self-Centered Wandering toward Knowledge

The desire to know is an attempt to assume rightful intellectual ownership of an ever widening world. Such an attitude implies acceptability of the world as a potential possession. To the extent that we achieve ownership of the world by knowledge, we become the caretakers and managers of our territory. We contribute to its improvement in the domain of our competence.

As long as the world remains unacceptable to the child and, as long as he is entangled in the dilemma of negating the world that also allures him, there is no apparent foundation for learning: He is too distraught by this alternative which he tends to solve by denial or by destruction of the source of discomfort. When a neglected child of good natural ability, left to his own resources, moves actively toward the world, his positive tendencies more than likely will lead to negative results. The case of Felix will attract our attention repeatedly. At this time we shall discuss his wanderings which finally brought him on the road to knowledge.

Felix was the first child of a mother who had five other illegitimate children by the time of Felix's referral, at the age of eight. Felix and his sister were conceived from the same man; the four other children had four different fathers. Felix's father soon married another woman, and the couple took Felix's sister into their home. He, however, was excluded from this family and constantly changed hands until his stepmother mentioned him to her girlfriend, Mrs. Byrd, who was moved by sympathy for him and took him into her house. At the time Felix had been living with a very old woman in a miserable shack. We learned from Mrs. Byrd about the state of total neglect and starvation in which she found the child, who had been left to his own devices most of the time. How he survived the first three years of life is hard to imagine. Mrs. Byrd said that Felix talked when she took charge of him at the age of three, but she had to teach him adequate articulation and verbalization commensurate with his age.

When he became a most appealing and attractive little boy, his stepmother suddenly wanted to keep him and interferred with the child's relationship with the adoptive mother, Mrs. Byrd. The boy became insecure and distrustful and, reverting to his previous "self-supporting" condition, he began to steal. Welfare workers returned him to his father and stepmother, but because of emotional neglect he had to be restored to Mrs. Byrd. He never recovered security again. She became just "the best lady I ever had."

Mrs. Byrd was a kind and intelligent woman but not an efficient housewife. The child artlessly depicted her as chatting with the neighbors and having no food ready at mealtime. Mr. Byrd was a competent man although an unskilled worker. His relationship to the boy seemed vague and abstract. He was described as never objecting to his wife's negligence about meals. Thus, from the boy's point of view, he was inefficient as a father and head of the family; but the boy was too appreciative to express this openly.

The Byrd family lived in a one-room apartment in one of those tenements which resemble a thoroughfare. Male roomers introduced Felix to homosexual activities. He slept in the same bed with his adoptive parents until they had a boy of their own. He, who was by then eight years old, was transferred to a mattress on the floor. In the neighborhood of Mrs. Byrd's home, Felix had had opportunity to play with children of a more privileged status and to be the recipient of toys they no longer wanted. Being extremely sensitive to his impoverished condition, he felt humiliated rather than favored. He therefore relied upon his own "initiative" by stealing to attain the social status which, to his way of thinking, was connected with ownership of new and representative toys. Although endowed with good abilities, he had rejected any kind of schooling until, at a later date in treatment, he had gained some sense of social acceptability. Then, he learned to read and figure so rapidly that, had his effort not been apparent, it would have seemed that he had mastered these skills formerly.

Felix worked out his problem with the help of toys; they were his mediators in learning about human and social relations and, in search of information, he began to read about them.

A bicycle and toy trains played an important part. The legitimate ownership of a bicycle, of a preferred, acceptable style and make, was considered the key to social acceptance. The special request in reference to style and make was based on former experiences that old, oversized bicycles do not fulfil the purpose of attaining the social status he desired. His foster mother gave him the coveted bicycle. On the first day of ownership he brought the bicycle to the Clinic and let another child, Jerry, ride it. Using the bicycle as a complement to his timid self and attempting to assert his superiority over Jerry, he lent him the bicycle as almost the first act of using it. Felix was the more substantial of the two boys but felt quite inferior to Jerry who tended to brag with exuberant verbosity. Jerry knew nothing about the reciprocity of obligations at the time. He stayed out all day riding the bicycle. Felix bravely ignored the insult but finally was afraid of having to return home with a total defeat, the loss of the bicycle. Though Jerry returned it eventually, it had not achieved its purpose of giving Felix a chance to convey favors on his own terms, as a privileged child like the kind he had envied. Jerry actually outsmarted Felix and prevented him from getting even with fate by using Jerry as an underdog in need of charity. The incident was a valuable though painful lesson to Felix in realism and fairness. He was helped not to react sensitively and to learn that equality is not a one way proposition.

As time went on, the bicycle failed him further. One of the older boys had been working for a year and a half, until he could finally fulfil his dream of a luxury bicycle. Felix's, no longer the best, unfit to claim regal status, became a symbol of inferiority and an object of his rejection. He "had" an accident. He also exposed it to the other children's destructiveness, unable to struggle any longer and desirous to see the end of a tool destined, but futilely, to establish his superiority. He left the bicycle somewhere in the streets to be taken by anyone who cared. Responsibility for that piece of deceptive goods could no longer be borne.

The lesson that ownership means responsibility and serious struggle was, however, slowly understood. Felix therefore withdrew upon a less exposed position previously conquered. Not long before this such a self-healing attempt had been successful—the play with a little wind-up train, an accepted substitute for the real thing—a " 'lectric train." First he had played with it by himself in the psychiatrist's office, then with her. When he had felt safe, he invited other children to play with him; all had recognized him as the owner of the train. When fate had thus been ameliorated and his self-confidence somewhat restored, he had no longer needed to play with the train, though he had spoken about the experience at intervals. Now the need to repeat the play was newly aroused because of failure with the bicycle, on a more exposed forum, outside the psychiatrist's office and with a more dangerous tool. However, he did not revert completely to the original stage. For the sake of his self-esteem, he needed this time a tool of higher standard, a real electric train. Still obsessed by his need to live out the role of the privileged child, he had to let other children come and play with him and accept him as the one who granted privileges. Unless in a tantrum, Felix was most careful in his handling of objects, whether his or other people's. The other children, on the contrary, were extremely destructive, some of them subtly so. They, too, retaliated against the pre-eminent role Felix hoped to play.

In order to help these children take an interest in preserving intact the precious train, he had, in sharing it, taught them to share. The toy, no longer a stranger between them, representative of an illicit ambition, became a friend that inspired their imagination. The train then needed its landscape which was provided by constructions made with an erector set. Felix acquired skill, legitimate pride, and status. His interest was engaged, and he began to read instructions and catalogues. From there he turned to books on the third-grade level. Felix was now nine years old.

One might raise the question whether, under the circumstances, the play here described still deserves its name. Are we allowed to call play the manipulation of objects which serve the definite purpose of providing the child with greater security, social standing, and successful rivalry? Should the question be answered in the negative, one would not be too far from a generalizing conclusion that play in its proper meaning loses its right and its very character whenever misery becomes extreme and stringent.

## Difficulties of Communication

It is only recently that therapeutic contact by means of ultra-lingual interchange has been explored systematically.[5] Language, the most immediate and explicit gauge between human beings, serves as the most obvious medium for obtaining therapeutic results. The gain of one session can be carried over to the next only when conceptualization of experience is possible. These gains can be retained for further elaboration of early, although repressed, material and serve to furnish new insights to patient and therapist. Verbalization, therefore, is of fundamental importance. But it does not include all communication, nor is it its sole and sufficient vehicle.[6]

It is consistently taken for granted that the child-patient milieu has to be manipulated in view of the child's object relation, the resulting specific pathology, and other basic concepts. However, when relations have become so traumatic as to make the child uncommunicative, the task seems impossible. Resistance to transfer of emotions then becomes overwhelming, and no positive effect can be obtained.

Traditional psychotherapy as an answer to the problem of emotional and mental disturbance on a certain level presupposes a balance in the cultural development of patient and therapist. This method, however, cannot reach a child who is so profoundly deprived that conceptualization of his experience is at such a minimum that he is unable to translate his inner reality into comprehensible terms.

To promote true intercommunication, the therapist has virtually to enter into the child's experience to the fullest possible extent and observe it in the state of becoming, as a reality in action rather than in thought. The child is an integrated person on the level of his specific condition; all of his present acts reflect his total range of experience. The therapist can learn to read the child's past, in particular the specific elaboration of his past traumata, through observed reactions, instead of verbal intercommunication. The child's deprivation is not one of circumscribed areas of experience which can be abstracted, classified, and retained. These deprivations are all-pervading and total; they are so pressing and confusing, coming from without and within, that even simple orientation might suffer. Thus confused about reality and himself as a reality factor, we are not surprised to find the child aimless, either helplessly erring, awkward, or blocked altogether and practically devoid of a communicable experience. In other words, he is isolated.

To try to establish a specific experimental setting such as a therapy or a play-therapy, would not be sufficient. A total panorama must be opened to impress upon us all facets of the inner reality of the child. We shall discuss this aspect of our approach in the chapters devoted to treatment.

From the information thus gained, we try to establish a complete picture in psychological terms.

## Main Overt Attitudes of the Child

As would be expected, two fundamental attitudes are displayed by the children treated in the Educational Therapy Center: either hopeless withdrawal from a world of pain, or an aggressive reaction to it, which represents an ambivalent or negative approach, a means of coercing the world into paying attention or an attempt to get even with it. Either communication is perverted into a warlike, predominantly destructive mode of behavior. In the first case, the child may reduce his verbalism to almost nothing; in the second instance, particularly when his condition is serious, he uses mainly emotional speech containing idiomatic phrases of a hostile character. This has been known as inner language.[7]

Depression or a *taedium vitae*, the challenging of the hostile world of the adult, cause them to exhibit a dare-devil attitude. They risk any kind of danger or punishment by stubborn inaccessibility to the point of muteness. Pleasurable experiences can be discounted altogether, unless derived from the satisfaction of obstruction and counterattacks.

These children may not even be communicating with us by their behavior. Their asocial acts may be no more than an aimless expression of profound discomfort. Any attempt to approach them by the means suggested by an aroused public is not only useless but, considering the children's inner experiences and lack of emotional as well as social maturity, is undeserved. These children may not only be unable to reveal themselves by words, but they may also be unable to accept the gift of words, kind as they may be. They are meaningless to them, confusing, annoying, and above all, utterly revulsive. They are the bitter or envenomed food served to them since they were born. In their inarticulate and low-voiced speech, they offer in return the same food which has been a false promise rather than a gratification. Distrust of all that the adult world has to provide, say, communicate, and teach is one of the many subtle reasons why such children shun learning and even avoid contacts with people, though these contacts are inevitable in school attendance particularly.

Despite the apparently insuperable difficulties implied in these children's isolation, which is due to family relationships and the rejection to which the community frequently exposes them, they are not necessarily lost but can be saved for themselves and for society.

When they are exposed to the therapeutical milieu, we may expect initial resistance, distrustful wavering, provocative testing and suspicious interpretations. But slowly they yield to the lure of life and the risk of giving in to love. Finally they reciprocate intensely. Feeling no longer singled out or exposed to rejection, indifference and neglect, they may discover values worth preserving rather than destroying. Curiosity is released. Intrigued by "secrets" everywhere, they try to become interesting by being themselves a source of exciting suspense. Starting from a small platform of experience they tend to discover and settle territory by learning. Preferably using their own methods they begin religiously to shape and master the world. They remain difficult for some time. They tend to be resistive to any intrusion upon their territory and to hoard objects for fear of being deprived of this tenuous hold on and ties to the world.

We shall endeavor to demonstrate that healing depends on a multi-dimensional endeavor that must be atuned to the very complex inner experience of these children. It must take account of their ambivalent relation to the mother and their general ambivalence. The negative role of the father has to be considered as well as the children's reliance on their own age group, with its multifarious meanings, notwithstanding dependency needs in reference to the adult. The children's ambivalence causes them to fear what they covet because they have known the mother's love to be deceptive, and pain has come from the very source that should have given delight. The father's negative role has either discouraged active tendencies which could have helped overcome the fear of a delusive goal, or it may have made the approach to life altogether forbidding, in particular when an exhausting competition with one or several stepfathers had to be upheld through the years. Companionship with their age group is fraught with similar problems. Friends sought for comfort and support prove to be inconstant. Having been led astray and into more difficulties, the children learn once more to fear what they covet and, in awe of the gift which is life, turn away from it altogether.

## Conflicts and Afflictions of the Child

These children who have been considered to be not only psychiatrically untreatable, but in need of punishment, were thought to be devoid of conflict and thus not in want of relief. Accordingly, it was held that they would neither covet treatment nor benefit by it.

However, we are convinced that potentially moral conscience is universal and can never be totally absent or silenced; its specific vigilance and direction has to be developed in reference to the milieu to which the bearer feels responsible and accountable. No indebtedness is incurred where no credit has been given. But no human being can survive, sorely deficient as his surroundings may be, unless he has received a minimum of care sufficient for survival. Neglect has cruelly marked the children with whom we are concerned, but even a rare token of love and care, once received, brings them relief. Even neglectful parents may be assumed to have given their children more than they have received from other human beings. In return, whatever else the children feel, they cling to their parents, obsessively reaching out for gratification; they try vainly to coerce the mother into granting it and, when they are consistently disappointed they may dream up gratification, and then forgive and glorify her. They cast their resentment upon the unnamed and the unknown. This is not possible without conflict, because resentment is primarily kindled in the home, by the very parents the children feel a need for, and want to love and to respect.

Relief, however, must come from him who brought distress; it must be the undoing of a hurt. This is the basic reason why the parents are the sole possible and the sole acceptable healers of the blow they have struck. Therefore, the children's longing for the parents is extreme. It is repeated failure and disappointment with the parents, the child's search for comfort in deception, and his denial of reality that prompt him to cast resentment upon the unnamed and the unknown. In therapy, hostility is transferred to the psychiatrist who becomes the one who struck, but therewith also becomes acceptable as the healer.

These children live in two worlds dominated by two systems of values. One is the everyday world of our visible culture, which in its superficial aspects does not reveal convincingly a reason for existence. The other world is the universe of their childhood, which even under its more or less abhorrent surface has preserved the immortal substance of man.

Thus a child who communicates already may anxiously advertise day in and day out, deviously or plainly, the tribulations his home inflicts upon him; yet he may still not want to leave the home for a more adequate placement, or if removed, may request ardently to return. He is motivated by the urge to continue his pathological interaction with the parents, and also by his need to redeem both himself and them. Above all, the child will resent intensely any implied criticism of the parents, particularly of the mother; he will also resent any implied or sensed refutation of his milieu.

Most of the time the children want to be held personally responsible. Despite complaints and resentments, they shield the family. They have reasons of their own, not easy to understand; they like "my mother and everything about her, her house, her town, her people." Perhaps they recall the great hours of relief and security whenever they were allowed to fold up upon themselves and their childhood atmosphere—be it only with the joy of pouting. They like a home where threadbare shades and curtains are hung with clothespins, just because it is home, remembered, and familiar. Children speak lovingly and with the depth and delight of a poet about rags and tatters because they were their own in their invisible world of eternal values.

There is much meaning in the early relations to material objects. Those clothespins, for instance, may have been a symbol of a spontaneous resourcefulness; they may represent to him his level and his way of coping with existence; they may have been a token for his particular ability, and therefore some motivation of desire to go on living with some conviction. A child in this state of mind is a soldier at war; in his daily battle he may enjoy moments of poetry, and the pouring rain may be comfort in those minutes when the strife has receded; inside a dilapidated shack, he may contemplate the elegy of his fate. Such feelings, such discord with realities, cannot be denied the children. They represent their most sacred, their most ancient anchorage in life itself.

## Unrest and Aimlessness in Space

More deprived and much harder to reach is the agitated child; the motor phenomena of children growing up in extreme destitution and exposed to serious neglect are hampered by the fact that there was actually nothing worth reaching for. Their impulse to grasp for something would not have been discouraged if, at critical moments, stimulating objects rather than void had surrounded them from infancy. A total lack of objects in the house may become a lasting impediment to the early and future experiences of touch and proprioceptive sensations. Without the stimulation by objects, no sufficient points of reference are available for differentiation of one's own body from other objects, and the child is not aroused to manipulate them. Consciousness of self and self-confidence are very poorly developed. Such barren milieu reflects an atmosphere of hopelessness and indifference which inhibits outgoing vital tendencies.

Only a poorly controlled and apparently aimless agitation remain when longing for life and experience are not altogether lost. A futile search and erring, the urge to touch indiscriminately, express an inappropriate trend toward orientation. By testing reality a child finds and defines. But unless a gentle maternal voice lends words to the fugitive sensations, helps the child to hold on to the idea of objects and to remember perception, the child cannot slow down for discrimination and recognition of sensations that remain but a shapeless lure. Frustrated attempts for cognition, the exposure to an abyss of nothingness each time the child reaches out for experience begets intense anxiety and renewed agitation.

These children are driven into the streets, to see things, to hear and touch them, to grasp, to control, to co-ordinate, to throw, to push and to pull, to own. Here is their opportunity to separate themselves from the world outside, to verify their being and their capacity for functioning.

In a world of innumerable protective hideouts, these children are less reluctant to deceive and less menaced than in the home. The young boy goes into the street badly prepared. He has not been taught the gentle ways to approach things. He has not been initiated to the alluring sound of his mother's voice who mitigated her refusal or to parental playfulness that alleviates its severity. He has to learn belatedly on the outside that which inside the house would not—and should not—arouse problems.

Restlessness can be observed as a manifestation of the want for the love objects, or as the symbolic expression of an ambivalence. O'Bryon was torn by indecision over which of his separated parents he wanted to live with. The father lived under well-adjusted middle-class conditions in a northern city; the mother had to contend in a southern town with less than the bare necessities of existence. Mutely he used to express his unsolved dilemma by untiringly mounting up the steps and gliding down the ramp to the exclusion of any other activity.

The aimless agitation of a nine-year-old ward of the Social Service Bureau could be explained in therapy as the child's unrealistic and illusionistic search for his father. The father was needed to find the mother. She was not only harder to find, but it was harder to redeem her status. Only through the restored community of the parents could he hope that it could be done. His own salvation or doom depended on it, as he saw it.

Despite the moorage in their miserable environment these children are intensely deprived and isolated individuals. Therefore, symbolically speaking, they hold out a hand clumsily and angrily. A humiliating dole of token interest will not satisfy their wants; even less will our reprimand of their aggressive inroads into our territory diminish their need for martial attack on our protected treasured possessions. The stronger we militate against them, the more we provoke their proud and irate counterattacks.

Unless these children can be made to feel that we are able to sense the poetry of their childhood pains and pleasures, we will remain strangers to them. But they must be included in our world and made to belive in us; they must be fondled into the will to change. By necessity this will entail a change in ourselves because these children have much to teach us. Our readiness to learn will encourage their willingness to reveal their feelings and convictions; the particular knowledge they have to convey will help us to impart our knowledge which is so difficult for them to accept.

# III

## *The Home the Child Calls His Own*

There are two significant conditions which characterize the homes from which the children come to the Educational Therapy Center: They are crowded with people but barren of objects. These homes make impossible the proper development of strong and sharply defined personalities. For some time now purposeful people have limited the size of their families; however, where large families have resulted from planning, and where they function harmoniously due to integration and fellowship, there is usually an opportunity for the children to test reality, to learn self-control. There is also a reasonable defining of individual rights and duties. But such large families require full-time and mature parents. Their activities have to be part of an integrated end. Their guidance of their offspring has to be continuous and intelligent.

Contrariwise, large families that spring up haphazardly fail, as a rule, to develop well-defined and strong personalities. But it is from these crowded homes, devoid of any apparent purpose, that stem the children in our care. The parents of many of them have failed in elementary education. Several generations often live together by necessity. Their unrealistic kindness opens the door to any of their kinfolk in need, regardless of space or the lack of even the most elementary furnishings and supplies—beds and bedding, chairs and tables, food and kitchen utensils.

Acting without thought about their own children, guided by indiscriminate benevolence, these families pool their meager resources in the face of insuperable odds and of impending emergencies. Unable to anticipate the emotional, social, and economic consequences, they increase the baggage rather than the forces for combat with their inadequate environment.

With this baggage train of dependents these people are constantly on the move. They are resented by the more affluent and less numerous families of the neighborhood. The quality of the quarters they can obtain declines with each change that circumstances impose on them. They become undesirable to the landlords because they allegedly cause the value of the property to decline, or they may be unreliable in paying their rent. They can be considered martyrs who share their fellows' burdens, often relieving the community of this burden; but when they are crushed under their excessive load, inevitably they involve the community in the end. Moving about incessantly for the purpose of evading their creditors may be just one symptom of their collapse. They often break down under the burden carried for dependents who are unable to cope in any positive way with the practicalities of life.

## Crowding as a Way of Life

For that matter, overcrowding becomes not only a way of reactive adaptation to single, or recurring individual situations, but a positive and constant attitude which these families try to defend. It is a way of life which is opposed to the envied habits of the strangers on the "right" side of the tracks who "pretend they know everything." The children as a result become involved in a confusion of antagonistic attitudes, humiliations, a sense of personal and family indignity, manifested by depressed or aggressive reactions of every imaginable description.

The story of a brother and sister, Edward and Caroline may illustrate such adaptations to crowding. Moving for Edward meant escape from an overpowering reality. It also gave him opportunities to take as baggage something familiar to cling to and sensed as his possession. His package of collected "familiar objects" supported an illusion of autonomy and of independence. Moving from place to place, Edward would take along his wife, his parents-in-law, two brothers, one of them married, another sister and her infant, and, not content with these many dependents, Edward would also lure his young, unmarried sister, Caroline, to move into his one-room and kitchen apartment.

Edward felt very important as the benevolent ruler of this clan. This founder of a kind of gypsy dynasty made it clear that he would not let anyone intrude into his business, except on his own terms. An apparent but actually non-existent co-operation made his home a prac-

48

tically impregnable stronghold. Edward tried to prove to himself and to others that he and he alone wielded real power, and he was indifferent to the existence of social order and civilization. Moreover, the group moving around with Edward seemed to derive a feeling of importance from being part of his clan.

He feuded with an aunt who had attracted Caroline. This aunt was the only conforming member of the family and delighted in flaunting her position in a snobbish, haughty, and rigid way. Such behavior, of course, served not only to diminish Edward's personal position in a world which he feared Caroline was ready to desert, but also to make it unacceptable to an unresponsive Caroline.

Caroline came to us at the age of fifteen, and was diagnosed as a schizophrenic. She was hostile, withdrawn, and verbally uncommunicative. She was placed with the aunt, the sole relative of good standing. Caroline's overt behavior improved to such an extent that after a few months an attempt could be made to enrol her in the public school, where she made a good adjustment. Treatment and occupational therapy were to be given twice a week in the Center, after school hours.

The girl came from a rural family of seven, including the parents. The family deviated in their standards, whether educational, social, or moral, from the surrounding community and ostracism against them was acted out by all the children on the road and village streets. When Caroline was six years old, her mother died suddenly. The father soon became involved with the law in a way which made him permanently unsuitable for the education of his girls, and the children were placed in the homes of relatives. Because of ill-treatment the children's new placement proved equally unsuitable, and a second placement was made for the girls.

Within a few months, while Caroline was still under observation, Edward had moved three times, to very different sections of town, living always in so-called two-room apartments, actually a living-bedroom and a kitchen, with a population of nine, partly unrelated people, of both sexes. Caroline's baby niece was reported dependent and neglected at the time Caroline was referred to the public school.

Edward had remained in touch with their father, and while Caroline still lived in the country she had been allowed to see him. Caroline's complete maladjustment in her very adequate country foster home was the immediate result. She became ambivalent about whether she wanted to continue to live in the country or go to town to live with the brother. Rejection of the foster home and what it stood for manifested itself in an increase and intensification of her symptoms.

After placement in town with the aunt, the girl lived in sedentary, as well as socially and economically adequate, circumstances. Her devoted aunt, though rigid and reluctant to accept needed guidance, cared for her, but the brother tried repeatedly to interfere and to lure her into his overcrowded home, supporting Caroline's ambivalence and tempting her to return to the less acceptable standards she had been used to. For a short time she maintained a state of indecision between the two ways of life. Profiting from the opportunity offered in the aunt's home, she played the role of the sweet girl, because everybody insisted on placing her in that role, and bided her time. No assistance for continuance of therapy was received by the family. Contrary to psychiatric advice the aunt withdrew Caroline from therapy. Anxious to forget and cause everybody to forget that the child was not well, she maintained that as Caroline's closest relative, she could and should assume full guidance of the child's life. A follow-up study revealed that Caroline was removed from the dilemma of her situation and returned to a foster home in her rural home community.

## Attitudes to Moving and Its Consequences

Even in the cruel anonymity of our cities, two basic cultural attitudes are still with us. They represent opposite principles of man's contribution to his survival on earth but are also complementary. The individual during his evolution shifts from one attitude to the next at various periods of existence, both attitudes at times overlapping. We are referring to the tendency of exploring the resources that are serviceable to survival either by moving toward new ones when the existing ones are exhausted, or by tending to create on the spot new resources mediately or immediately. Once sedentary habits have been established they are not easily relinquished. When, for a number of reasons (pressure or overpopulation, for instance) or motivations (of an ideological nature, for example), such human groups resort to moving toward new horizons, the sedentary mode of living is not necessarily sacrificed.

There are those elements in our population that tend to move toward seasons and harvests rather than to conquer the seasons and store the crop. We are not talking here of pioneers who venture out to new horizons, and, on an inhospitable spot, build a new sedentary culture. We are concerned here with the parents of children who graze to barrenness their puny pastures, moving from place to place, leaving behind them material disorder while they take along emotional disorder. Therefore, unwanted and distrusted wherever they go, they move on "regardless," hostile, withdrawn, and angrily defensive against anticipated rejection. Necessarily, they oppose their children's preferences, if existing, their potentialities for adjustment to the surrounding "sedentary" culture.

Tendencies toward stability, such as the sound attachment to the house, neighborhood, school, grandparents, or friends, are disrupted cruelly with the family's every move. Parents lure their children into the nomadic camp, irritated by any objections. Such parents can never be reached, a factor which may inhibit the children's co-operation under treatment totally or may cause a long stage of uncertainty, but at times the children permit us to convince them, in spite of what seem in the beginning insuperable odds.

## Moving and the Schools

Truancy from school may be but a symptom of the child's total or ambivalent lack of co-operation with an antagonistic and menacing world. The standards he is supposed to meet and the level of performance he must maintain can be intimidating indeed, particularly when, simultaneously, he is silently committed by his parents to oppose the requirements of the hostile environment represented by school; but he has to move on for his parents' sake, while they angrily discourage him from moving on. If children are not yet entirely set in their antagonistic social ways, if doubts have arisen in their minds due to adversities connected with their own way of life, and if satisfactory contacts with understanding adults have been made outside the family, a state of confusion, mental anguish and emotional anarchy may result. The children's most positive approach is tearful complaints to the therapist. One of these complaints is particularly about the changing of school, which makes studying hard and life miserable, especially when as a result the children lose all their friends and sometimes a beloved teacher or principal who knew them and their problems. The greatest difficulties arise when moving does not coincide with the end of a school term.

It should be noted that more than half of the people of the greater Richmond, Virginia, area own their homes and that the majority of the tenants in the middle-income bracket lease their apartments on a yearly basis. Most of these leases start September 1, and the middle-class children attend their new school from the beginning of the academic year. However, the monthly lease, and even more the leaseless rental, tends to reflect a lack of mutual regard between tenant and landlord, indicated, for instance, by a relative neglect of the property by the owner and often considerable unconcern on the part of the tenant and entailing increased safety and health hazards. Innumerable frictions deepen the cleavage between the social strata and thus add to the cycle of mutual rejection between family and community.

It is precisely in this milieu that the Center's children grow up. They are aware of and are infected with cynicism and defeatism, feeling dejection and rejection, as well as obstructionism everywhere. Surely these children have no motivation for constructive participation in a society which they despise because it has not given them confidence and opportunity.

We remember one case of a white landlord's failure to repair several splits in the walls of the house, even after having been informed that the housewife had been striken by rheumatic fever and a dangerous cardiac condition. When the woman died, one of the children expressed hatred of "the white man who killed my mother." It should be stated in all fairness that while such harsh attitudes intensify racial antagonisms, they are just instances of a general lack of concern of the one who holds the reigns toward him who is bare-handed and helpless.

The story of the Smith family is told here to illustrate the real danger and causal nexus of school difficulties and frequent moves. Four children, out of this family of six, ranging in age from eight to fourteen, were referred to the Education Therapy Center for learning difficulties and behavior disorders. The mother was allegedly promiscuous. The father, a laborer, had left the family six years ago, and since that time they had been moving between city and country,

either living by themselves—which meant in a house with strangers—
or at the homes of grandmothers or uncles, as only a temporary arrangement "because it was always so crowded there." In those six
years the older children had attended eight different schools.

This inflicted particular hardship on the oldest boy, who voiced
utter discouragement. His mother kept moving on and on. Every time
he was transferred to a new school, he lost one year. The erroneous-
ness of such practice was demonstrated even more blatantly in the
case of a very superior boy. Failure to assign him to the grade for
which he was actually qualified indicated, after a long struggle by his
mother to have him reclassified, that the class to which he had been
assigned evidently was one year below his chronological age but four
years below his actual ability for study. The oldest girl in the Smith
family, a very short, stocky child of fourteen years, missed the father
intensely. She had been raped at the age of eight and denied reality by
fantasies. Therefore, she also denied discouragement through these
many school changes and indeed bragged proudly that she attended so
many schools.

However, all the Smith children were bewildered about the charac-
terological identity of their parents, their mutual relations with them,
and other relevant persons in the home. Each child produced different
facts when asked for the ages, sequences, numbers, and even names of
his or her siblings; one, for instance, was significantly called "Eat-
more." They were equally confused as to remote and immediate goals.
They cried when they came to the Educational Therapy Center, ran
around aimlessly, unable to say what they would like to do instead of
being with us. Actually they were afraid of everything other than
being left alone to drift on their own. Everything else might mean
imposed interference and change.

## The Street and Inner Migration

In cases such as these, the street has an extremely strong attraction.
The child is nowhere, to be sure, but at least he is not in a house
where he cannot feel at home because his mother is absent or with
strangers, or because there are "so many nervous, nagging people
about." The Smith children cried anxiously because they did not
clearly know where they belonged, or to whom. To be nowhere, un-

der the circumstances, is safest. They lagged in self-identification yet they felt dimly that among strangers they were not met with excessive expectations. Anxious and utterly insecure, they were unable to make a contribution which would have been a creation from nothingness. To be active and purposeful as is expected among people thus was a deadly menace. As a result of migratory living the child has to adapt to many changing circumstances. He is deprived of the benefit of a persistent interaction between himself and his environment which would enable him to structure and master existing circumstances and to test the existence and quality of his own metal. Exploration of relationship in depth is prevented. A problem arises for these young nomads as an out-group in a sedentary society. Unlike gypsies, who wisely and with fair success, attempt to achieve isolation and a definite style of existence, children like the Smiths are not integrated in an organized out-group. They are not protected by their own, though primitive institutions. They do not have their wagon and wagon park, nor their baggage of people gathered under the clan's chief. They are nomads due to parental improvidence, usually by necessity, not conviction. Therefore, even at a later stage of life, they cannot be expected to create the means for defining their own world and, like gypsies, ignore ours. Their situation, should we fail to include these children, will indeed remain one of isolation, but for fear only and therefore devoid of any longing to come over to a shore to which there is no conveyance. To communicate, be it by getting into trouble with other children or by fighting, has its advantages. It satisfies a number of needs beside the fundamental one of hitting a target or a scapegoat. It is an evident justification for crying as a release of tension, for complaining as an outright expression of misery, for clamoring for help, compassion and attention, particularly toward nightfall when the last defenses have been broken down and loneliness can no longer be endured. Fighting in the street satisfies the need for outside stimulation particularly in a child possessing few inner resources.

## Family Incohesiveness and Insecurity of the Child

When a cohesive family group does not exist, the home situation is materially aggravated and everything is indeed on the move. The natural father's traces may be lost. Numerous legitimate and illegitimate "daddys" of very different characteristics and attitudes may have moved in or visited. Some may have been drunk and violent and stayed on with the family when the child hoped they would leave; others may have disappeared when the child had just taken to them. Soon the child will feel at a loss whether to wish for a father or for his disappearance.

Not only is the child menaced by the man's role as the mother's sex partner and the replenishment of an unprovided home with an average of two abiding pawns of his passing interest, but also by the changes in the mother's personality affected by each new relationship. Moreover, each separation is preceded by violent dissensions and multiple symptoms of asocial or antisocial adjustment. The child's liberation from a usually unwanted father substitute is at the price of a deeply resented humiliation of the mother, whatever the causes of the breach. Gratification forever is at the price of wrong and guilt feelings and to be relieved is tantamount to being bad. This promotes a new ambivalence, a new motivation for fearing gratification, and a repression of guilt feelings and a weary indifference to being bad.

Each time the boy is liberated from the father substitute, a new motive for defeatism has arisen. He also misses the man as a protector and resents that he deserted and exposed him. In his exposed condition he turns against the mother. Hate now has become the defensive barrier needed between him and the mother. To becloud the real meaning of his hostility, which as a barrier he must protect and cannot face, he displaces it on earlier phases of traumatization and pretends that she neglects to feed him. The son needs to promote the mother's hostility to justify his own hostility and to assuage his guilt feelings. Some boys display the described dynamism with the mother permanently, and may accept the stepfather as a substitute if the slightest opportunity is given, so that he may relieve his problems with the mother.

The emotional problem is complicated by the economic difficulties. The common-law husband may be costly rather than a relief from financial stress, as hoped. When he leaves, the family economics may have deteriorated to an all-time low. Necessarily this has slowly built up the boy's anger to a white heat which he will turn either outside or inside, paralyzing himself in order to prevent an explosion of some kind. The financial catastrophe may have occurred only after the man left and the mother is likely to project her despair on the boy. That the child is there, instead of the man, is sometimes cause enough to resent him. His helpless attempts to offer emotional and economic comfort to the mother contribute to further impairment of the relationship. The offer to substitute for the man who has left is irritating not only as a reminder of the child's inadequacy, but of her own in reference to a grown, and as such, a desirable man. Moreover, the child's eagerness to "jump into the hurdle" is justifiably sensed as his secret delight in her bad fortune. Under the guise of tending the mother a gift, he actually tends to absorb and consume her. Only by such behavior does the child resemble the man, as known to her from a disconcerting experience of a lifetime, and it is as an image of the male that the child once more has to be rejected. But the boy who also has fought for love and life, ready to trade in all that he had to offer, once more writhes in mortal pain. For the sake of mere survival, emotional eruptions of volcanic proportions may then become inevitable. Their specific manifestations should be interpreted as symbolic of the child's insistence on harmonizing his relationship with the mother by coercion.

It is under the guise of protecting the children that at times they are shifted around to and from the countryside, to and from the state, back and forth between distant cities, to and from a grandmother or some other relative. Often these "grandparents" are no kin at all but elderly people who have raised one or the other of the child's parents, people who enjoy children regardless of their parentage.

But for the children themselves, grave conflicts arise from such exchanges. Deep-rooted obligations are incurred by them without their volition, and strong bonds of dependency must be endured for which they do not feel responsible. The foster parents may contribute their share by rigidity, righteousness, and hypocrisy. The children may complain that there is as much drinking, carousing, and marital infidelity rife in that family as in their own. Only the economic status might vary. The adoptive parents may stress unendingly the conditionality of their acceptance of the child, thus they do not tell the child only "I shall love and keep you if you succeed in convincing me that you are mine," but also that they need to be convinced and at least doubt the child's acceptability. The foster parents in turn cannot understand what they did to deserve ingratitude. The benefactor only knows or remembers the noble part he took in a desperate situation and feels that he is entitled to credit for his willingness to help.

In the case of a conflict between parents and grandparents, children will often cling to their grandparents in an emergency, when neither generation has sufficient insight to look upon the narrow straits of its age limits, or when neither can muster enough patience and affection to try to understand each other in terms of the other generation.

Under these tense and menacing conditions, the pre-psychotic child may be threatened to the point of being totally uprooted by any change from the home of either the parents or grandparents. Any move may thus be feared as permanent separation. When the need for clinging to another ego is imperative, its manifestations may be more readily tolerated by older, maternal figures whose gentleness has been gained at the expense of the more vital and aggressive propensities of youth and its imperative demands. These, however, provide the very source of conflict between an instinctive, driven mother and a child barely equipped to endure life, even in extremely sheltered conditions.

It is a remarkable feature in unstable milieus that somehow the grandmother, who in extreme cases may be no older than thirty, has gained some stability, perhaps by moving less often, by refusal to change life mates or companions, or by solving her sexual needs in ways which represent a stabilizing rather than an upsetting element to the family group, especially to the child. This kind of grandmother is less perturbed by the struggle for existence, by an unsettled and inadequately satiated love life, and by continuous swaying between acceptance and rejection. This kind of grandmother, therefore, may answer more readily the child's dire need for reliable and stable relations. Although she may not be accepted without conflict, reluctance, and resentment, she may be the only motherly figure left to the child.

Stephen's story may provide some insight into that phenomenon. He was a very short boy of eleven when he was referred to the Center by the Juvenile Court for setting fire to a number of cars and pulling the fire alarm. He had refused to attend public school but accepted schooling in the Educational Therapy Center.

Stephen had moved repeatedly from one end of the town to the other, together with his large family group. His family, however, was not cohesive, and Stephen had to resort to meaningful maternal affiliations, in particular to an outgoing elderly saleswoman in a candy store. He missed also the children of the neighborhood, his old school, and the beautiful city park. When he had to move once more, he continued to run untiringly to this elderly woman.

The third of eight children, Stephen came from a more stable home than did most of our other day-care patients. At least his parents were married. However, his mother was an impressively capable perfectionist. She "loved the house" more than its inhabitants and her nurturing, tending, and unfolding talents were overshadowed by her compulsive needs. She ran an impeccably clean and neat home. Her ability and concomitant righteousness had a depressing and inhibiting influence on a weak husband. Stephen's father revolted by withdrawal into weekly alcoholic sprees. He kept things "rolling" though frustrating all her ambitions. This difficult home situation was aggravated by a local economic slump. Stephen's mother, however, was not able to evaluate fairly the degree to which her husband could be expected to control the economic situation.

Upon referral, Stephen was totally withdrawn, rigid, inhibited, and inarticulate. But his setting fires to cars was a symbolic communication, and a signal. Each time he had learned to warm himself at the hearth of a new house and it had become a home, it changed into a conveyance and disappeared. Cars were the symbol of the rolling home. The spark he painstakingly had lit at the hearth of the beloved home was converted into an incendiary torch and turned on the "houses on wheels."

Subsequent to treatment, the boy improved; he himself requested to return to a public school. However, a few months later he had a bicycle accident in the street and fractured his skull while working as a paper boy. Strangely enough, the family seemed unaware of the seriousness of the boy's condition; no doctor was called, though the mother was advised to do so. Stephen was found dead, alone, on the floor of the bathroom the next morning, although he had shared his room and bed with his brothers during the night.

In view of the frequent effacement and even more frequent absence of a father, the relationship between mother and grandfather is of predominant importance. A great deal of confusion may result from the fact that uncles and aunts are of the same age or younger than nephews and nieces. Mutual love and fraternity or mutual hostility will depend on the role which is assigned to each offspring by his own mother, and by the predominant mother figure of the house, whether one child is rejected by one or both, or whether more than one or all of them are rejected and neglected. If mother and grandmother are united by a common hatred of men, the boys may unite in common hostility, and their emotional problem may be aggravated by subtle hostile interaction in the family and be acted out ubiquitously by each child individually, or the paired or teamed-up youngsters' group.

Further complications are caused by the fact that several daughters with their offspring might live in the house. Some of the children might be legitimate offspring of an unfortunate marriage. Their legitimate status might cause the illegitimate children to react to this superior status in a sensitive way. A grown son might be living in the house with problems relating to the mother or sisters, whether he is married or a bachelor, or whether his marriage is whole or broken. We can only hint at the emotional assault from every direction, varying in pitch of intensity only, to which children from these milieus are exposed. What can they do but wthdraw with stubborn sullenness or explode under the momentary impact of almost imperceptible excitations because the breaking point has already been reached? Children who have been subjected to excessive stimulation in areas where a child needs to be spared are extremely vulnerable in these specific areas, usually those of hostile family interaction and multiple sexual involvements.[1]

First, circumstances force the children to see what terrifies them, then they become obsessed to see, to alleviate anxiety; they do it themselves and sex becomes an obsession for a second reason: known to them from infancy it is, and has been, due to utter resourcelessness, the sole tranquilizer for all loneliness, anxiety, and irritation. It is a recognized means to please and be temporarily accepted, but finally it will be developed into the most powerful weapon for vexation and revenge.

Walking through city quarters inhabited by these children and their families, one cannot escape observing the omnipresence of sexual preoccupations at all ages. No reserve, no differentiation is displayed. What we could observe most frequently is foreign to any person-to-person relationship, enchantment, and choice.

The agencies who refer children with sexual problems to us usually call it sex play. This is an improper term. These young, unfortunately, do not know a thing about the grace of being attractive, an expression of human culture and as such reflected in poetry, great music, and painting. What these poor children have known since their lonely days in the cradle is play with the body and the sexual organs. Only at times does a child with a genius for tender and gracious, as well as passionate, love, stand out in an untended wilderness like a flower from foreign soil. The emotional refinement of such children will, however expose them more cruelly. First they may have been in search of something intangible, with no eyes to perceive the crudities around them. The touch of the fingertips, extended toward a companion of like age, to an outside observer may seem as productive of poetry as a fine pianist's touch of the keyboard.

If our child is a girl who comes home half-awakened to the crude realities of life, expecting a fatherless child, she is again more cruelly exposed. It is our experience that whoever the girl's father is, if he still lives in the home, he will have had some furtive awareness of his daughter's quality and loved her reverently, hiding his adoration behind a rough indifference. The apparent ruin of this idol and the violation of what may be the man's sole sensed cause of pride will create a deep rift between the father and the guilt-ridden daughter; the similarity of the hurt inflicted on both of them from without will certainly not promote a greater closeness between them now than did previously the father's sensitivity to the daughter's charm. The father might regret his previous positive feelings for a daughter who proved to be just like everybody else. Nor is he likely to find out that it was his lack of experience in showing love and affection that prevented her from identifying with an adored mother and adorable womanhood. It also failed to convey to the daughter, in the delicate terms of a father, the awareness of her charming personality. He is not likely to find out that her exposure to her improper experience had its origin in family relations.

Whether the father is at home, whether his relationship to the daughter has made the relationship between mother and daughter difficult, it is our experience that the mother from now on will take over, rule the daughter and annex the child. She has innumerable motivations for doing so. In appearance the daughter's behavior is a repetition of the mother's behavior, and the mother now will like to dispense the bitterly resented medicine she once received from her mother. If the mother has come from a more self-respecting and ambitious milieu and once has been exposed to a strict rule by her mother she may never have ceased to resent her loss of freedom for youthful fun. She may have remained undecided between her own mother's conviction with whom she believes she now identifies, and her resentment of it when a young girl. Of these convictions she now suspects the daughter. Under the guise of censuring her, the mother may create an obsession in the daughter by starving her, by prohibiting any, even usually accepted, youthful distractions. When the daughter finally has succumbed and acts out the very experiences the mother once was forced to bypass, the mother will be gratified by identification with the daughter's objectionable behavior, or a form of voyeurism. But the awareness of gratification will have to be denied or repressed and therefore the girl will have to be censured and punished. If the daughter brings home a child, enjoyment of the child will have to be denied her.

Due to the lack of opportunity for maturation, the earlier born children of a girl or at times a couple are just by-products of "sex play." The children's rejection and neglect reflect the mother's lack of readiness for motherhood—its responsibilities and enjoyment. While the teenage mother is avid for sex gratification, the thirty- to thirty-five-year-old grandmother is an insatiable consumer of grandchildren, regardless of what it does to the child. Overprotection and neglect will alternate, and the basic realities such as available space, food, or privacy will be disregarded. The seeming insatiability for infants, whatever else it means in each case, or in more general terms, represents a form of promiscuity.

The young mothers do not grow with the child and the experience never deepens or widens beyond the early and helpless stages of childhood. The grandmother's greed for babies is one of the reasons she condones the daughter's sexual licentiousness and for her candid confession that she has no problems with her girls, while the house abounds in fatherless grandchildren. The parents of two boys referred to us, one of them having manifested murderous tendencies, discarded five of their ten young children but collected around them instead their elder daughters' five illegitimate children.

In thus adopting the daughter's children, usually sending the daughter to work, the grandmother stifles any expanding maternal feelings in her daughter. One grandmother went so far as to give away the child for illegal adoption without asking her daughter's consent.

For the experience of womanhood, the disarmed young mother will rely on mere sexuality at the expense of a more complete experience of femininity which includes motherhood. Usually this frustrating development entails depression and, on the rebound, the need for sexual gratification is enhanced by the need for some comfort. The sexual obsession leads to a sense of self-depreciation as well as an apparent indifference to it. The young woman becomes usually rapidly self-rejecting and engages in sexual activities without discrimination, at times in disregard of gratification or in actual denial of it. Hostility is developed against the young woman's mother, whose function is more or less dimly understood. The hurt is usually so deep that the teenage mother cannot verbalize it directly. Actually she may not admit to her consciousness the meaning of her mother's behavior.

This emotional upheaval maintains a vicious circle and interferes with maternal feelings and expressions at a time when the mother-child relationship should be at its prime. In a decade and a half, the daughter will have to catch up with the experience of motherhood and regain a more complete experience of womanhood, as well as idea of self, at the expense of her own daughter. Hardened by frustration and a life reduced to struggling for existence, she will in turn intimidate her daughter and thus irretrievably deprive the child of the unfolding power of maternal devotion. The closed circle of chastisement through generations of children for the sins of their elders can be interrupted only by a liberating act of generosity. Only the mother who rises above the confining experience of her own miserable existence can help the future generations gain entrance into the abounding gratifications of life to which her unselfish devotion holds the main key. It is at a hearth like hers that children will be inspired to master adverse circumstances in a way truly uplifting to behold.

But in the Clinic, we see at best a maternal grandmother at odds with her daughter, who in turn rejects her child, usually the boy. He therefore increases the rift between the middle and oldest generations, while the first and third generations join hands.

When the fear of loss has not been overcome by the grandmother since the days of her frustrating young motherhood, she will cling to the daughter's children, indulge and overprotect them. The youngest offspring glued to her body wherever she goes, the grandmother will flare up with irritation at the child's first centrifugal intention. The very moment he makes a move to grasp an object she slaps his hands or shakes him angrily. It is obvious that a child thus treated will be impeded in all areas of growth. At a time when he is but a promise of his future self, he is made the victim of an insecure woman, who on the contrary should be for him the focal point of a world unfolding within and outside of him. Instinctively the daughter becomes aware of what is going on, whether because of his unavailability to her, his passivity, or his tendency to show discomfort, usually by crying.

The child affected by the atmosphere of violent discord between the two women will hardly escape the temptation to play one against the other. Helpless in the face of unconquerable odds, the mother yields to weariness and indifference; or she will try to liberate herself, taking the child along, if she can. At times she will see no escape and in her despair desert her children. Due to the ever present interference between them, mother and child have never reached each other. The forever unanswered longing between them has prompted a tendency in both mother and child toward oversensitive interpretations of each other's behavior. If the mother takes heart to leave at a moment when interest is shown her by a man, the family will accuse her attraction to him as the motive for desertion. Actually the man may have been but an opportunity to escape somewhere rather than nowhere. Whatever happens, the child will suffer. Some of the traumas suffered by children in such families can be illustrated.

There is, for instance, Lester's case, where the great-aunt played the part more frequently assumed by the grandmother.

According to Kubie, the family is an autocracy ruled by its sickest member. A widow in her fifties who had lost her husband ten years earlier, this great-aunt was also the tyrant. Since the death of her husband, she had suffered the loss of a daughter fourteen years of age, and of a grandson eighteen years of age. She liked to be called "Miss" and insisted on using her maiden name.

She suffered from a thyrotoxicosis with cardiac and a number of nervous and emotional symptoms. She had an unsolved Electra complex, and she was economically dependent upon her father, for whom she had kept house since her mother's death. The love for her mother and the distress over her death, which lay years back, was conspicuously empasized.

Her grand-nephew Lester was referred to us by a county public school because of irregular attendance, which was excused by ill health, and because of a tendency to cry a great deal, a habit which could be traced as far back as infancy. A most attractive eight-year-old, he was the youngest of the four children of his uncongenial parents. At all times, four generations were crowded in a house which would have been adequate for one small family.

Lester's father, the widow's nephew, was sufficiently dependent on his aunt to allow her to interfere with his marriage from the start. She was passionately jealous of Lester's mother. She responded, in our first interview, to the question whether the child was breastfed with the statement that the mother had plenty of breast but no milk. She denied her the very title of mother and finally drove her out of the house. A few months before we saw Lester, she had finally succeeded in wresting the child from his mother.

At the time of Lester's referral both parents had deserted the home and the children. It should be noted that the father promised to come back provided his wife would be first to return to the home. Apparently he was aware of the aunt's role in his life and in reference to his marriage. Lester, however, could not escape the overprotection from which his father finally tried to liberate himself.

On his first visit to the Center the eight-year-old boy, well-built and mentally well-developed, sat crying and fearful on the lap of the aunt. She explained the situation in these terms: "You know how it is with other people's children, you must not make them feel that you don't love them."

Since infancy the boy was in the habit of crying and throwing things, a victim of the mother's cornered and weakened position. Though the child loved her, he dared not admit it; thus, he had to transfer to Santa Claus this dangerous and forbidden love. In his initial interview Lester said "Santa Claus loves my mother best of all people." The fretful child soon developed psychosomatic disturbances, featuring the aunt's thyrotoxic heart trouble. There existed between the aunt and the grand-nephew a kind of communal bond connected with the home, the embracing mother to whom they both clung. This became a decisive factor in his truancy problem.

The aunt actually did not want the child, but she was under the compulsion to deprive the mother. However, she could not face her role as the one who had systematically cornered the mother until she had but one choice, to give up and leave. As the great-aunt saw it, "the mother has dumped the children in my lap." Her real motives were revealed when she deplored with bitterness a destiny that would have her children dead, whereas Lester and his siblings were alive. To let the boy leave the house promoted anxiety, and in her ambivalence she "hatched" him into sickness at home and inadequacy at school.

Willy Mathew's problem involved both grandparents. This story is told in order to shed some light on the complexity of the motives that might animate the total family group. The grandmother's need to keep all of her daughter's children was her compensation for having been demoted in her marital rank by the emotional vehemence of the father-daughter relationship. The grandfather had a number of reasons to support his wife's tendencies. He wanted to appease her with these compensations, assign to her the role of the grandmother, while he played the part of the children's father and emphasized that he provided for them. To have the children in the house also served the purpose of holding the daughter on the leash. The daughter's vain attempt to liberate herself had led to the birth of three illegitimate children, the eldest boy being Willy, our patient. She finally got married, but this attempt equally failed. She married a depraved, violent alcoholic and a non-provider, and as a quarrel between father and daughter revealed, a disfigured replica of the father. She accused him of having himself all the shortcomings that he censured with hostile vehemence in her husband.

In this session she declared emphatically that she was going to request official custody of her children in court. Actually she already had custody of her children. The court was only a symbol of strength to be borrowed, since she was unable to liberate herself from bonds welded out of dependency, resentment, and a deep sense of guilt. These bonds still kept her confined at the parental home all day long, neglecting her own home across the street. It increased the husband's sense of isolation and rejection and intensified his addiction to alcohol as well as his desperate need for brutal aggression.

Willy was referred to the Clinic by the public schools. The reason for referral was his most irregular school attendance and the habit of constantly crying when in school. When absent the child was usually excused with the same excruciating headaches he gave as a reason for crying in school.

This twelve-year-old boy, a most attractive, solidly built child of average ability, stayed in a baby crib until noon time. When no more danger could be expected from school attendance or the attendance officer, he got up and sat in the grandfather's arm chair "taking good care of myself" as he said himself "so that nothing will happen." When he came to his second psychiatric interview, a number of weeks had elapsed. He was then in a habit of shading his eyes with his whole hand, like a child who has not yet discriminate use of his fingers. He cried profusely. He was anxious and infantile, but remarkably non-juvenile and "elderly" at the same time. When we tried to interest him in attending the day-care group, the whole family got up in arms to keep their "baby" (sick) in the home. The grandmother herself was so menaced that she entrenched herself in the home and could not even be seen when visited by the psychiatric social worker. The grandfather was her vanguard and was often sent to excuse the child for sickness or to hold him in the Clinic office at his side, crying and in a helpless condition.

Willy, aided by the anxious family, developed a new symptom at the time. He suffered great pains when urinating and had prevailed on the physician who treated him to operate on him for a phimosis. Our inquiry about the child's condition, however, revealed that the treating physician had been at a total loss why the child should suffer so intensely. In the weeks of preliminary therapy that preceded the enrollment in the global therapeutical endeavor, Willy would sit with an anxious and painful expression, covering his penis with a protecting gesture. He already announced that he expected an operation for appendicitis in the near future because he had pains in his abdomen. He also confessed that he rather wanted to be sick than join the dangerous crowd in our day-care group. He reported, bathed in wet tears, that he had been afraid to return to public school because the teacher had answered his request to go to the bathroom with the outcry: "You will go out of this room only over my dead body." This alleged exclamation by the teacher proved so shocking because of a phobic reaction concerning his leaving the room in his own home. Leaving the room (or liberation from his enforced confinement) meant walking over a woman's dead body. In his mind a confusion arose, the woman being the grandmother as well as the mother. All of this boy's symptoms were over-determined and he struggled for life to preserve them.

If he left the room to go to school, he stepped over the dead body of the grandmother, in reference to whom everybody had guilt feelings and at least one time or other expressed death wishes. But the child also intensely identified with the grandfather whose seat in the house he liked to occupy. Not only as the mother's son but as her father did he resent the mother's relationship to her husband, and it was because of his own resentment of the mother's desertion as well as to the grandfather's violent verbal attacks that he felt guilty.

Willy and his grandfather were terrified by that husband's violence and angry at him because they feared he might be the executioner of their ambivalent desire. Without him the mother would not be condemned by them and there would, and need not be, an executioner. Willy thus had developed a phobia that stepping outside he might walk over her dead body and he convincingly said, with great emotion, that he was obsessed by his anxiety concerning the mother as soon as he left the house. He had to watch her permanently; the fear for his mother's life was the reason, the child admitted, for his crying and failure to attend school. He said he could not take his mind off the vision of the man hurting her. The mother actually died a few months later from a hemorrhage in premature childbirth, a consequence of the husband's cruelty to her. Willy and his family weathered this loss surprisingly well. Apparently everybody preferred her death over sharing her. She herself seems to have exposed herself to danger as the only way out of her dilemma. Her death was actually the fulfillment of a commitment by all members of her family. Her husband was everybody's tool.

Hostility between mother and daughter through three generations was the reason why Stanley was referred to us, for incorrigible truancy and vagrancy.

Stanley's grandmother, Mrs. Samuel, was said to have been a victim of maternal rejection and to have run away from home. Her child, being born before marriage, was intensely resented by its grandmother, and the daughter was permanently censured. She grew up under such stress that she in turn raised her child, Stanley's mother, Marie, in such an unfriendly atmosphere that she too ran away at adolescence. It is most noteworthy and a typical observation that Mrs. Samuel now fully identified with her own mother's attitude toward herself, treated Marie with the same righteous inflexibility, censure, and rejection. The father, to whom Marie was close, had died early and left Marie in an unappeased state of longing. Stanley's father was an elderly man. Marie pretended that deep love had united them mutually, but the mother had interfered constantly so that the man finally left. Marie returned to the mother with her child and went to work. But the mother's hostility finally drove her from home. Then the grandmother obtained custody of Stanley, convincing the court of Marie's maternal incompetence, actually an incompetence of her own doing. After a few years of struggling during which the mother tried to obtain reversal of the court verdict, the grandmother died and the child was retured to her but too late for both. Marie had no daughter upon whom to retaliate, nor was she identified with her mother's dominant role and her overprotective attitude, rather with her mother's censure and rejection of her. Discouraged by guilt feelings and because of all the battles lost against her mother, she already felt defeated when the child moved to her reluctantly, never admitting the grandmother's death or his longing to be with her. The mother interfered between Marie and her child even now.

Stanley actually wanted to be nowhere and went to nowhere. He could not stay with the mother because he felt disloyal to both her and the grandmother. The mother's continued associations with older men and the birth, out of wedlock, of two additional children, provided associative material of a kind which prevented the grandmother's censure of her daughter from being forgotten. Nor could Stanley live away from the mother. He felt as disloyal and guilty away from her as away from the grandmother. Actually he finally had transferred his love of the grandmother upon her, but he only felt it when separated from her. To be able to go to the mother he needed to rationalize that he wanted to see his little brothers, whom he loved for her sake, but of whom he was jealous, which increased a longing he could only ambivalently admit.

Stanley was very depressed and withdrawn, very uncommunicative and irresponsive to treatment. He was much in need of love but afraid of it. When the daughter, in the parental home, has remained under maternal domination, although being a mother herself, her child is under unfavorable conditions for establishing a primary relation to her. Having experienced her in a passive interaction with the grandmother, or no more than as part of a whole, her image is only dimly outlined. Due to the vagueness of her character, and an emotional ambivalence nourished from numerous sources, she remains at best an unrewarding lure. The grandmother is needed for substitution of maternal functions and the availability of a center for orientation. The children impress one again and again with their habit of confounding the two mother figures, calling both of them "my mama" and "my mother." They only distinguish them when positive emotions are transferred temporarily to the one while the other carries the burden of all negative feelings. But the relationship being intensely dependent, the child becomes deeply involved with the grandmother's or grandparents' emotional annihilation of their child. Ambivalently the child is torn between love and hate of both. In Willy's case the mother's death finally became a relief.

It is an extremely frequent occurrence that the grandmother's hostility is used as a tool for punishing the mother, who is not likely to be as overprotective and condoning, and who promotes problems in view of her youth and sexual life.

Therefore, when the mother moves, failure to adjust to a new milieu represents a retaliatory measure for past as well as present maternal failure to which the child persistently contributes. The feeling that the mother is the elusive fortune is painfully enhanced each time she herself is deluded in seeing fortune at hand, fascinated by a new sexual relation. Deeply troubled herself, always between the Scylla of failing her children economically or the Charybdis of an unacceptable way of life, she may be compelled to move from one section of town to another.

For the pre-psychotic child, any kind of change, or the mere tendency toward change, as is well known, may be intensely traumatic. Life must be reduced to its simplest terms, specifically adapted to the disturbed person, familiar situations, identical routines which can be coped with almost automatically.

## Exhaustion of the Screening Function of the Nervous System

It may be useful at this point to refer to a concept of the nervous system[2] and the sensory organs as an apparatus for screening stimuli which would overwhelm us if all possible stimuli were to be admitted at once.

In accepting this concept of resistance we can understand certain symptoms of excessive unrest due to an incapacity to resist stimulation, one of the most obvious symptoms being sensitivity to noises. Or on the other hand, we notice the warding off of the assailing impact of stimulation by displaying rigidity, withdrawal, blocking off.

Similarly, when a child is exposed to excessive and chaotic stimulation or to a task which exceeds his tolerance, emergency reactions ensue. Thus, one can hardly expect the rebirth adjustment to new surroundings of an excessively exposed and traumatized child, defective or not. The impact of newness and the adjustment to it cannot be sustained any more. The stress of change, and even the temporary departure of figures important to the child may be the apparent cause for the manifest outbreak of a psychosis. Speech development may regress or cease completely and all the familiar symptoms of loss of motor and visceral control may develop with the alternation of states of aimless restlessness or total inertia.

## The Child in Search of His Place

In those homes where shelter is given indiscriminately under overcrowded conditions people come and go. Even intelligent children become totally confused as to who all these people are, whether they are related or not, and if they are related, to whom they belong. The meaning of the family to the children, and of the children to the family, is constantly changing. The children are so weary of all these harmful moves and emotional swaps within their home that they do not make the effort to know, or even refuse to know the people who increase the hardship of family living, no matter who they are.

Austin, an overgrown, sturdy boy, was no longer able to ward off the confusion aroused in his mind by his grandmother's aunt moving into the home after an extended stay in a mental hospital. That house was already overpopulated by a large family and by an itinerant crowd of undesirable masculine roomers. Austin resented intensely one of his aunts who provided for a steady influx of the home population by a growing number of illegitimate children, the responsibility for whom she joyfully referred to the Social Service Bureau.

The psychiatrist who visited the dark and uninviting home was admitted to a small living room. A crowd of people was sitting on chairs packed together along the walls. A baby carriage with two babies stood in a corner. Every now and then a door sprang open and a silent man appeared, to the embarrassment of the grandmother, and the matter of fact indifference of the remaining crowd.

Austin had been shifted around all of his life, within the city as well as to distant places, back and forth from mother to grandmother. He had the opportunity among a number of others to emulate a Virginia pastor supposed to be his father and another man for whom the mother had an unfortunate passion. He was Austin's heroic ideal. The man was in the habit of taking jobs as a butler with a maid as a regular partner for no other reason than to deprive his employers of their valuables. For his activities he had incurred an extended sentence in the penitentiary. Austin's mother travelled hundreds of miles to visit him. Austin had the opportunity to see his mother in much distress at all times. The love objects to whom she was partial, none of whom she ever fully forgot, showed her to have too many heterogeneous identities. The grandmother's home, a most disquieting place for Austin, was the only abode that at least remained identical with itself and where he felt he could be himself in his own room.

When this room was given to his great aunt, his capacity for tolerance was broken. The boy spoke incessantly about this unbearable deprivation and revealed it by spontaneous drawings. He roamed the streets aimlessly regardless of the inclemency of the weather. Finally he became so confused that he ran around naked in the streets in need of exchanging his own with the great aunt's room in the mental hospital.

The children may confuse the therapist by talking about newcomers or people who have returned to the family, without introducing them, at times being in search of an orientation while they talk. Introducing members of the family, perchance inadvertently, may be a sign of a child's embarrassment about irregularities in his family; it may indicate these intruders' undesirability, and the child's reluctance to name them. The child may, on the contrary be wont to talk about them as a new threat. A new competitor for the mother's love and attention was introduced, a new person who may upset her, cause irritation and further maternal ambivalence. When they recover years later, they find the words for their worst hurt, the loss of the mother's dignity by promiscuity with drunken men. New hopes and disappointments may uproot the child. We understand the child's difficulty to know who he is, what he is, and who and what these people are. The child asks himself: "Who is mama, does she love me, do I love her?"

Whenever there is a ray of light, if a mother, even in an angry way, shows interest in her children, these may and often do grasp for the straw that she extends. The children will feel guilty that they do not always recognize her love, enjoy her voice and sympathize with her headache and her stomach trouble.

## The Barren Home and the Development of the Child

We saw that the overstimulation of crowding and the ever repeated deprivation inherent in changing residence lead, in final analysis, to mental and emotional impoverishment. Life in a meager home to which many of the children are exposed whom we could observe, does not represent, as in the cases previously described, a way of bereavement by a distracting profusion of disconnected impressions. The child in the home devoid of necessities is deprived even of deceptive stimulation. Due to the mother's depression or lack of interest, emotional gratification has been wanting and therefore early sensory stimulation and the prompting of sound responses by the infant. The absence of physical objects in the house then intensifies the child's plight. This void is sensed as another denial by the mother, parents, or guardians of joy and opportunity. Some of the children were raised in so barren a home that they were not exposed to as much as the exciting shock of objects opposing them in the room.

Development of a self, well-defined against an equally well-defined objective world, is impeded; hence, unless the child is dulled completely, there emerges a will-o-the-wisp agitation, an aimless search, an obsession to touch and resourcelessly release everything; or the child is under compulsion to handle and "experiment" with everything promiscuously in the most inappropriate and dangerous manner. Whether among the scarce opportunities for observation they had occasion to see somene in the habit of taking a drink out of a bottle, or simply because of the persistent oral needs, they will tend to carry to the mouth anything they can lay hands on. The oral cavity actually is their predominant source of experience or pacification. The relatively high incidence among these families of children's death by poisoning thus can be explained. The pleasure coming from a sense of mastery over one's own or extraneous bodies is never experienced.

Obsession to touch, however, may lead to obsession to take. Gratification of unsatiated tactile needs has to be secured. A sense of mastery has to be gained by the freedom to touch, to do what is wanted, whenever it is vitally wanted. This is necessary under the circumstances for reference of experience to previous experience and tactile orientation. The child who has reason to doubt that he owns that freedom, needs to verify it and to ascertain it continuously. Every child is in a permanent search for himself and concomitantly of the world. When he can see no special reference to aid him at home, he will explore and find the way out of the home, usually to the trash can. This is his universe of inspiration and emotional satisfaction.

At a later stage, a grocery or a five-and-ten-cent store might be the lure. On the way to recovery from an obsession to take objects in the stores, the child might return to the trash can as a legitimate source of pleasure and inspiration. He may fully indulge the need to touch and handle, and to keep what brings proprioceptive satisfaction.

## The Dilemma of Ownership

The legal concept of ownership is not easily imparted to a child who because of absence of material things has not been confronted with the privilege of owing objects at home. He is faced with the necessity for collective or consecutive use of the very few objects in the family, even clothing. This may hold an element of mutuality, but in an atmosphere of extreme deprivation it is a source of frustration and hostility, quite plausible in a society whose foundations rest on an economy of plenty.

In such cases the imperative urge of the moment will take precedence over a transient enjoyment of privileges, thus emphasizing that ownership is casual and subject to distribution according to the momentary prerogatives which are warranted by necessity. Insofar as manipulating objects outside of the barren home is a need for complementation, of shaping and fathoming the child's self, these objects are necessarily taken by the child as his very own. Without the opposing things of the world he would not be a thing to himself.

Censure of tactile exploration of those objects is tantamount to a sentence. As long as there are life tendencies they will make the child do the forbidden thing. It will become an obsession fraught with anguish and guilt feelings. "To be" thus becomes identical with "being bad"; "being bad" then becomes closely associated with existing and being happy.

Here we find the sources of hopeless indifference to usual standards. For the sake of survival, they have to be ignored. These experiences are causes for the development of perversion, delinquency, and refusal to reform. "Something must be wrong with me," often proclaimed, is as much a profession as a confession and a legitimate excuse for not having to change. Guilt and anguish increase the need, and what the child must not enjoy he will have to carry furtively to a safe spot; that may be his pocket, his home, or any other place. These are some of the reasons why a child may be running back and forth between the house and the street. He will be in search of a shelter, protection and peace at one place; in search of life, complementation of self through adventure at the other, furtive and guilty wherever he runs and confused about which place answers which of his imperative needs. The movie theater may be a very important resort, a place where he can live and enjoy existing without being compelled to be illicitly bad, a place where he can be free to experience, by identification, a relief of tension. The mother who has nothing else to offer may have no other recourse than to strain the family budget further. She then helps the child escape from his obsessional impulses by sending him to the movies daily. Both mother and child may have the same terminology: To keep me (him) from stealing.

This solution may be the result of faulty and hence precarious education of mother and child which caused an agency to refer the family for treatment. Actually a hostile interaction is coped with symptomatically. It consists in the mother's need for an excitement and her use of first the father, then the son, for providing it. The helpless and passive tool using the passivity promoted in him, allows things to happen which actually are retaliatory "accidents."

### Sharing and Possession

If a child has been raised with the idea that he possesses nothing and owns an object only as long as he holds it, he has difficulties in developing respect for other people's property. Permanently, under the stress of anxiety, he cannot even conceive the idea of property; therefore, the idea of sharing cannot take proper shape, in particular when claims are announced constantly by others in a position quite as endangered as his. No one can actually share, unless from a secure position. Only a distinct self can take a definite attitude toward the owned object; only in the secure position of ownership can it be decided whether that object is at the present moment part and parcel of this distinct self, which is sensed as being continuous and permanent. Thus, the object will be either desired or not for temporary or permanent use. Then, if the problem of sharing arises, the object will be either sacrificed or not, depending on its actual purpose within a long-range plan. Where circumstances trammel an evolution of attitudes, the needs themselves do not have their history. They are kept unaltered. They are not left behind to remain but the dreams of the past and an individual's treasured heirloom, reference and resource material and his iron reserve.

The child under permanent stress may struggle for an object for very different reasons than those suggested by its apparent use. To be forced to give up an object to which he has to cling for reasons of his very own may produce an emergency situation and reaction. Communication between him and the other contender is immediately interrupted because none is aware of the meaning of the object to the other, nor that there are two different meanings for it. Being deprived of the thing may be sensed as an amputation of a vital organ and thus reveal to the child the precariousness of his whole existence.

Secure ownership and the experience that the world of objects can be relied upon nurtures a feeling of friendliness toward a friendly world. When, however, everything is shifting, the precariously owned object has gained neither enough stability nor enough reliability to become a safe tool of self in relation to a world which in its turn has not enough stability to gain body and structure or reliability to be trusted.

When the concept of property has not developed, the tool is abandoned and forgotten; neglected from the time that it serves no purpose to its user any longer, its preservation becomes irrelevant. Sharing presumes conserving a tool regardless of its continuous usefulness to us, but rather for its potential usefulness to anyone. Many of the habits of our children and the causes of their dissensions unfold their meaning when we consider these relations to the material world, for instance, the hiding of objects of relevance, forgetting them when they could be useful later or to someone else, hoarding as an expression of excessively securing one's self in a precarious world, the convinced arrogation of objects which serve to complement the self, and the dissenting report of siblings, each of whom in this regard has good reasons to consider himself the owner of the coveted object. The lack of a concept of ownership and of the tool character of an object in a group of individuals equally deprived of the thing itself as of its concept, increases the tendency toward destruction of those evasive, deceptive, and intolerably frustrating objects. The constant struggle and even fight for objects that one can never hold in peace for any length of time, devaluate the thing. It is destroyed because of its unbearable, unnerving character and also because it becomes a nuisance the moment it is unnecessary. Future uses cannot be foreseen or taken into account. Destructiveness serves not only the purpose of annihilating the resented objects, but also the purpose of depriving or punishing those who, in vying with the child for ownership and enjoyment, have caused it to be a trickery, to make life precarious and the world itself unsafe.

## Early Relations to Material Objects

Lack of co-ordination due to lack of opportunity and practice in the child's handling of objects will readily provide a rationalization for any "mishap" when he has to answer for the damage to objects of others or, once his anger is vented, to his own conscience.

However, the child's play partner and competitor for the object may not tolerate appeasement; now it is he who is unbearably frustrated, not only by pure deprivation but by the sensed hostility and the competition which was mastered by the other child in a powerful way. The struggle goes on and on; "I hate him, I could kill him," "I'll get him anyway," are outcries often heard in observed fights between the children or uttered in their interviews with regard to their real or symbolic siblings. Bob, one of three brothers, had bought himself a toy gun which he entrusted to his psychotherapist for safe-keeping as many of our Clinic children do. The gun mysteriously must have found—in a jealous symbolic sibling—another owner, but reappeared after a few weeks to the pathetic joy of the boy. That very day his sibling broke it intentionally at home, creating intense distress and further embittering their hostile and competitive relation. Unlike the child who illegally secures material objects for emotional survival, a child who takes food because he is hungry and has to keep the body alive is, though "wrong," more readily assured of compassion and tolerance.

A child who searches, touches, and takes objects because they answer a psychological need of equal importance, the need for self-definition and the clarification of the awareness of existence, has to contend with an additional embarrassment. He conceivably is considered undesirable by whomever he encounters, a being who causes trouble constantly for reasons one does not understand. Those adults who try to appease their own frustration and relieve their own suspense by trying to eliminate the child's disturbing symptoms have a doubly denying attitude. They understandably reject the child as he is, but refuse to examine what his needs are in order to gratify them and to liberate him from "necessity" or from the unacceptable road to fulfillment.

Anguished and confused by denial and by interference with his imperative demands for orientation, the child may lose the limited sense of identity he possesses and show increasing aimlessness and restlessness, sensing dimly the illogic of not being allowed to do what necessity commands. Any direct change of the child's behavior or, in other terms, the elimination of his symptoms attempted by the educator's prohibiting attitude will be doomed to failure. Frustration increases and with it the intensity of the impulse which at times leads to catastrophic reactions or total block and withdrawal. In such grave cases it is best to let the child be as he is, gratify him to the extent that it is possible and legitimate, and give him a framework within which he will live for a time without menace, failing to the extent that it is inevitable. Slowly he will learn to discover himself as something constant in reference to something predictable and will test his acceptability under requirements increasing with his capacity to meet them.

Permissiveness for the child's elementary needs will first relieve anxiety and slowly promote the joy of existing as well as trust in his tactful and unobtrusive guides to a simple and primeval state of well-being. Limitations imposed by inevitable necessity will soon be accepted without resistance as the means to preserve and deserve the cherished state of security.

Robert, a pre-psychotic eight-year-old lived in a tenuous reality. He was agitated, incoherent, ambivalent, suspicious, evasive, and slyly deceptive. His achievement in any of the three R's was nil.

At the time of referral, the child was trying to intrude many times a day into the psychotherapist's office. Inside the room, he would seek no immediate contact, but would run around restlessly touching everything obsessively, each time unlocking a lock that protected nothing, opening all drawers and his psychotherapist's pocket book, snatching snips of papers and pamphlets. Then without giving as much as a glance, he would fill his pockets with these papers, and often, after having secured permission, would leave in a hurried way. He seemed unable to wait and was apparently afraid of a negative answer.

At times this risk was not taken and the objects were furtively stuffed into his pockets, mostly in the back of his pants. At other times, he would manipulate these objects hurriedly, fingering them, laying the palm of the hand on them, beating them slightly; all these manipulations were accompanied by furtive elation.

These habits were soon given up, yielding instead to the habit of bringing a gift he had made, such as a water color picture eagerly painted before his interview, as if it were a ticket of admission.[3]

In the initial stages of treatment, Robert would draw spontaneously, not copy, all concrete objects he saw in the room, representing them in a totally abstract fashion by a neat, varied alignment of circles. Without his interpretation it would have been impossible to glean what they were supposed to express. Disregarding, at this point, the obscured, yet obvious, emotional content of these drawings, these pictures had to be considered as manifestations of the child's tendency toward orientation, a tendency which in his early days he did not have adequate and sufficient opportunity to exert, due to a lack of practically all relevant object relations, human or material. The mother, having developed a psychosis in her pregnancy with the boy, was hospitalized soon after his birth. He then became the object of the collective good-will of a struggling and working respectable family consisting of the maternal grandmother, an unmarried uncle, a divorced aunt and her two children.

The child's lack of direction, his aimless restlessness, his fixation on early sensory-motor patterns of experience and his indiscriminate tactile approach to everything, his habit of discovery, predominantly by touch, can be explained by his greed for unsatiated early needs, the satisfaction of which are the prerequisite for the discovery of the world as a frame of reference to the self, and thus, to consciousness of self.

(At a later stage, we encountered similar tendencies for discovery and assertion of self through kinesthetic and proprioceptive sensation in deprived adolescent boys. They express an imperative need for physical exercise, manifest an exclusive interest in ball games and are prone to act out violently, by physical action or exertion not only emotional problems but physical disease, in reality, dis-ease.)

Later Robert discontinued this purely abstract alignment of circles and would draw a house high upon the page, still displaying very few details. However, he did not cease when the house was represented but continued to draw straight lines crossing one another at various angles as though he had lost purpose and direction. But it was obvious that the house had to disappear in this structure of irregular geometrical figures. Though reality now was registered and retained more appropriately, his hold on it was still precarious; "his" object had to be hoarded and hidden behind an abstract unreality or undone, because it was as unsafe as his trust—and closeness—to the therapist. He was ambivalent whether to "give" or not and what he gave he also withdrew. Departure from reality into abstract regions occurred also when he was sitting, patiently drawing cursive letter-like characters. The more he drew, the more he showed a tendency to depart from accepted forms of letters, exaggerating parts or adorning them with flourishes.

It is interesting to note how many aspects of Robert's problems were unfolded by this behavior and how adequately it answered a variety of his needs. Although he seemed to desire contact with the therapist, he went on a hunt for "nice junk" immediately after entering her office. In view of his uncertainty about himself, and also in view of his early emotional experiences, Robert became frightened when he finally obtained fulfilment of his wishes and withdrew into a world of things.

At times he even prevented the closing of the door, for relief from his ambivalent suspense, when he submerged himself in important and satisfactory activities. But these were equally fraught with contradictory emotions; he was uncertain of their legitimacy and his elation had furtive connotations. However, in the psychiatrist's office, all of his manifestations were acceptable, those which were his specific and at the moment only possible ways of reaching for and attaining the fruit of life. Permitted and helped to "find nice junk," he could through the medium of material objects, proceed safely with his task of orientation toward people and in reference to himself. In particular, the pocket book was not forbidden, since it represented the mother's enfolding arms, a crib, and the availability of elementary knowledge from a secure position. Moreover, his teacher helped him throughout the day in manipulative activities. Later he was exposed to careful doses of contacts with children and other adults. The collecting of junk and the intrusion into the pocket book spontaneously subsided.

From a restless, incoherent, manipulating, asocial and evasive little creature, Robert became self-assertive and aggressive enough to test adults and children in a playful, mischievous and impish way. He followed a line of conduct by his free consent, co-operated well, gained contact with people and finally wished to return to public school, and succeeded there.

We should also like to report an observation of a group of six children, eight to eleven years old, all of them from fatherless homes. Two had lost their father through death, one of them had a father on a chain gang, another's father was being sought by the FBI, and two had been but incidents in the mother's life. Like Robert, they had been deprived in early life of adequate stimuli and reacted similarly to Robert on superficial observation; three of them were exposed to undesirable overstimulation resulting from the disquieting home conditions created by the alcoholism of the fathers one of whom perished as a result of his addiction.

At the beginning of each treatment session, the six children would place the furniture, especially the chairs in the room, into the very same position; they would always sit in the same order, close to the psychotherapist. They wanted to be read popular fairy tales, always in the same order; some of these stories were called for as many as three times in a row, though some children protested.

Once the stories were read, the children would tell their own. One of the boys, whose mother gave "parties" together with a male "friend" regularly turned out some pornographic tale. He embarrassed those children who were in search of a nursery paradise and who tended to terminate the session by asking whether they could close the shutters and sleep in the Center. Their embarrassment caused him embarrassment; he looked around, felt out of place, and adjusted to the group. He gratified his need of expressing anxiety in his particular way in individual therapy.

The furniture arrangement obviously served the purpose of shaping the office into a place of fond associations. Once it stood its test as a protective cloister, walls widened and encompassed the whole world, the children's dream as well as their yet limited reality. Where children have none of these lovable auxiliaries to hold on to, humble as they may be, none of these passive, mute, obedient servants of wood, which to them constitute home, their status as eternal foreigners will not be changed and they will remain restless travelers on this earth. They will feel an inability to be satisfied by the pleasures of the moment and be driven anxiously from one instant to the next, and from one object to another, with no past to collect and resort to for the anticipation of the future, which in its turn, determines present behavior.

Through habits, through the possession of familiar objects, and through repetitive situations, we acclimatize ourselves on this earth. An excess of habits may be dangerous; but a minimum is needed for the realization that we exist and that we own a plot of this ground upon which we tread and from which we proceed and advance. Owning, having, handling, acting, make us feel that we exist. This experience precedes the conscious awareness of being, of self; if self-realization is denied, we are unable to acknowledge the involved interrelationships which make up our world.

## Honor among Thieves

Barrenness of the house and the lack of stimulating environment in early childhood were similar for Chester as for Robert, though the latter boy came from a struggling family. Both were in the habit of stealing and both showed emotional indifference to children and adults. Both were unable to engage in a purposeful occupation; both were permanently on the move in an aimless search.

Chester was less able mentally. He came from a home of destitution and remained there until rescued from it through our care. Exposed to terrifying traumata, he turned his face away from the mother-Medusa which life represented to him. He did not feel the urge to discover himself and the world in order to experiment and to live. His performance remained poor and solely at the service of his illusions, his stealing in stores, at the service of experience on a most elementary level, coincided with equally elementary impulse gratification. He was shy and ashamed and had established intense emotional ties with his dead father. He had built up an ideal of the father in his mind that had not the slightest resemblance to the original.

Chester had a romantic, highly emotional, and regressive attitude and showed very little inclination to action. Robert, on the other hand, when insecure, flew into action and into a search of experience, while Chester withdrew into a dream world of sentimentality and inactivity.

Chester lived in a little brick house which the therapist and a teacher had visited some time ago. The house was located at the edge of town. It stood off by itself; there was no pavement. Apparently the surrounding houses had been torn down. There was no electricity, not a single piece of furniture in the house except for a metal cot, without bedding, standing at the entrance. There was no equipment other than one tiny stove. The mother was at home and a little girl sat on the cot. A few minutes before we entered, a drunken man went into the house. Although the relationship seemed unmistakable, Chester's mother assured us that the man was her brother. If that should have been true, it would also have been a problem to the child.

The boy was the third of eight children that his mother had borne up to that time. The two elder and three youngest children were not by Chester's dead father. The oldest daughter had disappeared. Although loud and coarse,* the woman was distinctly a well-intentioned mother. She had a fourth-grade elementary education and apparently no ability for any kind of work. Her promiscuity was a means of increasing her income, though by an infinitesimal degree, without having to account for it to the social service bureau. The children seemed to take this situation for granted.

The tiny, unfurnished home was extremely dirty and unkept. Chester too was neglected at all times. His mother considered the time when her husband was alive as the best in her life. Her husband allegedly was a contractor and a good provider and was particularly fond of Chester. However, as a matter of fact, the father had been under treatment and died in a mental hospital and also suffered from Paget's disease of the skull. He was described as confused, irritable, and violent whenever a situation did not suit him. Chester's father never got beyond the second grade and could never hold a job, he depended on relief off and on for six years. None of the children of this couple seemed to be able to work. One of Chester's brothers was referred to the Center for a learning difficulty; a shy and slightly depressed boy, he attended regularly, co-operated in a reliable way, and made a good adjustment.

Chester would articulate like a small child and talk in a high pitched voice, almost as if he were a baby. His overt behavior was extremely silly. One day the therapist told him the story of Christopher Columbus, emphasizing the phases of distress in his life which might suggest to Chester some identification, and indeed he began to shed ample tears about Christopher Columbus, and to tell the story of his own life as he saw it. He depicted his father ideal, as he imagined it. As so many orphan children, he saw the solution of his problems in past glory with close communion with the dead. The differences between life and death are largely effaced. Life and an active approach to its challenge are lost, and what remains is a vision modeled on a delusion of the past. There remains a wish to return to a total undoing of existence, a longing for primeval nothingness and a state of consciousness imagined as a painless, dutiless, totally protected human condition.

* This is a qualitative, not a pejorative term.

The boy spoke of the time when his father still lived. He used to sleep in one bed with him; this was confirmed by the mother. His father, Chester pretended, had died at his side one night at 2 A.M., although actually he died in the hospital. Apparently forgetting his father's actual death and the resulting transition, he added that his father went out with him as he would do at that hour, took him to the train of which he was the engineer. His father could drive any kind of engine, freight engine or streamliner. Chester then would continue to sleep on the coal of the tender without being afraid of the other men who were with his father. His brother would not go with the father because he was afraid, but he, Chester, was not afraid of any man and would go out at night with any of them. These allusions to frightening men were suggested by a fusion of the imaginary men who shared the defunct father's coffin with men who came in from the street. He feared they could be pall bearers of the mother as they had been of the father. Chester wished that these frightening men who visited the mother would be with the father instead. It was his way of making them inoffensive by the father's power, the power of death and the father's glory.

The child showed his intense confusion by identification with the mother's suffering from the dangers she was running, as well as with the father with whom he shared the bed and hearse (in his fantasy the coal tender). Identifying with her, Chester was full of anxiety; identifying with the father, he was ashamed of anxiety and projected it onto his younger brother. But the younger brother he was talking about is in reality Chester himself; he took refuge with his father in the past, a glorified and idealized reality which became identified with death and future. Death is connected with his father's departure.[4] Thus Chester kept running to find an escape and remained suspended between life and death until he could be helped.

His conflict was further revealed by his building with colored blocks. He would build spacious mansions, neat, high, and lofty. The houses were of brick because "wooden houses burn down so easily." In all his mansions, there was a wide hall and two bedrooms at opposite sides of the house. In one bedroom lived a man, in the other one lived a woman, both unnamed; no children were mentioned.

In this manner, the child expressed again his denial of the real situation, his objections to his domestic status, his resentment of other men sharing the dead father's privileges and his anxiety aroused

by the father's death and the present home situation. Sexes are isolated from each other; children do not interfere with the loftiness of
the place. And for once, Chester retained for himself the fulfilment
of his wishes in disregard of reality and fear. Thus, there are among
these dismally traumatized children those who are not totally inhibited by the confusing conflict between necessity and its denial,
and not altogether discouraged to the point of having become too indifferent to seek such a solution of the problem of self, even by
dream and fantasy, or to venture out in quest of the world outside.
On these frail tendencies the pillars of assistance can be raised and the
bridge of communication will stand.

The low mental rating of the majority of the children from barren
homes and their poor performance can be only partly explained by
emotional attitudes. The lack of opportunity for sensory stimulation,
particularly tactile stimulation and experience, and the concomitant
lack of propriosynesthetic development find their expression in poor
motor co-ordination and a strong sense of inadequacy. Curious and
active exploration of challenges for gaining experience are inhibited.
The original absence of opportunity has led to an inhibition and
inability to avail one's self of opportunity. At best, interest may be
expressed explosively.

There is a further handicap in conquering experience by sight. No
visual ideas of objects are formed and no idea for their handling is developed; a preparatory mental stage for knowing how to perform is
needed. Such a stage would represent stimulation by visual imagery
and imagination, and motivation for activity. The source of so-called
laziness, inertia, fear of being active, and lack of manual dexterity
lies in mental resourcelessness and the inability to anticipate what
could be achieved beyond what already is; the tragic continuity of
such deficiences through generations thus finds an explanation.

The parents of our children are usually relatively inactive by force
of circumstance. Perseverance and inertia are much harder to overcome than obstacles encountered in an object world. Objects impose
their own order and thus present a challenge.

*From the Empty Home to the Prohibiting Outside World*

Inasmuch as objects for manipulation are generally found outside
the empty home, the small domain of the child's immediate neighbor-

hood becomes naturally his to explore. Here he is let alone as long as he does not invade the sphere of interest of the adult human. But he soon becomes a trespasser, and a clash with society teaches him that the outside world is rigidly bordered and divided into provinces which no one is allowed to invade without punishment. Venturing out for the pleasure of living and learning, he will understand with dismay that this world, replete with intriguing and lovely things, must remain to him a desert and the objects he yearns for and dares to touch are thorns to his exploring hands. The fear of learning and the subsequent rejection of all educational bait offered in school to the child from the barren home may indeed have taken root at the time of such early forbidding and confusing experiences.

# IV

*The Psychosocial Economy of The Family:*
*Its Normal and Abnormal Aspects*

## Freedom in Dependency

Living is a continuous movement, alternating between outgoing experience and the return to the inner self. This process is essential; only by tidal withdrawal upon himself does the individual have an opportunity to integrate his relationships into a conscious experience and thereby benefit from them. Thus, in a relationship of long duration, this miraculous shifting between mutuality and recession evokes the repeated charge and charm of newness.[1]

Each partner in a marital relationship, for example, has so changed and grown in the course of outgoing and withdrawal, that he returns for the new process of fusion as another, altered self. Hence, change is an inevitable consequence of relating to another. Each partner has become the other's builder, resulting in a growing dependency of one individual upon the other. However, this fusion opens up an important wellspring of conflict, for each partner may now come to fear the impact of the other, and to seek intensely a new identification with the former self. Conflicts may arise whether the partners are fervently united, whether they are strong, undeviating personalities, or whether they are weak and in danger of vacillating identifications.

Such inner conflicts arise, of course, notably in adolescence, particularly when the growing youngster is confronted with a powerful parent or educator. Each contact produces a change within the self—the self which the child seeks, builds, assesses, and which the child must protect from adulteration. Changes may come to the adult as an animating experience since they are perceived as differentiation and intensification of his own past. Wordsworth says:

> Hence in a season of good weather
> Though inland far we be,
> Our souls have sight of that immortal sea

> Which brought us thither,
> And see the children sport upon the shore,
> And see the mighty waters rolling evermore.

Insofar as maturation consists in the proper utilization of whatever experience may come our way, by whatever channel and from whatever direction, the grown-up's contact with youth, unless under unusually destructive circumstances, will revive

> the strength in what remains behind;
> In the primal sympathy which having been must ever be.

Given such a state of maturation of the adults, the impact of the younger will, moreover, ultimately aid the older in bringing in the harvest, and the hue of autumn will seem as bright and glorious as the tints of spring. Whether the youth has willed it or not, he has thus abundantly repaid the strength imparted to him long before "the shades of the prisonhouse" have begun to "close upon the growing boy."

Outside influences can be of immeasurable importance to the young. Their experience is vague and, if they are vibrant youngsters, they anticipate far more than they have had opportunity to verify. They are likely to feel an urge to explore reality at one moment in one direction; at the next moment, they choose other goals. Such outside relations are often unselected by the child or may be imposed upon him. At times the child himself exhibits an amazing adequacy in choosing his contacts, either unconsciously or through brilliant apperception.

Such fortunate opportunities may occur within the family. Contrariwise, the specific influence emanating and radiating from a highly differentiated and specialized adult may produce shattering clashes. The young person, moving in a definite direction of his own, may be dimly anticipating his own future differentiation and specialization. Driven toward that intriguing goal, he will be impelled to reject anything that threatens to lead him away from his particular path. But once the goal is apperceived, and the youth no longer has to embrace the cosmos as a whole but can begin to penetrate it sharply and discriminately, he will find unending revelation from wherever he may stand; he will have learned not only to tolerate, but even to integrate into his own specific outlook on life the specific approach he formerly rejected. In this rebirth, this rediscovery of what once was strange and unacceptable, generations are reconciled and a continuity of human strivings and efforts is established.

## The Search for the Self

Yet, before that time has come, while the youth is still in search of his self, while he still assesses his vaguely understood relations with the rest of the world, he must protect a yet fragile inner structure whose foundations have been newly set; any interference, and especially a masterly and powerful one, may be felt and rejected as an adulteration of the self. Since ambivalence and contradiction exist in all human behavior, other contacts, being weak rather than strong, and yielding rather than compelling, will offer no challenge to his strength and provide no opportunity for measuring his power of resistance to obstacles. Precisely for that reason the child will find these contacts antagonizing and intolerable.

Apparently bent upon gratifying some immediate and superficial need, the child may be testing in reality the confines of his individual cell, exploring his power to tear down the barriers and widen his horizon; conversely, he may simply be extending his willingness to allow some of these barriers to persist. At this point gentle guidance can be a forceful influence; the perfect guide will be that adult who, not beset by obscuring complexes, will sense what is proper at each individual moment in each individual case, being ready to act or to bide his time, speak when advice is longed for, but is not explicitly requested, and be silent when counsel is demanded but tacitly unwanted.

Wisdom of this kind may also dwell in the abode of those who are accustomed to the presence of sorrow and affliction. A parent "tempered in the furnace of sorrow and adversity" is not always ready to try to guard his child against outside evils. His insight into the profound involvement of all human experience, behavior, and relationships, as well as his knowledge of the limitations of direct solutions, will inspire that delicate balance in attitude that serves the child's purpose, paradoxical as it may seem, but with a sweeping and generous view of the future protects a "wholesome" outcome. Such an imponderable communion might represent the sublime moment in a parent-child relationship, or may convey to a treatment situation a quality which transcends the specificity of a rationalized and verbalized approach. Yet, such moments of perfect insight depend on inspiration, which is whimsical and elusive.

The awareness that the mutuality of a relationship can be achieved only if each partner can withdraw within himself, develops out of objectivity and discloses to each partner the separateness of individuality—a separateness which is a source of inescapable isolation and yet a stronghold, safe from intrusion. Respect for each other establishes a sacred zone upon which no one may trespass.[2] In this manner, the dignity and equality of the partners is mutually acknowledged; regardless of excursions into the heights and depths of emotion, there will always be a return to the safe and serene ground of mutual esteem.

## The Need for Withdrawal

Exhaustive experience of one another's identities would, by complete dissociation from the personality, preclude living as an individual. The need for seclusion is as essential as is recuperation during sleep. The impact of the other self must be laid aside as would be an arousing book or the concrete presence of a work of art, which we must escape lest it overwhelm us.

If, however, the family is not aware of the necessity for such temporary refuge into the self, suspicion is apt to arise when such needs and habits are discovered in some member of the family group. Guilt feelings and anxiety on all sides may result from this awareness which enters as a wedge into the relationship. Temporary withdrawal indeed does not imply abandonment. It may, on the contrary, indicate a supreme union within the family "community," though in abstract, sublimated terms.

Yet, withdrawal is not always possible. Among the economically depressed classes this situation may be due to crowded quarters. Crowding hinders the child, not only in his studies at home, but in his flights of imagination which help him develop necessary abstract attitudes. It is above all a dissociative element because the individual becomes a function of the family collectivity. Intense mutual irritation is the result of this inescapable confinement. Withdrawal then is perceived in terms of escape from the home, and perhaps into the oblivion of alcoholic intoxication, as is often the case with fathers.

Where there is no conscious awareness of graver implications, the family group quite naturally accepts the temporary withdrawal of its members provided there is a relationship of trust and inner security. Withdrawal then becomes a routine by which family members take each other for granted and are not constantly enmeshed in vivid conflicting associations.

The one-year-old child may sit forlornly, exploring the physical and spatial relations of his playthings and their eventual value for satisfying his oral libido. The parents may read or indulge in hobbies or specific occupations of their own. Adolescent siblings may scurry about, each concentrating upon his own very personal and private goals. At these moments, the family is but a local community. This kind of preoccupation with self is felt as comfort and relaxation.

## The Tidal Movement of Tension and Solution

In a harmonious relationship, these neutral phases serve not only to keep each individuality composed, but they function as creative pauses. In less harmonious relationships, the neutral phase does not compare as it should to the whole of the mood, similar to that rhythmical silence in music where the preceding sounds still resound and where, bound by the inherent rhythm, new sounds are anticipated. To become a creative phase and the stage for integration, a state of neutrality must be endowed with kinetic energy or, in other words, with a dynamism derived from past experience and impregnated with visions of the future.

Within the family the lack of harmonious oscillations between its members is the result of unreflective living. The individual cannot find himself. Since he does not integrate his experiences, he fails to mature and his resourcefulness is diminished. His ability to relate to others becomes grossly inhibited. Human relations are then merely incidental and do not bear the imprint of the person's authorship. Spontaneous reaction to profound mutual experience, be it intellectual or emotional, with its intense animation and elevation of the joy of living, is absent or negligible; so are the relaxing moments of integration and contemplation. No substance has been harvested for assimilation. Stagnation within dries up the flow of communication with the family.

There is an analogy to the rhythm of fusion and diffusion in the tidal gratification of purely instinctual desires. Such tidal movement, unless embedded in higher human thought and feeling, recedes, leaving no trace, tending to interrupt the continuity of the relationship. Since the rhythm cannot revive itself in a non-existing relationship it must derive its new stimulation from without. When this happens, the need for reunion is no longer necessarily mutual. In contrast to a union where each companion contributes his individual share, no interplay of personalities occurs in the moment of fusion. Interaction of personalities is a precious means, not only for knowing and sensing distinctly the nature of the partner, but for sensing and knowing clearly the self. Similarly, some of our significant potentialities are not realized unless stimulated by significant relationships.

We shall now illustrate, with some case histories, disharmonious family relationships which are devoid of the fulfilment of the dependence and withdrawal from dependence process, so essential for maturation. We shall similarly depict the vicious circle of revolt against dependency and the need to cling to it by the tie of hostility. Futile and costly attempts at substitutional fulfilment will be outlined. In all such cases inertia will be in evidence whether by restless motions of distraction and various expressions of disregard and antagonism or by the inert display of devastating hostility, all resulting in the loss of the capacity to relate, to love, and to embrace life. We shall finally allude to the tragedy of the underprivileged member of an ostracised sub-group who, because of induced doubt of the worthiness of his sub-group, cannot unfold to his next of kin for replenishment nor to his distorted self-image for integration of experiences. We had abundant therapeutic results demonstrating that the observed disturbances in the children were due to causes which when eliminated also eliminated the effects.

## The Cycle of Mutual Rejection

The individual who craves sexual fulfilment may indeed be familiar with all the external stimulations that make the needs of two partners crystallize if they have no other community of purpose. But moments following sexual gratification are of great mutual dissonance and isolation; as time goes on, due to anticipation of disenchantment, they are intensified and carried over into the periods of mutual intimacy. Hostility enters the moments of expected relief, and resentment of the anticipated depression prevents even momentary gratification. Perverted stimulation, usually of a sado-masochistic character, will be increasingly resorted to and not be followed by relaxation. Hostility and resentment at that time have established ties of a dependent nature between the partners. Neither partner at this time has freedom to be sensitive to the need of the other, to delay an answer to his quest until a mutuality of desire has developed. Coincidence of want can no longer be achieved. This makes the relationship increasingly unbearable. The demands, at times obessive, of the most ungratified of the two partners increases in the other the tendency to reject him and frustrate his desires. These have become repulsive not only because of their relentless obsessiveness and the exhibited weakness, but because this repulsiveness, caught by the rejecting partner, can be used as a defense and returned to the self-humiliating and humiliated one, intensifying steadily the vicious circle.

In the family marked by an obsessive need for mutual punishment, the children inevitably are recruited as instruments of chastisement.[3] They are prolongations of the arms of the parents—deadly weapons to intensify the agony and ordeal of the compulsive struggle, limited only by the necessity for keeping the adversary alive for another round. Whether the child allows himself to be set against one parent or whether, because of ambivalence or generalized antagonism, he exercises his destructive power against both, the weapon thus fashioned by either parent becomes a boomerang which, when it finally returns, has not yet exhausted its ballistic energy and can be fatal to both.

This was the case with Mary Smith, the eight-year-old girl, whose story we shall tell here. The mother was irritable, hostile, and self-righteous. She burst out in tirades of hatred and contempt against her husband, reviling particularly his rages of temper and his excessive sexual demands. In a more restrained manner, she also criticized her little daughter and her sister-in-law, who until recently was Mary's foster mother. Mary's mother expressed complete unawareness of any part she herself had played in contributing to the girl's difficulties.

The girl's father, who had a long and steady employment record, when interviewed, showed antagonism which apparently represented a transference of his usual reaction to women—submissiveness, a realization of his own weakness, and then revolt. He was not of the same ethnic stock as the mother, had a different religious background, and was more immature. As a child, he had run away from home and school, earning a living as a woodcutter. He retained a violent hatred of his mother, female teachers, and his religion. His marriage, that in his conscious awareness was to promote his self-esteem, cast him in the home of his wife's parents with a divorced and an unmarried sister-in-law. The latter, very similar to his wife, was involved with her homoerotically. However, he appeared to be gentle, in need of acceptance, contrite about the outbursts that so annoyed his wife, and eager to control them. He reiterated his sincere attempts "to be a good husband and father" but lamented that "no one ever seemed satisfied" with him. The child rejected all his efforts to win her affection.

The past history, as told by the mother, revealed that from the day of her birth, Mary's father had openly rejected the child "because she was a girl." Instead, he lavished his paternal affection upon a nephew who resided in the same household. Mary was a pathetic and appealing youngster; she attracted the sympathy of a childless uncle and aunt.

Mary remembered that, at the age of three, she went to live with this couple in another state. Although the father had originally consented to such a plan, he periodically demanded that she come home. Yet, once returned to her parents, Mary demonstrated such uncontrollable behavior that she could no longer be tolerated and was quickly sent back to her uncle's home. After five years of this uncertain arrangement, Mary's foster parents decided to adopt an infant son, asking at the same time to adopt Mary as well. Mary's parents flatly refused to consider this request; accordingly, she was returned permanently to her natural family.

When Mary came to live with her parents, the mother, pretending to restore Mary's health, insisted that they sleep together, thus dislodging the father from the marital bed. She thus denied him all of his male prerogatives, as a husband and the progenitor of the child, as well as the ensuing paternal privileges. Thus, mother and child were equally and conveniently included in his resentment and irritation against them. The child was made to feel that rejection of the father was the price to pay for the only token of love received, sleeping in the mother's bed. The father was denied love of the child for which he was longing in his pitiful isolation and insecurity. His bitterness and rage enabled his wife to accuse him with apparent justification of having been the sole cause of Mary's maladjustment and her rejection of the home. The cornered father, driven beyond control, retorted in the one way that gave him complete mastery over women—by affirming his sexual superiority regardless of the child's presence in the connubial bed. In so doing, he dragged his wife from her throne of infallibility and associated her, in the eyes of the awakening child, with his own complete debasement.

When we first saw Mary, she spoke of her aunt as "mother," unconsciously rejecting the role of her true parent. She mentioned how her "baby brother," who had come from "City Hall" had "grown much too fast." "At first he was just a tiny thing," but now, Mary recounted, he was "already ten years old." Thus, very obviously, he had grown not only into her place within the family constellation but had actually surpassed her in importance. A few weeks later, Mary's brother had become still older in her mind, attaining the age of her father. Here was a symbolic expression of final and utter condemnation. Yet, insofar as Mary felt cornered and rejected like her father, and humiliated because of the reactive defense mechanisms she displayed, she identified with him. Her mother had observed the same change previously by saying that the girl was the very image of her father.

Thus, we see how the boomerang completed its flight and exacted its toll.

An instance of some of the consequences to the child of an unresolved Oedipus complex of the mother is presented in Albert's story.

Albert, a twelve-year-old boy of dull normal intelligence, had started to steal at the age of three. His mother, an epileptic product of a broken home, rejected and neglected, was animated by profound resentment. Her father had been married four times, three times to women much younger than himself. Her own emotional and erotic life was tempestuous. Even her common-law husband, with whom she had lived for many years, complained continually of her promiscuity and of the fact that she burdened him with the care of the children. Eventually he became an excessive alcoholic and finally abandoned the family. Frequently thereafter the woman hailed him into court for non-support, well knowing that under Virginia law he could not be held responsible.

This woman was a splendid talker and with clever conversation she wilfully dragged her two daughters—Albert's full sisters—into the abyss, drawing them into her ways of hatred, of torturing men, and of defying the accepted mores.

Albert had spent his early days with his grandmother. Their deep affection for each other prompted the grandfather's sudden request that Albert, then three, be returned to his mother. The child recalled that from thereon his life was an unending series of terrors, the epileptic spells of his mother, the alcoholic orgies of his father, and the violent battles between the two, slashing madly at each other with knives while Albert watched in hypnotized fear. For stealing he was punished by the burning of his fingertips. Seven years after separation from the grandmother he still ran back to her, barefoot in the snow, self-gratifying and self-punitive at the same time.

When we met Albert he was ambivalent in his allegiance to both his mother and the grandmother and obsessive in repeating the trauma of separation. At one time he was intensely involved with the grandmother, living at her house, joining her church; then, just as suddenly, he returned to the mother's home, degrading the grandmother in the mother's favor, only to return once again to make amends. Albert asked repeatedly whether the therapist could not help the two women to agree that he must not feel guilty toward one for loving the other. With his suppression of hatred toward his mother came suppression of all emotion resulting in his loss of the capacity to love.

However, the mother's fight for him, for the sake of depriving him, and her cruel rejection once he accepted the lure, were the main reasons for his fear of showing his feelings. Stealing, which started as a compensatory mechanism, was overdetermined in its motivations, but in the foreground stood elements of resentment and revenge. He pretended never to be sorry and never to regret the trouble he created. He pretended simply to have a jolly time as he once had when he stole the life savings of an old woman and spent the money wildly at a carnival; or when he had filched his grandmother's church funds, hurting her where she was most vulnerable, and depriving her of the respected status in the community which he and his mother could not achieve. This also served to bring about the equalization of status of the two women, which he sought. Raising the mother's status and giving her the place she obsessively desired, he well knew, was impossible, but lowering the status of his grandmother and disowning both grandparents seemed to be within his reach.

In the human relationship there is then an oscillating movement wherein each partner brings his entire being into moments of common experience and, carrying this experience into a moment of cogitation, withdraws unto himself. The inherent motion of the relationship is lost where it lacks relevancy. We saw how the relationship can be sustained by hostility and we understand the stagnant, leaden, Strindberg-like situation where, as in the case of Mary, no one can be freed from dependency because hatred has become a need, a link, and a way of life. Even Mary realized her involvement, remarking, although with ambivalent meaning, that now she wanted "to stay with my parents forever."

In family relationships devoid of harmony, yet where dissonance, annoyance, and irritation have not taken over entirely, the relationship derives its main energy from the exigencies of daily living. As has been said, the routine of life, under harmonious circumstances, is an element of that relationship, a joyful and relaxed opportunity for contacts. Contrariwise, the daily routine in a family where there is no intrinsic relationship becomes a purpose in itself, a greed, a substitution. Thus, we may see family members on a shopping spree, attempting to bring trifles into the house to make up for the lack of substance in family relationships.

In a similar way, children may take objects home with them from wherever they go. If a child has a positive relation to his therapist such a habit may hold symbolic significance. It shows the child in a still dependent relationship and in need of a concrete, reassuring token for sustaining the emotional tone and extending it beyond the hour of actual collaboration. Facing a return to the emotional void of the home, the child clings to the symbolic mother and an object representing part or all of her; the insecure child cannot postpone gratification. The future is nothingness; what is not now the child feels will never be.

Obsessive stealing may have one of its important determinants in the vague and persistent malaise which is due to inharmonious intimacy or to the emotional dullness reflecting meager and irrelevant communion. Blunted emotions and compensatory stimulation was one of the sources, as we have seen, of Albert's delinquency.

## From Past Discords to Future Terror

It is a known fact that children are apt to develop positive relationships with the parents, provided that the father exercises his responsibilities in full, but especially under the condition that the mother fulfil a concrete, perceivable function in furnishing or attempting to furnish the most elementary needs. Any inclination toward mutuality seems to concentrate almost exclusively on her. When the mother—a basic anchor in life—has been "lost," depending on the age of the child and on the specific circumstances, the child may either stiffen and be blocked by shock, anxiety, or resentment, and stubbornly withdraw, or sway shiftlessly through a confusing world.

Observation of the spontaneous behavior of these children reveals that either approach or withdrawal is impeded because of this basic insecurity. (We are not discussing here those exceedingly severe cases of children clinging to the adult in need of a symbiotic coexistence. The behavior here described is clinging indeed, but for *basic attributes of existence* rather than existence itself.) These children, for instance, fear to leave the psychiatrist because this is associated with the mother's desertion and it gives them a sense of isolation of cosmic dimensions. Similarly, afraid that other children might drive them from the sheltering love, they are unable to leave her for one single moment, although due to the intensity of their anxiety they are unable to make any significant use of her presence. In other instances this inability may be a part of the life-time role assigned to them in sibling competition, and confirmed by the annoyed reactions they may have elicited from a teacher lacking proper understanding. These children are similarly impeded in their approach to the psychiatrist, for fear of being hurt and of renewing their usual experience of rejection in the home and elsewhere. The dissonances of the past are projected as terrifying reverberations on the future.

When the child is thus stifled by fear, his attitude is likely to be of a static quality. He may sit inert, even appearing at times to be relatively content, or he may display a stubborn, resistive tenseness.

Yet, whatever his mood, nothing else will happen. Between the past and this present contact with the therapist, the child has not had its phase of active integration, and he does not return full of energy for an exchange of experience. If the child produces anything at all, it is likely to be a story of some interference and resulting anger provoked by other children in the Center, at home, or at school, or a complaint about a teacher or parent. That is, the child shows that he is very easily disturbed in his state of being and becoming, in other words, of "self-determination." The process of assimilation of experience, or integration, has to be aided by the therapist and used as a basis for inducing a beneficial mutuality. When the session is over, a great deal of skill is required to encourage the child to leave without hurting his feelings and increasing his insecurity and re-activating his fear of a void of experience.

We recall the day when Mary, leaving her therapist with a spontaneous expression of affection, felt like extending some of it to her mother, who was taking her home. The girl tendered her hand to help her limping mother walk down the steps. The mother's instinctive reaction was to withdraw her hand.

It is not surprising that each time Mary arrived at the Educational Therapy Center, she darted around aimlessly, saying "no, no, no" to herself without apparent cause. Slowly, she began to concentrate on an activity of her own choice, chatted happily, and filled intervals with gay humming and singing. When the departure bell finally sounded, however, restlessness and negativism re-awakened and she began to murmur her "no, no, no" once more.

## The Picture of Regression and Integration

Children possessed by pent-up hostility, are not devoid of guilt feelings. The sense of unworthiness caused by the child's rejection in the home is assumed by the child as his own responsibility. The reluctance to integrate, and thus to structure an inner experience, can be seen as an amazing analogy to Hamlet's state of pangs and lassitude, as a longing "to die, to sleep, no more," and "by a sleep to end the heartache." What keeps the child wavering, increasing rather than diminishing his inertia, is the "dread of something after death." Yet, while Hamlet "is sicklied over by the pale cast of thought" and paralyzed by the awareness of his conflicts, these children may be too weary to bring them to the surface; they allow themselves to be overwhelmed and submerged.

In some children, the refusal to integrate their experiences expresses itself by flightiness, shallowness, and evasiveness. It is an escape from an unpromising and unrewarding self, too weak to harbor, hold, and thus protect from exposure of all kinds. This may be but a phase in his development. We remember an orphan boy who had undergone a phase of intense revolt, manifested by gangsterism and delinquency which was the cause for referral to the Educational Therapy Center. It was followed by a period of contrition, extreme weariness, and self-rejection, to the point of loathing life altogether. This in turn yielded to a stage of flightiness and shallowness. Then, there appeared a last vestige of lassitude, an evasion of inner discourse, and skepticism, and a doubt that perhaps he was ridiculous to involve himself with life, a life evidently not worth struggling for. Thus, a temporary crisis in treatment resulted.

When a child shows this symptom, the therapist has nothing to hold on to except her awareness of the state of the child, with warmth and insight. His not wanting to hurt the therapist by his rejection of life and his longing for love prompt him to hesitate to inflict upon himself and others (in this case, the therapist) hurts which he has often experienced. Now, in a rebirth of candor, he again reaches out toward life and trusts the solicitude of the therapist which hopefully leads to self-recognition and acceptance, and an embrace of the world whose promise is no longer denied by him.

At the time of the birth or rebirth of hope, a certain clumsy spontaneity may develop. The child will find his way in and out, to and from the therapist, he will try to attract his attention by a smile, a coquettish, and at times silly and regressive giggle. He will intrude at the most improper moment and rumble as noisily as possible among the toys; he will try to exclude others from the therapist's presence, or withdraw in a way which expresses a need to have the therapist to himself by lying down on the couch and feigning sleep.

In the same way, he will have learned to announce his readiness to leave when he is saturated for the moment and in need of being himself. He may start to topple down his blocks, or put them away untidily, or suggest projects for the next time, or announce plans for a future outside the therapist's office. When the child's behavior in reference to the therapist becomes dynamic and phasic, it has become a living relationship.

We have seen how the illegitimate child, Cyril, had deep feelings of rejection and frustration. His neurotic symptoms developed out of repressed hostile wishes against his mother. He ignored his stepfathers and confused their names with his true father's name by corrupting the sound of all these names in such a way that they all sounded alike. Discussing his parents, Cyril frequently shifted the locations of the father he had mentioned, so as to lead us further astray—a negativistic symptom widely used by these children.

This mechanism seems to evolve out of their own experience of confusion and a tendency to retort in kind. Actually Cyril's mother, with whom he lived, was constantly on the move and was hard to trace. The first behavior displayed by Cyril was extreme negativism, inertia, regressiveness, enhancing the manifest state of immaturity. He indulged at such moments in inarticulate, hardly audible, semi-baby talk, and a concoction of ingenious tricks designed to manifest his hostile withdrawal or his longing to occupy the place of his younger siblings, who, he felt, were loved and accepted. His inertia was a performance suited to stress his part as a victim. The child seemed to say; "I am resisting passively, but I know it is to no avail. I am not in a position to gain the status I covet. Do what you deem fit; I am tired of it all, anyway." This attitude constitutes a means of soliciting pity. One of Cyril's neurotic symptoms served the same purpose— a forced, noisy swallowing of something he felt obstructed his throat and for which he had been taken from one hospital clinic to another. Moreover, by demanding his mother's constant attention, it separated her from his siblings and revealed that he could not "swallow" the situation in the family.

The psychiatrist approached the child in a way that would not impose upon him, but rather would give him, the privilege of feeling free to respond as he chose. She wanted to meet him on the same level of maturation to which he had regressed. To her friendly and expectant, yet passive, attitude, he replied, to her surprise, by going to her library and selecting a daintily illustrated edition of Anderson's "Thumbelina." He wanted to be read to.

This action was infinitely revealing. It showed the first release of tied-up, negative activity into a spontaneous and living form. What he chose was, as with so many of these children, a new start, way back in the past; a revival of a dreamed-of childhood paradise where things are delicate, and where a mother gives her child a whole universe by the simple device of reading him a story.

It was deeply impressive when Cyril, sitting cozily as though protected in a nest, looked up with a glance as if to say that, like the swallow, he felt grateful. He was allowed to feel that indeed it was the therapist who was indebted to him for making this day beautiful. He had shown that he could be happy. This led to a desire on Cyril's part to enhance his value by giving something of himself again. He did it in the way he thought would please the therapist best— by reading to her. (It was quite evident that his reading deficiency was intensified greatly by an emotional element and due to the ungratified needs that still had to be satisfied.) Thus, we sat together like the most intimate of friends, each time he was unable to read a word it was told to him in a whispered, gentle voice, almost concealing his mistake from him, and as though sharing a secret.

Accordingly, the fact that he was giving was subtly emphasized, enriching his self-esteem. That he was also receiving was allowed to penetrate just to the extent that he needed to feel it, and only insofar as it could promote the child's maturation and, in final analysis, his independence. Reading provided an opportunity to talk casually about his problems. His principal difficulty proved to be his feeling of insignificance and rejection arising from his illegitimate birth. While Cyril was actually accepted by his stepfather, as he later revealed, he identified with his unacceptable procreator as one who did not belong and who was of lesser status.

When the child became more secure with his therapist, no longer having to be repeatedly convinced that he was wanted, he lost his inertia and his inability to leave the treatment room spontaneously. He was now unafraid of hurting the therapist by the desire for certain boyish associations which developed at that time. He no longer needed to solicit her attention by his forced swallowing, and when he arrived at this stage, he felt free to disclose his problem.

When his relationship thus gained vitality, it became phasic. This represents a liberation from dependency needs. The child becomes free to "come and go," or to withdraw upon an integrating self and to choose renewed object contacts. These phases may be hidden at some point in the therapeutic, or for that matter, in any human relationship, because their inner rhythm differs from the one imposed by the necessities of the realistic, external situation. *But it is doubtful whether a very sick patient at the climax of transference could ever accept repeated separations from his therapist, if these did not represent an intrinsic element of the relationship and its elaboration.*

Yet there are times when the situation seems beyond repair. The traumatism may be of an appallingly complex character, and usually involves the child in the totality of the family situation, extending obviously over at least three generations. Moreover, to be constantly exposed to an example of improper handling of family relationships is in itself habit-forming.

Children will know only provocative or aggressive family relationships if they come from homes in which the members of the family are paradoxically linked together by their constant need to act out mutual antagonism; these children are trained to believe that every encounter is an act of hostility under an infinite number of disguises.

Under such conditions, their approach to other children is rather unfriendly. To become acquainted may mean to kick and pinprick. It may mean to wrest some precious object from the hands of a child who himself has a dire need for it in order to fulfil some inner demands of his own. Thus, the reaction of the attacked child, cruelly yanked back into reality, may be a terrible one. If children are questioned about their motives or the need for establishing relations in this way, their almost universal response will be that it was "just for fun." It will be a truthful answer, the child being unaware of any ill intention or of the pleasure and satisfaction derived from his violence. It is taken for granted that turbulence and tears may be the results of this instinctive behavior, and indeed the child in need of tumultuous emotions might find certain gratification.

When the Center is attended by a few children suffering from this emotional reaction pattern, activities of this nature may be the only unprompted ones. The need for unrest is so great that, as though addicted, the children cannot resist slipping out of the room for a little fight. The attack on another child may also be aimed at the teacher or the therapist. Old modes of reaction toward parents are tried out again, at first with the anticipation of a "mean," unfair, rejecting reaction; but later, hoping for a relaxed and understanding response. At such time, the hostile struggle recedes and yields to the "play of love and chance." The child has matured for the phasic polarity of confident and reliable human relationships. Although a relationship may still be broached by a challenge, yet its form and meaning has changed and the tournament may well end by a chivalrous handclasp and a devoted friendship based on mutual respect.

## Sociological Differences

We have been impressed by the contrasting attitudes toward objects assumed by extremely deprived children and disturbed youngsters of the middle class. Life has been so deceptive in all of its phases and all of its aspects that the deprived child of the economically depressed classes, unless already improved by therapy, cannot postpone gratification. Nothing is sure but the present moment and what it actually holds. The children of the middle classes, on the contrary, can be observed to live for many long months with the dream of future ownership of an object, as a bicycle, with which they converse in fantasy, which in their mind they manipulate and love, for the future possession of which they work, and for the sake of which they are aggressive in soliciting economic help from adult friends, hoping that they will enrol them as employers for odd jobs. They may be very imaginative in finding remunerative occupations.

According to our experience, even in extreme cases of deep-seated family conflicts, certain areas of existence are spared from direct traumatization. Food is usually, if a subjective problem, not an objective one; the same holds true of clothes. Even where the relationship between family members is replete with hostility, the middle-class parents cannot afford to deny what the lower-class parents cannot afford to offer. The improvident parents of the lower classes will, at best, promise that which they can never fulfil. The frustrating parents of the middle classes will stall, delay, but usually compromise in the end.

Whatever his individual problems might be, the man in a permanent position with a predictable income will derive from it a measure of self-assurance and self-reliance, because he can identify with himself as a person of permanent status, a worker, and a provider.

Not so the man of the lower classes who struggles on, week by week, or day by day. Often he feels like a tolerated tool, subject to a daily approval under the inclemencies of the economic market. To be subject to a daily revision of one's status is sensed as an enslavement to which a man may react by showing that he has freedom, the freedom to stay away as he pleases, or, in other terms, that the job with the boss, too, is subject to a daily approval or acceptance. Every new employment necessarily modifies his consciousness of self, since it requires a new adjustment which is predominantly unilateral. The man is not wanted personally, but anonymously; he is wanted precisely in disregard of his characteristics as an individual which, therefore, he has to conceal and to repress; in the process of self-concealment and constriction, self-assurance and the joy of living are lost. He will feel a cleavage between himself and the casual employer who does not see the man but the hand or the tool.

An enormous strength of character is required to keep up an optimistic view of life and to uphold a continuity of purpose when self-respect in the occupational sphere is profoundly and persistently menaced. When the merciless struggle continues without reprieve, we may expect depression, hostile, aggressive expression, sensitiveness and compensatory self-aggrandizement which may lead to paranoid adaptations.

## The Role of Work

When the head of the family has no specific and personal role to play in his employment sphere, and is but an exchangeable tool, or is but one of the required numbers of a kind, the children show lack of interest in the father's pursuits. Even if he does not change jobs frequently, which confuses the children who cannot keep up with them, being inquisitive about the father's occupation entails touching upon areas very sensitive to all the family members.

Contrary to the middle-class man who talks about the mental challenges of his work and some of its unpleasantness, if he has an interested and sympathetic audience at home, the lower-class man tries to recover from the monotony and vexations on the job and at home submerges his personality. Unless the relationship of the middle-class child to the father is quite negative, the child will probably speak with pride about the father's work, whatever his occupation, and benefit by the father's knowledge.

The Negro children who have been treated by the Clinic (most of whom are of the lower socioeconomic strata), provided they have a father in the home, rarely talk about him and almost never about his work, even when prompted. They do not know what he is doing. In many an instance the father's relationship to his job resembles that to the distasteful source of distasteful food, and he is therefore prone to quit impulsively when his tolerance has been exhausted, unconcerned about the availability of other employment.

The father's example may be one of the reasons why work becomes unpalatable to the children, and why they do not even care to try it; his aversion and need for abstaining may be so great that no other considerations can be thought of or accepted. The children sense that the bread they eat costs the father too dearly, and to be able to eat they must repress everything concerned with his work and, with it, the father himself. The repression of the father is also suggested by the hostility of the mother, who often does not understand, for she cannot afford to understand why her man has to let the family down, interrupt his work, and often takes to the bottle, less distasteful to him and sweetened by assurance of oblivion.

The man in the middle-class position of employment is more apt to grapple with difficulties, because he is made to feel and actually is part of the enterprise and his interest is therefore engaged. Severance of the relation because of obstacles that cannot be mastered represents a loss, and at times an economic calamity. If this results in an emotional crisis, the children have at least opportunity to be impressed by the greatness of the loss that severance from employment may represent. If adjustment to what seems severance is rapid and complete, the children will have opportunity to benefit by the father's aptitude, versatility, and courage. They can familiarize themselves with conservation of possessions and acceptance of substitutes.

In a happy middle-class milieu, the children remember fulfilment of desires granted with the joy of giving and the pride and thankfulness of being able and privileged to pass on joy. Without undue anxiety they may desire a wealth of necessary as well as luxurious things. These are legitimately available and potentially obtainable. They do not have to break through the realm of possibility in order to enforce obtaining the impossible. There is no need for opposing, contradicting, and combatting the frustrating consistency of the world.

The loud lure of our immodest economy may enter a pressing wedge into the family harmony by the unreserved exposure of its enticements and through competition and rivalry. We concede that our economy promotes insatiability and a concomitant fear that the neighbor might take away the apple of fascination in a paradise of bounty. Anxiety due to the disproportion between the family's greed and the provider's relative insufficiency will tend to bring about a state of cold war in the family. Mutual intimidation and alienation will become a retaliatory weapon for frustration thus inflicted and incurred.

In this psychiatrist's experience, unemployed mothers will tend to identify and align themselves with their children, disregarding their real interests. They often use the children as missiles against the husband, in resentment of their economic dependency, emotional frustrations, and complexes. Needless to say, genuinely disinterested feelings toward the children are lost in such a state of hostility, regardless of the inevitable tendency of hostility to become generalized.

## Hostility and Deprivation

Dedication will insidiously be infiltrated by defensive maneuvers. Constantly renewed endeavors by either side to use the children will almost become a necessity for support in loneliness, anxiety, and the need for alleviation of guilt feelings. Hostile impulses against the children, spurred by their naturally wavering loyalty, have to be overcompensated as well as guilt feelings due to conscious or unconscious misuse of their filial role. Condoning and indulging procedures will be practiced so as to relieve the one partner at the expense of the other. Deprivation in an economy of plenty is only relative. Gratification of appetites is altogether excluded and the firebrand of hostility will be kept alive. The father is punished for his financial prerogative as the sole provider, which he brandishes with intensified terror, until he stops exhausted.

Threatened by incessant assaults from the total family group, the father will cling with an increasing fascination to the delusive power his money can yield, and, anxious to be depleted and deprived, he will sit on it, like Fafner, the dragon of the Volsunga Saga of the Edda. Finally he will refuse to part with any of it except the bare minimum necessary to meet his basic obligations to the family. The longer the father remains attached to the money as a supportive part of himself, the more it develops into an aggressive weapon in his defense against intensified family assaults. His own fascination for, and in particular retention of, the treasure causes a fascination in his family members for whom that money gains a wealth of meanings. He may wonder why it is that for his wife or child money seems to be everything. The two parties will engage in a pointed fight, the one attempting to retain, the others to extort a release of the cash, until the fight gains murderous proportions, and the father may yield the hoard to save his skin, but punish the victors by losing his job and producing no more.

At this time, deterioration of family relationship and family economy may undergo a total decline, but depending on insight and the capacity to assume responsibility, love and pity may reappear and the family may be reunited in a common struggle for existence. The "curse" coming from the "goal" has vanished, everybody will have to put the hand to the wheel to get the family in motion, turning away from the obsession to *possess*, literally the power to sit, and moving onward to harvesting profits deserved by "labor."

While anxiety in the economically more secure classes is usually fostered by the seduction of being seated at the luxurious "banquet" prepared by our economy of plenty, anxiety of uninvited bystanders is due to resentment at being excluded from the festival of life in all of its fundamental, as well as uplifting, aspects. However, it is obvious to the child who has a father in the home that it is not in his power to grant or withhold the festive offerings that attract the child's eye.

There exists an ambivalence in an economy and a society where standards are set in terms of economic success. The father is a nonentity; unless he is economically successful, it is hard to admire him. But the child, still struggling for integrity and self-respect, is in need of admiring and respecting the father. Unless he can do so, the child feels that he will become a nonentity himself. How else would the self-respect of the child be bolstered, if neither the father, nor he, nor any member of his family is eligible to be guests at the official "banquet." In the absence of joy and an active community, and in the presence of depression and deliberately imposed resourcelessness, there is every likelihood that the child will have no choice in the end but to attribute to the father a lowly position.

Sometimes the child will turn to an uncle, whose superhuman efforts have resulted in some measure of success; but to maintain it, the older man cannot allow himself to be fettered by the burden of a distraught child clinging awkwardly to him. Again the child will be informed of his ineligibility. To be able to hold on to the uncle, the pride of the family, the child has to look elsewhere for people who can be blamed for his deprivation, those who beckon to everyone but leave him out: the stores, their owners, and all that is associated with them. Only in returning disrespect and in disregarding the rules of society can the child get even with those whose acceptance still remains his goal.

## The Mechanism of Violence

Hostility of children is sensed and acted out violently against material things. Unless there exists an intense emotional problem regarding the parents, hostility takes the form of contempt and disregard rather than of physical violence against people. The danger of physical violence against people is minimal when these people have but an abstract existence in the child's mind. Only if a transference is made from the parent to a particular person reminding the child of the parent and provoking the child's vulnerability, can it happen that violence is physically expressed from man to man. However, violence against the house as a symbol of the unrewarding mother, whatever the child's stage of libido development, may be used as an everyday occurrence in the Educational Therapy Center.

The obsessive longing for the fulfilment of the mother's role is liable to promote a displaced or impotent violence. Need of the mother, the lure of her love and of the role attributed to her present a last barrier to physical violence. The necessity of preserving the object which keeps alive the obsession represents a deterrent to physical violence, which would eliminate the target altogether. The danger is greatest where there is no interaction between mother and child at all, and where there is no gratification of any kind, not even by mutual, chronically manifested hostility. The chronic futile struggle tends not only to give vent to the emotions but also to exhaust the capacity for action. In those cases where pent-up tension becomes overwhelming and is finally acted out, because of an acute exacerbation of a chronically endured vital menace, the victim could well be the mother, original source of the child's suffering. Displacement of violence, however, is possible because of the need to spare the mother as a source of gratification, even by hostile interaction. Where there has been no interaction, the source of pain, the mother, has remained so abstract a feature that violence can be more readily placed on any cover figure, or any male or female person to whom an emotional transference is made. Due to the abstractness of the mother and the total evasiveness of her, even as a target, anything and anyone can trigger the pent-up ubiquitous hostility into action.

Lindner's masterly description shows how a box used by his psychoanalyst on a prison round was associated with a box belonging to the patient's mother. The patient was obsessed by the idea that the mother's marriage ring, which he used to remove from her box for his secret marriage rituals, was hidden in the box carried by his analyst. Due to this incidence (we disregard at this time other elements of the transference as revealed by the author), the psychoanalyst became the denying mother who withheld the symbol of union from him. The unleashing upon his psychoanalyst of the patient's murderous impulses against the mother was triggered by the presence of a box, and a chain reaction of associations.

The need of deeply hurt children to inflict pain is not only a means of retaliation but is, as is well known, more a perverted and angry attempt to elicit love. Any way of "having it out" with someone is more tolerable than indifference and neglect. Provoked expression of active rejection at least justifies angry manifestations. Mother and child may at this point have an interest in maintaining each other as necessary targets and objects needed for rationalization. It is their only way of reaching each other, or feeling that they have any emotions at all, and that there is at hand an object for triggering the release of tension.

A young girl able to express her feelings once said: "I know I should not use my sessions to shout at my mother constantly, but this is the only way I feel I am living, that is why I feel relieved when I am here. I feel I am living. When I am violent with her and throw things, I am fighting to be living, when I appear calm near her I have given up, she has finished me up again." Thus, fighting the mother becomes a desperate attempt at eliciting life-giving energy as well as a struggle against the mother's rejecting tendencies and her annihilating power. As long as life tendencies remain in the child, the mother is protected from total annihilation; when these life tendencies are exhausted, exterior aggression is spent.

## The Racial Differential

The Negro child of the destitute classes is so traumatized that his anxiety and almost cosmic isolation narrow down his perceptiveness to the needs of the moment, as well as to the area of most intense sensibilization. Such a constricted attitude is reflected in the fact that to living subjects, no less than to inert objects, is attributed only an instrumental or functional character.

Rejected in the community regardless of personal merit and individual traits, only a strong independent mind can rise to a relaxed self-evaluation and a sense of dignity devoid of resentment against others or one's own existence. The problem is intensified when a child or growing youngster is unwanted at home due to his parents' self-rejection, notwithstanding their individual problems which are usually injected in, and inextricably enmeshed with, the general community rejection to which we are here referring.

A child cannot gain any conception of a disinterested relationship between self-respecting people when he has been deprived of the experience of being valued for his own sake. He has no motives nor does he possess clues for scrutinizing with genuine interest another person by reason of his or her existence. Characteristic individual traits are not and cannot be retained. Knowledge of another man's traits would be worth gaining only if it served an immediate purpose, as a means of defense, and only as long as the other fellow has but a momentary function which can be replaced by anyone of his kind. If one has recourse to him again, it is for the sake of expedience, the way—at times to be taken only literally as easily accessible—is paved already and the approach facilitated. Only slight doubt is felt that the "guy" might not function again. But the child's fundamental distrust will cause "that guy," as insecure as he himself already is, to fail or to be made to fail after a short stage. Then a new nameless creature will be needed to fill the ill-defined function and provide another "pick-up job." No motive, therefore, could be found to retain the name or traits of a fellow who is but an unspecified tool.

If pressed, destitute Negro children may have one specific characteristic to call to mind, the hue of a person's complexion. Rejection, self-rejection and projection, with all of their ramifications, are symbolized in terms of color. The white culture imposes itself as the model for both valid and non-valid reasons. If the Negro child thinks of his color as a fundamental mark against himself and if he feels that he has to justify his very existence rather than to fulfil it, we can blame, in part, his school books, which ignore his existence totally. The books showing the ideal white family, the family as it should be, suggest to these children, who come from a deprived and troubled milieu, that in their quality as Negroes they cannot make the grade. The longing for perfection becomes the longing to be similar or identical with the white people, rather than the striving to acknowledge in his own specific terms man's universal purpose.

If this longing actually represents, in final analysis, a tendency toward sufficiently abstract ideals, it may be highly motivating and lead to a positive and proud concept of the self, as in the more successful social strata among the Negro people. Ideals are our own when we have conceived them, man's universal opportunity, unmarked by origins. But if this longing develops no further than to mean concretely the white-skinned man and his privileges, it leads necessarily to a fundamental ambivalence in reference to the white man and to the Negro himself. Not only is the ideal figure itself disappointing, because in reality he denies his own principles which therefore become fallacious, but the same ambivalence concerns himself, and, unless he is totally paralyzed, self-affirmation in the most deprived and least resourceful group is achieved in opposition to what the culture establishes as its goals. Where there is enough strength left for revolt against the ambivalence, the search is made for one guiding light; religious answers are often sought, without alleviating all of the torment.

Among white people in a mixed population, the conflict is not in terms of rejection, self-rejection, and projection, but more liable to be in terms of rejection, self-acceptance, and projection. It is not permanent and ubiquitous; though it begins in childhood, it confronts the white child at a later stage. The conflict is fundamental to the individual only insofar as it is a moral conflict, repressed and full of projective defenses.

But with the Negro of the lowest socioeconomic group this conflict starts with the mother. The specific brand of illegitimacy which is such a frequent occurrence in this group is due, in addition to more general psychological motivations, to this ambivalence in racial matters. When opportunities for full participation in the surrounding culture are denied on racial grounds, a sense of total disarmament results; when otherwise the odds are overwhelming, condemnation by a culture comes as a universal shock, particularly if the official value system is, however ambivalently, accepted. This fosters the destructive feeling that to this world there can be only a negative response.

In view of inhibited maturation, pathetically reduced opportunities, and the resulting lack of resourcefulness, as well as the frustrations of instinctual life, sex represents one of the few experiences available for gaining a sense of being and of self-affirmation. People under those circumstances are comparable to the infant abandoned in his lonely crib, gesticulating aimlessly, who happens to discover that he can play with his own body. At the stage of maturation where the instinctual life still serves overwhelmingly narcissistic tendencies, the sex partner becomes predominantly a means for experience and specificity is fairly irrelevant.

## Life, Death, and Sex

Life and death, however, may be at stake in the experience but in a profoundly different acceptance of both terms. Under auspicious circumstances life and death as implied in sexual abandon are not mutually exclusive. The individual gives up his particular existence to merge into another. The merging is so complete that it outlasts the climactic moment and conveys in the intermittent periods a sense of wholeness to the individual and of permanence to the union. Neither of the partners to such an inspired match is conceivable as being just incidental to the experience. The abandoning of individual existence for a moment implies rebirth and animation; it renders possible the active attitude toward the choice of partner and gift of self. The intensely vital elements of the experience become liberating rather than binding.

Sexual abandon, therefore, does not imply self-devaluation or denial of existence, since a positive gift is made. Self-esteem must precede the act; he who wants to give must feel that he has something worth giving and something acceptable; he must also feel that the other is worthy to receive the gift. The partner to such an immense act of total abandon is sensed as something treasured in itself, for itself, but also as a representation of an integral value. Thus, under fortunate circumstances, each partner to a sexual act gives all of his life to receive all of his life.

In this respect, the sexual union is life-giving and creative independent of its procreative function. The union is an opportunity for the individual to reach out beyond his own limits into nature, its immensity and promise, and beyond it into the sublime. Under tragic conditions, however, there is no actual abandoning of one's individual existence, no actual merging and subsequent rebirth, but destruction or indifference, indifference meaning a helpless neutrality and indecision in reference to both life and absence of existence.

In extreme cases, self-assertion and self-realization are missed, shame, depression, and anxiety follow, and renewal of the experience is in the nature of a standstill, an obsession, the ever repeated tendency toward an elusive goal by improper means. Temporarily or permanently, the subject may not be reflective enough to recognize in himself a specific object capable of selecting another specific and complementary object which under ideal circumstances is the only possible one. Because of the immature level of integration and the lack of specificity the sexual experience is not actually retained and does not survive itself; in cases of temporary regression which has to be repressed, the conflict tends to promote symptoms. If the relation is continued with the same partner, it is not because of the bridge of inspiration which stretches from one point of culmination to the next; if not due to resentment and hostility and a dim community of shame, the relation is maintained because of inertia, convenience, and the enslavement of routine. Life is not lived, but it is undergone, on a vegetative level of integration for the sake of eliminating bodily discomfort. A general passive release is in operation, which to the extent that it is geared toward pleasurable relieving of body disturbance, is at the service of life, though by passive and inappropriate means. Relief cannot be subordinated to, and integrated in, the higher purposes which are absent, but the whole process is submerged in the metaplastic overgrowth of the partial sexual function.

The rejected and self-rejecting person is actually in an absurd status of negation of existence while life, and necessarily some affirmation of existence, are proceeding. Life is lived in a permanent contradiction to itself and an intolerable burden of ambivalence weighs it down and constricts it. For those to whom the world is a longed-for mother which turns to them nothing but a hideous medusan front, the sex act may embody a suicidal tendency resulting from generalized hostility and aggression.

Sex may become delinquent in purpose, and one of its rewards is that it is oppositional to what is accepted or to what is positively identified with a rejecting world. Satisfaction may be derived from its delinquent nature.

The child may be taken as a corollary to the sex experience; we have seen girls as well as boys make the gesture of rocking the baby in their arms as an invitation to sexual intercourse. But the gesture gives double connotation to the word "baby" as well as to the rocking and the embrace. Associated with the lust of love and life, the child is taken for granted, a corollary and symbol of sex. He may be loved instinctively as a reminder of it, particularly in infancy. But this kind of love holds few elements of responsibility. The child is subordinated to the parents' sex needs and resented when in their way. A new motivation for rejection arises when the child stands up as an inadequate erotic competitor for parental love. Since sex is most obviously lived in total disregard of the child's existence and needs, the child reacts by intense intrusiveness and is repulsed with corresponding violence. Sex itself then may be used as a terrifying and shocking weapon of expulsion.

Louis, an eight-year-old boy, was referred to the Educational Therapy Center because he could not be kept in public school. He was in a state of confusion, roaming restlessly around the premises of his school or the Center as well as on the streets, crossing them disregarding traffic. He was evasive and seemed almost incoherent in his constant irrelevant verbalizations. In therapy, he immediately turned to the doll house and was profusely verbal and fantastic. His stories concerned fire and incendiaries, burning mattresses in particular, which were thrown into the street.

As time went on, he told about the totally inadequate nutrition he was getting; there was no milk for him but whiskey for his mother and the married aunt with whom they lived. The father, not married to the mother, lived across the street and accepted him partially until he became involved with another woman. At that time he withdrew from the child irrevocably. Crossing the street in disregard of traffic became uncontrollable. The child reported finally that his mother had been a chronic alcoholic, as was his aunt, that the mother was promiscuous and when drunk exposed herself unclad in a provocative posture to his view.

Louis developed sufficient ego strength to want foster home placement. He adjusted well in the new home, and the mother was relieved to be rid of him.

To overcome their intense anxiety, the children in turn may use sex as a frightening, even terrorizing instrument of hostile aggression. Dayton, whose case is extensively discussed elsewhere in this book, is one of many. At a period of his life where he was most intensely traumatized and at the threshold of pre-adolescence, he developed voyeuristic habits at home and in the Center, where he interpreted all staff relations sensually, hid behind doors and corners to catch his suspects *flagrante delicto*. He then verbalized aggressively what he thought he had seen at home or in the Center, to which actually he had transferred anxieties, at least partially motivated by the actual conditions at home. By intense verbal aggressiveness, he exposed all the sex delinquents he saw, particularly at home, and, by actual sexual exhibitionism of his own, frightened his sisters, whom the mother indulged in their less obvious feminine exhibitionism. He thus attempted vainly to convey what anxiety his sisters, with their less provocative exhibitionism, promoted in him and how it affected him. In the mother's mind, the sisters' exhibitionism was not directed toward him, and she failed to appreciate that it affected him even doubly, as an observer as well as a jealous brother; that he in turn exposed himself she considered to be grossly pathological, while in his own mind he simply took the same license as the sisters and was as inconsiderate of them as they of him. Retaliating against the mother's sex and business relation to an elderly man, he pretended loudly that he had sex relations with an old lady roomer of his mother's. There existed an associative link between this woman and the mother's emotional involvement. The mother's dependent relation to her elderly employer was threatening to him, and similar to the one to her elderly male partner, though not because of any personal sex relationship. Both rejected him and deprived him of the mother's love, the mother sacrificing him because of her dependency on them. Provoking sex offenses, though in imagination displaced to another person and carried out in this particular instance only verbally, was his way of punishing her. In the group, tendencies to use sex as a mutual threat, with suicidal-homicidal intensity, may become apparent.

Amos, a nine-year-old, overgrown, obese, dark-skinned boy, from an intelligent, striving, and highly educated family, all of whose members were light skinned except for his mother and him, was referred by an out-of-town child guidance clinic. The child and his mother had long been subjected to individual psychotherapy and the child was said not to have improved. Elimination from the family situation and treatment against the background of our day-care program were considered desirable.

Nothing in the transmitted case history, nor in the discussions with referring agencies and the mother, prepared us for the pan-sexuality of the child, nor did he display any obvious symptoms of it in his initial interview. Amos' breakdown was due to his sense of defeat and total exclusion from the family. Though overdetermined, his symptom complex was strongly motivated by its quality of being an unfailingly shocking tool of aggression, the existence of which would justify exclusion and make it more bearable. Moreover, to be a part of the family, the child had to pay the heavy toll of excessive conrol imposed by the father. According to observation by his former therapist, not a misplaced auxiliary verb escaped his cold and strict reprimand, either in reference to this eight-year-old or to the younger children. Therefore, once motivation for precarious control was absent, the explosion was complete. Exhibitionism was mentioned in his record, stammering, intrusiveness in the form of constant questioning without actual interest in the answer, abandoning indifferent attempts; disobedience and temper tantrums at the rate of two a month were reported, as well as violent sibling rivalry transferred to extra-familial relations.

The house in doll play was considered too crowded to accommodate all the children, the mother was regarded as belonging in the house, the father as an obligation that must be accepted and who is fed ahead of the children. The father's gifts are not taken for granted but treasured. Motor phenomena such as poor co-ordination were mentioned in the clinic report, as were clumsiness and slovenly performances.

The initial interview with this psychiatrist, which preceded by four months the actual intake (a foster home in Richmond had to be found by a placement agency), revealed, in addition to the symptoms already mentioned, a child well conditioned by previous psychotherapy, who played comfortably but showed a tendency to clinging relations and iterative signs. The drawing of a house with a door were but scarcely outlined; there were no windows. Observation at a later date suggested that the child's outside position in the family as suggested by the drawing was partly due to his dark complexion in a light-skinned family, a color variant which happened to coincide with his relative mental inferiority in a gifted family.

However, the accident of pigmentation had deep implications. The mother was of illegitimate birth, and her family, before finally raising her, had considered giving her away for adoption. Her father, with whom contact was established when she was already seven years of age, was the only dark-skinned member of her total family group; she resented him for having misused her mother. He also was less ambitious and less studious than the others. He failed to continue supporting her in college, a factor which compelled her to work her way up to the third year, in the course of which she married. The mother, being dark skinned, like her father and Amos, caused dark complexion to be associated with an illegitimate status and a form of illicit intrusion in the various families involved.

The mother's history pointed to her conflict in her first pregnancy, the one with Amos. It occurred after two years of marriage when the father was still a student and she the provider. Actually both parents rejected the child and the paternal grandmother appeared to have overindulged him, rejecting him later overtly as a product of the mother's inadequate education. The paternal grandmother had vainly opposed the marriage, to the point of threatening to commit suicide. The father, raised in a broken home by his mother and grandmother, at one time had undergone treatment for paranoid schizophrenia, but he continued his studies until he had acquired his master's degree. This implied that Amos' mother was pushed around in the house of these domineering women and elsewhere, subjugated to them while the father was absent during the school semesters. Actually, it meant that he was still committed to his mother, whose major object was to see him become a graduate professional man. His marriage was not acknowledged. Marital difficulties arose from the parents' diversities of opinion in reference to birth control, or sterilization, as suggested medically; five children were born to this union. Though the father's motives were consciously religious, we are inclined to believe that they were not devoid of an element of suspiciousness, hostility, and domineering tendencies.

The mother felt insecure and inferior due to her illegitimate birth. Intense conflicts were felt in reference to Amos, who, like her father and herself, was the only dark member of his generation in the family. She felt disinclined to breast-feed him but showed some signs of rejection toward all of her children, none of whom she desired to breast-feed.

From the child's own history, one additional factor stands out. He was sexually traumatized at the age of three by the request of an eleven-year-old white boy to perform an act of fellatio with him. The mother happened to catch the boys in the act and, intensely shocked, she traumatized her child a second time by her reaction. The consequent rebound taught the boy the power of shock to be achieved by sexual misconduct. To the mother, the abusive incident represented an additional hurt, reinforcing racial implications.

In the Educational Therapy Center the child was an excessive eater, exceeding by far other children with a similar symptom. He was avid for the other children's food. The same observation was made in the foster home. This symptom again was overdetermined and, according to observations and the child's verbalizations, it appeared to be motivated also by pregnancy fantasies, due in their turn to his need for incorporation and being the mother as well as turning the tables against her threatening fecundity by taking her place. Self-indulgence also was suggested as a regression to his early days when the grandmother indulged him (before rejecting him frankly), on his return to her house following an intermediary stay with the father.

Amos was intolerably demanding and tried to exclude the other children from the use of objects, and from the attention of people except when he himself enrolled them instrumentally. He invited the children's physical or sex aggression and then screamed with stentorian voice. He constantly tried to retain undue attention by stuttering stridently and with a whistle. When he had nothing to say, he would reiterate the name of the person he thus harangued, introducing long intervals and appearing to be on the verge of enunciating his communication. The way he stuttered was meant to be tantalizing, as he retained his victims without reward for their prolonged and sustained attention.

Though revealing his intense frustration by inflicting it, the stuttering also increased his own torment, and hence the fury to strike. Amos was capable of working himself up to such intensive excitement that he almost passed out. In this tragic condition the grip of life escaped him, even in its painful aspects. He used the same technique for aggression in reference to his passive sexual needs.

He asked for extracurricular individual interviews to complain about alleged sexual aggressions of any description by other children, or he complained loudly and stuttered in a strident voice when in the presence of other children. He allegedly reported all actual or imaginary experiences in every detail to the foster mother. Although the children on the whole were inconceivably tolerant of him, he was too disturbing an element to be kept in his group and was assigned to one individual worker all through the day for activities and outings, a routine interrupted only by his individual therapy sessions.

## The Enemy as Friend

This child was engaged in a sado-masochistic relation to another boy, Freddy, a very light-complexioned adolescent whom the psychiatrist found in an intensely irate condition. He said he had been insulted by Amos because of his, Freddy's, light complexion. Although his motives were well known to this psychotherapist, he was given opportunity to express his reasons for reacting so sensitively to the other boy's verbal attack. All that he could proffer in an intense verbal outburst was self-rejection and his profound ambivalence against both his white and his Negro origin. Freddy's mother was intensely self-rejecting in a way which implied his own rejection and showed it in particular by manifestations abhorrent to him. All of her devoted, competent, and willing service she gave to an upper-class white family and a Catholic institution, though she remained Protestant. She neglected her home to an unbelievable extent and was drunk throughout the weekend.

Freddy hoped that, as if by magic, his mother would carry her more respectable identification into her home. He once pretended he was a Catholic and asked the psychiatrist for a rosary, thus making himself, through the mother image in therapy, the recipient of blessings denied to him and to his existence by the real mother. Later he asked the psychiatrist for an amulet which he first wore only on Sundays, afraid he might lose it, but subsequently he never parted with it. This one he wore around his neck and close to his heart, another one which he had bought himself, he carried in his pocket, in order to make it a sacred place where he would be in awe of putting any unacceptable stolen goods.

The father, a white man, had left the mother and the three children he had with her and married a white woman. Freddy, the youngest child, continued to run to his father, until the door was closed to him unceremoniously by the father's new wife. For an extremely long time he pretended having no recollection of his father, but within two weeks of the incident here discussed, confronted with the anxiety of a visit home, he mentioned that he had one white friend in life whom he had lost in an accident, but he had a negative attitude toward further discussing him and particularly concealed whether it was a friend of his age or of the previous generation.

The rejecting attitude of Freddy's father prevented him from recognizing the white man in himself and the mother's self-rejection prevented him from acknowledging in himself the Negro. Therefore, he was neither; and he did not find out that he did not have to be classified but could be *self-identified*. As the human product he was, society forced him to live nowhere and that was inevitably impossible. This was an important factor in his very precarious hold on reality.

Both Freddy and Amos had a tendency to show hostile complementation of which the individually motivated sex problem was but one element. Freddy, who had been subjected to treatment for some time, benefited readily by the psychiatrist's interpretation and easily understood and accepted that the other child tried to solve a problem of his own, in attacking him as light skinned.

The dark child saw in the light-skinned boy the image of siblings who threatened his proper place within the family unit. The light-skinned child whom he attacked and successfully tried to offend was reminded of a condition that caused him to feel off bounds everywhere: a negligible nonentity to his father, a negative entity to his mother. When, however, the common element was pointed out to the older child, he identified himself with his previous enemy, Amos, and despite his own tragic condition, all of his human charity was aroused.

However, in all families, white and Negro, the psychosocial and sociosexual relationships follow the same pattern. The problem of self-identification of each family member with twosomeness and the group feelings are largely the same. The eternal change from the extrovert to the introvert and back are necessary for all family and group life in general.

Such life must bring opportunity for solitude to the individual, it must give the family group an opportunity to recover from the special stresses introduced by each individual member, and it must give the individual member an opportunity to recover from the stresses inherent in group life. In fairly harmonious families and groups and among well-composed individuals such opportunities set in motion a permanent cycle of love and new acceptances, a higher emotional fertility in an unending spiral of development.

In the absence of these intermissions and creative pauses, a chafing family experience tends to replace an auspicious cycle of an ever renewed mutual understanding and encouragement. If the fortunate rhythm toward and away from the family community is interrupted by the vicissitudes and humiliating experiences connected with the social structure in which families live, then it is difficult for the individual as well as for the whole family group to maintain their integrity, their self-identification, and to feel the need as well as the value of solitude and contemplation, or have the material means to satisfy this basic need. Anxiety and strife will prevail and hostile dependency will develop if it is carried into the community or infiltrates the network of our social structure and menaces its security by seemingly submissive betrayal.

However, such is the unnatural environment in which our Negro children find themselves and such are the disturbances promoted by their environment. The treatment, as we shall see in subsequent chapters, consists in the creation of a therapeutic milieu which liberates them from the bonds of dependency, interrupts the vicious circle of hostile interdependence, the implied contempt and self-contempt and the strain of enduring the absorbing tension of hatred.

# V

## *Parents*

The story of these children's parents may help us understand how absurd is the idea that by means of punishment or short-term separations the child's conformity to social and moral standards can be achieved. The story of the parents and the understanding of the deep-seated mutual interaction with their children, although highlighting the serious intricacies inherent in such an interaction, also may represent a challenge to assist these families. Patiently we might follow Ariadne's thread and in the depth of the labyrinth annihilate the monster it harbors.

SOME BASIC FACTS[1] AND COMMENTS

### *Family Structure*

Over 60 per cent of the families of our children are one-parent families by death, desertion of husband or wife, divorce, separation, or because there has never been a marriage. A number of the marriages were consummated after conception or birth of one or more of the children. Most frequently, with few exceptions, the children live with the mother. The father has deserted the family and his whereabouts may be unknown, or he is deceased, not infrequently slain. He may have perished in a car accident, an accident on the job, or died of pneumonia incurred by excessive zeal at work in disregard of health hazards. A small percentage of the fathers are in penal confinement; some of them are on the road gang for non-support of the family.

Non-support may be due to simple self-centeredness and refusal to take responsibility, to hostility and alcoholism, promiscuity and the involvement with one or subsequently several women. These involvements may not be of a passionate but dependent nature. The man may want to be nursed but he provides economically, or he may depend with all of his needs upon a woman until she gets tired of being exploited. One of these men who invariably repeated this behavior pattern was religious, zealous, rigid, and self-righteous. A few of the fathers who have disappeared may make a temporary reappearance after many years. At times the man's place is taken, or he is made to fail because he was never forgiven and his weakness never forgotten. His return is met with suspicion. Another father returned after almost a decade to his family of five children. He had remarried and apparently reformed his former ways. He had become a preacher. He still rejected his son who tried with ardor to gain his interest that in the boy's mind would have amounted to a blessing of his existence. But the father was adamant in reserving his interest solely to his eldest daughter. At the time she was sixteen years of age. He lavished dresses and frills upon her. Did he come home to his little girl, to his growing girl or to his wife of olden days? In telling Dayton Peterson's story, we shall report the dreams and longings the boy had nurtured in reference to the father through many painful years of his total absence.

## Why Do the Fathers Desert Their Families?

When we meet the deserted family the absent husband is always the sole offender, but the accuser is not always convincing. At times, the remaining partner seems a person hard to live with, hard to satisfy, demanding, self-indulging, rigid, nagging, and harsh. In treatment she may become self-searching and tend to improve.

In other cases two dependent people had been matched who may return to the domineering parent or the man may leave town under commitment to his mother who is glad to take him from his wife. She may permanently conceal his whereabouts and conceal from his family his short-lived returns. Two inadequate people have become incompatible because neither could complement the other's inadequacy as both had expected. Rather did they mutually multiply their inadequacy. The man knew at least to defend himself by escaping a further impairment of his condition and the excessive ballast of his poor caravel. As usual, the simple facts need to be explored; they do not always speak for themselves. Nor has a bitter, emotionally and physically withered woman necessarily been the same before being hurt, and the hostile expression of her distress may only reflect the reversal of an intense investment of feelings in a woman of limited resources for recovery.

## Unmarried Mothers

A high percentage of the mothers in the one-parent families is unmarried and the children in the home have different fathers with no meaningful contact between the parents or the father and his children. These women are most impressive. Their inadequacy in defending themselves in the sexual area can be due to mere identification with their unmarried grandmother and mother. That no other issue could be found than such an identification with a milieu and with a behavior the young child sets out to loathe and to decline is due to a dependency they cannot outgrow in that milieu. These women are driven toward sexual indulgence and are avid for the presence of men. The pleasures surrounding their company with men as feasting parties seem to be their only relief from the bondage of living and their only forever ephemeral grasp on joy. They are too depressed to have the strength to be hostile or revolt. They hang on to their children as they did to their two mothers, because as mothers they still remain the dependent and helpless child. They call it love but are unaware of the children's needs and their neglect. Being the ones they are, they are less able to understand and promote the needs of a growing child. Not only by their frustrating helplessness and aridity but for mere fear of an inadequacy in reference to the growing child do they impede his growth as did their elders. Above all, their need to indulge in their way of life is soil and nurture of their existence and necessarily has to take precedence over the child that does not cement, merely serves to prop up their warped structure.

Usually great-grandmother, grandmother and the young teenage mother are alcoholic. When we see the young mothers as patients, they are hopelessly listless. Some of them seem inseparable from the child who hangs passively rather than rests in the mother's uncuddling arms. A pervasive sadness takes place of what, in a less helpless woman, might be guilt feelings. Irritability with the children alternates with gentle sadness; it is their weak and undefined reaction to the injury caused by their bondage to this adversity. These young women have a conspicuously sensuous character. Sensuousness does not enter as a motivating factor into the higher purposes of existence. We are helped to understand what happened to the mother when we see her hold her child passively without as much as a tendency to express any acceptance. We may see her children or the children of another young mother like her in the Clinic when repeated desertions have become final by total disappearance or when the protective services have assumed responsibility for them. The mother may have been committed to the state farm. Some of them return improved. They needed their children as an incentive for improvement but may not always be able to maintain the necessary effort. The child's role as an incentive is but an illusion. As the passive instrument he was made to be, he lacks vitality himself and the power to inspire and keep up the illusion.

We observe young mothers who slipped into promiscuity of a very different connotation, resulting from a spiteful relationship to the father and a love against which both, father and daughter, defended themselves by hostility. The mother equally may be involved in this hostility in condoning the child's "faithlessness" to the father. When she comes home with a child who has no father of his own, her own father may withdraw in a deep and painful disappointment. Identified with the father's rejection and hopelessly depressed she persists on "throwing away" her depreciated self, using her contrition for a motivation of further instinct gratification. The Oedipal problem is maintained by its perversion. Father and daughter connive in despising and defeating her. The young mother is being condoned further by her own mother in indulgence of sexual impulsivity as well as in her depressing contrition, both factors contributing to the rift between father and daughter. The mother meanwhile finds comfort enjoying the daughter's children and the fruit of the daughter's indulgences.

When the father lives with the family but neglects mother and daughter emotionally, the daughter may fall prey to substitutional father figures who "love you but give you also all that a father should give his girl, nice dresses and other things." The girls talk about these "things" in an enamorous way, as though they were dolls representing the girl herself. They betray by their behavior as well as by their verbal explanation that they are the child as well as the woman and act out longingly and resentfully an Oedipal involvement with their father. Often these young girls' relationships were procured by female "matchmakers" to whom the girls listened rather than to the mother because they deeply resented the mother's position as the family's underdog and revolt against the brand of feminity it represents.

Not only resourceless children are subject to such behavior. Girls of good intelligence may deny it in time of crises and be infantile and irrational or they may rationalize an extremely unreasonable behavior.

The case of Frances, like so many of these young unmarried mothers who are the mother and the child and who become finally obsessed by the psychological complexities of their situations, illustrates the inner experience of a young girl deserted by her father. When her father disappeared Frances, a girl of dull normal intelligence, was ten years old, physically and sexually premature, and emotionally dependent.

Frances was referred to us at the age of thirteen by the State Industrial School. She came from a home of extreme misery. She was the fourth of eight children. She was promiscuous, had acquired a venereal disease, and was an incorrigible truant. The father had disappeared intermittently before he finally vanished.

According to the girl's mother, he was supposed to have had spells of amnesia. We do not know whether he himself used to feign amnesia and the mother was too ready to believe him or whether this diagnosis was of her own invention because she wished to exonerate him from blame and save herself from rejection. The welfare worker in her community was inclined to consider the amnesia an illusion which the mother needed to uphold and which intensified Frances' problem.

Information about the character and the dynamics of the relations between the family members was hard to come by. All our attempts to enrol the co-operation of the mother or May, the older sister, were in vain. Our objective knowledge of the family situation is based solely on a factual welfare report and on Frances' communications.

After a few months of treatment, Frances was released to her mother, contrary to what we thought advisable, and soon had to be returned to the Industrial School and to us for further treatment. This time she had become pregnant, and therefore was transferred to a foster family in Richmond. However, after a few days, and before treatment could actually begin, she ran away, accompanied by another girl unknown to us, who apparently had made a very satisfactory adjustment in the foster home. She was again placed in the State Industrial School and received one treatment session a week.

Frances would talk of her father with eyes focused dreamily upon infinity, either smiling happily or, when disgusted with him, pressing her lips together, her eyes betraying stern hostility. She reported how nice her father had been to her at all times and explained that once her father had left, the home had lost all its glory. She refused to stay home, became a truant, and kept late hours, because "she did not see why she should not enjoy the same freedom" as her father and her brother.

The distance at which the father dwelled necessarily eliminated all conflicts. The girl's inner explanations could thus be pursued unimpeded by reality-testing. What drove her into the street was an identification with the deserting father and his rejection of the mother. Frances' admiration for the father's independence included a search for the enchantment that had left the home and had remained with him.

Leaving the home appeared a liberation from all serfdom and execration of a miserable, barren, and over-populated abode which had become hateful by the father's disdain of it.

The girl's identification with him was so complete that she attempted to imitate his faithlessness in regard to his loved ones, using it as a weapon wrested from his hands and returned upon himself. The girl reported the story of a "boyfriend," "quite a bit older" than her. She "loved," him but was "unfaithful." She did not know his whereabouts, nor he hers, nor was she aware of the nature of his feelings toward her.

This boy, she later confessed, was the product of her imagination and a cover figure for the father whose whereabouts was equally unknown to her as her whereabouts was to him, as well as the nature of *his* feelings. This fantasy, though actually confused with the father of her child, permitted her to punish her father by "faithlessness" for leaving her and leaving her forever. By this means she no longer appeared to be a victim of his treatment. It placed her in a situation where she could inflict the torments which she resented. Moreover, in having a lover to whom she was linked by permanent feelings, she succeeded in satisfying her need for legitimacy. While her promiscuous activities were her resentful answer to her father's devaluation of her, she felt a need for redeeming herself in raising one of her sexual affairs to the status of a durable love.

The clinging to the father as an ideal figure, perilous as it had been to her own standards and to her own valuation of the home, served the purpose of redeeming this home from its fatherlessness and its rejected condition. As time went on, her attitude became spontaneously one of guilt and need for redeeming herself in relation to the mother, an ardent wish to help her in every way, and for the father to return to the home and its care and obligations.

However, this relationship was established at a distance from the mother and in as illusory a mood as had been her idea of the father since he had left. Upon her return to her home, as mentioned, she had found it to be so distracting that she felt unable to cope with it. Rather than help the mother, Frances felt in need of help herself, in a position of humiliating dependency and threatening failure. This suggested renewed identification with the father, whose needs the mother had not met. Thus the mother became responsible for the father's desertion, as well as Frances' failure. The vicious circle once again was closed.

When Frances returned home for the second time, she became involved again with her child's father, the relationship with whom was tied to the unsolved complexes she fostered in reference to the father. She asked the psychotherapist whether she should marry him, knowing him to be unsuited for her and not intending actually to become permanently involved with him. He was only a cover figure, but as an individual he meant nothing to her. He represented the father and legitimacy, as well as a tool for identifying with the father, a means for justification of faithlessness and retaliation. She actually married this man, lived with him only occasionally, but had five children by him in short order and then divorced him. Not to become the mother had become a vain dream.

These young girls may have one child after another but never get married. They are eternally in search of a solution but too ambivalent to find it. We may see their adolescent sons withdrawn and mute because of the unspeakable hurt of the mother's relationships to men. These come and go and leave her pregnant with another child. These women usually keep a home, some of them have an income. Their love affairs may contribute to an obsessive tendency to relieve their emotional misery or to alleviate the pressure of a marginal income. The boy may shrink from benefiting from such profits, recoiling further upon himself. If he cannot resist or cannot possibly avoid it, he despises himself for being really her son. If the men expose the mother's inadequacy, he will refuse to be different, unwilling to learn or to work, refusing to offer the mother gratification when she turns all of her attention elsewhere. She also is punished for her inadequacy by a retaliatory inadequacy.

We should like to leave the mother for a moment and show how the children's problems tie in with her condition.

### Reviling of the Mother as a Symbol

Verbal attacks on the mothers of other children, especially with regard to their sex morals are frequent among pre-adolescent boys. It is here that the carry-over from the natural milieu is particularly noticeable. The mother of the attacked child is often completely unknown to him. She may long since have deserted the child or may have been dead for many years. This type of assault expresses the hatred of the attacker towards his own mother, a hatred he dare not admit. He therefore displays it toward some other child's mother. It is an embittered revenge for the attacker's own indignity, but it provides him with a momentary elevation of status.

The child strikes with the very weapon which has wounded him. Out of his own inner experience he can localize the most sensitive spot of any child, the depreciation of the mother's dignity, as a person and as an ideal figure. The mother, whose wickedness he deplores, is an inescapable part of himself, and the fact that she is the source of his being implies a compelling fatal and material affiliation.

At least as frequent as these attacks are the imaginary accusations by a child that such an insult has taken place. Often retaliatory measures are being started for a verbal assault that has not actually occurred. This behavior has multiple motivations. Evidently, it is a means of venting pent-up hostility. It may be manipulated subtly in such a way that one who has said nothing, actually the victim, appears to be the aggressor, and the first child has gained an alibi for his own aggressive impulse. The victim may respond by defenses characteristic of his problem. He may cry, leave the room in a peeve, fight wildly, or bide his time and hit from behind at an unexpected moment.

The first child, or both, have made a strategic gain by creating a confusion, disturbing the purposes of the classroom situation, and symbolically a momentary breakdown of the orderly world at hand. The origin of the trouble is forgotten in that most welcome confusion. The inexperienced worker, convinced that he saw with his own eyes who started the fight, may further discourage a child's confidence in the perspicacity or fairness of the adult. The victim may therefore have lost his hold on the continuously shifting ground he has tenuously gained. But the aggressor, through the triumph of the moment, through the encouragement of his subtle aggression and the pleasures of deception, may also sense a loss because the adult could not match wits with him.

If the quarrel has remained localized, at this point it is almost certain to become general, motivated by identification with people or the roles they play at the moment, or by the possibilities of creating the greatest possible confusion for the greatest length of time. Should this happen during class hours, it provides a welcome opportunity to use the time for satisfaction of instinctive and emotional needs rather than for study.

The obvious reactions to home, the relationships and origin of the child can be aired in treatment and day-care. The disruptive behavior, on the other hand, may indicate a wish to discuss family relationships and alleviate anxieties. Often the children reveal an obsessive need for talking about matters of deep concern; in profound doubt of the meaning of all values, they may complain indirectly if they have somebody left to be proud of—the father, perhaps, or the grandmother.

One child confided "I am hungry, my mother is too tired to get up and feed me and there is nothing in the house to eat." The implication was that she conducted herself sexually in a way which precluded attention to the needs of the child in any way. Another child appeared almost entranced by the sight of a bit of food, but when asked whether he had had breakfast or lunch, he replied with an air of defiant pride, "I had chicken for breakfast." Obviously, while the former child may have been trying to evoke pity as his way of arousing sympathy and fondness as a basis for assistance, the second boy was certainly hungry, ashamed, and bitter.

Repeated outcries about "mother," though unmotivated from without, may be motivated in many ways from within. It may be a confession of unworthiness, an admission of self-depreciation, a tacitly expressed "look at me, I don't even have a decent mother."

Without any detectable cause, Felix one day cried out that the children, in referring to him, had called: "Little Black Sambo has lost his mother." Such an outcry may be an appeal for solace and assistance, a hand stretched out in hope of an escape, or the manifestation that he feels stigmatized and persecuted. The resulting sensitivity to anything short of total acceptance is extreme, since the child feels that in his indignity, exposed to his scoffers, he is stripped and naked. Vexed to the core, he breaks out in desperate, destructive rage, regardless of the consequences to himself. At a later stage, when rage is no longer diffused, children may aim at window panes as symbols of their confinement. At times their dreams reveal the meaning of their day-time manifestations.

Whether a child accepts or rejects the standards of living with which he is constantly confronted outside the family, he cannot fail to have been impressed by them. Faced with these new ideals, together with old unsatisfying parental identification, he finds himself in a desperate and insoluble dilemma. Living in two such contradictory worlds seems to establish insurmountable and ever renewed conflicts. It is not surprising, therefore, that these children have been considered untreatable. Their perplexity is truly great. It is difficult not to deny a world which has excluded them from all desirable goods, whether mental or emotional, social or economic.

Between destructive and self-destructive moods the child may want to refer back for comfort to the very ones responsible for his confusion, especially the mother. These conflicts are bewildering and paralyzing. The child is rather like an insect sensing danger—frightened, yet not knowing where to turn. His involvement with his inadequate mother becomes one of a thousand needs. Shame, guilt, and revolt torment him. The mother on whom he depends is not the ideal he can accept, that he has wanted and longed for. He is ashamed, because his need for a person whom he cannot respect is humiliating. He feels guilty because she has made him wretched and aware of his helplessness, and thus he revolts. But if he can glorify her, bestow upon her all the attributes he has dreamed of, then the conflict vanishes, his needs are gratified and he is at peace. One of our children will illustrate these points for us.

An eleven-year-old and the fourth of five illegitimate children, had been rejected by his promiscuous mother at birth and by the maternal grandmother, who subsequently raised him. His mother died when he was six. Benjy never returned home from school until late at night. Apparently, no one knew or cared about his whereabouts or his welfare. Although he had never had contacts with his mother, during interviews with his therapist he said that he missed his mother very much, but that her ghost watched over him all the time; that sometimes when he was out late at night, her ghost whipped him so that he would remember not to misbehave again. He created in fantasy the star that could guide him to decency.

When children in this way have built up an aesthetic or poetic image of their mother, just one shattering word from a companion can make the vision disappear.

Those inconspicuous acts of annihilation of the other child's imagery, erected in honor of the ideal mother, symbolize a form of assassination. It denies to the victim the very ground on which he treads. The attacker knows it because he himself has a depressing sense of this negation of his own existence.

## Hatred and Self-Hatred

Teddy, a sixteen-year-old high school student of low average ability, whose progress in school was satisfactory, was referred to the Educational Therapy Center by the school, for disobedience and inability to get along with his classmates. Simultaneously he was referred by the court for driving a stolen car.

He was the illegitimate son of a deteriorated alcoholic father and a promiscuous mother who had had eight illegitimate children. He was reared by kind people, neighbors of his father. Though his contacts were actually with them and not with his parents, who showed no spontaneous interest in him, his conflict was in reference to his parents.

Teddy revolted against, but identified with, the father as the doomed man, at one time feigning drunkenness, at another time coming to school after having consumed a small amount of alcoholic drink. He glorified his mother, depicting her with intense emotion in his earlier remarks as coming demurely from church with "his sister," when at that time there were actually six siblings, four of which were sisters. They found the father drunk in bed; he became violent and abusive.

Teddy pretended that then and there he suggested that his mother leave the father, which according to him she did. At the time of treatment, Teddy emphasized that he was his mother's legitimate son and actually returned to her home, where she lived with a man and his children. This attempt, which resulted in a dramatic lesson in realism, precipitated an intense crisis. He felt that his difficulties with the boys at the high school had been caused by their degrading his mother, whom he tried to idealize at that time with the result that they ridiculed him. Actually he had laid himself open to such hurts by his sensitivity and lack of realism. The cruelty of the other children was invited. They were his tools for sealing his self-rejection.

The nature of his problem with his fellow students was not recognized at school, and his social status being against him, Teddy could obtain a legitimate status nowhere. *To hate himself was his only road to conformity*, and it necessarily weakened his active tendencies for adjustment.

Adopting goals different from those prevailing at home implies, as a first step, denial of parental standards, which represents another form of self-annihilation, an inevitable death which, however, precedes new life. Liberation can be accomplished only by investment in a completely new reality. The old one usually seems forbidding.

Actually, one of the most impressive and most constant findings, with the majority of all of our children, is their confusion between hatred and self-hatred. This compound attitude is based on a reciprocal rejection by mother and child. The child at first is unwanted as a *corpus delicti* of one's own, though denied unworthiness, as well as the pawn of a man whose role was negative or indifferent. By identification with the mother's attitude, the child becomes self-rejecting, and due to her discouraging educational approach his hostility against her is aroused. He is made to be alert to all of the liabilities which his origin and way of life impose upon himself. Outside the home, at an early age, he will be everywhere in the position of Teddy. Children and grown people will cruelly kindle the embers of hatred against the mother and simultaneously against them who hurt her and him. But self-hatred equally will grow by identification with the mother's status and by the experience of himself as hateful and bad. They pretend they belong to the devil and to hell. "I want to be punished. I want to die. I'm mean." Thus, they exclude all hope and grant themselves all liberties. In this way they keep a vicious circle in perpetual motion until someone surprises them with unexpected reactions of kindness and understanding that finally, in a patient process, may halt the perpetual turning of Ixion's wheel.

When emotional vehemence is at its climax, any attempt at self-control by the child may place before him the alternative of annihilating versus self-annihilating tendencies. To be good and conforming means deserting the mother, and the elemental lure of life to be bad excludes him from all realistic and noble privileges that others have.

The conflict elaborated by these children on an amorphous and unyielding medium is the consequence of the eternal problem of man's duality and the duality of the mother and the woman. As the one who procreates and mothers, she has to be earthy, sensual, passionate, and strong. As an educator, she has to partake of the sublime and be able to point the way to those infinities man is able to conceive and is forever yearning to achieve. In view of that goal, the child at all times needs the pure and sublime mother; he cannot bear to be deprived of what is the attribute of man in his uniqueness. No mother, of course, can achieve such pinnacles of purity, for to do so she would have to dwell in infinity, unobserved as woman, wife, or lover. Yet, in reality, in her true being, she gradually imparts to the child through love and its vicissitudes, through the contingencies and exigencies of the objective world, the awareness that his vision is not to be fulfilled and enables him to accept joyfully the imperfections within his own nature and to integrate himself without guilt in the great cycle of life.

The tragedy of the children we describe is derived from the fact that the vital aspect of their nature is devoid of the powerful beauty and poetry which originates from the deep and intricate infiltration of the sublime into the woman's nature. To our children and their mothers there has been given the intense ambivalent longing for and fear of nature, as well as the divine. A young girl gave as her reason for not joining the church as shame in reference to her past experience, "with what I went through I cannot see myself walking down that alley." The longing for the sublime may be repressed and denied, as a defense against the painful awareness of hopeless inadequacy. However, it is ever present even where treatment remains unsuccessful.

The mothers of one illegitimate child as we see them, those who do not get married or make only a short-lived marital experience, are usually extremely lonely and embittered women. Their attitude toward their children is harsh and unbending. It takes many long months before we can arouse them to a point that they can broach a smile, a smile that may seem artificial enough. It may die again at the sight of the child.

We will presently offer an unedited and uncorrected autobiography, the spontaneous product of Aaron Enesco,* his mother's only illegitimate son. He was referred to the Educational Therapy Center at the age of fourteen by the public schools.

Aaron was at that time in the throes of a schizophrenic breakdown. A pervasive anxiety prevented interpersonal rapport. Not enough healthy affect was preserved to help him venture out toward or sustain an effort in view of establishing a social community. His thought processes were flighty, his perception of reality quaint and strange and narrowed down on an impoverished, self-centered world. His mind was "enfeebled" to quote a passage of the psychological test to borderline intellectual functioning. While his verbal IQ was still 91, his performance rating was 54. A previous school test had shown a full scale rating of 91, twenty points beyond the one achieved at intake.

The beginnings of treatment were exceedingly difficult because of the boy's paranoiac traits as well as a refusal of any dependency other than of a material type. He was begging constantly, evasive unless lying, with his head on his arms, on the therapist's desk, refusing to leave because he was too weak to walk home. He needed carfare.

The mother was extremely hostile, projective, and defensive of her own way of living which she refused to amend for the sake of the boy. It was impossible for a long time to obtain her co-operation. The boy, having a problem with both his mother and with father figures, was assigned to first a female, then a male therapist, with no apparent basic result. One day he requested to talk to the psychiatrist, his first thera-

* All names only are fictional.

pist, to tell her that he refused further treatment. This significant request, and the session that followed it, led to his and the mother's acceptance of a "family treatment." For about one year mother and son were seen together. Then the son was taken into an adolescent group, which he had feared previously. He is holding his own extremely well against prejudice, rivalry, and aggression.

The following autobiographical statement is a way of reaching out to all men for recognition of the seriousness of hurt that caused his breakdown and an appeal not to let his "disgrace" stand in the way of his "rehabilitation." A note of exhibitionism cannot be discounted and a beclouded demandingness of a most deprived child not only emotionally but materially. The lack of realism, the implied self-centeredness on his own importance, are in themselves not necessarily seriously pathognomonic for an adolescent in discomfort. In a positive sense it is his recognition that he needs help and a justified fear that his record will follow him everywhere and discredit as well as discourage his impressive efforts.

I, Aaron Enesco, was born May 5, 1944, in Richmond, Virginia. As far back as I can remember my mother was working in a tobacco factory. She had a woman, by the name of Mary Miller, to keep me while she was working after my grandmother died. At the age of three my mother sent me to live with my grandmother's stepmother because she kept insisting to keep me while mother worked. She lived in a small country town in Virginia. She was very kind to me and gave me everything a child could possibly want. I grew awfully fond of her, but by the time I was getting to really love her, my mother met a man by the name of Alexander Granger who promised her happiness and a home for her child and they were married about ten years ago. Alexander, was a farmer in a small country place in Virginia.

Just before my mother's marriage I became ill with trichinosis and after my dismissal from the hospital Alexander carried mother and me to his residence to live.

At the age of 6–½ my mother enrolled me in the elementary school. I stayed there five years. During my stay I became fond of the school and my teacher's, Mr. and Mrs. Thomas. After they left Mrs. Trusdale came to teach. I am not bragging but I was real smart in school and Mrs. Trusdale was awfully fond of me and my elementary academic ratings.

I was leading a terrible home life compared to what I had been leading. First, my stepfather was an alcoholic and sold corn whiskey during the week and week-ends and just before he went to work everyday, he would drink at least a ½ pint. Being a child I detested all alcoholic beverages and since this was done in my presence I grew to dislike his ways of bringing up a family.

Many a time he would fight mother, for no reason, when he had been drinking. This caused me to grow to despise him. This went on for five years constantly. Finally my mother and I left him and moved back to Richmond where mother had been living for 22 years.

We moved in with one of my mother's best friends in South Richmond, where I was enrolled in an elementary and junior high school. I maintained my good scholastic record during my 2–½ years' stay. During these two years my mother was working and by being separated from my stepfather and being a woman, she became the girlfriend of a man who was no more than a strange face in my life, but being young I did not understand sexual relationships and sharing mutual feelings. I disliked the man because he was a drunk. Just like my stepfather. Strange men kept entering into my life. I couldn't understand why mother could have so many men.

At the age of 12 my mother and I moved to another part of town, where I entered junior high school. When I grew accustomed to the pupils and teachers, everything was fine for about a year. Then I started getting into arguments with the students which led to fights. The students called me sissy because of my light voice and were jealous of my good report cards. I just couldn't understand why the fights always involved me.

At the age of 13 my mother and I moved to a rough part of town, which I despised. I continued to go to the same school and still confusion was still coming my way.

At the age of 14 my mother and I moved closer to school. My cousin and his friends were envious of me because I made good grades in school, so therefore they persuaded me to play "hooky" from school. My grades fell. The school truant officer came to my home to see my mother about my absentee's and naturally this worried mother.

During these years I had seen men in my mother's life for instance Alvin who was no more than a friend to me who mother had met after we moved from South Richmond. A man named McCully was trying to take my stepfather's place, but he was a drunk, just like the rest. I began to understand sexual feelings and this made me feel sick to know.

The school said I was becoming a problem and referred me to Dr. Hertha Riese who have helped me to rehabilitate myself. My life has caused me to become emotionally sick and this went on for three years.

My high school record, during the 9, 10, 11th grades has been terrible, but I am a senior now and I have started to make good grades again, but I am not completely well.

In other words I was neglected during my childhood and early teens and this caused my emotional setback. With Dr. Riese's guiding hand I think I will pull through.

What I can't understand is why mother did these horrible things to me because she is very intelligent academically. Sometimes she can answer more questions from the college bowl series than the student's because mother reads so much.

I want the world to know just what I have gone through and one day I hope to take my mother out of this kind of life. I love my mother dearly and since I am 17 and almost through school I can understand these things.

Personally, I think my mother never got over the death of her mother. I transferred from one high school to another to get a fresh start and now I am doing fine. When I apply for college and my job, I hope this is not held against me.

Written by

AARON ENESCO

Presently I am living in Richmond, Virginia. I would like to go into the theatre one of these days. I have good recommendations here in Richmond.

In the case of one of the striving middle-class families whose eleven-year-old girl was referred to us by the juvenile court as dependent and neglected, it was said that the illegitimate birth of this child had broken her grandfather's heart. The child's mother was her parents' only daughter and the apple of her father's eye. She had six brothers, all respectable men in respectable positions, who never forgave their sister, nor the child for having been born. She was regarded as the family's pillory. When her mother died, at the time of the young girl's referral to the Educational Therapy Center, none of her uncles were willing to offer her a home. The child and her mother had lived in the grandmother's home.

The rejection among all three of them was annihilating. Not even on her deathbed would the little girl give her mother a drink of water. The girl, who had suffered from frequent and violent temper tantrums and a tendency to muteness and withdrawal and who did not work according to capacity in school, recovered fully when placed in an accepting foster home and forgot to hate the mother and herself for having been born.

Rejection of the child, whatever its motivations, can be annihilating by intent or effect. When the mother turns her hostile expression of despair against her illegitimate daughter as her own perennially personified failure and stimulus for self-reproach, the young victim's condition is truly tragic and may be reflected frequently by schizophrenic reactions of one type or another.

These mothers never forgive themselves nor the child that it came into this world "to mess up my entire life." Mothers may foster all sorts of dreams about the glorious education they would have gotten and the resulting careers they would have had. The mother resents that, because of the child, she is made to pay through a lifetime wages for an experience meant to be the fun of but a moment. The child is the scapegoat for all the mother's failures and frustrations. The mother's bitterness does not necessarily preclude an extramarital sexual life into whose existence the child may gain an insight and at times may become involved as a real or feared competitor.

These women are blinded to their human and attractive feminine potentialities. These may be denied or reduced to the controllable minimum. Discrimination is not developed and the incentive to choose coming from the self-assurance that one has titles of one's own are lacking, titles that in a permanent relationship reassure a woman that her "eternal summer shall not fade." Those women, however, are aware only of their instinctive need; they have to show their want, that it may be fulfilled. Knowing nothing about their dormant and agonizing qualities, the sole awareness of their unredeemed instinctive urges gives rise to a depreciating self-image. It then determines the behavior by which the need is advertised and gratification is received—receive implying the man's behavior and the woman's inner experience. All the censure of self is passed on to the child, all self-hatred and all hatred of men, all of them who have not helped her and were not equipped to help her rise above her "degraded self." "Just like the rest" means to the mother that the father is emerging behind the mask of any man. The child does not understand the mother's painful motivations and the cynicism by which she tries to wipe away pain. He resents the temporary lack of modesty connected with advertising her needs. The daughter turns away from the other sex until she yields under the same terms with which she had been familiar throughout her life. The mother's anxious protection will bring about opposite results. In her latency period the girl may have co-operated with the mother in becoming a live corrective figure or the ideal of the mother's former self and with her obsession of restaging and reconverting the bygone opportunity. But the mother's anxious watchfulness will slowly become the child's motive for refusing a fulfilment of the assigned role.

The mother's coercive watchfulness teaches the daughter to doubt herself. It is sensed as the mother's distrust. Anxiously and resentfully she rationalizes that she will give her mother some of her own medicine. Such reactions may be the result of an anxious, self-righteous education even in those cases where the mother is in control of her instinctive behavior.

One of these cases of rejection was noteworthy because the little girl had an older brother who suffered from infantile paralysis. He was blind, deaf, idiotic, and his lower limbs were flaccid. His little sister was referred to us because she was regressing to the same condition and behaving like him. This was her way of reaching out for the mother's devotion which was invested exclusively in her son. She made him the director of the family stage. He was privileged not only as a boy but as an eternal infant with whom this intelligent but dependent single woman could identify. She was tied fathoms deep by guilt feelings to his crippled existence. We assisted her in liberating herself from the dependency on the boy, who was committed to the mental hospital, and in devoting herself to a most attractive daughter, promise and renewal of the existence of both. As a result the little girl made good progress in treatment. Until we could soften the mother who was petrified by hostility, we had to tend to her own needs for dependency and acceptance. She was forbidding in all of her reactions and her voice sounded like a rattle, a sound used by the child in group therapy to express rejection.

Despite the occasional incidence of the one-child family, the average number of children is six or seven.

The large number of children is due to a number of interlocking factors. We have discussed various aspects of dependency, of sex impulsivity—sex being from the days of infancy a main source of solace and comfort. At an early stage sex activity is considered a necessary expression and support of health. Improvidence may account for the failure to control the number of children, an inadvertance of the role of children in a rural community, from where many of these families come, versus their role in a municipality, and finally the reluctance to reduce the intensity of the sexual experience by introducing the conscious elements inherent to control. On the other hand many children may be wanted or rationalizations may be used to justify the great number of children born into misery and discord.

It is interesting to note that "a surprisingly large proportion of the total group . . . had no knowledge of birth control prior to the birth of the first child.[2]

Approximately four-fifths of the parents have been dependent on their parents for housing and care during the early years of their marriage or during the unmarried mother's pregnancy, or through indefinite or extended periods of time.

Roughly a third of our patients in the third or fourth decade of life are still living with their parents.

Ten per cent of our children are full orphans by desertion or death of both parents. They are living with grandparents, other relatives, friends, or foster parents.

In the case of a third of our parents, usually large families, both parents work. Only a few of our mothers can afford to or tend to stay at home.

## Inadequate Adjustments or Maladjustments

But contrary to the young women described, who may finally disappear or even die as victims of male violence or jealousy, these married women have enough strength to subjugate the world to their purposes or emergencies. They are not ignorant of social and moral requirements or standards. Some of them compromise their standards of morality to raise their economic standards. Such was the case of Nathaniel's and Daniel's mother as well as Aaron's, though the compromise could not meet the son's avowed or silent disappointment in the mother's morals and could not alleviate the children's deep sense of loneliness. Other deeply dependent mothers like Dayton's, whose case will be described extensively (in the Appendix), will inadvertently be caught in the nets of their helpless and stubborn attempt to improve an economic condition that compares unfavorably with that of their masters.

## The Antisocial Mother

A third group disregards standards and will do so increasingly. They manipulate institutions, ideals, and people whether a passive, slowly ground down husband, whether the children or the workers of organizations that they attempt to enrol into subservience to their needs.

Whether young or old, attractive or homely, they are delusive like jack-o-lanterns. A promise thus held out is almost never fulfilled but holds the victim in its vise. Since they do not have the usual resources and are profoundly deprived, they cannot help depending on these crafty defenses which they have mastered at an early age. Their defenses they consider highly satisfactory, even essential, and therefore they are resistive. These women's children and their husbands sense that by nurturing the flame it will go on burning. Its deluding scintillations are in demand, and the mother's defenses become the children's, who depend on them for her sake and for their own. Like her they will be resourceless and have learned to master life by craftiness only. These women may not escape feeling confounded. They can never be sure whether they can reach their own evasive feelings or thoughts or whether these will remain but words and tools for manipulation of others and of self-deceit. In the latter case the self-deceit and indulgence in contrition and apparent striving for a better status represents a longing for feeling human that is imbued with simultaneous incredulity. At such a time inadequacy is felt but dealt with by new illusions or self-delusions. The tragic character of such a harassed condition is beclouded by its apparent coldness and the total insensibility of the person to other than her own vital concerns.

The mother may waste away and drink away the husband's honest earnings. He will be disarmed and while he goes on striving he may have to ignore knowingly that the mother enrols his children in every deceit and stealing. As he is involved with her or suffers from an inertia with which he pursues the routine of working and living, he becomes passively involved with the family delinquency that keeps the mother's whiskey flowing and the family's food supply at a bare minimum.

The mother's harassed condition may be reflected more obviously in the children who are the ones who go around gathering, stimulated by exterior solicitations, without grasping the meaning of things or their quality as objects. Later they will be stealing for self-complementation and complementation of a mother who is demanding of complementation. Unable to reach it she will need many children. Each of them will be a product and tool of her obsession and will be deprived of the opportunity of self-fulfilment and simultaneously of the longed-for complementation necessary to substitute for it. Hapless gathering in the family group goes on and new and forever starving little vampires are being born and enrolled.

Only a deep-seated therapy could hopefully contribute to a fundamental change of personality. The initial attitude of the patient is not compatible with the treatment but with satisfaction inherent in the patient's present status which is adverse to change. Any emotional investment and any acceptance of commitment or compromise would be weakening the actuality as well as the sense of their power. These conciliatory attitudes would interfere with the delusions about solidity and validity of their existence and with the justification of being the ones they are and living the way they live. The delusion therefore is essential to their existence. Moreover, these patients cannot be regarded or reached as entities. They live in symbiotic colonies similar to the symbiotic relationships observed between the mother and her children. The mother was raised under similar or identical conditions and in each of these families and their collaterals the same pattern of complementary existence prevails and is fostered through generations. These families are as solidly cohesive as a coral reef. In its interstices settle other passive beings as for instance the husbands or those depending on concealment. In a way similar to the one observed between mother and child, the members of the family group cannot isolate themselves and find an individual existence nor, for the sake of survival, can the group afford to release a part of itself. Economic advantages may further contribute to the dependency. Economically successful members of the large family group may take the part of acceptable citizens. In the face of success society may not be too inquisitive about its origin.

In addition to the serious or even forbidding impediments that parents impose to change, the worker himself stands in the way of such an undertaking, the realism of which is always doubtful and which can only be attempted with the hope that utopia is not a land of dreams. To reach an objective attitude is not an easy task to achieve. The fear of not being able to match the patient's craftiness and therefore to be inadequate as a helper may deprive the worker of the conviction necessary for the initiation and pursuit of assistance. The contradiction which exists between the patient's dependency and the frailty of her emotional condition on the one side and the lack of juvenile guilelessness on the other, make great demands on a worker who, while concerned with one of the two faces, is being exposed to attacks from the other. The helper, moreover, has constantly to ride on the fluctuating grounds of wavering factual evidence. As long as he longs for solid ground under his feet, he will be exposed to further and even more eager use of deceit because the patient is reminded of the power of deceit.

The therapist's approaching all information, unprejudiced by its factual or imaginative evidence, by mere study of its dynamics, might help the patient learn about the futility of his or her own approach, and while his problems at hand are studied objectively, he or she sees that one can be caught at one's own game. These patients may even lose, not simply with the usual lack of embarrassment, but with some sportsmanship depending on intelligence, the need to lean on stronger support, the enjoyment of the gamble more so than the asset or the fantasy and play that the patient has been misled by education to invest in antisocial behavior. In this pseudo-artistic departure from realism we might have to look for the roots of the fascination that these jack-o'-lantern personalities produce. The helper is far from being protected from succumbing to such a lure. It appears in terms of deception in reference to therapeutical achievement or assurance for collaboration if the child be returned home, a return which if achieved would toll in the child's doom.

Those patients bowed under the yoke of need may respond to warmth and may not be insensitive to their growing feeling of adequacy. Those others who have unused potentials for sublimation may enjoy the challenge inherent in the therapeutic tournament, but doubt is indicated that they will outgrow that stage and seriously go to war with themselves.

The approach then presumes a high degree of invulnerability because of insight, a capacity for gratifying the patient's dependency needs in symbolic terms. Concrete needs must be answered immediately by very good and effective guidance to the proper sources and to successful and acceptable self-help. Hopefully the joy inherent in achievement may supersede the pleasures of gambling and impish destruction.

The mother's chances to change are greatest if she is made to reach out for her children who are placed at a certain distance. The children's helper must remain alerted to the fact that these mothers' crafty strategy and tactics will continue unabated and tend to undermine the child's road to freedom. But the tenor of what she longs for may change and meanwhile her child may gain strength for liberation.

The story of Mrs. Sherwood and her son Spencer illustrates the case of such a mother who stands in the way of her son's emotional, social, and moral adjustment because of imperative needs of her own. The story may highlight some of the real difficulties encountered until a child progresses, protected from the mother's haunted and haunting pursuit. Mrs. Sherwood was capable of gaining an insight into her actions and could even express it, but for years she could not resist her destructive impulses, and she used her confessions ambivalently. By surrendering her arms, by exposing her defenses and her strategy, she gave herself a chance to rise above destructiveness. But simultaneously she was seductive and used the exhibition of her illicit actions and her way of life as much to weaken the helper as to strengthen herself. Her surrender therefore was used simultaneously as a means for deceit and self-deceit and a combination of guerrilla warfare with those arms that were still concealed and which she had no intention of relinquishing at that moment.

Spencer was an attractive seven-year-old when first referred to the Educational Therapy Center by the Catholic school. His uncontrollable, attention-getting behavior upset the work of the whole room. He had been unresponsive to any attempt made by the school to help him.

At the time of the referral, the family of seven, the parents, two girls and three boys, were in a chaotic situation and a vain attempt was made to give treatment to both parents. The father was not providing and was gambling in the company of men who fostered hostile feelings toward the other sex. He accused his wife of homosexuality. Actually she liked to visit with professional and semi-professional women for gain of prestige. There was no evidence that she was actively homosexual, but she admitted marital infidelity with a number of men and, when we met her for the second time, she was living in a common-law marriage, where the same polygamous behavior was repeated. One of her lovers at this time was her former husband whom she still visited at intervals at a distance of several hundred miles. Her common-law husband displayed personality traits of irresponsibility similar to those of her first husband; the other gambled, this one was drinking. His problem of alcoholism, however, came to our attention only after she had bolstered his hopes for marriage, permitting him to grow fond of some of the children, as well as to buy new furniture, appliances and costly toys. Before the marriage could be concluded Mrs. Sherwood discovered her "conflict between the man and the church" and, for her own edification, made the "good" choice at the expense of the emasculated man. At this time he was saddled with his gifts which, without losing face as a loving devotee, he could not withdraw. By drinking, however, he could withdraw himself and even retaliate for her deceit. It is worth noting that homosexual activities had been going on for some time between Spencer and his younger brother, activities which we have reason to attribute to Mrs. Sherwood's debilitating influence on the opposite sex. Her husband seemed to have in mind this hostility of hers when he spoke of Mrs. Sherwood as homosexual.

Mrs. Sherwood was attractive, intelligent, a highly verbal woman with a powerful imaginative personality and a two-year college education. Her predominant trait was the need to rule and her predominant tool consisted in deriding in order to rule. She tended to build hopes up to a climax, then break her promise at the time of expected fulfilment. Breach of promise was always rationalized by her. In view of her need to rule she resented owing something to others and humiliated the donor. The church was equally a victim of this attitude of hers. At a time of misery, when the husband had left the large family, a priest worked hard and successfully in order to obtain in the nick of time scholarships for all of the children. Mrs. Sherwood, who had accepted the priest's dedicated endeavors, left them unaccepted and suddenly placed all the children in the public school. She excused her decision by asserting that the scholarships had been awarded too late. This motivation hardly seemed convincing. The children, who were used to the Catholic school, where they returned later, should not have been exposed to such unnecessary changes. Mrs. Sherwood was in a constant state of indecision between verbalized ideals and contrary acts. She seemed involved with her own self to the point of actually believing what she said and of finding good and valid reasons for what see did.

Mrs. Sherwood was a clever and not particularly scrupulous business woman. She had relationships of a personal nature with a variety of officials whom she tended to use for her purposes. She insisted on being on good terms with the juvenile police as a means to dominate her son. On the surface, these men were recruited as father figures. Actually, however, she was just adding to her collection of weak men, thus depriving the boy of any moral, social, or legal authority to respect.

At the time of the first referral Spencer had made an unexpectedly fine adjustment in the Educational Therapy Center. He enjoyed the reliable and disinterested fondness he received and responded to it with genuine devotion, which was reflected also in his good work in class. At first we were aware of parental resistance only in reference to their own treatment. However, when the boy ceased to be an obvious problem and apparently lost his exclusive dependency on the mother, and when he chose us for love and guidance, he was withdrawn from the Clinic.[3] This happened quite suddenly. The mother placed him with an aunt about forty city blocks away from the Clinic under the pretense that he could not adjust in his own family. The family insisted that Spencer go to the public school but he sped to us secretly. In view of the family's attitude, which would preclude treatment unless we could hope that the protective services and the court would recognize a legal motive for committing the child, the public school seemed the logical agency to work with the child. As could be expected with women like Mrs. Sherwood and her sister, the school overlooked the complexity of the case, and we abandoned our endeavors on Spencer's behalf.

Four years later Spencer was returned to us by the mother. The parents' marriage had broken up. They were legally separated. The father lived in a large northern city. The mother at first concealed her relationship with another man because it involved her dependency on city welfare. The boy was happy to be returned to us, but at that time he was beset with old and with new problems. He had become untruthful and took or destroyed everything in sight; nothing in the Clinic was safe. He had become wary in his communication and extremely restless; he could not control his impulse to run home when he knew his mother was there. He could not benefit from his treatment schedule at a time when he knew his younger siblings had returned home from school and were with his mother. He was extremely disturbed and constantly fought the younger sibling figures in day-care. Concentration on his studies was impossible. He was fascinated by the mother who kept him bridled, in a state of bewilderment and insecurity. It took time to help him overcome his uncontrollable impulse to run home and to comply with one of the few strict rules which, as a prerequisite for treatment, requires that the children be made available for it. Had we not been in a position to master this situation, we would have been cast in the same inefficient role assigned by Spencer to all other potential ideal figures and the Clinic too would have become effaced behind the force of the mother's will.

Spencer still longed for a warming and glowing hearth to return to. He would run to his therapist promising spontaneously that today he was coming for his session. But at the time of his interviews he was gone already, driven by the anxiety that his younger siblings could spend a short while with his mother in his absence. His relationship with his therapist was disturbed by his fear of a conflict of allegiance and an emotional attachment that once before had not been sanctioned by the mother. The boy knew by now that the mother spoke of cooperation while at the same time defying it. He felt that involvement with us might entail the danger of complete severance from the mother, who might again become a need. He had learned that in a number of ways, as he reported when an occasional impulse prompted him to unburden himself. Spencer's way of revealing facts showed that he understood their implications. Actually he had co-operated with his mother on innumerable instances. He had learned that the mother glorified her second marriage joyfully before the whole family until even Spencer looked forward to its realization, a realization that originally he had good reasons to loathe. The future stepfather had become involved in the discrimination against Spencer and was the mother's tool for striking her son as an object of her hostility. But the man's involvement with her was punished by demotion. The real father's return was always pending. Spencer knew that his mother's decisions were unpredictable and that everybody else was powerless in the matter. Therefore he remained undecided and fatalistic, not knowing whether or not to wish for his own father's return. He could feel like an actor, not just a helpless onlooker, only by identification with the mother. This attitude, which had multiple determinants, also had a sexual connotation. As we know, Spencer and his younger brother, the one next to him in age, were indulging in mutual homosexual activities. The second boy was brought to the Clinic for treatment but not enrolled in day-care.

The failure of his foster home placement which was arranged shortly before the marriage was obviously brought about by Spencer. He ran to the mother constantly, finally entering through the window at night which, according to the mother, just "happened to be open." Thus mother and son demonstrated the nature of their mutual relationship. The mother revealed later on how, in being constantly alluring, she had contributed to the failure. This confession was made at a time when she asked to be trusted with being more co-operative in a new attempt to place Spencer in a foster home, this time at her own request. Actually the Clinic was aware that Spencer was again acutely in the mother's way. He had repeatedly interfered with the mother's intentions by divulging her secrets. She, on the other hand, assumed, in order to support the boy and to cause him to connive with her, that the objects he took home with him from the Clinic had been given to him. It was extremely hard to enrol her co-operation for a return of these objects. She condoned certain of his acts so convincingly that you were no longer sure of what you had seen with your own eyes. She would be very hurt at the "undeserved" suspicions. She would motivate her child's distrust by pointing out the lack of trust we had in him, appear to be very generous in forgiving and allegedly help him in exercising forbearance. Spencer did not steal elsewhere but in the Clinic, which quite apparently became an object of his ambivalence, transferred from the mother to the Clinic. This is what caused him to vent his aggression against his own siblings on sibling figures under treatment. He acted under his own impulse to please for the sake of being gratified by the mother's condoning his acts and offer the tokens of his partiality to her rather than to his helpers. Such forms of manipulation are very typical for these deep-seated disturbances and were characteristic of Mrs. Sherwood's whole family group as it could be traced two generations back.

In spite of these difficulties the child developed sufficient need of the Clinic and sufficient loyalty to it to motivate his regular attendance. He revealed his problems by profuse speech and his acting out. For the sake of not losing the symbolic mother, he learned to control his impulses to such an extent that the Clinic's tolerance limit was not exceeded. Warmth of feelings slowly superseded the perfidious friendliness and uncommittal attitude at the time of his return to the Clinic. His potential for love and positive strivings were quickened to such an extent that a foster home placement in a rural area at a sufficient distance could be carried out successfully. Welfare and school now equipped with the necessary insight to protect the child from renewed temptation so far have prevented the mother from interfering. Her interest at this time has been invested in her business sufficiently to give up the son who has become a menace to it. Time then will favor a severing of the dependent ties, the enjoyment of growth, and the freedom from the mother's manipulations. Simultaneously the mother is being weaned from a relationship, the concrete experience of which is interfered with by distance. Because of omnivorous and possessive tendencies, release of the child is not readily acceptable, but for the same reasons any dependent object can fulfil dependency needs. Because of the concrete nature of such dependencies they cannot thrive at a distance and relationships close at hand must be resorted to. The child's new dependent relationship on suitable parental figures then may come into the open.

We usually make an attempt to have the child enrolled for treatment elsewhere. The children at that time having co-operated with the placement are adequate objects for therapy but frequently therapy was denied to them. The child's progress then depended on the quality of the placement, the social worker, the understanding of the school teacher or at times the child's maturity to continue therapy coming from great distances by himself and to master the temptations inherent in his previous condition.

In contrast to these mutually dependent relationships ruled predominantly by the mother, we may see the mutually committal ones. These leave the child open to the world and the transference of mutually committing relationships. Such a child may be anxiously compulsive, he may have almost a magic fear to fail his benefactors, but he is at liberty to acknowledge that he is receiving help and feels the need to reciprocate. Contrary to the dependent child who has only the one-way road back to the deceptive protection of the mother, the mutually committed child feels he has a choice. The chances are that he was raised in a two-parent family. If he is in conflict about his new reciprocal commitment, it is because he feels he is indebted to give more but not that his own wholeness is endangered by loss of the mother who exploits this dependency.

Therefore, if, for reasons of parental inadequacy to help the child master his problem, a child needs to be placed elsewhere, we can count on both the child and the mother. In raising him, she has endowed him with sufficient independence and ego strength to choose his relationships and use them for the mutual benefit of the individuals involved. She has enough of the same qualities to share them without feeling endangered and in need of interference. She is capable of seeing or learning about benefits to each individual and in genuine terms the child's education and welfare.

We have seen, in rare cases, increasing improvement in these dependent mothers, but when the children, contrary to our advice, were returned to the mother, she was no longer capable of maintaining the effort of coming herself for treatment or sending the child. She knew to keep the appearance unaltered and thus protect herself from further interference. At times such an attitude may reflect a sound tendency to reach independence. But often the children's tragedy is great because they actually had changed and the ax was struck again against their roots.

One half of all children in the Clinic are in foster homes. Few have been abused by severe beatings, burning their fingers for stealing, etc. Foster care children come from one-parent and two-parent families in about even distribution. Most parents are interested in their children but cannot sustain their interest, or they are not aware that their concern is self-centered. Care is by provision of concrete things; discipline by yelling, strapping, depriving the already deprived child. They frequently resort to ignoring the children when they are incapable of disciplining, too busy, or too indolent.

## Education

The majority of these families come from rural areas in Virginia or North Carolina and 70 per cent of our parents have attended these rural schools, at best to the sixth or seventh grade. Twenty per cent have some high school education and an additional 10 per cent have attended college or business school.

With few exceptions the *mentally able parents* are intensely preoccupied with status-seeking and for long periods in their lives fathers and mothers will attempt to improve their education and acquire professional degrees. While studying either during the day or at night, they may work for the balance of the day. Their strivings are not matched by opportunities to use their education in a satisfactory way. Parents with master's degrees in highly specialized fields are working as mail carriers, porters, or at other menial jobs. That both parents work, the father at two full-time employments is not an exception, nor is one full-time and one part-time job. Some parent may have a business of his or her own, in or out of the home. They might give each other mutual assistance on the job and in the home or compete in an unfriendly way.

The fascination may be concentrated so exclusively on either social or economic standard or education, that is, on the areas of most painful denial by the surrounding culture, that love life is reduced to instinct gratification and parental devotion to decent care of the children's material needs. A stern unsmiling attitude is excused by fatigue which the child, unless frozen out of mental and emotional life, registers as rejection and answers by serious forms of "monkeying" verging on or having grown into prepsychotic or psychotic mannerisms.

In view of the longing for social status many parents overspend their credit, buying attractive houses whose exterior, including the front yard, are tended in preference to the interior. The adolescent children will complain and censure the economic pressure, the parents' anxiety and the neglect inside the house. For their own standard within the adolescent group they tend to the interior themselves. This behavior is in contrast to the depressed youngster of the inadequate families who struggle listlessly from day to day outside of society and the world on the whole. The striving families try further to be well represented by expensive cars and clothes, a factor that reflects their identification with the general culture which they are ambitious enough to embrace against a most frigid resistance.

Three-fourths of the respondents in a survey of our families,[4] had personal property valued at less than $250.00. One-fourth had no real property. Savings accounts were extremely limited. The majority of the respondents in this study had incomes between $100.00 and $300.00 per month.

## Health

The tension underlying such a struggle that starts in early childhood is reflected in frequent vascular disturbances, the much discussed high blood pressure of the Negro which need not be explained by constitutional vascular weakness. *If we remember the constant need to repress, disregard, forget, and forgive the rejection and limitation to free movement and access to self-realization, we see a picture which deserves a great deal more scrutiny to be properly appraised.*[5]

In all socioeconomic and educational levels we may find obesity in both fathers or mothers, in a number of cases of an extreme severity, predominantly among single parents. On the other hand extreme height and emaciation are not infrequent. Alcoholism or excessive use of alcohol by both sexes on all socioeconomic levels must be regarded as an escape of tension as well as a negative aspect of culture identification. As easily conceivable, hypochondriacal complaints are frequent.

## Age

The majority of the parents are between thirty and forty-five; 15 per cent are under thirty. These rough figures do not include the teen-age mothers who are referred for their own and not their small children's problems and are therefore not registered as parents. Their parents, however, figure under the majority group just quoted.

## Religion

With few exceptions the families are protestants, merely by denomination. The 15 per cent who practice their faith belong to religious sects and are overzealous. Their church most frequently gratifies dependency needs and supports arduous strivings against unruly instincts. A relatively great number of the fathers and even the mothers preach or have important church or missionary functions. They claim their vocation was suddenly revealed to them. The religious function is fulfilled on Sundays and humble jobs may be the economic resource of the family. One family of five children was deeply impressed by the father's vocation as a minister, which overshadowed all of their economic misery. In one instance the father who thus worked and preached also went to college to become an ordained preacher.

Religion covered in one of our observations a father's compulsion to coin money out of any possible resource. He used his son as a miracle preacher from the age of three to the age of fourteen. At that time the young boy was referred to us for forging checks. The boy was very verbose and flighty. In a slightly incoherent manner and very much in need of communication, he dictated his life history for a whole hour and could have gone on, if not interrupted. He said until his adolescent years, he had been naïve, he had believed in his vocation and had always something to say, but the older he was, the more he began to doubt himself. He was increasingly anxious and prayed for ideas, not to be exposed, and not to be made ridiculous before the congregation. The father was angry, nagging, and denigrating and made him feel desperate. He began to have less appeal on the pulpit and earned less money. He began to accumulate debts because he had to pay his father the cost of transportation to churches as far as thirty miles distant as well as other expenses. At that time he "still owed his father twenty dollars." "Nobody knows how this worries me." He explained that he had no other resources, and the father made it close to impossible for him to earn it at his father's store. The boy became the father's scapegoat and was held responsible for every error in the father's store which may well have been made by his brother next to him in age. The father was extremely jealous when the mother tried to come to this boy's rescue and interfered anxiously with any contact.

We have young adolescents with obvious sexual problems stemming from such a religious milieu. More frequently the child's neglect or rejection is due to the righteousness by which the parents dissociate themselves from their instinctual selves.

The mother of Ada, who is discussed elsewhere, rejected her child in pregnancy considering it the fruit of an indiscretion since it was conceived twelve years after her son, both from her husband. She was particularly eager to conceal it from the members of her church.

Therefore she refused to nurse her, let her mother tend to the child whom she helped with the ancillary tasks.

At times the pastoral function is used to cover up a double life. The pastor and a girl's mother may be associated as zealous matchmakers. The young girls thus abused are referred to us usually by the juvenile court. The mother usually files the petition when the girl acts up beyond or outside the realm assigned to the girl, a behavior which might endanger her economically, undermine her reputation, or deprive her of her lover, who becomes attracted to the daughter. In one of these cases the young daughter thus abused was also exposed to the use of drugs, the only case in our whole experience.

The following letter was written by Zenobia, the daughter of a woman who resisted all our efforts to help her not to reject the charming nine-year-old girl. Zenobia reacted by a serious behavior and conduct disturbance. Dreams and delusions about her family brought her very close to a break with reality. The young girl was also in the habit of writing longing letters to imagined people which she never mailed but accumulated in her chest of drawers. After the father's death the mother had replaced family love by a righteous ardour in one of these religious sects. The child had to be placed in a foster home. This letter was written in the last months of the girl's treatment when she was close to fifteen years of age.

DEAR MOTHER,

I don't know how to say this but I'll do my best. Being without your love is only putting me down it's not helping one bit. But maybe that's what you want. Why can't we act like mother and daughter. Must religion come between two people as it did us? I don't think God made any religion that says mother and daughter must be as far apart as we are. Sure I go to a Baptist church, but mother am I that sinful that you can't be in my presence? Mother I've changed a lot I have a mind of my own. I'm old enough and mature enough to know right from wrong.

Mother use common sense do you think if God was to come down to earth in the form of man do you truthfully think that he would praise you for not being in the company of your daughter. Please mother be reasonable, look at this establishment from all angles. Even if it proves you wrong be truthful about it. I'm not going to ask you to answer back because I know you wouldn't. All I'm asking of you is to be the same mother you was when daddy was living.

Your loving daughter,
ZENOBIA

But we may observe forms of deep religious experiences of the Dostoevskian type. The mentally limited mother of three children, two of whom were our patients, was the wife of a mentally retarded alcoholic who deprived her and the children not only of all of his incidental income but also of hers. She had the reputation of walking the streets in a section of town where she was unknown. She claimed that this was her only resource for providing for her children, being without any ability or education. She also claimed her behavior to be an immolation: she deserved to drink her fill of bitterness for disobeying her late father and marrying her husband. She was never going to divorce him, since this was her promise to her father, who placed before her the alternative of renouncing the man before marriage or never. Since her father was dead and unable to relieve her of the commitment, she could not make a one-sided departure from it. Neither the masochistic nor the compulsive element in this attempt to solve her difficult problem can be overlooked, nor can a possible rationalization of instinctive behavior. But this was not the impression this woman gave and her daughter was a dutiful and reliable little housewife in spite of an imitation of some of the less demure elements of the mother's behavior.

## Parental Ambivalence in Reference to Standards

A profound bewilderment in reference to standards necessarily invades those of the children's parents who do not have the superior equipment in energy and endurance to cope with the duality of a world which they are taught and are supposed to respect while they are comforted with an incomplete example, with the condemnation "to live outside the temple" and deprived of the initiation and the objects necessary for the "cult." If, longing to belong inside, a mother identifies with accepted standards in spite of great odds in the family, she will represent a supportive structure to her child. However, if she remains ignorant of the child's unanswered needs, and of the profound meaning of the lack of fundamental satisfactions, she will not be able to offer security and peace. Her standards, unsubstantiated by the realities of a true home, are similar to a foreign language. They are audible, but meaningless to the child; they cannot actually be retained or integrated, nor take root and bear fruit. The unconscious awareness of his inadequacy will embarrass and confuse the child who needs a unified, comprehensible world. The mother's conscious awareness that, try as she may, she cannot convince her child and make him belong to a world with which she identifies, may lead to desperate frustration. A state of hostility will come into existence between her and her child and result in a vicious cycle of mutual rejection.

If her trouble is derived from the choice of an inadequate mate, she will be on the defensive against that reborn partner that she brought upon herself. The child will stand up permanently as a reproach to her error of choice and its effects. The child will sense that he is not taken for what he is to himself but as a representation of an unknown evil. He, in turn, will take her as the representative of a hostile world, a menace wrought of femininity and of dependence upon it; also he will, with anguish in his heart, feel that after all he is also the father's child and cannot escape being it, try as he may. The obscure causation of his behavior, of which he himself disapproves, leads him to the mystic idea that his father is in his blood and cannot be expelled; he feels that he is under a curse.

Longing vainly for a unified harmonious world, the child may regress in his behavior by an uncanny instinctive knowledge that his formation has been misshapen at an earlier stage of his development. His attitude is clear to those who can understand the call of helplessness. He may undertake an aimless search, staying away late at night, fearing the requirements of that foreign world within the home, which makes the home a strange place and not a familiar abode. If his behavior, which is adequate in view of the child's condition, is viewed as inadequate by the child's teacher, the parent does not have to reject him explicitly to cause a sense of worthlessness, isolation, utter loneliness, and distrust.

The situation is worsened if identification with accepted standards is overt only and the mother preaches "water when she drinks wine."

One of these mothers, Mrs. Peterson, a former model domestic, identified with the refined forms of living in which she had served with mutual satisfaction. However, she suffered intense resentment for being denied or excluded from a social group in which she was allowed only to serve. Her role was felt as that of an outsider to the play. That someone should perform an essential part on the stage, and still be only a bystander, represented a cleavage to her for which she found no corollary in a discrepancy of merit. Her resentment brought emphasis on community of demerit and identification with those elements of conflict in her masters, which found expression in excessive drinking. Though dependent upon the social service bureau since her husband had deserted her and their five children, she would give drinking parties in her neat home. Apparently those drinking parties served the additional purpose of illicit sources of income. Frustrated again in her ambitions, she extended her hostility to the investigating social worker, who served as a symbol of the world she deceived. The worker, she said, begrudged her everything, even to the wax on her shiny linoleum. Her ten-year-old son, Dayton was supposed to achieve for her the coveted higher standards, but he was totally confused between the two contradictory attitudes pursued by his mother and the secrecy which accompanied her hostile behavior. Accordingly, he himself would unfold two different expressions of fearful identification with attitudes connected with those drinking parties which so eminently occupied his mind. Dayton would alternate between violent gesticulations, declamations of horror stories and fearful visions of animals and varied vermin. He would shift suddenly without transition to whispering, at times shielding his mouth with his hands. What he whispered was inaudible; actually he said nothing. Whispering was a gesture, the imitation of an observed phenomenon, the meaning of which was only partly understood; however, the child used it as an expression of his conflicting tendencies to communicate what caused anxiety to him and to suppress what should be revealed. An element of hostility in his whispering was evident in the deception which held the observer for a few seconds in a state of hesitation, wondering whether she had understood or not or whether there was anything verbal to understand.

Mrs. Peterson's child, Dayton, was in a pre-psychotic condition when he was first seen in the Center. Because of theft he had been referred by the juvenile court, who had not made an intake interview of the obviously and grossly disturbed child. The mother had taken the child to court as an alibi for her righteousness, with the intent of forestalling an investigation of her own illegal activities. Thus, when the child greatly improved, she withdrew him prematurely from treatment, because as a recovering and communicating, as well as a recovered child, he was again a menace to her, a witness, from another world, who would no longer be able to endure certain aspects of his mother's immoral life.

## The Conflict between Parents and Children Regarding Home, School, and Church

If, on the other hand, the home tolerates and even condones asocial behavior, or if the inhabitants live so chaotically that the child's asocial ways are not noticed, the child misses the supportive structure which should help him at least to live in one world of well-defined requirements, similar or identical inside and outside the home, such as prevail in school or church and including his parents in the world of accepted standards. This would boost his self-confidence as of one who somehow belongs in the world of acceptable people.

Through the absence of such standards in the home he may never be exposed to an acute inner conflict capable of making him aware of his shortcomings and giving him the strength to face them in combat. Sad and listless, such a child will conform to the ineffectual behavior of his parents without confidence in himself, his family, or his society and its opportunities. When, however, the child fosters strong identifications with the standards taught at school or in church, a struggle for harmonizing the home with school or church may ensue. The unanticipated immensity of the task may provoke frustration, irritation, and an increasing revolt which may represent a moment of crisis, making possible exhausted surrender to, or general revolt against, a forbidding world that resists conquest.

All of these problems are reflected also in the child's and the parents' attitude toward church, which is a very vital factor in our sphere of observation. The number of children who do not attend church is minimal, the attendance of the mothers is nearly as good, but there are many fathers who do not go to church.

Church attendance may have a concrete, tangible motivation. Evil instincts are more readily resisted when censure has to be feared and faced in a group of equals, many of whom are struggling in the same bog. Still the head is kept raised for fear the neighbor might guess the misery. This seems a deep-rooted tendency; avowal of distress does not come easily from the lips of either children or parents among our patients, though the parents usually are more explicit.

To show them compassion could be taken as exposing their wounds. Church is for them a place where they succeed in forgetting inadequacy. Comparison with their equals lessens the distance to the abstract goal and alleviates the fatigue that befalls them in anticipation of the road ahead.

Faith and a longing for redemption seem a predominant motivation, particularly since in the majority of cases it is the only abstract and noble endeavor available to our group. Church is above all a place where one can belong and be accepted, regardless of the lowliness of his condition. And we have seen impressive reactions and a deep symbolic insight into profound problems by children to whom the usual world of learning was closed. Church to them has an advantage which no other source of knowledge possesses. It is not solely a conquest of life and a positive approach to things, but one which tends toward and beyond life and thus attenuates life's cruelties and gives them courage to endure it.

It is because of this need for a better world that children may choose other churches than the ones their parents choose, often at a great distance from home, though this may not be the only motivation. Churches with ecstatic services to which the elders might cling with passionate ardor do not always find favor with the children. They are, after all, too deeply identified with the surrounding culture, whatever their good reasons in finding fault with it. The grandmother's church may be preferred or that of a friend or teacher; the popularity of a church or its clergyman may prove attractive; churches with a charitable and a social program may be sponsored by a mother who wants the children to have all the good things which are denied to her. The lure of a charitable church program might be great even in hostile families who reject church as an element of society to which they do not belong, or as a symbol of a God who has tried them beyond endurance and rejected them.

### Parental Attitudes toward Treatment: General Consideration

Parents who have sufficient affinity for life and for the new life incorporated in their children, enough faith in our institutions and a lively sense of responsibility are also the children's opportunity for developing similar attitudes; thus the children will reach out for help. Nevertheless, parents who jeopardize their children's treatment should not be burdened with the full responsibility for such failure.

Actually, the parents we have in mind often are not in a position to take their children to treatment centers. They may not be able to comply with the schedule because of their own economic limitations. Their working hours may be excessively long, the security of employment precarious. Other parents, no less disturbed than their children, may not be relied upon. The whereabouts of still others may be unknown, or the child is removed from his home.

Therapeutic interviews of the parents have to proceed under their accumulated stress, physical exhaustion, or excessive preoccupations due to socioeconomic pressure and its consequences.

Parents are not always ready to recognize their share in the causation of the child's difficulties and their own part in the possibility of surmounting them.

To trace difficulties back to their involved origins and to face responsibilities which so far have been denied may be an overwhelming task when the sheer struggle for survival absorbs or saps all the parents' energies and all their mental potentialities.

Children of the middle classes also may be untreatable and permanently or temporarily resist changing. This is true in particular when parents engage their children in a pathological interaction. A serious dilemma results: should the parents' liberty to jeopardize their children's mental health be maintained, or should this liberty be curtailed in such individual cases where neurotic or psychotic motivation turns it into license? The private physician will be in the same dilemma as once the practitioner who treated patients affected by communicable venereal disease. Only the obligation to report these cases where parents, due to their own pathology, interfere with their children's mental soundness would place the human society in the position to prevent serious emotional or mental disturbances or disease in children and the future generations. We do not advocate an arrogant and omniscient intrusion into family affairs but interference with the pathological indoctrination of one generation by the other. Contrary to the parents seen in our Clinic, the parent in the average child guidance clinic, belonging to the middle classes, is usually culture-identified. Family maladaptation is in coping with the trend of the time and the surrounding culture. The specific symptoms of their maladjustment represent an often deplored but accepted expression of defense against the evils of our civilization, or of an aggression which at least recognizes the existence of this culture. The parents' disturbances, therefore, can more readily be treated on an individual level, under at least partial disregard of the cultural setting in which the treatment is cast. A psychiatric approach to their problems, as well as institutions suitable to assist them when the pathology of their defenses militates against them, belong to their own pattern of life, whereas the parents of the children who specifically concern us are all too frequently made to feel that they are—and are to remain—hapless and hopeless outsiders whether they like it or not. Thus whether or not they admire our culture, are ambivalent or hostile and negate the world itself, they are bound to be suspicious of its institutions, and stand aloof or resist.

Actually what appears to be negation is rather a stymying ambivalence resulting from rejection by the prevailing culture, a rejection absorbed as self-rejection by its victim. The compulsive maid who is trying to be deserving wipes from her masters' household her own deeply sensed and deeply repudiated "blackness." Returning home, she finds her own house "unwiped." Having adopted the "pale-faced" children of her masters and "being" their mother, she will be faced at night with the ever renewed shock of her untended mirror images. With bitterness and distress she discovers that her blackness is an "original sin" that she cannot redeem and that her children are perpetuating it. It is they, the most innocent links of a chain of undoing, who will incur her wrath. How can she want to give up having a target, a target that may help her becloud that it is against God himself that she is revolting? How can she foresee or even accept that in the Clinic Eve's purity before the downfall is acknowledged, strivings are supported, and error considered inevitable?

Even when the middle-class parents suffer intensely outside the area of family or occupational problems, for instance with regard to political or religious convictions, cultural integration does not seem greatly affected. The denial of certain aspects of our present political or religious order may still presuppose recognition of the dominant cultural principles, as long as specific constructive counterproposals are advanced. Political analysis of the evils of our culture, for example, indicates mainly that the critics are very interested and preoccupied by cultural problems, whatever their motivations may be.

The least constructive and therefore least integrated elements of any culture are its indifferent "witnesses"; they live inertly on the fringes of our culture, from where they fail to contribute their own share.

Such a role of assumed detachment from the community context may be justified under extreme conditions when the stress of living completely exhausts the individual. Often such withdrawal will be connected with the feeling of inadequacy and shyness. These parents, for instance, would not think of engaging in any form of social co-operation. They cannot realize that a partnership with the Clinic in principle could be established on equal terms. These parents would be too hopeless about the world and their own role in it or too angry to co-operate. Parental co-operation in the treatment of their child, therefore, is often reduced to the minimum compatible with his survival.

### Reasons for and Patterns of Resistance

It is interesting to scrutinize in some detail by what means some of the parents resist the Clinic—a resistance which may reflect their active and positive struggle for a raised and respected status in the community. This resistance was observed in the early days of the Clinic as an unconscious opposition to its willingness to take the patients as they were and to help them to achieve a more liberated status. It took the form of a partly justified and partly feigned devoted assistance to the Clinic.

A small community group that met regularly in those early days of our endeavors had a tendency to be diverted into airing concerns about the Clinic and the community at large rather than staying with the discussion of the parents' emotional problems in regard to their children. In spite of the familiarity of the parents with the character of the Clinic, they tended significantly to redeem it by associating it with a school. Thus, in their discussions they were inclined to avoid a conscious awareness of the character of their children's disturbances.

Once more, concern had been conveniently shifted away from the child. As a stepping stone to an illusional rise of status, the Clinic had been placed in the position of the child, his competitor for attention. It was now, therefore, a sibling or substitute beneficiary of parental interest and devotion and thus an object for the parents' assistance. Treatment and advice were now avoided and the roles between the parents and the Clinic were momentarily reversed.

For many of the parents, whatever the seriousness of their own condition and their actual social behavior, school is a major symbol of our society and the child's adjustment most frequently is conceived and measured primarily in terms of adjustment to public school and in "getting" one's self "an education." Whatever the pathological interaction with the child, there remains a conscious tendency to see the child conform and achieve in this area. This represents at times not so much a hope for a future career as a present gain of status for the total family group. Education under such circumstances is an escape from more profound personal and family issues, a borrowed cloak for masking unresolved and unattended tasks of importance.

A raise in social status is frequently sought by co-operation with the Parent-Teachers Association. It may, as in the case we shall soon report, be applied dogmatically, and, despite the public service rendered, it may become an element in supporting the parent's pathological symptomatology.

Four of the five children of the Gable family came to the attention of the Clinic in relatively short order; the school referred one of the two daughters, in an acute amentia-like condition. Her adolescent sister came to us of her own accord. Two younger brothers were referred by the mother on the suggestion of the school principal. Both boys were pre-schizophrenic. We mention at this time only that the father, a menial laborer with good ability and understandable ambition, succeeded in gaining status in the community by discovering one day his vocation as a clergyman as well as by zealous work in the Parent-Teachers Association. He was totally blinded to his children's obvious and serious material deprivation as well as to their emotional condition. All the children reached out for treatment eagerly, the boys running to the Clinic in any weather over a distance of more than fifty city blocks, and regardless of any obstacle in their way. Although the children's need was explained to the father as well as the nature of the gratification the children were reaching for, although the anticipated traumatization by denial of such gratification was carefully explained, he was unable to accept the facts. At that time his relationship to the world was abstract, devoid of warmth and expressed by means of the role he had assigned to himself, a role he fulfilled in obedience to God's call on him. The Parent-Teachers Association was for him, at the same time, an intensely rewarding forum, where he could mirror and admire himself in all of his importance. Because of this need he insisted that his children remain in public school. Public school was to him not just the usual highway to education, but a sacred door and the only one to the heaven of social conformity and acceptance.

Tragically the boys had finally to be committed by court action to the Richmond Social Service Bureau and for treatment to the Educational Therapy Center, in disregard of the hurt caused to the father by the shattering of his illusions. However, this proved an advantage to a genuine co-operation with the Clinic and to his gaining a deeper view on life and his relationship to his children.

Mr. Gable began with the release of tremendous hostility toward all those instrumental in removing his children from his home. He was especially hurt because the commitment happened to occur when he was out of town, leading a Parent-Teacher Association group meeting. He was outraged at the treatment he received from community agencies. He denied the need for therapy for himself but stated he would continue to come to the Clinic as the only way he knew to get his children back. The first change in his relationship to the Educational Therapy Center was noted in the decrease of expressed hostility and growing enjoyment of the exchange of thought and the scrutinizing of his motives of action with his therapist. He denied knowledge of the subject of psychology but was always ready to engage his therapist in a verbal battle over psychological motivations in general to prove a point that was in his favor. He was encouraged gradually to talk about himself and was able to discuss his early deprived emotional life.

It is interesting to note that in the early therapy sessions he always came in superbly dressed, but after his boys were returned home he came in wearing his work clothes. He finally was able to let the world, his therapist, and himself see him as he really was.

*The Family's Unpreparedness—Further Motives and Patterns of Resistance*

Our conviction that any case referred for diagnosis and treatment or recommendation should be attended to with the least possible delay and should receive promptly an offer of help to the child is based on a reasoning which motivates an aggressive approach in psychiatric social work.

We do not take the attitude that the patient or the parent must be ready for treatment. Such an attitude might determine the doom of a yet redeemable condition for both the present and the future generation. At least too many precious years may be lost and with them the favorable period for treatment of the child may pass. What are the possibilities of treating a child who does not want to be helped and whose parents are recalcitrant?

There are a number of ways to be or not to be ready for treatment. A change in attitude in reference to treatment may be possible or not if we base our approach on the awareness of such variables. All workers in the field are familiar with those applicants for treatment who are actually unaware of the meaning of treatment and what it implies. Necessarily, at the beginning of any clinic's contact with these parents, there should be a stage of preparation for such an undertaking. When at least three generations of a giant family cluster together, even though they may not live under the same roof, the danger of their pathological interaction must be foreseen and an attempt made to avoid their interference, aimed at maintaining the family pathology. This implies evidently that in taking a case history one endeavors to round up an even wider range of persons than are usually relevant to the child's emotional condition and obtain a report about the nature and closeness of such relationships and their complex interactions.

We were called upon through the years to treat a few of the antisocial offspring of a large-sized family "clan." A whole section of town was infiltrated by a village full of kinfolk interacting in a typical and repetitive manner. Although they clustered together and were dependent, they deliberately left everybody in the dark about their close blood kinship. We could observe particularly two sisters and their families. They were immature, dependent women. They, like three generations of their womenfolk, had had their first child in their teens. They married passive husbands who impregnated them about every year with an infant kept permanently in a close mutual dependency on the mother. These mother-child relationships (in one case there were five sons), made the father superfluous, except as a progenitor of and provider for the mother's offsprings. The unrewarded fathers were not recognized or appreciated and, in their isolation, would indulge in week-end drinking sprees. The mother's ties with her children and the feuds aroused by any kind of interference by the fathers in favor of severing the mutual bondage, as well as the concomitant irrationality, disarmed them in their role of the head of the family. As a result authority was conceived in the image of the inefficient father and reacted to with irrationality, complete resistance, and obstinacy as taught by the mother. All the elder brothers of our boys and, as our information goes, practically all adolescent boys or young men of these families have delinquent records; first committed to the industrial schools, they later incurred criminal penalties. Both cousins whom we accepted in day-care, at that time ignoring their natural kinship and mutual dependency, were referred to us because of persistent truancy and total lack of co-operation of the families with the school. The father's lack of co-operation, we found, was sensed as a necessary condition for his survival in the family; the mother's non-co-operation was a condition for maintaining the children's dependency on her. One of our boys would stay in the house, in bed half of the day, symbolically in his crib, waiting for the mother to return from her employment as a domestic worker. In the afternoon, when school was out and no visiting teacher in sight, he would watch television. At adolescence, the two boys began to move around town in groups, engaging in petty antisocial acts, which they reported defiantly in the Clinic.

A tremendous and patient effort was made to enrol parental co-operation. Neither family could ever be reached. Letters remained unanswered, there was no telephone and the door would not be opened to visitors. When the visiting teacher attempted to put pressure on the families, one of the mothers accused us of calling the school authorities.* It is worth mentioning that the boys gave as a reason for their chronic absenteeism that there was no opportunity at the Clinic

* It should be mentioned that Virginia has given up compulsory education.

to learn anything, and later, when they ran regularly as a pair from the training school for educable mentally deficient children, they alleged the same reason. They ignored that previously they had found the public schools also incapable of conveying necessary knowledge.

When they finally attended the Clinic they formed dependent relationships to two maternal figures, one being their therapist, but were totally unspontaneous and practically non-verbal, with unpredictable exceptions. A program was outlined that seemed likely to attract and interest them. They consented to the plan, as their mothers were in the habit of doing in reference to plans, but without the slightest commitment. The two boys moved together as if they were Siamese twins. They would just sit it out, the one like the reflected image of the other, though they would never stay to the end of the day but slip away around noon time. They were imbued with such a pent-up hostility and were so withdrawn that we finally had to commit them to the training school to protect them from an antisocial career similar to the older boys in the families, and to help them obtain some form of vocational training. Therapy was available in the training school but never made use of by the boys. Each time they ran from the training school, the parents would keep them hidden at home. One is still in need of help. Success may yet be forthcoming.

It took us another year to convince the mother of the other cousin that she was the key figure in bringing about a turning point in her son's life. She began to come for her sessions. Finally, her boy stayed with conviction in the training school and improved. He changed his attitude to such an extent that quite spontaneously he wrote a fond and appreciative note to his former therapist. His attitude was followed by some improvement in the attitude of the other. But mutual dependency seemed to be loosened.

## Making Scapegoats of the Children

A mother's avowal of helplessness in the face of her child's or her children's chronic resistance to her ardent educational endeavors, from which most frequently the father is actually or supposedly excluded, often conceals from herself and from those whose services are requested what actually prompts her to go out for help. Whether a family is socially ambitious as Celestine's, of whom we are going to speak, or only afraid of being caught for outright antisocial behavior is not necessarily relevant to their attitude at the time of referral.

In either case the mother or the parents may go through the Juvenile Court for a gain of status under the guise that they desire advice for a child that refuses to go the straight way as required by them. The children usually have been ostracized by the family for a number of reasons. Their isolated position has made them more vulnerable to the family pathology and therefore intensely anxious and rebellious. A vicious circle results which the family group can no longer master. Help then is sought as a defense, not as care or concern for the child or children. When we meet these families, they usually see in the child a problem, hence the aggressive, critical presentation of his disturbance and the total oversight of the child's good qualities. These may be at a minimum at the time of referral because the child's self-esteem, his self-confidence and his vital energies for struggling have been ground down. We can observe how any of the children's positive gestures are cruelly discouraged. They are not noticed or are received with icy coldness; the response may be by remonstrations, reminding them of past failures. Demands may be made for an immediate improvement, improvement being a condition to whatever may follow, but improvement is simultaneously discouraged by parental weariness and depression which convicts the child. An obvious exhaustion of hope is emphatically displayed. At the time of referral the ostracized child is usually made the scapegoat. The families come for assistance in the cure of a symptom while wishing to maintain the fundamental and underlying family pathology. The children are to be freed only of those symptoms which disturb or endanger the preservation of this pathology.

In unsuccessful cases the parental resistance to change is overwhelming. The parents come to the Clinic with a tacit expectation that they will be joined in the discrimination against the child and that everything else will be left untouched. In one instance they adamantly refused to reveal their own family history, which was obviously the source of their immaturity and revolt against their paternal function. Unless the parental interest in working with the Clinic can keep pace with the child's treatment, parental anxiety may cause withdrawal of the child from treatment. The parents become aware of their failure and inadequacy and due to a competitive attitude, they deny the

Clinic the opportunity to help and to the child they deny those gifts that the parents have been begrudging or incapable of granting but that the Clinic can offer. When the parents have not risen to the generosity of facing their own share in the child's failure, they are afraid of the child's confidence in the therapist and the revelations that the child might make. Moreover, as elsewhere, we have to face the problem that each time the child improves, the family pathology is endangered and a more or less successful attempt is usually made to withdraw the child from treatment or to silence the child while supposedly treatment is still in process. The parents' inhibitions in facing the opportunity to help themselves, aside from the vital importance which their symptoms have for them, are supported by the fact that their pathology involves the whole family group. It is therefore as difficult for a single member to extricate himself as it is for a criminal to escape the grip of his gang.

In the case of Celestine Lorray, a brilliant young girl of a socially ambitious family, the mother and all of her sisters were in the habit of encouraging each other to drink to a state of drunkenness with the tacit aim of stealing money from the purse of the one most drunk. For their "protection," the children would be taken to the party and thus initiated early to the family pattern and enlisted in its underlying pathology.

The children were isolated from the social quarters sufficiently to be aware of what was going on, frightened and excited by it, tempted by curiosity and so disturbed by horror that to spring into the flames of the identical behavior presented a major lure. Celestine's anxiety was intensified by her father's religious puritanism and his total abstinence from alcoholic beverages or any recreation outside church activities. The girl had a deep-seated primary problem in reference to her mother, but felt threatened additionally by the father to the point of refusing to be baptized into his church. She wanted to join a church which would "understand a tortured soul and help it by forgiveness."

Tragically the parents' exposure of their children's failure and punishment may be successful not only with the child, who acts out, due to his subservience to the parents' needs, but with agencies and the court. These may be misled either because of the child's obvious problem, his antisocial behavior, in an apparently well-organized family or because the child is involved in a sado-masochistic interplay and helps in beclouding a home condition that is harmful to his emotional wellbeing. Necessary assistance to the child can be unduly delayed if the law is willing to recognize parental neglect only in its physical and material aspects rather than in its expressions of subtle emotional rejection and inducement of mental pathology. These cases are not infrequent. *The child is the more exposed, the securer the parents' socioeconomic position, with which they veil and becloud doom imposed upon their children. We are confronted here with a primary problem and a preventive task of all concerned with a prophylaxis of mental and emotional illness, in particular when fostered by generations of pathological parents and their respective children.*

We present the case of Nancy McLead as prototype for the subtle grinding down of a child's emotional soundness, in the Appendix.

## Evidence of Parental Hostility Assessed at Intake

It is important, at intake, to assess the intensity of the maternal or parental rejection in its proper dimensions. The assistance requested by the family might be aimed at defeating the child or at recruiting justification for an unconquerable rejection. Reporting the child's symptoms does not serve the purpose of providing the necessary information to those who will work with the child but serves rather to enrol sanction and support for the urge to punish, as for instance by egging on and nagging the child unendingly. This solicitation by the mothers, at intake, of alliance for the practice of hostility, reflects an uneasiness in reference to the rejection for which justification is searched everywhere and at any time. The children report that their mothers give them a bad name "all the time," meaning everywhere, with the neighbors, the wider family group, etc. When the father is in the picture, he may remain in the background, in no way available to the child but causing an anxious mother to win her spurs with him by persecuting the child.

The marital relationship may depend upon the possession of a target in common and the parents may make an over display of a dovelike wooing affection, as in the early days of love-making. Depending on whether rejection is total or ambivalent or whether the sado-masochistic interaction prevails, the child will be an obviously unwanted onlooker. A boy may be incited by the parents' display of love also to make love to the mother and to be more intensely involved in hate with both of them. We saw a girl under similar conditions masturbate without reservation in the waiting room. Sexual indiscretion as well as hostility increases the eroticism and the need for its perverted manifestations. The parent-child relationship may be transferred to siblings or sibling figures and acted out sexually or as sado-masochistic substitutions for it. That we witness a pattern of the family's way of relating is obvious, when one sees that it is a familiar expression and a language between the people, an observation that will readily be confirmed as we continue working with the child and his family group.

When the child is thus made to feel fundamentally insecure about his place inside and outside the family and whether his or her existence has any justification of any kind, the parent may hold it against the child that he is isolated, lacks the ability to make friends, that even his movements are awkward and that he has a tendency to withdraw or on the other hand is avid for attention, invasive, or clinging. Evading their responsibility, they may suggest that his troubles are of an organic nature, referring to the poor motor co-ordination.

The means by which the child is isolated and ostracism against him is promoted are usually extremely subtle. Under the guise of love and care, the child is coerced categorically into behaving contrary to general habits. To be allowed to conform to these habits and customs as to wear a hat or not, a suit or a sweater like the other children, would help the child gain a sense of belonging that he covets with more ardor, the more he is made to live outside the paradise of parental love.

Because of this denial of the liberty to conform in those areas where conformity is in order and connective, the child in his anxiety feels pressured into a rigid and compulsive attitude toward the parents. Unless equipped with apparently minor tokens of equality, the child may not be able to venture out into the group of other children, meet people in general, or go to school.

There exists a whole science in the use of clothes as means of defeating the child in the specific direction of an emotionally sick parent's needs. We shall report the manner in which one boy's mother, in having the son go around in squalid and tattered clothes, exposed the father to censure and the son to a delinquent acting out as the father's son, while actually the son had to fulfil the mother's own needs. We shall allude in another boy's story to the role excessively fine clothes played in isolating the boy from age companions and himself because this was the magic by which the foster mother tried to redeem his sordid origin and make him wholly her own. When this boy and his brother subsequently came into therapy together, they revealed that the foster mother, taking them in her confidence, had admitted tying them so closely to her by exaggerated tokens of love because of lack of closeness between her and her husband. Both boys were intensely involved with the foster mother. To cope with this emotional upheaval, they resorted to a mutual incestual homosexual relationship. In this case the foster mother's motive for dealing inappropriately with her concern for the boys' interests was not hostility but self-centeredness. Both she and her husband enrolled the Clinic's assistance in order to help each other and the two brothers.

Other children tear their clothes, deeply hurt that the mother is not familiar with the right size, interpreting it as a lack of interest in their growth, or, as the case may be, in an interest in their precocious maturation and their outgrowing the need for care. The children will be aware of their undesirability when the "mother dresses like a queen," while the children are wearing clothes several sizes too small until they are entirely too short and ridiculous and the shoes hurt their feet. Excessively fine apparel may be not only a display for the public eye causing the child to revolt against the false role he has to play as the beloved child, it not only represents substitution for closeness with the child in person, a substitution rejected by the child who longs explicitly for the loving presence of the mother, but it is used subtly as a means of denying to the child carefree play and company with other children and of holding the child under the thumb constantly, exposing him to failure and punishment. Clothes may be used to "sissify" the boys, making them feel awkward and exposing them to ridicule by covering them up with overly warm and protective clothes, allegedly because the child catches colds easily, actually to drown out the real meaning of the fear that the child might be sick. They blind themselves to the fact that the clothes may be the cause of colds rather than the means of preventing them. To prove his male valor as well as to retaliate against the parents and finally to force them to show him concern, the child deliberately will expose himself to the inclemency of the weather. In short, everything can be used as a means of isolating and of coercing the child or of deviously denying him gratification. Time and schedule must not be forgotten as a medium for a sado-masochistic interplay. The management of time is one area by which the child can retaliate successfully from the time of toilet training on. After soiling or wetting is outgrown and destructiveness has become distasteful even to him, mutual annoyance in reference to a rigid timetable, imposed by the parents and ignored by the children, will keep motives for hostility or constant irritability alive.

Failure at the very beginning of the therapeutic endeavor to assess appropriately hostility and its implications, may make the suitable approach ineffective. The parent who is frustrated in the need to deal with his or her hostility and with the concurrent anxiety will be incapable of co-operating. Hostility against the child is intensified and, in reference to the Clinic and its workers, becomes prohibitive. There will be no end of rationalizations for subtle hostile acts by the parents if one is not on guard to disclose at that period a friendly interest in the child or anticipate a possible improvement. Much time will be required until the parent can face his or her hostility. We mention only in passing parental rejection, expressed by a depression which silences and freezes out any vital tendencies in the child. In the early treatment of a six-year-old boy without speech development, the child began to enjoy his treatment intensely and showed a tendency not only to utter sounds but produce situations which promoted this tendency of his. The father who usually brought him could be observed to respond so listlessly to the child that one could witness this behavior only with concern for both. The mother who participated in group therapy was cold and aloof.

The mother of Ada, an autistic nine-year-old whom we met already, informed us at her intake that she had been extremely ashamed to become pregnant at a time when her only son was already twelve years old. She concealed her pregnancy everywhere particularly in church. Although she had a great deal of milk and had to be treated by shots for a time because of the abundance of milk, she refused to breastfeed the child in order to be able to move around freely and hide her existence. She raised the child together with her mother for whom she had an unusual devotion. Her husband had married her despite the fact that she had declared her mother would always come first. The grandmother attended to all personal care of the child; the mother's co-operation was reduced to ancillary tasks as washing diapers, preparing the formula, etc. The child was halfway acceptable only as the grandmother's concern. When we met the child, the grandmother was dead. At the time of intake the mother considered the effort to come to the Clinic and the expenditure of bus fare too great an investment in the treatment of her speechless child who had but a tenuous hold on reality. Only the father's intense reluctance to institutionalize the child caused the mother to co-operate and subsequently to respond to the child and the Clinic.

This woman's liberation from considering motherhood as a yoke cannot conceivably be achieved by simply bringing together two people, the mother and her child. One is emotionally reduced, tied by the specific direction of her longings; the other is silenced or at least aimlessly groping because the object of her desires has turned elsewhere and is unobtainable. The mother's basic immaturity must be taken for granted at the beginning of the treatment. The therapeutic relationship to her therapist can be relevant only if the patient's mother can be accepted as a mother's child which she actually is at the time of referral. She would come to her session taciturn and angry. She would feel imposed upon for having to go out of her way for her child's sake whom nevertheless she thought she loved. Obediently she would fulfil her duty toward her like a child who consents to do her homework. The duty is accepted because of an infantile subservience to her mother's guidance as well as to society, "a school" of standards. But the fulfilment of duty does not well exuberantly from the deep fountain of maternal experience, and tasks that have not been memorized cannot be visualized or understood readily.

The therapist, the new symbolic mother, has to point the way to the mother that leads beyond the stage of a dependent school child in need of parental guidance. It must go beyond the period where powerfully outgoing feelings are still dormant and the meaning of life has not yet been perceived in its fullness and therefore has not been invited into the emotional household. Marriage was by permission of the grandmother, a permission that in the mother's mind had a deadline at the age of dignity. That age she believed she had reached, when the second pregnancy revealed to the mother church and its representative members that she had not conformed to standards. These at least were her childlike fears.

Enrolment into her child's treatment meant to the mother that obviously she had not passed the grade of maternal maturity. She needed to be comforted by her own mother figure for failure. One of the positive aspects of this therapeutic endeavor was that, once the mother could find a motive for her co-operation, she also tried faithfully to offer her childlike contribution in order to pass from now on the test of well-performed motherhood. To show up adequately for approval, she had to know her daughter whom she was to discuss, animated by the interested inquiry or the quest into the daughter's way of being. The mother's own inquisitiveness and her curiosity were aroused, observation became a means and the discovery of the child an astonishing result. The discovered child necessarily uncovered herself, though awkwardly, by initial attempts to communicate, encouraged by an unexpected and "shocking" adventure in expectant observation that emanated from the most ancient source of the child's longings. The mother's attitude of the good girl who recites to the maternal teacher her lesson of good motherhood was bound to change because of the intrinsic rewards reaped from the new mother-child relationship. It began to be a lived experience. This development had to be sponsored by avoidance as well as stimulation. The approval demanded initially must not support the little school girl's dependency on good marks nor teach her the alphabet of motherhood as an opportunity to memorize it. Instead the therapist has to descend with the awakening mother to the sources of her experience and, sharing it, help her recreate its creative elements.

This mother had rejected her child. She concealed it at the time of pregnancy as a fruit of an assumed indiscretion and she refused to breastfeed her in order to becloud the child's impure existence, but this case had good auspices for improvement because of the mother's artless and non-resented subservience to her own mother. The relationship was comparable to the master-apprentice co-operation and the mother had remained unaware of her own mother's denying function and of any element of revolt against her.

This revolt became apparent, however, as one motivating element in the mother's initial resistance to accept guidance herself. This problem was overcome by the early emphasis laid on gratification; the need was so great that for its sake the girl's mother had once endured her own mother's constant surveillance. This problem was further brought under control by the avoidance of a domineering attitude by the therapist and on the other hand by supporting or sponsoring all liberating and creative tendencies of which the mother was capable. At such a time she was struck by and could face the insight into the implications which her dependency on the mother had on her relation to Ada and its bearing on her condition.

In learning to yield to the experience of motherhood, the mother also learned to find the rewards of a more complete and deepened existence and to discover her own self as a source of joy to herself and others.

Many of the difficulties which we encounter are well known to all workers in the field. In particular they are known to those who do not limit their service to patients already aware of their needs for therapy and anxious for them.

Success in enlisting the parents' co-operation can be expected from single women, unmarried or formerly married, and, at times, from men who tend to lean on help and to be dependent on guidance. Those co-operate who are troubled about their feelings toward their children, or those who are concerned about current recurrences of their own emotional involvements with detrimental consequences to the children or their family constellation. Some long for relief from the pains of hostility, others come only because they are concerned about their children, either totally unaware of their own need for help or only theoretically prepared by the general assumption that problems with children usually are consequences of educational errors.

Mothers or both parents may be anxious to interfere with the treatment because of general distrust; driven by guilt feelings or suspicion, they aspire to bring matters under their control. Some are frankly competitive and try to use the assistance intended for the child. This was the case of the mother just mentioned, who under the urge to be mothered herself became eager to come for treatment during the time set aside for her child. In the early stages of treatment, she would misunderstand that the child also had an appointment.

In such cases the child may be sensed and depicted by the mother as her vampire. One mother expressed it plainly. The pregnancy and nursing of her son had depleted her to the point that she could never recover, consequently she was clutched to his infancy and clawed anyone who would attempt to help him grow up. At the age of sixteen, a handsome young man, he was still a complete nestling. What the mother discounts, however, is that the child's condition originates in his total lack of gratification and the resulting obsessive and angry insistence upon having his thirst quenched at the very source which is dry or turned from him. Though not necessarily so, some of these women are excessively obese and the children report that the mother eats or drinks coffee continuously. She constantly chats with neighbors, neglecting the house and the elementary care of the family, including the preparation of the meals. Some women admit their own inadequacy, though not necessarily with humility, which entails the striving for improvement, but as a justification of failure as an unalterable fact which precludes action.

One area in which our endeavors exceed what is customary in child guidance clinics is the persistent attempt to involve the mother who has given up striving altogether, the discouraged, depressed, and neglectful woman, the one who indulges in promiscuity to the exclusion of any action and any constructive life. In other clinics such mothers are regarded as untreatable and service is refused them and their children.

Albert Miller, a most attractive eight-year-old son of one of these women, was referred to our Clinic by the juvenile court for having raped a two year old girl in his community. He committed this act as a leader of a small group of his age companions, all of whom abused the little girl. He was innocently proud of his feat, seeing it in terms of his sub-culture as evidence of his adequate masculinity and bravery. The boy was committed to the mental hospital by court order and later placed in a foster home. The mother was outraged, hostile, and projective but could finally learn to appreciate the gain in understanding her own life and her own son's behavior, as viewed by society at large. The mother reformed her way of living to the point of being eligible for one of the homes in the city projects which removed her from an undesirable neighborhood to which she had clung stubbornly for a long time. In this city project she engaged with conviction and leadership in community activities. Her emotional life became controlled and acceptable to the extent that Albert, a fine ten-year-old now, is about to be returned to his maternal home.

Furthermore we have succeeded in thawing resistance to treatment by persistence of long duration. We have been able to make friends and work with hostile mothers whose evasion of the child's treatment reflects a generalized resentment, isolationist tendency, and intent on denigrating anyone who might lend help. The child's failure usually is seen in his inherent wickedness, due as a rule, to the inherited traits from an inherently evil father. When these women finally respond to our endeavors, they may still be so ambivalent that they let us "have" the child and pretend that they are incapable of co-operating in view of their working schedule and imperative commitments. Actually, at that stage, they are half conquered, but afraid of contact and what it involves. *We do not refuse to begin the treatment of a child in need of it, when his mother is not yet ready to co-operate in reference to her own problem.* Actually she is already tied to us in two ways. She has dropped her child in our lap and *acts out a symptom* by rejecting personal contact with the child and by providing only for his immediate needs. But since we are already useful and since she will want to use us more to express her wishes or complaints, a dependency of her own develops which will be the opportunity for the Clinic slowly to give the relationship a therapeutic direction.

Finally, we may work on a long-range treatment with the psychotic mother of a psychotic child. In cases of a child's interim hospitalization we may continue to work with the mother and the child's eventual return to the community. In the case of Hezekiah Reynolds the mother, who once was delusional and projecting, progressed to the point of being self-searching and concerned about her attitude toward her son, whom she began to try to understand. Her sensitivity still exists and flare-ups of distrust occur, but her distrust can be expressed and aired.

She is able to have all three of her children with her and, although our patient considers her difficult to live with, he is recovering remarkably from his own hostile and suspicious withdrawal. He is able in psychotherapy to discuss actual and remote experiences openly and face them squarely. He shields himself realistically against the mother but faces friends with trust. He also is brave enough to comfort himself with the fact that the "mother has never changed her attitude toward any of her children since the time of their birth" and can explain in his terms that her motives for discrimination are irrational.

He attends the Center in day-care with satisfactory regularity and has a hobby of training pigeons, which was one of his slow ways of coming closer to living beings and people in general and to his therapist in particular, with whom he shares this interest. At present we are working with good results on the mother's Oedipal involvement with the elder son, a problem our patient has learned to master by an increasing liberation from the mother and greater trust in a community of interests with the brother. The attitude of both the mother and our patient have changed to the point that both can accept the elder brother's enrolment in the family treatment. Progress achieved so far finds him imbued with sufficient confidence to co-operate with us.

When a mother who tended to relinquish her duties to us becomes herself dependent on our services, the therapeutic relationship and its gratifications may soon bring about a boost in self-esteem and self-confidence. Concomitant is a feeling of well-being, that, in addition to releasing hostile tension, distracts the mother from the obsession to pursue her child with persistent unkindness. Since the children, particularly those in day-care, are developing intense affiliations with their therapist, their teachers, and the milieu (close friendship with their peers is usually a remote result of a child's adjustment), the mutual dependency of mother and child is sufficiently loosened at an early state of treatment to alleviate that agonizing strain. The treatment therefore usually can be pursued.

When, however, the predominant problem, as in a number of cases, is the mother who cannot relinquish her need or morbid interaction with the child, even as work with her is attempted or pursued for some time, steps will be undertaken now or later to instigate foster home placement. The majority of the younger children in need of it will desire it, some of them taking the initiative to ask for it and, when it has taken place, they prosper under it. Others are too involved with their mothers to respond readily. When actually committed to their public guardians, they might run home repeatedly, in constant contact with the mother, and promote in the foster home the same frustration as at home, that is, they are attempting to transfer the mother-child relationship to the foster home. (The foster mothers are under supervision of the city social workers who in turn are in close contact with the Clinic. Moreover, the Clinic itself works with the foster mothers, either in session with the worker assigned to the case by the city, or alone with a group of mothers or foster mothers. We usually succeed in preventing the foster mother's involvement in the child's problems with his natural mother.) In spite of this care and the corresponding therapy with the child himself, and work with the natural mother, a few rare cases remain for a long time recalcitrant to improvement.

## Foster Parents

The city wards, who are the Richmond equivalent of those formerly referred to us from all over the state, are usually placed in better *foster homes* than those which were available to the state children in the postwar years when we had opportunity to observe them. In contrast to the state at that particular period, the city had a very active Foster Home Intake Service. Not surprisingly, we found the quality of foster homes to be superior in those agencies which actively recruit them and create a sufficient pool for proper matching of foster mother and child. However, small agencies cannot afford to do this, and the results are often damaging to all concerned. Since these agencies handle only a small number of children, the foster mothers may be kept in a prolonged state of expectancy and when the time comes may no longer be available. The agencies therefore recruit foster homes they believe to be singularly suited to the particular case, but the test of experience may reveal deep-seated incompatibilities, such as the foster parents' rigidity and incapacity to understand the child's problems or mode of expressing them. The agency then may be more concerned about the precious home than about the child, who may be given up. Also, unless the child can be assured of a suitable home, he might engage his new home in the identical neurotic interaction from which he was supposed to be liberated. Similarly, when a social agency has no sufficient pool of foster homes to resort to, it will be at the mercy of the few; the outstanding homes must be called upon too frequently for the benefit of children who promote hostile-aggressive interaction. The exhausted foster mothers then lose their standard and the agency is inhibited in their inevitable appeals to these mothers' disinterested dedication and abnegation. The desperate agency may be tempted to institutionalize the child or find reasons for returning the child to his unsuitable family. The small group of intensely frustrated and resentful foster mothers will congregate and advertise a child's shortcomings and discourage another perhaps more suitable foster mother from giving the child an opportunity. The group rejection is finally sensed even by the most artless child and his undesirability and status of belonging nowhere is cruelly brought home to him again.

Homes which were studied skilfully and conscientiously can be retained practically on a permanent basis. The foster families become very experienced. Some impress us by great wisdom and a total investment in the task they have undertaken. The children feel secure and enclosed in the human society. Not all families who have self-centered motivations for taking a child into the home are unsuitable.[6] These motivations are subject to change. The experience of parenthood under the assistance of expert advisers can promote greater emotional depth and insight. We consider unsuitable for foster care rigidly righteous men and women, those who graciously consent to take a child into their home that they may raise him to their own standards. They may trust their motives and the value of charity. But they may be in want of the reverence that the deep-suffering should command. Young children usually betray more readily their humanity. Their suffering and defenselessness is obvious and convincing. The growing child, however, buries it in cynicism and roughness. Condescending foster parents' want of humbleness of devotion is what causes foster children to run away. The child knows only of his humble condition, but it is out of his unregistered nobility that he refuses charity and the implied depreciation of his parents. Under humiliating conditions, he "does not care" for help, and for the sake of self-respect he becomes aware of his loyalty to his parents. We should not like to be misunderstood to mean that the foster parents are supposed to make a cult of the children. We mean, however, that a condescending approach is not in order. The foster mother can expect to be beneficial in her approach if she is ready to learn how the troubled child feels, to be "child-centered" in her attention and offerings, discreet, expectant, and available. She supports the child's tendency to unfold his own potentials and tends to inhibit distortions from developing.

Righteousness is the crutch of the intensely threatened person. A child displaying but slightly antisocial tendency might already arouse anxiety in a threatened foster mother and provoke her angry and rigid defenses. An interaction may develop where the child is made to act out the foster mother's or the foster father's antisocial needs and to suffer subsequently from their acting out hostility against him. Compulsivity as evident is a quality adverse to successful child-rearing. A frequent tendency is seen to make out of a living little girl a doll, a neat little toy to be dressed up. What then grows up is a robot-like creature whose sole animation is expressed by narcissistic exposure. Not all of these women are permanently unsuitable for their task.

The case of Daniela and Vicky Middleburg is one of many illustrating the salutary results of good foster home placement. It is given in the Appendix.

### PARENT–CHILD INTERACTION

The description of devastating parental influence on the children we are portraying would be more than incomplete if we were to omit the following cases of pathological interaction. They were chosen to unfold before the reader's eye a few of the designs by which a mother can hold her child in bonds, preventing his fulfilling his own human vocation, however humble it may be. The cases we shall present are particularly tragic not only because of the inexorable hold of the mothers on their children but because of the annihilating results. Society gives up these children, considering their cases hopeless. It is our impression that no brave and bold efforts have yet been attempted. For instance, Martinez and his mother might have learned to relate more soundly had both together been exposed to intense psychotherapy. In the absence of such an opportunity for people of her social and racial situation, she never reached a sufficient awareness of her condition to look for specific help, nor did she ever become aware of her problem and her share in the child's emotional malformation. We could not work with her at a distance of 200 miles. Whether a more aggressive approach by the mental hygiene clinic of her home community might have led to success cannot be decided. In the case of failure long-term therapeutic institutionalization and a program that keeps in motion positive life tendencies should be attempted. At the time no such opportunities were available. Extreme difficulty is seen in helping a boy in Furny's circumstances. The father's effacement and the mother's domineering attitude are very resistive traits. Being complementary they tend to reinforce each other and to become increasingly entrenched. The child being involved with the parents symptoms will resist whatever tendency the parents may show to change. Had Furny's problem been recognized at an early date even a placement in a country group home and enlightened social work might have sufficed to relieve the agony of his bondage. Liberation from the mother's forced educational feeding with food yet indigestible could have been Furny's opportunity to befit his own size and strength. The mother will need help lest she resist insight into the child's need to be himself. His hollow overgrowth will remain her need as long as she is afraid of real manhood in the form of a husband or a growing son. A son returning home able to fulfil his innate masculine vocation, which includes embracing the world outside home, would be sensed as a menace.

Emanuel's is the only case in which a long-range treatment was attempted and contacts with the mother went beyond the intake interview. At the time we were not equipped to invest enough effort for overcoming the mother's adamant resistance to change. She was obsessively driven to run her own course. It is likely that at no time we could have reached her. It is likely that Emanuel could not have been better protected from her interference if her pathology and her specific voyeuristic interaction with the child had been understood by the placement agency and the hospital. Her manipulative ability might have aided her tendencies too well. These are the cases in which the child's hope seems to lie in long-term therapeutic separation from the mother lest not long after the opportunity was missed the penal institutions bring about these long-term separations with a corrective but not necessarily therapeutic intent. As long as the heir of his mother's antisocial needs has not learned to understand his problem he has no clue where to point his resistance to temptation or malady and he invests at times a major and painful effort in the wrong direction.

## The Case of Furny: The Female Procrustes and Her Two Hosts

At the age of fourteen, Furny was referred to the Educational Therapy Center by the attendance department of the public schools, for disobedience, unruly behavior and truancy. He was referred again at the age of twenty-one by the probation department of the penitentiary, for assessment of his sanity. At that time he was married, had a child, and had been in the armed forces.

## THE FAMILY AND FAMILY DYNAMICS

He was the only son of Furny Burrows, Sr., and his wife Violet. He had four older and two younger sisters. He knew only two elder and two younger sisters. The sister next to him in ascendance died when he was four years of age.

Motivated by dreams, hopes, and longings, Mrs. Burrows, Furny's mother, had come from a state farther south where she had been teaching school. Her discursive mental ability, her capacity for discriminative observation, her vivid imagination, and, when emotional complexities did not interfere, her leadership quality as displayed in church and community activities made credible her assertion. The absence of specific teaching requirements for her ethnic group in that part of the country at that time also emphasized the likelihood of her statement.

When Mrs. Burrows met her husband, she was twenty-five and he was forty-five. She was then a maid and he a cleaning man at the same private home. She was attracted to him because in spite of her youthful charm he remained reserved and aloof. The most desirable thing about him was his complete lack of domination over her. She loved her independence and disliked having her actions controlled by others.

She overlooked Mr. Burrow's shortcomings in education and the realities of his employment situation. In spite of a courtship that extended over one year, she was surprised after marriage to find that Mr. Burrows was not a steady worker and really had no job at all; he just did odd jobs, nagged about material things, and was inclined to pout.

That he might feel inferior never occured to her, except for the age difference. There was, until a few years ago, a barrier between them; he was often sick with a heart condition for which no organic basis could be found.

At the time Furny, Jr., attended the Center, the father was generally described as a self-effacing, weary man. He had persistently failed to contribute to his son's education. The father never made decisions and took refuge in sleep when difficult situations arose. When the Educational Therapy Center tried to approach him, he would refer everything to Violet and retreat from any form of responsibility. The mother reported that the father could not understand why the boy was so "devilish," and that his assumption of paternal responsibility consisted in reprimanding Furny when he failed. He had no patience with his son until recently, when Furny was already a man. Self-righteousness, extremely puritanical moral concepts were further traits to which the mother objected. The father denied actual occurrences in terms such as: "A Burrows could not do that," or "You have to measure up to a Burrows." Mrs. Burrows asserted that Furny, Jr., was beginning to do the same thing without, however, quite measuring up to the father's achieved standards. From childhood onward, the father appeared to him as too perfect, and as expecting too much of him. The son felt that he was never allowed to be a boy, by that meaning mischievous and boisterous. The mother thought that the father begrudged Furny everything and did not properly provide for his needs. Unaware that she was causing the relationship to become less meaningful and more antagonistic, she secretly provided clothes instead of insisting that the father learn to play his part. The father, on the other hand, never faced his children directly but always approached them through the mother.

Mrs. Burrows was an attractive, intelligent, and representative woman, an excellent church and community worker. She has contributed to the family economy through her own earnings. In contrast to these qualities stood the neglect of her household, which is said to be cramped and disorderly, but not unclean. Though not without a tendency to keep the reign of government in hand, she has always co-operated with our Clinic and much of what is reported about Furny is due to her search with us for the secret cause of Furny's behavior.

Mrs. Burrow's father deserted his family when she was six years old, and her mother died when she was eleven. The tragic lesson of the irretrievable loss of the father taught her "to love a man and not to lose him, to tolerate, forgive, humor, minimize a whole lot of things, to express admiration when he was in want of it, to treat him and love him like a child." She had learned this not only because she herself was deprived, but because "she deeply felt what the mother had missed." Often when her husband thought Mrs. Burrows did not care, she was actually showing composure in order not to hurt him. She and her husband were incompatible. She did the best she knew, but the father "pouted" constantly and the children "took it in."

Mrs. Burrows and her husband were never in agreement and never co-operated. She felt the father tried to press Furny into his mold. this meant he tried to shape him into a person devoid of strength and stamina. Her own ideal was heroic. However, she admitted at the time when Furny was a stranded man that her husband was more ponderate and had a deeper insight into things than she. She did not know boys and thought that the extraordinary behavior of their son represented a boy's usual ways.

According to the mother, both of the parents had wanted a boy very much, but the father was "not nearly as anxious about it" as she was. Pregnancy occurred during the years of the depression. At that time, the family was almost destitute and extremely troubled. The father lost his job at Thanksgiving. Offered a menial job at Christmas, he refused. In March, during these economically and emotionally critical days, a week after his sister's death, Furny was born. The mother disapproved of the father's attitude toward employment and considered him conceited and irresponsible but was disproved. Through his own endeavor the husband soon found work as a janitor's aid, was soon promoted, and has been steadily employed as chief janitor of a fine apartment building for nearly a quarter of a century.

Mrs. Burrows feared contacts with young and normally aggressive men, and so had overlooked her existing, though abstract needs for enjoyment of masculinity. Therefore, she came to resent in her husband the very qualities for which she had reached out. She also lacked experience in family living and in the relating between parental figures. Fearing the child less than the man, she was trying to raise in Furny the oversized image of masculinity for which she had longed all of her life. Due to her childhood experiences "she considered the man a child," but of the child she gave us a history of such extreme precocity in development that it is most likely that it corresponded to a needed myth of her own. While fostering in the son extreme needs for independence from and ascendency over the husband, she herself clung to the son. He became, and was to remain, a part and parcel of herself and her triumph over her husband, who had disappointed her by being just what he had been and was supposed to be. At eleven years of age Furny had to be economically independent and was allowed to make "big money." The mother's urge for using her young Samson's strength for outdoing "the father" was readily available to her consciousness. She was, however, totally blinded to her role of the Philistine who simultaneously bereaves Samson of his power when it serves his own independence and growing manhood. She was unaware that her son had remained consistently ungratified because of an assigned precociousness. It had deprived him since the days of infancy of the unconditional mother love usually enjoyed by the infant, when nothing is expected of him, while the mother showers her child with a universe of delicate tokens of her thankfulness for the miracle of his existence. Nor did she notice that her child thus unquenched would be weakened by subservience to and the working for love on depleting commitments. Pressed by the mother's unconscious assignment, Furny was doubly deprived of a lesson in reason and an opportunity to reason it out for himself; therefore, his judgment remained untrained. Further confused by his own manifestations of daring boldness which were his vainglorious attempts to fit the assigned role of an oversized man, he had no chance whatsoever to see his way clear to any form of independent orientation and liberation.

Actually neither of the two male members of the family, thus placed under a definite role assignment by the mother, were free to reach each other and to discover individual or mutual needs of their own.

In view of the symbiotic relation between his wife and his son, any interference by the father would have promoted catastrophic reactions. Had the husband refused to play his passive part, he would have become a menace and interfered with the vital needs of both. Necessarily the relationship between mother and son would have changed. The father was not able to assume this threatening role, nor was he able to face her panicky reactions. To Mrs. Burrows it seemed that it was the father and he alone who should be incriminated with his son's enigmatic behavior. The uninspiring image of man he presented was held accountable for both Furny's weakness and his hollow display of supermasculinity. Furny, Jr.'s, boss appeared to her a much more suitable father figure. He swelled Furny's masculinity outside the house in an area where its substitutional function was acceptable. Mr. Snyder's admired bold and vital masculinity was exerted not only at a safe distance, but also by mediate rather than immediate influence on family relations and affairs. Mrs. Burrows therefore succumbed to overlooking the dangers of Furny's associations with his boss. That something was unusual would otherwise have struck her, due to Furny's conspicuously overbearing behavior toward him. This same boss introduced Furny, at the age of eleven, to the illicit liquor trade and traveled around the state with Furny riding a truck.

Mrs. Burrows belatedly realized that she may have expected too much too soon from her son. Unfortunately, she was too involved to benefit from her insight.

Liz Burrows, Furny's wife, complained of her mother-in-law's habit of sitting around in her home and begging Furny to help his eldest sister and her six children. Significantly, the sister's husband was alcoholic. For delinquency in providing for his family he was committed to the state farm. By her intrusive behavior Furny's mother would insist that Furny deliver the majority of his income to her for his sister and her family and retain a pittance for his own family. She is said to have returned for another $5 in the afternoon on a day when she had already received $10 in the morning. Thus Furny was retained as the provider for her and her daughter and a title to an independent married life was denied to him. Liz was convinced that her mother-in-law had caused the delay of her marriage. During the first eight months of her marriage Liz held two jobs while Furny was irregular at work. The money, however, was always given to Furny's family and, with the mother's support (so we are told), even to Furny's girl friend. The mother seemed as unaware then as when he was a child that her requirements were excessive and that her son made strenuous efforts to meet them whether by hook or crook. Furny's in-laws were fully aware that Furny's mother not only condoned everything but silently promoted her son's delinquencies.

Furny had threatened his mother repeatedly that he was going to perform a robbery, if she did not recognize that he needed money for his own family. However, the mother remained unaffected by the emergency under which he and his young household were laboring, and the danger to which she exposed Furny. She thought that he was "just joking." She objected to expenditures for his family declaring that they were luxuries. "If he bought anything for his child, it was just the finest." That Furny's in-laws found fault with Furny's total inadequacy as husband, father, and provider was, according to her, due to the fact that he was wanted only as a soldier. Devoid of a uniform and an income, he was uninteresting, she said.

When the delinquency was performed Furny did not blame it on his subservience to the mother but on his subservience to a friend. He could not get rid of him and his inexorable appeal and reluctantly consented "to get it over with."

### FURNY'S PERSONAL HISTORY AND DYNAMICS

Although breast-fed for only two or three months he was said to have been "very aggressive" and have often bitten the breast. He lifted his head at three weeks, sat up at three months; at the same age he began to stand holding himself. He ran around in his crib at five months, skipping the crawling stage; he walked at seven and a half months. He fed himself at an early age, was very clean, and an excessive eater all his life.

From his second year he was always in mischief, precociously manly and mannish. He imposed his whims on the whole family, in disregard of reason or consideration. He made an extremely poor adjustment in school, and contrary to his assumed former precociousness and the resulting expectations, he did not learn well. His failure was in contrast to his sisters' excellent achievement and success. Contrary to Furny's, their development was not jeopardized by excessive and inappropriate expectations. A poor reader, Furny liked to play rather than study. The teachers described him as "trifling, loud and noisy, most antagonistic to the group, not easy to handle, always a nuisance." His school attendance was poor and very often he was tardy.

Until Furny came out of the army none of his sisters accepted him, except the youngest. The oldest sister used to say, "I don't know why we have to have a boy." He played too rough, and the girls were gentle. In the house as in school he was extremely loud, boisterous, overbearing, and constantly annoying. The mother admits that although she loved the girls, the boy had "a unique place with her by being but one of his kind." The father, she said, did not mean enough to her to prevent her from putting a great deal of her feeling on Furny, Jr. In spite of her preference, the son always felt neglected and resented it. He was jealous of the girls. The mother mentions one significant instance when she had brought them washcloths. Years later, shortly before going to the army, Furny mentioned to her that he had been left out. She then bought him two big ones which Furny treasured so much that he took them to the Far East and still has them.

Furny repeatedly warned his mother that his father would hurt her. Before going into the army he specifically told her to be on her guard of him. Father and son became companionable only lately. Furny had tended the fires for the father in order to avoid his exposure to bad weather. They even began to go to church together. The son expressed a dislike for the mother's pastor who "yells." When we talked to the father two years after Furny's sentencing to the penitentiary, the father recalled only the son's kindness, and expressed his extreme surprise that he could have committed a dishonesty.

### OBSERVATION IN THE EDUCATIONAL THERAPY CENTER

Furny was a good-looking, harmoniously built, overgrown fourteen-year-old when he was referred to the Educational Therapy Center. His face was devoid of expression except for a motionless sadness; a weary and embarrassed passivity pervaded his huge structure that seemed to belie his lack of stamina.

For a short time his attendance at the Educational Therapy Center was regular, and Furny made a surprisingly good adjustment. He was so happy that he hoped his two companions in truancy could be enrolled. He worked religiously with his understanding and motherly teacher and communicated with his psychiatrist. Furny was submissive, but excessively demanding, and acted out when not in session in order to concentrate as much attention as possible on himself, as well as to show his power and independence. He was extremely sensitive to being imposed upon and had transferred his repressed problems with his mother to his public school teachers, as he revealed in therapy. He felt observed and thought that one of his teachers in the public school looked at him reproachfully.

The absence of his teacher in the Educational Therapy Center, due to sickness, caused him to act out with extreme violence. He demanded insistently to go to the bedridden teacher's house to be taught there, or at least to see her. He acted out by carrying downstairs furniture up to the roof, and upstairs furniture down to the basement as though reversing basic relations and demonstrating his own topsy turvy family situation. Though extremely rigid and disturbed by the slightest change of routine, he was himself unpredictable as well as insensitive to the disturbances caused to others. His judgment was extremely poor and his behavior irrational. In a grandiose manner he promised jobs to all the boys. He gave the appearance of taking an active share in planning his treatment, his studying, recreation, and work but was unable to carry out the first step. Actually, he did not have strength to mean what he said.

The absence of the teacher occurred at the very same time that Furny's work at the service station suddenly ended, after more than four years' duration. His boss disappeared. What was not revealed to us at that time was the illegal character of the trade in which boss and boy were engaged, that is the antisocial source of Furny's spurious potency and the specific behavioral motivation derived from his job. The mutual dependence of the man and the child, and dependency in common on offenses against the law, was and remained connected in Furny's mind with a restless "drive" for "big money" "which you cannot afford to forego." Years later, when seen again, Furny still felt that it is legitimate from one's own subjective point of view to earn as much as possible by any means.

The boss, Mr. Snyder, had filled perfectly the role of a father fitting into Furny's relationship to the mother. The community with his substitute father lifted Furny to the status of a provider and of male predominance in the family. The companionship between the father figure and Furny was based on work and interest in common. The man's illegal status, on the other hand, weakened his character as a father and gave Furny a power that he had never been able to exercise in reference to the real father, who was protected by his evident integrity as well as by a dignified and, in view of the circumstances, wise withdrawal.

The natural father, though a man of integrity, failed him because of an uninspiring righteousness and his lack of involvement with life, love, and action. The substitute father failed him by unworthiness and the direction of action toward worthless objectives. The latter had the mother's approval.

Mr. Snyder's sudden disappearance provoked a serious deprivation of power and a state of panic. Instinctively he revolted against the mother, the ultimate source of his tragic dilemma. But he beclouded the painful issue, depreciating "the women" anonymously. That the relationship with Snyder was fraught with homoerotic elements was demonstrated by relations to his friends, which later were reiterations of the forever unfulfilled and interrupted community with Snyder.

In his acute state of complex deprivation, Furny came to the Center with a gun. He was violent and intruding. The therapist invited him to take the gun home. Furny disappeared, but returned three-quarters of an hour later and shot into a classroom from the back-yard. It seemed a miracle that no one was hurt.

But was it actually a miracle? Furny needed to assert himself as a man and manifest his revolt against the mother he equally needed to spare. The Educational Therapy Center represented the mother suitably, and he shot "her" from where he dared, that is from the rear. It was his ambivalence that directed the bullets to by-pass a human target.

It was tragic that the Educational Therapy Center had, however reluctantly, to fail him and to insist on the recommendation of a more structured therapeutic milieu. Because of the mother's involvement and the father's effacement, recommendations were not carried out and Furny came repeatedly, asking for readmission as though asking for support against his own impulses that involved him in a number of illegal acts and loss of his short-termed employments. He was always dismissed for his sensitive reactions, his flaring up, unruliness, and lack of respect for authority. He was never able to actually dissolve the ties to any relationship he had thus forfeited. His delinquencies were always of a nature to show he was not through and still needed to drink from the source he had so violently rejected. But they were also revelatory of his Oedipal attachment to the mother and of a desire to reach out for hidden treasures not legitimately his. His failures were followed regularly by discouragement and contrition. It took quite some time until he recovered his weary spirits and applied for new employment. "Putting up his age," Furny finally enrolled in the army, in need of paternal protection and guidance. Many of his pathological needs were gratified during his years of service, but he got tired of it. When courting his wife Liz, he was repeatedly AWOL, and finally was dishonorably discharged but pretended the contrary. In one instance he asserted that he had requested the undesirable discharge. Furny did not enlist in the army alone but in the company of one of the two friends he had once wished to enrol in the Educational Therapy Center. While in the army on the West Coast, Furny was introduced to the use of cocain which he sniffed and of heroine which he finally injected. Feeling that he had become intensely addicted, he finally gave it up at the time when he was already married and dismissed from the army. Economic conditions probably contributed to this achievement. At that time Furny was dependent on his wife's earnings and she refused to provide money for this purpose.

### FURNY AS SEEN BY HIS WIFE

According to his wife, a gracious petite woman who appeared sound, purposeful and still dedicated to her husband, Furny was "all right" in courtship when still a member of the army. She denied that it was for her sake that he went AWOL. He was just tired of the army. He had been in a great deal of trouble before he knew her. While he lived with her, he never worked for more than a few months, pretending he needed a vacation, whereas she held two jobs at a time. She could never understand why he so often got tired of working. Difficulty on the job she attributed to his lack of a sense of humor, his sensitivity, and tendency to fight. He could seldom be gay at home with his wife without becoming offended at something. Often he could not be talked to or even looked at. When he felt offended, he would beat her mercilessly with his fists, once even kicking her down the steps. He was always armed with a gun and knives, once threatening his wife with a knife. He was unpredictable in his moods, startled by the slightest noise which made him "shake all over" and scream with anxiety. A car in the street could cause him to crawl under his wife's arm and grab her, like an anxious baby. His sleep was gravely disturbed.

His friends were promiscuously delinquent, selling whiskey, stealing, gambling, and taking dope. Furny boasted about his own cheating and playing with marked cards. His friends called for him in the evening, and he would not be seen at home until the next morning. At times he would return spontaneously; at other times his wife had to search for him. She would find him at taverns or other places, sitting up all night. Often he would be riding cars and his whereabouts would be unknown, Furny pretending to have been out of town. The origin of the self-injected dope remained unknown to his wife. Under the influence of dope he seemed to be "walking on clouds." He then felt as though he could "take the world and tear it apart." He would sit around snoring as though asleep but denied the obvious fact. Seven or eight months before he committed the delinquency which brought him to court, he gave up his addiction although he felt quite sick.

His wife adamantly refused to give him money for narcotics. He smoked doped cigarettes but never at home. He drank, but not heavily, and seldom to the point of intoxication.

The company of smaller children pleased him and he played ball with them. He was fond of his baby and enjoyed taking it along when he played with other children. But his affection did not prevent him from seriously neglecting the child, even when dangerously ill. He preferred to believe that his wife was just imagining the illness. His wife's complaints were countered by him with a blunt statement that his mother and any of his sisters had precedence. Wherever Furny went, for instance to a dance, he chose the company of his sisters. The household money was used to take out his sister's friend, Bonnie, who was his girl when he was already married. Bonnie was the mother's protégée, and all these women joined in ridiculing Liz's and Furny's marriage.

While Furny stayed away, neglecting his wife, he felt excluded from the home. While Liz seemed interested only in Furny, he used to come from his mother's home, searching jealously for his wife and threatening all members of her family. Liz explained the mother's opposition to Furny's marriage as due to economic interests. But Liz overlooked the fact that the mother was at all times more tolerant of

Furny's relationships with men and even promoted these in disregard of the men's real character, which she seemed to ignore. The mother herself represented one of these relationships as having started in child-hood: "Rud had a real fascination for Furny." She admitted she liked the boy a great deal and always approved of this association. She equally voiced the opinion that Furny "had an overdose of skirts all his life." In support of her own views on the mother's motivation for interfering with Furny's marriage, Liz reported that his family leaned on him for assistance; the father was in need of help at work due to the weakness of old age and the mother was clinging to Furny's role as the family's grown male provider. Furny could never rely on reciprocation of assistance, not even in reference to the simplest and most evident requirements of family courtesy. "They took from him and then cut him up." "Their refusal made Furny mad and he started fussing," and, as previously mentioned, he threatened that for relief from stress he would have to resort to a hold-up. Neither parent seemed in the least aware of his distress, the mother belittled the seriousness of the son's appeals and outbursts, and the father admonished him but to no avail. Both seemed to resent the side effect of a dependency they had fostered.

It is noteworthy that Furny displayed the same unpredictable behavior toward his wife as that shown him by the women of his family. At times unacceptant of his wife's assistance, he would at other times request personal services such as washing and cooking for him, even when he lived with his natural family.

The mother's and the wife's reports agree on Furny's excessive restlessness. He was obsessed by the idea of driving a truck and was never able to stay in a closed place. However, in the army, he cooked, because "that meant good food." It was the lack of opportunity to drive that caused his loss of interest in the army. Eighteen months ago, Furny had been twice convicted for speeding and reckless driving. He had lost his driver's license. When he drives with the mother, Furny is said to be in the position of controlling himself, otherwise something may suddenly "snap in his head," the mother quotes her son as saying, and he exceeds the speed limits. Having found no steady job for a long time, Furny is said to have become so restless that two years before Furny's brush with the law, the family foresaw a mental breakdown, though not delinquency.

### FURTHER IMPRESSIONS BY THE PSYCHIATRIST

One evening in winter, the psychiatrist sat working alone at the Educational Therapy Center, at that time an uncomfortable place in an uncomfortable section of town, when two huge men suddenly stood in front of her. They were Furny and his friend Rud. They both pretended they had been honorably discharged from the army and claimed they had unsuccessfully invested their money in a business. They had now bought a truck, had customers, and needed $200 operating capital, which they wanted to borrow from the psychiatrist. The two young men were persuaded to return another day and again arrived after hours, when the psychiatrist was again alone at the Center. Though their appearance was most disquieting, they behaved respectfully and left without further discussion when the loan was denied.

From all evidence they had been on the fence between borrowing material support for what they represented as a legitimate way toward mastery of their emotional and economic problems and a resort to to their own purely "male" devices, regardless whether "legitimate" or not. Their mention of the "trucking business" as their source of income, considering the total complex of available information, seemed to reveal that Furny was under compulsion to repeat his experience with Mr. Snyder and, as in the days of early adolescence, to act out under maternal sanction and support. The gratification of having caused the mother figure to fail and to have offered justification for acting out at variance with, and independently of her, might have allowed the young man to leave without the need of expressing hostility on the spot.

Furny was seen again only once, when the psychiatrist was in consultation with the staff of the mental hospital to which he was sent for observation following her recommendation to the court. He was in one of his listless and defeated moods and showed none of his hollow boastfulness by which, in order to delude himself and others about his deep sense of weakness and inadequacy, he used to defend himself in the past. The psychological test taken in the hospital showed that he was still using this kind of defense. He boastfully had mentioned cheating at cards and always winning, at a time when he had just been caught at one of his own games. He exulted his psychological finesse in evaluating the partner and "immediately attempted to establish an interview in which he shifted his role from "examinee to examiner." In the consultation session Furny, though honest, tried to dissimulate his pathology in his responses to questions. In his letters to Liz, also demonstrating love for their child, he mentioned his preference for the penitentiary. His friend was there, and it was a place for men as he conceived them—tough. But Furny was not devoid of a genuine need for punishment and atonement. He was not hardened, but neither was he in conflict. He was rather in a state of extreme discomfort. He seemed lost, a bewildered child in a labyrinth, not knowing how he got there, and too weary to find out or to consider that there could be a road to light and freedom.

## The Case of Emanuel

Emanuel Seminary was the fourth child and only boy in a family of four children. The father deserted the family two months before the birth of Emanuel. His whereabouts is still unknown. For five years the mother longed for her husband's return. Upholding the original standards and working as well as supervising the children became increasingly more than she could endure. First she became promiscuous, began to drink away a sizable share of the family's income, then she would obsessively repeat that to the father it mattered not whether his children were in rags and starving. When she kept Emanuel in rags deliberately she would taunt him with "your father is probably driving a Cadillac in New York or Chicago."

The mother's own father had deserted his family. Her mother died when she was twenty-one months old. She said she had a beloved sister and that the two little girls had had a happy childhood in the home of a grandmother who was widowed. In her original contacts with us she never mentioned her two brothers. Later it was observed that there were close family ties.

Help from different men was accepted. This entailed her engaging jointly with them in activities conducive to excessive smoking and drinking and she went to such an extreme that she was hospitalized for delirium tremens. The strain prior to this hospitalization and which contributed to it was excessive. The family's house burned and with it all of their few belongings. Her brother-in-law died.

He had supported his daughter, her dead sister's child. Mrs. Seminary had raised this niece. Then one of her own daughters was discovered to have a heart condition, still another, who like all girls of this family had been a good student, was expecting an illegitimate child.

Emanuel was referred to the Educational Therapy Center by his mother on the recommendation of the juvenile court. He was eight years old at this time. At the initial interview the mother was observed to be constantly nagging the boy. In her intense desire to love the boy, but unacceptant of his growing, she kept him in infantile dependency. She neutralized his masculinity. Although he was now accused of stealing, she attempted to relieve him of his inherent sinfulness by calling him her "little baby Jesus." But he also had to exercise the function of the missing male, be an object for exploitation as well as a target for intense resentment and aggression. He had to be crucified to expose her distraction and the father's neglect and his own male unworthiness. At the same time he was to redeem it by fulfilling the father's obligation and precociously assist his mother. When Emanuel began to help her and himself by stealing, she pretended not to accept the behavior which she herself had promoted. She literally performed a policing function, which she enjoyed demonstrating in the presence of others. She would question him methodically and firmly and usually succeed in "getting out the truth." The boy was made to feel very guilty. He did not yield the truth without resistance. The mother then as a regular occurrence changed her tactics. She would coax him, promise that if he told the truth "mama will not be angry." After this cajoling scene Emanuel would be made to sit on her lap and be stroked, held close and crooned as "her baby." Emanuel would melt and under great emotion and tears tell the story which would permit the voyeuristic mother to indulge in real or exaggerated stealing sprees. So she encouraged and rewarded him by these subtly graduated love scenes which one day we were made to witness. "Be mama's good boy" she pleaded "mama would not tolerate anything like this." She made him return that which he desired only ambivalently, because of the love scene which was his reward. Sometimes his reward was the clothing of which he was in real need. As she kept alluring him, she kept him weak and dependent and herself reassured of her own righteousness.

The eight-year-old Emanuel was frail, underweight, restless, and furtive and a constant thumb-sucker. He immediately responded to the psychiatrist with the result that the mother withdrew him for six months. Then when she needed an alibi for her righteousness and when therefore the boy was returned to us, Emanuel could no longer be reached emotionally. He feared a new painful discontinuance of contact with the psychiatrist and the therapeutic home. He was confused about his role assignment by the mother and uncertain whether she wanted him to make an attempt to get well. Emanuel was again referred to the Educational Therapy Center by the court. Again withdrawn by the mother without any consultation and then sent out of town for a three months' summer vacation.

Emanuel was now eleven years old when we saw him again. Again it was a court referral. We consented to take him for day-care on the condition that the mother co-operate with us. This was achieved to the extent that she did not again withdraw Emanuel. He came to us daily, though in such a ragged and squalid condition that the regularity of his attendance seemed a miracle. But now it seemed to have become his own symptom. According to the mother's commitment, he exhibited paternal neglect and his own unworthiness. Mrs. Seminary's own attendance was extremely irregular, but she submitted to personality testing and her reaction pattern was found to be of a sociopathic nature.

By now the entire family was dependent on social service aid. The mother's submarginal income had to be stretched to cover the niece's care. The niece was not legally qualified to receive help. In the meantime a second daughter had become pregnant. Mrs. Seminary by now a grandmother was giving in to her new role and was inseparable from the grandchildren. This was a hurt as well as a blessing for Emanuel. Released from the infant-like position which her possessiveness had demanded, he came to feel that she was no longer faithful to him and he was now free to accept his own psychotherapy.

It should be noticed that the mother pretended that Emanuel was her only "problem child." The reason for the mother's discriminatory attitude toward the boy was due to her general attitude toward the sexes. The behavior of the girls was an acting out based on positive identification with the mother's conduct and an approval of it. In addition, they gratified her need for infants by letting her take care of the children. The mother literally carried the children, in close embrace, wherever she went. At the same time, the girls also satisfied their mother's voyeuristic needs by gratification of their own sexual tendencies. When Emanuel acted out, at the unconscious bidding of his mother, he also had motives of his own, which represented a censure of his mother's behavior. As such it was not complementary to his mother's needs but represented liberating tendencies of his own. In censuring her, he was indeed the father. In providing for her, he gained title to her and also expressed determination to eliminate her partners, who were unacceptable to him. Thus did he provide for his mother's, as well as some of his own needs by what was also an act of censure and disapproval of her way of life. He exposed it by his apparent lack of concern over his ragged appearance.

Loosening of dependency upon the mother was slowly achieved, but to an extent sufficient to motivate his request for foster home placement in order to "break myself of stealing" and "come back as a decent boy to help my mother." His relationship to the psychiatrist was extremely demanding and dependent. To be able to leave her, he needed a nickel for comfort; and during certain phases of treatment he would return after hours. For the most part, this occurred after a stealing spree. He "ran" to the psychiatrist as he had run to his mother after having acted out, but the comfort he sought was of a different nature. Unable to be alone with his sense of failure, he needed support quite frequently during the months preceding his liberation.With great cunning he managed to enter the Center at night without breaking in. He held two parties in the Educational Therapy Center because it afforded him a home which granted him privileges denied him in his mother's home. He was considered "too young" to attend his sisters' parties.

Emanuel is of average mentality and, like his mother, capable of fluent, well-articulated, verbal expression. However, he withheld communication for long periods, preferring to use words only as one of the means of expressing his concrete demandingness and dependency. His quests for relief from his indecisiveness between admissable and inadmissable impulses were characteristically ambivalent. For a long while it was necessary for the psychiatrist to see him daily if she were to avoid being made to feel responsible for his having to leave the Center and "go stealing." On the other hand, he played most ingeniously, though averbally, like a tot imitating the noises of trains, bombs, and other missiles. His performance soon became even more remarkable. Every amorphous scrap of wood was used creatively, and its potentialities visualized with extreme rapidity. Summary comments revealed that the struggle between the "enemy" and the "friend" was resolved in favor of the latter.

Emanuel became more genuinely communicative as time went on, and the mutuality of the relationship was expressed by a display of affection and comfort which he derived from the gift of his affection. However, his desire to be like others was still maintained and expressed in such terms as "having what others have." His interest in stealing guns and rifles was substituted by accepting the use of those acquired in the clinic. When he later wanted a bicycle, he had become more realistic and also more willing to delay gratification. He not only determined sources and prices of second-hand bicycles but developed plans to provide for his share of the purchase of a bicycle.

His long-delayed verbalization had been caused by his dependency on his mother and by his need for performing the roles she assigned him. More specifically, he did not want to reveal anything that would entail relinquishing the gratification derived from his symptoms. As his liberation tendencies increased, he began to overcome this reluctance. However, even as he began to reveal his long-concealed plight, he continued to exonerate his mother. He realized that he had never had what he wanted, he was hungry, and he had no clothes, yet "mama couldn't help it." After the rent and the bills were paid, there was not much left for living. Unlike his mother, he never mentioned his father's delinquency, but like her, he ignored the fact that she spent an excessive portion of the family income to provide for her chain-smoking and drinking. With slow discontent he explained that his mother had every intention of buying him a bicycle but had always to postpone it. This coincided with his nighttime intrusion into the Center for the purpose of giving parties. He defended himself not only for what he had done, but from further deterioration of behavior, loss of control, and drifting away from standards originally held by the family. His symptoms, no longer an exposition (unconsciously promoted by his mother) of misery innocently incurred, were now an exposure of his own individual involvement and desire for liberation. Resentment of exclusion from his sisters' parties animated and reactivated a higher resolve. (He became his orphan cousin's defender, whom he said the other children, aware of her unprotected condition, attacked in the streets.) After having been passively isolated, he actively differentiated himself and attempted a rescue from his family's persistent lowering of standards.

The decline of his sisters' mores disquieted him profoundly. As girls with an acceptable way of life and a concomitant fine adjustment in school, they had redeemed, in his mind, his own inability to learn and his mother's illegality. Unable to exert influence on their present way of life, he tried to raise the sisters' standards and make their parties acceptable by elevating the men suitors to fine boys—one of them owning a Cadillac.

To equalize his home condition with that of the world, he carried on his illegitimate parties in the Center, defiling it as his home had been defiled, and punishing it for being inadequate to his needs, again as his own home had been. But he discontinued those secret intrusions when official parties were given for him and his friends. One evening he took the psychiatrist around the Center, showing her the potential and actual avenues for intrusion and instructed her in safe methods for eliminating them. In this way, he compelled himself to abandon this reproachable behavior. Though he remained dependent on the assistance of the psychiatrist for avoidance of digression, he actively and spontaneously offered co-operation. He wanted to redeem his symbolic home and soon reversed the established pattern. Rather than defile his symbolic home and thereby reduce it to equal standards with his natural home, he initiated an attempt to restore it. And in a long-range plan, he intended to bring the natural home to equal standards with the redeemed and trusted symbolic home.

He discussed this plainly in therapy, and once he had made his decision to recover under the more appropriate conditions of a foster home, he worked unfalteringly toward its realization. He was bent on being the one to talk to and convince his mother of the soundness of his plan, and to request her co-operation. He was now aware of his mother's influence on him. Emanuel was reassured that everything would be done for the mother during his absence in order that he may, upon his return, find the home where he could be and remain "a decent man who helps his mother." This was at that time his hope: to reinstate the acceptable male in the family and to restitute the role of the father, delivered of the delinquencies which Emanuel was called upon to expose and atone, a dependent instrument of inexhaustible resentment.

During the two or three days before the transference to the foster home—from which he would come to the Center for weekly treatment—he insisted upon being driven home by the psychiatrist. This was symbolic of his new way of life and of the help of the psychiatrist which would, in the final analysis, achieve his return to a home for which he, unlike his father, could not deny devotion and responsibility.

However, the mother continued to interfere consistently by telephone or intrusion upon the foster home, drunk and with a drunken party; or by failing to visit Emanuel when he longed for her, or when she, like the other children's mothers, was invited and expected to visit. Frustration and despair caused him to look for compensatory gratification of a kind which would artificially elevate his status to that of a man. He produced pornographic drawings in profusion, which he would either forgetfully leave in his pockets or present to his girl friend. His and his mother's displaced voyeuristic-exhibitionistic tendencies now were disclosed frankly. He again began to steal but would forgetfully leave the stolen objects anywhere. He instinctively incited the artless foster-mother to repeat his mother's coaxing and cajoling behavior, though hers was due to a different inner experience. The effect on Emanuel, however, was the same, particularly in that the foster-mother was cast in the role of the unrewarding mother because she could not condone his antisocial behavior. Hostility toward his own mother, he tended to repress, but readily transferred it to the foster-mother whom he could more easily "face." His mother, during this time, frankly competed with the foster-mother, pretending she could more expertly deal with his problem. Emanuel was exposed to the alternative of yielding to the lure of the mother, since hostility was not only repressed but inactive with reference to her, or be made aware of his feelings in transference to the foster-mother and be made to work through his problem.

This story, however, had a tragic aftermath. The mother never relinquished "making me nervous" as Emanuel put it. To escape her, Emanuel wanted to continue his treatment in a mental hospital where he might be afforded the protection of some isolation. But his mother, as before, succeeded in interfering with his progress by weakening his resistance to her influence. Contrary to the urgent warning of the psychiatrist, Emanuel was placed in the home of apparently well-adjusted relatives. They proved to be grossly antisocial and also connived with the mother, who feigned to be out of the picture (she had moved out of the state). Again the boy began to struggle doggedly. In trying to escape the family's net by earning a basic living, but poorly equipped due to a lack of education, he was made to feel harshly the inadequacy of his resources. Soon he was caught writhing in the mother's net, ran to her and was involved in an illegal act. Not considered to be psychotic, he was held legally responsible for his act.

## The Case of Martinez: Tantalus Unquenched

Martinez was born when his mother was twenty-four years old. She pretended he was very much wanted; however, his parents did not marry until he was four years old. It was his mother's contention that his father's sole purpose for the marriage was to delay, for a few days, his return to the army. During his furlough he was indiscriminately promiscuous.

Martinez' father, while yet an adolescent, experienced his first encounter with the law. He was arraigned to answer for a vicious assault on his mother. He later became, as had his father before him, an alcoholic. Non-support of his wife and child resulted in his commitment to the penitentiary. Throughout his life he continued a career of "entering and stealing," caching the booty in his mother's house.

Martinez' parents were divorced when he was eight years old. His father did not remarry. During such time as he was not incarcerated or a fugitive from the law, he took up residence with his mother. Martinez' grandmother, a religious fanatic, claimed she could not prevent the delinquencies of her son nor the misuse of her premises. Furthermore, she denied knowledge of the presence of stolen goods in her house, although her grandson and another son of hers participated in the stealing and storing of goods. This secret introduction of the stolen merchandise into the grandmother's house may be symbolic of an unresolved incestual tendency existing between her and her son.

A neurotic interaction between Martinez' grandmother and her son was carried into the next generation. It developed between Martinez and his mother, and was tinged with conflict and ambivalence.

Martinez' mother came from a respectable family. She was isolated in her family because of her lower mental endowment. Her problem became more obvious and painful in school because of her sister's outstanding performance. The social standards of the family and of the striving middle-class milieu from which it was rising were not sympathetic to the unsuccessful student. Thus her feelings of isolation from her family were consolidated into feelings of general social failure. This motivated revolt against her milieu, and prompted her association with the antisocial young man she eventually married. While he was unscrupulously delinquent, she remained ambivalent, due to an emotional dependence on her family, particularly her sister. Consciously she identified with her family and acceptable standards, yet she had unconscious antisocial tendencies. Because these latter tendencies could not be overtly manifested by her, she sought vicarious gratification through the antisocial behavior of her companion. She was aware only of his enigmatic attraction, despite her disapproval of his behavior. However, the combined pressures of her family, his emotional neglect of her, and his frequent brushes with the law were sufficient to enable her to divorce him. Yet her need of his function remained, and she raised her son in the image of his father. She constantly promoted actions which she sincerely believed she tried to prevent.

Her insistence that the child was bad from the *outset* served the dual purpose of identifying him with her former husband for reasons of symbolic possession, while at the same time making the father responsible for the child's badness. In telling the child that he had been bad, she was not only consigning the child to his father as the root of evil, but also referring him to a source of delinquent education. His father veritably had, across the street in his mother's home, what could be termed a "workshop of delinquency." Telling Martinez that he was evil fulfilled further the purpose of projecting evil outside her own conscience.

This unconscious device permitted her to feel different from the father and the child. Moreover, she could attribute their similarity to the mysterious and necessary causes of heredity rather than to causes so clearly fostered by herself. The son's morbid activities came to be perceived as inevitable in the minds of both mother and child. The mother's preoccupation with the undesirable acts of her former husband, promoted in Martinez the uncanny feeling that his father was a hero. He also felt that, to become important to his mother, he had to endeavor to become the equal of his father. His position was comparable to that of a mechanical toy animal attached to a string. It is released for a moment to venture abroad, only to be irrevocably returned to its master.

Aside from the alternatives of dependency upon and exploitation of his mother, he was further involved in the bewildering quandary of having to be part and parcel of his mother as well as her male complement. Martinez had to struggle for emancipation, while yet simultaneously fearing it, because of the new dangers with which it was fraught.

To the mother however, he was only a representation of the father and of his function. He was the tool with which his mother could reach out for his father and hold him in fulfilment of her commitment. When he did run to his father, he provided his mother with what she perceived as evidence of his inherent badness. For this, she censured the boy, who returned to her like a poor animal in need of love and forgiveness. He could not explain why he behaved in this manner, being under an order to do what the terms of the order seemed to forbid. Even had he been capable of analyzing his mother's behavior, his dependency upon her would have prevented him from acknowledging her role in his tragic existence, or her influence on his behavior. Her categorical statement that he was inherently bad was all that was necessary to complete his enigmatic situation. What drove him to his father was as contradictory as the assignments from the mother. He identified with his father not only because his father was the "desired evil," but also because he was the father and as such Martinez' refuge from fear of involvement with his mother.

To substitute delinquent behavior for instinctual drives did not prove satisfactory. On the conscious level it represented loss of the mother's love, the part of her which was identified with acceptable standards. It isolated him from the mother's family and the human community. But above all, it split him from that part of himself which was identified with average standards and which could call the other side of himself "evil" or "possessed by the devil."

Thus, she weakened the child's faith in any freedom of his own, and left him exposed and unassisted in his branded condition. When the child continued to run to his father and joined him in his delinquent pursuits, neither she nor the boy understood why he did it. But both were fulfilling her wishes in keeping the father alive and active among and within them.

She had had a suitor for many years, a respectable man who was acceptable to her family and especially to Martinez. His mother's pretense that she could never trust another man became manifest when she later visited Martinez in the industrial school accompanied each time by a different male. Apparently it was her unfortunate first love and its implications that stood in the way of serious and binding relations with men of a different character than Martinez's father.

After having described him as an incorrigible child, the State Welfare Department referred Martinez to the Educational Therapy Center. His most recent episode of antisocial behavior involved the choking of a girl in school. He was considered a bad child in infancy for throwing objects out of his crib. He broke things. Through the years he had run to his father and engaged in breaking and entering with him, helping him hide and store the loot. Martinez was a non-learner and a truant. He was a small stocky boy, who could be impersonal and aloof one time, friendly, submissive, and subdued at another. He was passive to the point that his movements seemed to be endured rather than the result of an active intent. He had no mimicry; his head seemed sunk into his shoulders as though to be less conspicuous, and made him look as if he were ducking. He stepped cautiously without swinging his hands. No organic basis for his motor behavior could be elicited.

In the early days of treatment in the Center, Martinez had a tendency to break objects by throwing or crushing them. He tried repeatedly to emit the devil, saying he felt sick and had to vomit and, mustering all his evilness, squinting as he imagined the devil would do, he expressly stated he wanted to get the devil out of his system. One day he wanted to jump out of the window because of his unconquerable badness. He again asserted he was "sick and disgusted" with himself. In that session he reported much of the material which helped to reveal to the psychiatrist his interaction with his mother, as well as her problems. He suffered from "terrible headaches." Also sickness and weakness were his escapes from his overpowering impulses, volcanic forces which seemed to sweep away the world and himself. At such times he would break into cars, and steal indiscriminately. He then hated himself identifying himself with the mother's judgment, saying he was inherently bad and possessed by the devil. After such exasperations, he would become increasingly subdued until his meek childlike and dependent attitude was reestablished for a time. Then he tried to use his manipulative ability—gained in destroying—for reconstructing, whenever possible, that which he had broken. He behaved like a dog who anxiously tries to discover in the master's attitude whether he is going to be petted or whipped. Being delinquent was actually being obedient and entailed uncertainty whether he would be rewarded or punished.

He tried to obtain additional punishment by taunting his companions to beat him mercilessly. He liked best those who punished him, but he also felt menaced by their insidious attacks. He gave a sensitive explanation which showed that when he attempted to strangle the girl, he foresaw an attack on him. At the time when treatment was interrupted, he spontaneously spoke of his fear of being killed by the other boys if he did not obey their orders to be delinquent.

A dream he had also expressed the ambivalence against the mother and evil forces, and the hope that "the shark" could be dead without his assumption of responsibility for it. "I dreamed I fell in a stream of water. A shark chased me but I was so strong, I dragged the shark up on the boardwalk. I saw that the shark was going to die without being in the water, so I kicked the shark back into the water, then I went home. After I got home, I heard the shark was dead."

He was very much afraid of walking the streets in the dark, believing he would be more prone to possession by the devil. He also thought he would be safer in the country. This argument was based on the realistic appreciation that temptations are more numerous and pressing in the city.

In the early phases of treatment, the mother was used as the ideal figure to whose standards he failed to live up. At one period it seemed as though the mother was going to marry the suitor who seemed such a desirable partner, and so fitting the image of a father for positive identification. During that period, Martinez was serenely optimistic and happy. He made plans for his life and adjustment at home. When the mother failed to marry this man and came to see him with other suitors, Martinez first tried to deny reality to himself and to the psychiatrist. He finally was confused and extremely angry and erected a totally unrealistic picture of his mother.

In spite of strong and repeated warning against committing Martinez to his mother's custody unless she first submitted to treatment and in spite of a number of other substitutional recommendations, he was sent home, a victim of the policy of his custodial agency against which the professional workers could not prevail. Shortly before his return, the mother, in letters which he showed to the psychiatrist, entertained Martinez constantly with his father's delinquent pursuits and his shrewdness in knowing when to leave the state, and in returning only after "his time was over." Again she had resorted to enticing the boy under the guise of deterring him. But it was obvious that her depicting the father in all his wretchedness was also a violent means of segregating herself from him, which however never fully succeeded. In his last sessions Martinez told his psychiatrist that he knew he would be a success at home. After school he would never leave the house in order to avoid becoming delinquent. As we know, he was afraid other children would kill him if he did not again join them in their delinquencies.

Because of lack of co-operation of both mother and son the recommended treatment of mother and son was not carried out in their home community. A few months after his return home we received the following letter:

We find that Martinez is not making a satisfactory adjustment in his home. He refuses to attend school except occasionally and on those few times he leaves at lunch. He stays out at night until one, two, and sometimes as late as four o'clock in the morning, and then stays in bed the next day until noon and often as late as three o'clock. When he arises, sometimes he eats and other times he doesn't, then he stays around the house tinkering with his bicycle or tearing it up, as his grandmother says. Later in the afternoon he disappears and is not seen again until sometime in the night. He never eats at the table with others, he will eat only certain foods. His mother says that often she will go out to hunt for him and that many times she will find him standing in front of a building by himself, perhaps with a stick in his hand punching the ground. This building is one that is used as a gathering place for the young people and contains a piccolo and a drink stand. His mother says "she seldom finds him with anyone else."

Two of these cases, Martinez and Emanuel's seen superficially would seem to bear out views on the heredity of pathopsychological conditions. We, however, take the view that whatever the physical limitations of these children might have been, their observable fate seems to explain sufficiently their tragic development. If we focus on the hereditary aspects of human behavior we might easily be discouraged from observing and reforming reality factors that must not be overlooked as necessary if not sufficient causes of personality breakdown. Emanuel's mother, whose Rorschach test showed her to function as a psychopath, unfolded the full picture of antisocial behavior only fairly late in life when adversity had struck relentlessly this woman who had become an orphan in early childhood. A similar steady breakdown could be observed in another mother to whose story we allude only shortly. She lost her own mother early in life. She came to the attention of the attendance officer when she was thirteen. At that time she was taking care of an alcoholic father and two brothers who were severe conduct problems. She kept a neat home and tried ardently to help all three male people to amend their ways. She explained her truancy with shame to come to school badly dressed and having epileptic spells.

She came again to the attention of the attendance department as the mother of two children. The family had no home. Mother and children moved into the place of any man that would take them in. She had to resort to having our little patient and his younger sister go stealing. The boy would fight the police doggedly but still hold on to the little sister. Once he was caught you could not take your hands off him, or he and the little sister would be gone.

The mother had become a deteriorated alcoholic and finally ended up taking a man's life. At the time our little patient was utterly distraught. Endowed with the same potentials that once distinguished his mother, he seems at this time to be on the way to a more promising career. He is no longer exposed to struggling alone against a stream which would be bound to exhaust his youthful resources and his strength.

Furny's mother, too, lost her parents early and was capable of indicating how it influenced her attitude toward men. None of these only sons had a father to assume responsibility for their training and education. Furny's father was aged and effaced, chosen to meet the mother's need for a fatherly husband and her need for independence. He is typical of the man who helplessly connives with his wife's objectionable attitudes. His passivity extends to the area of cognition. It is his defense to ignore what he actually disapproves of. The mother raised in the son the fulfillment of all her needs, above all an image of man that was similar to her and the opposite to the father. This automatically deprived the son of any respect of male authority. But as the mother's creature, stretched to fit the frame she had structured in disregard of his size, he was disarticulated. In his weakened condition he was made to feel inadequate like his father. While to the father was assigned the role to resign, the son was stirred on to spurious motion. Finally to entertain the illusion of strength or find rest for his restless and paining limbs, he had to reach out for artificial comfort through the use of dope. We see a special interest in presenting his case as an evidence of a mother's instrumental use of her son who was never allowed to be himself, who had to overreach himself, to be her man from the time of birth, her provider when he had barely passed the ten-year mark. She kept him bridled as a provider to his sisters and parts of herself. Her need to absorb him went so far as to identify herself with Furny's boy friend and his dependency or fascination for Furny. In Furny's mind the boy friend was a substitution for the mother.

The mother's own lack of a satisfactory family life in childhood apparently had left traces in an incomplete sex identification, which in turn was transmitted to her son. That Furny became delinquent was the result of his mother's direct commitments, the lack of the father's protection, and his own helplessness in liberating himself from extreme dependency on the mother.

Emanuel's father had deserted the family and Martinez's father neglected the mother. Both mothers attempted to retain the father in the shape of the only son.

Emanuel's mother used him as an anvil to substitute for the father who had known to escape. Martinez's mother used the son as a substitute for the father as the one who acts out her covert tendencies. Both boys were under an inescapable commitment by their inexorable mother, both struggled, Emanuel responded to therapy. But society permitted the mothers' influence to prevail. Both boys succumbed, the one became antisocial because antisocial responses to the mother's double bind commitments were rewarded, the other became asocial, undecided and blocked because carrying out his mother's double bind[7] commitments lead to censure and rejection.

# THE CHILD UNDER OBSERVATION

# VI

## Sex Education and Maturation

### The Parental Model as Factor in Sexual Development

There can be a surprising contrast between the stultifying, un-differentiated socioeconomic milieu in which the children live in dilapidated, unfurnished, crowded, disorderly homes and the elaborate dynamism set in motion by the process of emotional and sexual maturation. An astonishing lack of education, reflected in rudimentary speech, is in sharp contrast with the sensitive and subtle description of all stages of their emotional growth. Listening to the child's daydreams or nightmares, one is reminded of the wellsprings of literature and the universality of those mental and emotional processes all men will undergo. The imagery used by these children is of compelling beauty, and their language is true and forceful.

It is very impressive how they protect their parents though they owe them so little in terms of accepted standards. The majority of our children shield the parents and the muteness that many of them display is due to their reluctance to uncover the lurid faults of their kin. Criticism of the parents and identification with more desirable ego-ideals arouse guilt feelings and the desire to make amends.

So, for instance, when Robbie had begun to identify with adult figures who usually represented more acceptable ego-ideals, he showed great concern about his mother's mores and drinking habits. He was very much ashamed of his lowly status and miserable origin, which he wanted to change by helping his mother and his younger siblings. However, in the psychotherapist's office, he maintained an embarrassed silence and actually ran out; but he talked to a friend who was under stress for the same reason. The therapist happened to overhear the conversation. At a later stage, when Robbie valued the opportunity to live with his foster mother, a kind and maternal woman, he asked permission to pay his mother a short visit, emphasizing that he only wanted to see her but not to stay with her.

Such requests for home visits at crucial moments, when the children feel they are on the verge of deserting their delinquent parents, are quite frequent. They feel guilty when they have advantages from which their next of kin are excluded. They also fear to be punished for lack of active devotion which is expected by the parents in a complete disregard of reality. The children cling tenaciously to their own parents rather than to substitute figures, apparently overestimating the importance of kinship by blood. In reality they are sentimentally looking for parental attributes that are of a non-material nature and largely independent of facts. Often the child-parent relationship has been viewed in the light of the search for integrity and self-respect and in relation to adjustment by means of denying reality or common standards. The need to retain their parents at any cost is often expressed in pathetic ways. The children in a desperate attempt not to reject their parents deny to themselves their obvious faults. Finally they become confused in the vain effort to sustain the illusion.

The story of Isaac Jones is an example of ambivalence toward a parent caused by a very harmful tenacity to such an illusion. His story is given in the Appendix.

## Ideals of Womanhood: Venus and Elizabeth

In the old German saga of Tannhauser, the hero loves the pure maid Elizabeth. However, for many years he serves and is being served by Venus, the alluring goddess of sensual passion. To atone for the sin of infidelity to pure love, Tannhauser makes a pilgrimage to Rome. He is told he will be eternally condemned unless the branch in his hand will bloom anew. Tannhauser dejectedly returns to Germany. Upon his return he finds Elizabeth dead. But his sins are forgiven as the branch suddenly begins to bloom. Reward is inherent in man's untiring effort.

The exciting distance and differences between the sexes and the infinity of ways of dramatizing the differences and their extreme aspects in the many phases of love find their expression in the myths and literatures of all countries.

Man will be drawn to Venus or Eve; he will long for redemption through Elizabeth or Zenta, as in the Flying Dutchman. But he will long to re-enter the mountain of Venus and will be damned to sail the high seas, unable to die until again redeemed by the sublime woman.

It is the same with women: Alkmene, while in the embrace of man, would be confused and wonder to whom she actually belonged, her husband or her God. Whomever she believes she holds, she may be disquieted by a feeling of belonging to the other. Whatever the gap between the sexes, illusion and fantasy will still be used to increase it. Thus man succeeds in augmenting the intensity of longing that he may intensify its gratification. At times the glorified idol has to be raised to the stars, only to be, at other times, denied and reviled.

Bases for polygamy exist in the need for intensification of longing leading to the increase of gratification and for alternating between the experience of the sublime and the terrestrial, when these cannot be satisfied by the same person through the inherent polarity of the sexes in the potentially inexhaustible rewards of monogamy. Unless the need for steadiness of emotions and the yearning for heavenly tranquility are extreme, emotional polarities in each partner are a necessity for the fulfilment of love relationships. They are brought about more or less consciously in the love play of the sexes. The supreme moments of gratification and the temporary easing of desire will, through the miracle of love, eliminate the urge for promiscuity or polygamy.

In much the same way, the pre-adolescent youngster is still tied erotically to the father or mother whom he does not want to leave; he "never wants to get married," the parent is but a representative of a love object. Naturally, the parent as a person with a still active sex life is only vaguely known to the child and he dwells at an eternal distance, which makes the parent a suitable subject for fantasy. Thus fantasies in adolescence are most intense and persistent when the parent of the opposite sex lives far from home or is seldom, if ever, seen. When, however, the discreteness between parent and child is repeatedly violated, the elements of antagonism and dislike are sharply accentuated.

## The Fear of the Unknown

Fear results when the search for one's identity and the struggle for its preservation are faced with the temptations and threats that come from awakening sensuality. The young person has been striving for and is reaching a climax in the attempt to define his or her identity with increasing consciousness. If he is permitted to approach the potential love object (of self-complementation) and then withdraw at will in order to test and evaluate his differentiated needs of the moment, and if he can gauge the intensity and concreteness of the approach, each such attempt will bring the young man or woman closer to a discerning awareness of self. It will reassure him as to the specificity of his wants and will increase the sense of freedom in his approaches; that is, his freedom to choose. What is required at this age is a loose framework of opportunities and an absence of the compulsion to undergo concrete sex experiences.

The adolescent youngster must not be diverted from the slow, delaying process of molding, studying, and experimenting with his anticipated role in love and life, and conversely, the role which love and life are to play for him. Precocious experience thrust upon him from without will prevent him from girding himself for the great problem of love and life, which is the fulfilment of one's own self without loss of one's identity. His freedom to find his own orientation and the answers to his sensed needs will be impeded; he will be exposed to the necessity of reacting mainly to pressures from without, which are probably unwanted and which, for the sake of proper self-realization, he must or should resist. Almost more obnoxious are the uncalled-for intruding, even though seemingly positive, pressures in the direction the young person desires. They subtly deprive him of the liberating and inspiring experience of independent decisions and acts. Again, the youngster might lose sight of his goal and for the sake of preserving independence, he may take a course contrary to his own real needs.

The children whose problems we are discussing have been cruelly deprived of the freedom to try out in imagination and in innocent play what love should be and could mean to them. They have not had an opportunity to avail themselves of the joys of healthy amorous companionship among young people of their own age. Unlike the average youngster, they have either a lack of innocence, or an extensive experience in sex matters. Shame enters as hindrance in the establishment of a relation between these maladjusted and emotionally burdened children and more carefree and happier youngsters.

## *The Free and the Enslaved*

Indeed, youthful companionship generally is the necessary escape valve for gradual deliverance from too rigid and dogmatic an identification with the parent. Each of the young people temporarily attracted to each other may not only provide each other with an awareness of what is, or is not, satisfactory, but may in the latter case give rise to various thoughts of the ideal. A youngster will experiment with a combination of desirable traits in a love object; these traits he may have seen previously in a pleasing proportion in another person and they may eventually determine his final choice of a mate.

In spite of the stirring newness that lifts the taboo on sexual gratification, the new love model must be familiar, in order not to create anxieties which may overwhelm anyone in the face of the unknown. In the framework of persistent longing, the new model will represent continuous life and light rather than unforeseen pain and darkness; therefore, it will be desired, and therefore, it can be conquered.

In this connection we must remember the conditions under which these families live, their crowded homes, the economic hardships, the dissensions arising from the need to cope with unending problems, the strain of the perpetual exposure to what amounts to a public forum of a village or a small town within the houseful of people who know and often viciously criticize every one of the youngster's steps. The children are aware of everything that goes on between the parents, the lack of love and the lack of acceptance. When people are closely bound together in space, their frictions are produced by mere proximity. Neither partner is seen as an entity in himself but rather as an obstacle to the other, someone who is reluctantly dependent and intensely resented.

Sex relations between the very young are prone to occur in intense resentment and hostility because they are a degrading answer to a physical need provoked by a sex partner, rather than mate, whose humanity, whose struggles and sufferings, and whose ever repeated attempts to be attractive are overlooked. Neither does the lure of a vital, strong, and beautiful sex partner redeem the situation or lead to an elevating experience. If the girl displays good qualities or has good potentialities, the boy does not know it, neither does she recognize in him the gratifying or the redeeming man.

The idea of the complete communion of the sexes is never suggested to a child living under such conditions. Sex life is not integrated in an all-encompassing relation. All the circumstances observed are intensely depressing. At the conceiving of life stands not love, but usually hatred and contempt. Until disgust, cynicism, and despair take over, life tendencies might be strong enough to tell the child about more human relations. The knowledge, which is not provided by the outside world, will come from his inner longing. The boy will want to take the father's place and treat the mother properly, with all his childish passion.

For example, Emile said: "Daddy does not like mother when she fusses, but I love her, even when she fusses." But Emile came from a fairly orderly and organized home where the father, although henpecked, still had a part to play. Where conditions are less auspicious, even though the mother may remain a light and a beacon in the child's life, he may be able to "watch and look out" but not to follow it.

The children whose case histories follow have been traumatized at home specifically in the sexual area. Their cases are particularly grave, because the traumatization persisted through all their lives. Grave as they are, they are unfortunately not exceptional; the following pages give a short glimpse into their struggle before they either broke down or rose again because they were offered, and could accept, help. The case of John Martin McGregor is presented in the Appendix.

Seeing these children so differently from what they have allowed us to observe, we must ask ourselves: Who are they? Why is it that potentialities, which we must consider to be universal, take the specific shape they assume in these children, individually and as a group, children who have a characteristic way of mutually understanding and misunderstanding each other? In seeing the sweet and angelic aspects of the child's character, do we glimpse his unaltered virtuous and loving proclivities, the unspoiled founts of his peaceful and constructive nature? And do the more forbidding aspects of his character mirror an acquired hostility and destructiveness, discoverable when his personal privacy is intruded upon constantly? Is it at moments of solitude only that innocence and purity can be preserved or recovered?

These children have experienced few hours of undisturbed solitude, hours where they could be Adam before the fall. When the competitive aspects of life with one's fellow man take the shape of crude violence of one type or another, reactions of a similar or identical sort are facilitated, and control necessarily becomes more difficult.

Whether a child likes to identify with the parent models or not, he has no freedom in choosing, he cannot escape being shaped by their influence. Exposed constantly to the stressful observation of his model's active and reactive behavior, and to his own inner elaborations or behavioral responses to it, the child will have neither inspiration nor resources for developing attitudes of a different, more spontaneous and creative nature. That is, having formed habits due to a repetitive influence of a most monotonous, though explosive type, he has lost whatever potentialities he might have had for sound personal or original solutions. Insidiously he has become saturated with the mode of living of his disturbed surroundings; he has become theirs and is no longer his own. Who he could have been and become he will never know.

Unlike his privileged fellows, who have had some acquaintance with the sublime genius of mankind, he has no resources for such self-identification. In that austere company the privileged child has at times risen to lofty heights. Whether eagle or wren, in that high altitude a self-experience is gained which can never be erased and which creates repeated self-identifications with supreme moments of being.

## Trying To Escape the Inevitable

As a worker for the Juvenile Court, I have studied the problem of Theresa, a twelve-year-old girl who lived in a one-room apartment with her mother and an aunt, both prostitutes. Theresa slept in one bed with her mother and was made to get up when a customer came. Then she had to sleep sitting in the room, her head on the table.

Theresa was a gentle and depressed girl. Her school teacher had devoted a great deal of attention to her and had observed the girl in her conflict between instinctual drives and the longing for virtue, for which, however, the child could not resort to either a maternal or a paternal ideal figure. Her image of the male was fragmentary.

The duration, intensity, and the more or less exclusively symbolic nature of identification which was all that was possible with the teacher and court worker could not compete with the duration and intensity of the maternal influence and the gross experience in the home. The teacher could watch the girl standing at the entrance of an alley leading to a brothel and attended by young people of her age or slightly older. She was apparently experimenting with the thought of yielding to temptation, yet trying to build up a resistance by disapproval. The child had a sad apprehension of not being able to escape the destiny mapped out for her by her mother's disreputable way of life and by permanent exposure to its influence. Profoundly dependent upon her mother, witness to her sexual promiscuity, Theresa was deeply involved in guilt. Dimly she knew that she had no hope. Rather than being a means to an end, the behavior of Theresa's mother was an end in itself and barely transcended the sphere of vegetative living.

How could we formulate Theresa's fundamental dilemma? To see her, gentle, sad, and delicate, she did not seem predestined to an existence devoid of more idealistic aspects. The possibility that our society is at fault simply cannot be discounted. Acceptable or inacceptable behavior as judged by society does not reveal motivations. While society protects itself from undesirable and destructive influences, it must respect the outcast who has reasons of his own to "fail." While the impact of instinctual drives may weigh heavily in the scale of decision, particularly in adolescence, personality problems and emotions of the subtler and nobler order are still of high relevance in motivating and determining the outcome of the conflict.

While deplorable from the point of view both of the individual and of the human community, failure has its inherent logic, and under the circumstances was the unavoidable road, and thus the only solution at hand. Not unless we introduce new causal factors, such as treatment, for instance, to bear on the child's inner reality, can we expect a different outcome of any of these children's gigantic losing struggles.

## Fate and the Will

Theresa, deprived of a maternal ideal figure, hard as she must have struggled to construct one, and reared under the impact and bondage of traumatic sexual impressions, lost her self-respect.

Placed with an aunt who lived several hundred miles from the girl's home, Theresa escaped and returned to her mother once the case was released from court. When I met her again, Theresa was fifteen, sad and gentle as before, but now pregnant and diseased; she said: "You see, here I am, it caught up with me after all."

Theresa lived in a world where all her needs were satisfied at best at the submarginal level. However, she was confronted with the amazing contradiction of being supposed to conform with all phases of desirable behavior when every crumb of bread she ate, her very sleep, her need for her mother involved her in such misery and shame as to make her burst out in wild screaming one night, whereupon her mother had her arrested. To have to yield her place in the mother's bed to a strange man once more had proved to be just too much.

Such involuntary involvement in the wrong is the very basis of these children's isolation and their apprehension of other people's fear of contact with them. They are considered taboo. This is eminently true with regard to companions of their own age, whose parents indeed dread, and are bound to dread, associations with any youngster like Theresa, who knows so much and is so troubled. These children sense it and are made acutely aware of it by the active contempt and hostility of those others who have the opportunity to live acceptable lives and be accepted.

In Theresa's case we are dealing with just another variation on one and the same theme, the dilemma which traps these children. To make her bread edible and purify the spring which quenched her thirst, Theresa had to identify with her mother. This identification isolated her even more profoundly, weakened her self-respect, and hampered her conforming to accepted standards. Theresa became insecure and confused. Such is the unbearable situation which many a child will circumvent, whether by violent hostility or by despair or by compensatory inflation of his ego, as an expression of basic ambivalence: i.e., his acceptance of established values and standards, and his inability to uphold them. If, on the contrary, children like Theresa identify strongly with accepted standards, satisfaction of their most elementary needs and natural appetites is prevented; their self-respect is gravely hurt.

Dayton's reluctance to join the family meal, because his mother "tried to poison his food," was an obvious expression of that insoluble dilemma. He was not the only one of the children we could observe stealing food nor the only one who was unable to refuse food at home and who thus felt doubly trapped and humiliated.

Dayton, refraining at one period of his treatment from joining the family table, used to arrive hours late. But, ravenously hungry, he ate, throwing away those dishes he believed to be poisoned, the ones his mother had prepared personally with particular care but ambivalent feelings.

He would reverse an actual situation most humiliating to him, saying that the mother supported her "pretender," who actually made gifts of food packages in a condescending attitude. He repeatedly asked the psychotherapist how she would feel about such an acceptance of gifts by a conceited man who did not belong to the family.

It is not frequent that a child is as definite at a crucial time as William was: He turned away from his mother, an alcoholic and prostitute, who, like Theresa's mother, lived with a prostitute sister. Both women had been arrested a number of times after having been found drunk and unconscious in the gutter.

William was a poor learner; his intelligence rating was on the borderline of mental deficiency. But he stood up against the home condition and ran away from it repeatedly and persistently, spending the night under bridges and porches whatever the weather, until he was brought to our attention by his school principal and removed from the home. He stubbornly struggled for years to make his placement agency and the Educational Therapy Center understand just how far he could comply with average ways. But he finally made a good and earnest adjustment, though not without passing through an intense crisis of longing for what he had left and revolting against social conformity.

William's identification with the mother would have amounted to partiality to her, not immediate sameness, as was the case of Theresa. Moreover, what Theresa knew of men was likely to make her hesitate, when there was still time for running away, to sleep under bridges and porches. With the boy, the particular, precocious knowledge aroused revolt; with the girl it aroused fear. Moreover, the girl was more subtle and sensitive, "thus the native hue of resolution" was "sicklied o'er with the pale cast of thought," and whatever her inner struggle, it lost "the name of action."

The two alternatives, the anguish of refusing to identify with her mother and the anguish of yielding to this identification held her in a tormenting grip, and the impressive flight back to the mother and to that self which had invaded her slowly but ineradicably was but dependent and automatic behavior, without spontaneity and hardly deserving the "name of action."

Slowly even dreams of a state of perfect harmony will vanish and Theresa will give up any hope that she will be able to overcome the bondage to her tragic heritage. Theresa needed less than what she dreamed of and more than she had.

Paradisiac tranquility, and, in the area of beliefs, conformity, is not conducive to any fruitful human endeavor. The search and conquest of fulfilment must be challenged. In final analysis it is a matter of *choice* motivated by a confident acceptance of life and elaborated by discourse, whether it be an inner dialogue or a stimulating disputation with an inspiring opponent.

## Sensitivity and Sex Relations: Causes for Promiscuity

We should like at this time to cast a cursory glance at the art of love-making, which has interesting implications for these children's sexual behavior.

Before the climax in sexual relations, the partners experience an emotional evolution. The early stages of maturation have preponderance when the sexual stimulation begins and the later stages of maturation as the sexual relation is consummated.

This evolution protects the sex relation from degenerating into a routine. It has to be built up each time. Each partner generates in the other the state of maturation required for the climax, which is an expression of the all-embracing roles the partners play for each other in a relation which is completely satisfying. Although a biological process, it has to engage the total person and create a total abandon in order to be gratifying. The extent of this creative process in the art of love and on the part of the lovers will determine the completeness of the satisfaction. One element in this maturation process is the capacity to love one's own emotions, as well as the ability to partake intensely and sensitively in the feeling of the other. The increase of one's own satisfaction and responsiveness to the other's needs promote and unfold specificity, intensity, and harmony of satisfaction in and of both partners.

This partaking in the partner's reactions to the relation represents a particular form of self-denial which is immediately rewarded. It is in this phase that the sex act is most obviously deprived of the character of a purely self-satisfying lonely performance which would reduce the partner to a mere instrument of pleasure. A true love relation recognizes the partner, senses and acknowledges his or her presence, takes considerate account of it, and encourages being taken account of in equal terms. Communion is emphasized and enhanced by the exchange of words at every phase leading to the climax of sex enjoyment.

The final surrender is usually announced in the initial phase. Women expose it in their childlike innocence and helplessness. The child-wife is represented in various guises in various cultures and areas. She symbolizes the initial stages of love-making. An obvious example is the "Shepherdess," image of innocence of the eighteenth century; a romantic cloak which reached into the early days of Freud's influence on sex concepts was the shy and modest female who, with lowered head, looked toward the ground with half-closed eyes.

The corresponding stage in men may be an accentuation of boyishness, as characterized frequently by a form of dependency, a tendency to search for the protective maternal features of woman before meeting her on grounds where the extremes of trust are necessary in view of the totality of abandon and mutual surrender.

Each of the partners is the child, unarmed. What the other receives in his mind is the partner's alleged strength and maturity. From this discrepancy where each is the child and offers the comfort of an adult, derives the partner's confidence in the other's innocent and unarmed attitude, as well as in his strength which he trusts will never be ill-used. Unless such confidence prevails, sexual relations, being dangerous, may be exciting, but will be perverted and consuming. They will represent a hostile passion which has nothing of the character of love.

However, a partner's childlike features do not remain hidden. The woman's inviting helplessness awakens her partner to awareness of his male ascendancy, and from a child he becomes the man he potentially is, and as such he can also inspire confidence. In turn, his need of her arouses her sense of power which she may use for the practices of pleasurable delay, of the playful fencing with all feminine armour until mutual conquest and surrender are achieved.

This initial phase of love-making is as critical as it is exciting. It is the one most easily lost in the routine of a constant relation. Through repetition the transition of one stage to the next is facilitated and the creativeness of the experience is endangered. It tends to degenerate into a rapid and monotonous procedure; certitude may become deadly. Polygamous tendencies have their source in the stagnant waters of a relation which has lost the stirring tension and excitement of each initial phase of love-making.

That all literature concerns itself so predominantly with the initial stages of love-making is due to its significance for the completeness of sexual enjoyment and the quality of experience in the final climax.

This phase also plays an important role in neurotic conditions. The inability of the man's mother to release the son is not solely due to her jealousy of his maleness but also to the fact that his childlike features will be turned toward the younger woman. She loses both the charm of young manhood and son and the radiance of childhood and early youth that, through him, surrounded and animated her.

The father's reactions toward the daughter are generally less obvious but still critical and intense. Depression, withdrawal, fantasies, and even acting out elsewhere are not uncommon. After marriage, economic preoccupation and professional occupation usually prevent intrusion upon the children's quarters. These, however, represent a temptation for an unoccupied mother-in-law. She is not distracted from her preoccupations with the son's emotional relations; on the contrary, she is ambivalently attracted by him and his family, since her services are desired within the house and with the grandchildren.

Interference by the older generation with the younger one takes the form either of the former's attitudes in actuality or of the role assigned to it either in reality or in imagination by the younger. The feeling of being interfered with by prolonged dependency upon the older generation leads generally to complex patterns of irritation of all the involved members against all.

Continued dependency of the younger upon the older generation may interfere with the initial stage of the sex relationship. Fear of unfaithfulness toward the older generation might arise from awareness of being childlike in the new relation. It deprives the first relationship and seems to be alien to the new "affiliation." Confusion and associated guilt feelings may arise from the analogies of new ties with old fantasies; therefore, the new relationship can only be consummated with anxiety. It becomes a secondary Oedipus or Electra situation; the wife becomes the mother of the husband-father. The couple may jump into the final stages without sensitive and gentle build-up, avoiding the early stages, which are anxiety-provoking. Therefore, satisfaction will not be experienced; depression follows a purely physical sex act from which part of one's own "soul and body," and therefore part of the partner's, was divorced.

What is really sought under such circumstances is an "unrelated" person, lest the element of infidelity to the elder, which cannot be totally discarded, enter the relationship. Continued belonging to "the older" as his or her child degrades the marital relation into a purely sexual one. This explains why passionate, apparently satisfying relations may become interchangeable and still may remain intensely dependent. An element of hostility as well as anxiety intensifies the dependency. The marital partner has grown into the role of "the older," and "legitimate" love is hunted for elsewhere; but each time it becomes legitimate, it assumes incestuous features and has to be renounced. What is sensed may be only the partner's failure to provide gratification as well as guilt for one's own hostility. No consideration is given whether the partner has had an opportunity to unfold his or her satisfying potentials and whether the unrewarding relationship is the consequence of an unsolved earlier attachment. Thus ambivalent reactions of hate and self-hate, destructive and self-destructive tendencies arise. These attitudes stand in the way of the regeneration of the relationship and the building up of the confidence which leads the partners in "childlike innocence" into the protective arms of each other.

A permanent longing for fulfilment may keep them together, until both love and longing, deception and resentment have ended in the death of all emotions—resentment surviving the longest. Nor is the gain of independence the necessary consequence of separation. These are the cases where mutual tribulations may continue over time and space. Other answers are not sought anymore and, if they are, may not be found or may again be unsatisfactory. The second marriage might find the partners more weary, overtly more compromising and equally as unrewarded unless some profound revision of their whole life is accepted.

Rather than represent the enticing initial charm of the woman, extreme exhibition of childlike features may seem ridiculous, repulsive, or irritating. In men, rather than radiant boyishness, it may assume obstinate irrationality; the dependency may become so complete that the man will deny himself professional success, expecting the wife-mother to take over. Rationalizations will be called upon to justify, by the assumed need for self-realization in vocational areas, the morbid professional inactivity and the social dependency in practical life. However, actual vocations and self-realization may not be pursued because of the urge for keeping the dependency alive, as well as the resentment of the punitive and self-punitive needs that ensue.

Another motive for omitting the initial phase of childlike beginnings of the sex relation may be the intense anxiety retained from harsh, punitive, and rejecting parental attitudes. In these cases, to be a child represents a state of utter isolation and exposure, and it cannot be re-enacted as the initial stage of love-making that leads, in the final analysis, to utmost and confident abandon. This implies the trust in total reciprocation, which in these cases may not have been experienced, and in the partner's strength to let him find his way back to independence and the active renewal of the tie. Though momentary, the liberation is essential for the preservation of the vitality of the relation.

Necessarily, sensitivity has remained undeveloped due to early and chronic emotional neglect, a factor which intensifies the problem. Even if we disregard this phase of the problem at this time, anxiety at the thought of being a disarmed child again suffices to cause fear of exposure to this condition. Due to this anxiety, the preparatory phases of love-making will be deprived of their playful delight and promise, and the sexual act will be accomplished with the fear of not being acceptable. To secure its accomplishment the victim of such emotions will attempt to proceed with utter speed. Feeling unwanted and under pressure, thus on the defensive in an emergency, the man will be devoid of any consideration and tempted to be cruel. We have also been able to observe girls in such condition, who tend to give everything rapidly in order to secure acceptability, only to find that their very zeal has caused their acceptability to vanish as soon as the gift was handed out and that in their distress and emergency they have to begin all over again, emergency and distress increasing as their acceptability, and with it their self-esteem, becomes more dubious.

For the technique of love-making, early maternal rejection may be of fundamental importance. Sensuousness, such as gentle stroking of the skin and outlining the body contours, rooted in those earliest stages where the child is subjected to the tender acceptant love-making by the mother, may remain an unawakened need and thus a defect in the building-up phase and, therefore, prevent perfect consummation of each sex relation.

We have described the children's sex development in terms of their libido dynamics. In contrast to the children's lack of opportunity in observing refined and discreet expressions of love in its wholeness, and in contrast to their precocious and excessive exposure to mere sexuality, stands the way children flirted and "made love" among themselves in group therapy. All of our group therapists had identical experiences, whatever their own sex, age, or race. Contrary to experiences in the day-care group, where at times an epidemic of sexual unrest may break out, acting out in the therapeutical group showed these children no different from any well-trained and well-behaved child experiencing the first enchantment of early love. Some of them had been referred specifically for promiscuity, excessive sex interest and activities; few of them were lacking in knowledge as far as sex was concerned.

We shall disregard at this time the reasons for the difference in behavior in the general group from the behavior in the small therapy group. The approach of these children to one another was sometimes as delicate as could be described by an artist's pen or brush. This impressive charm actually was a fundamental reason for their promiscuity; in other terms, their "innocence" was the condition of their continued "culpability." The children could not benefit from experience. They were always beginning anew. Every fresh contact was like a new dawn of day. They were but a delightful piece of nature beyond good and evil. They just lived in the present moment without remembering or foreseeing. There were those among the girls who were totally narcissistic, actually enjoying their own charm as others would an accomplishment, and the observable play actually appeared similar to an aesthetic achievement. They knew how to choose the boy who would fit into that play and knew how to perform with him something completely innocent and gracious in appearance.

They are those who are in search of themselves and of a single lovable trait they might glean from the eye, the assurance or the behavior of a boy. This need is so important that it haunts them as urgently as sexual desire or self-hatred. Moreover, the hope that the man might redeem them causes them to throw themselves away. They are as timid and reluctant when approached and as delighted by attention as any inexperienced young girl.

Simultaneously, the boy feels enhanced by the gift of his approval and delight. The value he himself creates at the moment makes him the owner of a treasure, though he might not be devoid of doubt and skepticism which match the girl's insecurity.

These girls, many of whom had been deserted by both parents, are often raised by conscientious relatives, mostly single elderly women. Treatment revealed what had been missing in their upbringing, and the knowledge of their background and their guardians confirmed it. Neither father nor mother had been wasting precious hours of enjoyment on them, looking at them with enchantment, talking sweetly and sillily to them to solicit their first specifically human response which is the child's clumsily sketched first smile, unique expression of comfort in the presence of acceptance and the child's manifestation of assent to an inviting world.

In normal situations, such early arousal is preceded, and continues to be followed, by the parents' fond glances and gentle handling, thus tenderly developing the child's sense of being and self-identification. The supporting hand which is held under the child's back is comparable to the safe ground on which the adult stands. The child's back is his first base of contact with safe ground. In view of its eminent importance this "sole" is of enormous proportion relative to the total body surface, a signal announcer of danger or security. With his back the child begins to respond and to sense the responses he has solicited and elicited from the mother's hand, and in a dim way he learns that he is not helpless. Contrary to the neglected child who will whine in discomfort or lose stamina for action, the loved and tended child will learn to promote the proper responses to his needs. This means that he can, as time goes on, rise above the state of pure being into action.

At the same time, the world becomes motherly and satisfactory, a promise of pleasure. The mother's mobile hand simultaneously draws the child's outlines; she thus prepares the child for the awareness and acceptance of his bodily self, his bodily limits, and the many points of contact with the world. Through the mother's responsive support and through her gentle strokes, the familiarity with the world is established. His first adventures will be incurred by the tactile travels of his small hands on her bosom, her neck, and the most unsuitable places of her face. Infants who are given insufficient amounts of the delightful luxury of love, those who lie lonely on an unresponsive mattress with no sensitive maternal fingers lightly tracing their outlines, do not learn early about their being, its limits and its powerful capacity for producing responses, for changing unpleasurable conditions. Expecting no answer and fostering no hope to come from an inert world, they will be late and awkward in exploring, if not disturbed to the point of not responding at all.[1] We can see those children sit inertly, or rush and run blindly, some of them permanently imbued with good will but in trouble all the time because they are insensitive to the world and its concrete reality, to the other fellow's condition, and too impatient and anxious to learn about their own.

Sexual experience is used by the deprived children as a medium for a belated gaining of self-awareness, self-assurance, and pleasure. That this area should be chosen is due to its exquisite fitness to provide for the satisfaction of the neglected sensory needs of the past and the intense relatedness of sensory and sexual urges. It reproduces most readily the early state where responses and successes are achieved by a way of being, rather than any active endeavor and mastery through intelligent manipulation of matter. Efforts are small, urges intense, and rewards immediate, whatever the aftermath.

Very few of these children, if any at all, have been raised under conditions where they could witness the expressions of affectionate communion between the parents. These expressions we like to call play. They raise the parental relationship from pressing necessity to the loftier heights of imagination. The child thus learns to toy with charmingly unpredictable situations, to live in suspense with regard to what could develop from them. He will not be weighed down by a rigid clinging to concrete reality and what is immediately at hand. He who knows how to play can leave answers in abeyance; he includes the future in the enjoyment of the moment. When the parents play with him, identifying him with the partner delightedly seen in the child's cherished features, it feels supremely comfortable, gives in to both, and, in a sense, is begotten and born anew. Each time, through the joy of living, developing tendencies are enhanced and the trend to grow up is promoted. As time goes on, a strong awareness of being will give the child the tendency to react to those influences which will further self-realization at an early age; the very factors of spontaneity observed in the parents' love will arouse his own spontaneity. In his childish hide-and-seek play, he will reveal that he is not necessarily yours, but only if he so chooses. You must go and search for him, behind his little hands, or later by the sides of his crib or behind the door. Like his parents at play, he will be thoroughly caught by the thrill of suspense, and the anticipation that he will be captured.

Such an enchanting joy of laughter and life itself is unknown to the children who concern us in our work, children whose parents don't live together, who never really belonged together and therefore never included the children—unforeseen by-products of their sexual activity—in their community. Instead they are exposed to crude realities which are terrifying to them. To escape fear they experiment with the very thing that frightens them as long as it is unknown, as a self-experience. As an adult behavior, it also seems important behavior and the child believes it enhances his own status if he or she emulates adult behavior in this impressive area.

We shall tell the story of Queen Miller which illustrates these considerations:

Queen actually had three names—her mother's name and the name of the mother's husband, though nobody knew whether he actually was the father; she had a third family name because she was born in the hospital of a distant city, where the mother was confined under the name of a distant relative who had hospital insurance. She left the child with this woman, whom she barely knew, pretending later that she had thought she was a married woman in orderly circumstances. Queen was the third of five children; two elder sisters were illegitimate and there is every reason to believe that Queen was also.

Queen was referred to us by the Welfare Department because her temper tantrums and sexual behavior made it impossible to keep her in public school. She had been committed as incorrigible by her parents because she constantly ran away from home. But the school teacher believed she was ill treated and the school authorities had reported the father as cruel, because Queen came to school bruised from strappings.

Queen once gave a snapshot to her psychotherapist, showing a most gracious, smiling six-year-old, missing two front teeth. When we met her she was nearly twelve, a homely, stocky, short girl, who was never seen without her thumb in her mouth. She was sensitive, and her attitude varied between affectionate sweetness and a peeved, negative aggressiveness.

In the day-care group she had a tendency to stray away from the classroom and move around the hall and its darkest corners, her thumb in her mouth, in search of the boys who, however, good naturedly rejected her, pretending she was still a baby in need of a pacifier.

When she began to communicate, she talked obsessively about her father's hatefulness and violence, but slowly a picture of the total family was gained. It confirmed facts known to the Welfare Department, and it clarified the meaning of the emotional situation. The mother and grandmother were victims of circumstances, after the grandfather's death, both having a tendency to be helpful to the point of making people dependent and resentful of their help. Thus a group of people were crowded together, each in the way of the other, resentful of each other, and an imposition on the poor mother who was incapable of meeting the needs of a dependent mother, dependent siblings, a dependent husband, dependent children, and the starved illegitimate children of her elder daughters. These also had a serious problem with the mother's husband, who revolted against everybody's dependency but his own.

It is at one stage of this tragic cycle that the temptation arose to make Queen, as a new-born infant, appear to be another woman's child and forget about her.

The woman who raised Queen lived in a large northern city. She was a prostitute and lived in a one-room apartment in a tenement house. Queen remembered that while living with the substitute mother she never had milk and was always hungry. She recalled with delight a meal given to her by a kind woman who served her milk, chicken, and white potatoes. However, she was given whiskey and cigarettes by the woman she lived with, and to quote Queen "was taught nothing of what a child should know and all it should not know." In school she felt out of place and, as in the tenement house, preferred to be in a hall in search of comforts of her own.

It was with intense emotion that Queen, who had never heard of a therapeutical couch, after several years of an intense attachment to her therapist, one day took a garden chaise-longue standing in her psychiatrist's office and placed it in a convenient spot. Reclining, she began to speak with closed eyes: The woman who had raised her during the first years of her existence brought home men from the street or from an inn across the street, at the rate of at least three a day. Most of them were drunk and so was the woman. Until about the age of four Queen was a witness to the woman's activities and took them for granted. From then on it frightened her, and she usually was put into the hall of the house. At first she used to play and forget, but she became more terrified as time went on. When Queen was under five years of age, a boy whom she had never seen came through the hall, and to alleviate her fear she got him to join her and tried out with him what was an unknown thing, which intrigued and frightened her.

One day, the woman fatally stabbed one of her clients. She was apprehended and the police found the child. Subsequent to a search for Queen's natural family, she was turned over to them without inquiry into their suitability for her education. The mother, a total stranger to the child, came for her from a southern rural town. Queen reported the anxiety felt when she traveled—"alone," as she significantly recalled—to the strangers supposed to be her next of kin. She could never recover from the feeling of living among strangers, though she excluded grandmother and mother. She was at a loss to understand why, meeting family members on the street, she would cross over to the other side. She also mentioned fear of sexual aggression from any of the men.

Queen suffered from phobias. During the years of treatment she passed from an extended state of dependency and her stubborn symptom of constant thumb-sucking to an insecure competition with other girls, an attitude she gave up after a crisis of deep remorse, having been taught by cruel evidence how her denunciation could hurt and defeat another child. At first she built up a harsh and righteous conscience by criticizing others, revealing the inner menace she thus conquered by standing at the window, looking at the prostitutes and drunken men in the street, making despicable remarks. She developed a symptom of folding the curtain between her fingers and rubbing them against the curtain while sucking her thumb, and began to be concerned about her own problems in terms of her filiation to the devoted foster-mother (who had been appointed by the State Welfare), to the church she wanted to join, the children of the neighborhood with whom she associated. This implied problems of common endeavor and equality. But Queen was not yet able to reach out for the real issue. She needed crutches. She tested this equality by expressing the desire for ownership of a bicycle and attendance at the public school.

Having been unsuccessful with the boys in the day-care group of the Educational Therapy Center and in the use of lures copied from the woman who had raised her, Queen had gone through an extended stage of tomboyish behavior and fighting. Her dress was torn by a rigid and highly sensitive boy on such an occasion, and she was exposed in her slip. Although the boys, with kind firmness, carried the young fighter from the scene and behaved in a fond and surprisingly discreet way, Queen had a violent temper tantrum and was disconsolate for hours. Finally Queen's therapist managed to take her up to the office. There it was discovered that although the dress had been given to Queen by the Welfare Department, she considered it a gift from the foster mother. Queen pretended she had sewed it for her. To Queen it was a symbol of filiation with the loving and respectable woman. It meant virtue and wholeness; it covered her underlying indignity. The dress that had seemed ruined was perfectly restored, having yielded in the seams only.

Queen could grasp the symbolic meaning of this restoration in the therapeutic session. Much of her anxiety in reference to the irreparability of her past indignity and the hopelessness of her acceptability and integration into a less scarred human community was overcome step by step from then on. She became more generous with herself and others and therefore was finally able to confess what she thought were the worst indignities of her life, which she had feared would cost her the therapist's love. At this time she understood trustfully that she would be neither condemned nor deserted. She had matured to the point where, having gained a perspective on distance covered, she also became aware of her effort and sensed the achievement. This liberated her from her dependency upon the therapist and other supportive women in her life (foster mother and teacher). Though she knew she might not actually risk loss of love by her confession, she was capable of risking it.

A few months later, her foster mother had to go to the hospital, and Queen had to be placed elsewhere, with a woman who had two other foster children, one older and very successful in school and another several years younger than Queen. The foster mother was much more worldly and outgoing, much less protective than the first one. Queen made a splendid adjustment in home, school, and community, in particular she could live with the more mature and adequate child, and assume the part of a helpful elder sister with the other. She was a radiant, most attractive young girl when last seen, capable of analyzing her circumstances, her human relations, her own behavior and goals, with remarkable discrimination. She stoically took the disappointment of leaving Richmond, for which she had fostered a profound affection, because so much love, friendship, and genuine affection everywhere had contributed to the adjustment she had so ardently struggled for.

We may add here that Queen had been able to benefit not only from positive circumstances but also from adverse ones. Rather than succumb, she profited from frankly viewing the shocking conditions in her family. During treatment she had longed to visit them, beset by guilt feelings, particularly toward the mother's husband, a dependent as well as righteously religious man, despite his cruel treatment of the child.

## The Oedipus Complex: Help and Hindrance

Co-operation of child and parent in education should be based on the anticipation on the part of both generations that the child will one day embody all the characteristics of an accomplished adult. Identification with the parents and formation of ideals could not be conceived without such anticipation, and though implicit, the Oedipus complex can be regarded as the sexual aspect of such an anticipation. In this light we can understand why the child identifies necessarily with the person of his own age group. However, since the accomplished adult embodies an integration of the total attributes of man, which include all the evolutionary stages, the child will also have to achieve an identification with people from numerous integrative steps which lead toward the accomplished development, whether the modes of identification are with real or fictitious people. Thus the child finds interesting motivations for contacts and relations in general.

In other terms, these identifications occur because the achievement of accomplished adulthood is an abstract and distant goal. The love of the parent of the other sex is suggested by the very fact of this identification, if for no other reason. Such love is an experiment, whatever emotions may be involved, in the vast majority of cases. It is actually not destined to be carried out to its ultimate conclusion. The parents' general role of protectors and prohibitors is well suited to answer the child's need for inhibition. It provides rationalization of his normal reluctance for consummation of sex experience at this stage. The parents' function as representatives and models of adulthood in general is necessary but not sufficient. The specific parental function as loving and protective adults must combine with their will to refrain from interference with the child's goal of reaching accomplished adulthood.

All real love objects are conceived as admirable. They are "adored." Only when partaking of such quality can they be relied upon to preserve the ideal to be attained. Since high resolve is man's best share in all that is desirable, aspiring toward the goal of the perfected adult type is one of the happiest and most rewarding experiences for both parents and children. These experiences convey a sense of value and are prerequisites for identification with other ideals which represent other incarnations of the accomplished adult type. In a humiliated condition the child shuns comparison with these ideals. The child who is deprived of self-respect and self-esteem will try to restore those qualities by correcting the humiliating reality, either exalting his own status unrealistically or denigrating the status of the objects to be matched.

Further evidence that all real love objects are conceived as admirable can be found in the striking observation that sex-delinquent girls, when in a position to choose, tend persistently toward refined and intellectual boys. The need and longing for perfection exerts a protective influence on the loving person, who is sensitive and alert to the loved one's potentials even before they have been realized. However, every love object is bound to fall short of expectations; it must be reinstated again and again to uphold the love object's role, as well as the sense of values of both partners. Preoccupation with the lacks in the loved one's perfection and resulting censoriousness, rather than enjoyment and encouragement of positive qualities, exhaust the capacity of the loved person to strive for his or her highest potentials for self-realization, as well as fulfilment of the role of an "adorable" and "adored" partner.

## Love and Disillusion

Lynn's case is one of excessive reliance on the admirability and protective capacity of her father, which she tested excessively.

Lynn, an endearing twelve-year-old girl, the adopted child of an uncongenial couple, was used as a means of re-establishing their marriage. It resulted in a competition by the parents in overprotecting her.

Lynn identified with her mother. She expressed this suddenly one day, seeing a picture of a mother and child: "I am the mother and the child."

She adored her father; she would crawl into his bed, thus creating a conflict in the father. He struggled to uphold his protective role and to match the child's untarnished ideal image. But soon he found himself involved with another woman. She was an evident substitute, with attenuated incestuous traits, far younger than his wife and only a few years older than his little girl.

Lynn and the mother understandably saw only his failures. The little girl, who tearfully confessed, "I thought so highly of him," did not only love her love and her protector but also cherished her identification with the mother. Both ideal images were tarnished and degraded by their mutual rejection. The rejection devaluating the mother included Lynn, who identified with her. Moreover, the vulnerability of the mother, her initial despair, and later the comfort accepted from other men, made identification inadmissible to a child who had idealized her. A tragic side-aspect of this case was the fact that the child chosen to bridge the gap between the parents innocently became the instrument that cut the last ties.

Lynn's trauma occurred after a number of years of opportunity to build up an ideal. Most children we could observe were not fortunate enough to have a model of striving parents to follow; they had to deny reality early and to retouch their parents' portrait beyond recognition. Such touching up, however, is generally necessary to define the goal. Too many individual variants would become confusing, the identification with what is common to mankind would be impossible. What differs from case to case is the concrete material available and used for the molding of what each individual envisions as the accomplished type.

An intellectual boy of twelve once told his psychotherapist, "I hope my father does not have shortcomings I am unaware of."

A little eight-year-old girl, concerned about her father's dissenting creed, raised him to the status "next to Jesus." The illusion needed for definition of the goal also serves as a means of detachment from disappointing concrete realities.

The process of growth and of a stepwise growing detachment from the parents can be achieved by way of many adverse complexities. Indeed the detachment cannot be accomplished unless discriminating elements of the relationship are emphasized. If the relationship is too satisfactory, one of two alternatives will occur: either the detachment will be delayed, retarding the process of maturation, or the child will be antagonistic to the bad features of his milieu until he becomes absorbed, felled, and defeated in his vain struggle to uphold ideals.

Whether the child is poorly equipped mentally or fairly alert, whether crude or sensitive, the process of sex maturation will be extremely subtle and complex. We shall further illustrate the complex and subtle experiences of sex maturation observed in children of varying intelligence and raised in extremely deprived families.

## The Importance of Legitimacy

At the age of sixteen Emmett, a feeble-minded boy referred by a policewoman for truancy and being a public nuisance, was still inching along on the first-grade level, extremely proud of any achievement which he could display for admiration. He was very sensitive to the fact that, as he said, his mother had entirely too many children, multiplying their actual number by five. Although born out of wedlock, he attributed legitimacy to himself, denying it to his mother's other children who were identified with their fathers. These children equate legitimacy with prior rights to their mother's love; as this contains an element of self-love, they consider all fathers as intruders.

Emmett's various sex difficulties became serious enough to warrant an attempt to expose him to some form of individual psychotherapy. One day he requested sex relations from his young female psychotherapist, one of the aspects of such a request being his need to feel adequate and accepted. When his blunt request did not lead to the imagined result, he tried a number of devices to make himself acceptable. He tried to find and hold a job. Moreover, to convey to himself, as a male, superior status and threaten the psychotherapist as a female, though simultaneously trying to encourage her, he stated that heterosexual contacts had been more exciting to him than homosexual ones. He pretended to have had most satisfactory experiences with mature women, which, he said, conveyed to him a feeling of greater security. Thus he appealed also to elements of protective love.

Actually this entire elaboration was an almost literal transference of problems lived and acted out previously to punish his mother, whose experiences were too much for him to bear. While the boy experimented thus with problems of general and sexual maturation, his own mother, a feeble-minded woman with many illegitimate children, sensed the child's transference of Oedipus fantasies on to the therapist and became jealous of the boy's attendance at the Center. At a time when Emmett matured visibly and displayed improved posture as a manifestation of a sound self-realization and self-assertion, as well as a certain relaxation of his excessive sensitivity to his family problems, his mother pretended that Emmett did not want to come for treatment anymore. The child then requested commitment to the training school for the retarded children, in order to have opportunity for growth and education.

Another child, John, thirteen years of age, was almost as blunt but even more subtle in his transference of Oedipus fantasies onto his psychotherapist.

John was of dull-normal mentality and a persistent truant. He came from a barren home in the slums. He would bluntly inform the children at the Center and all visitors that the therapist was his mother, and that he was going to marry her. In order to erect the barriers this relationship required, he would mention to the other boys that she had a husband who loved her very much. Thus he enhanced her value as much as he increased the distance. The husband, said the boy, might object to her consenting to marry him. At a later stage, he wished he could marry the therapist's daughter, thus showing increased reality adjustment in dreaming up love objects closer to his own age. At the time when incestuous fantasies concerning his siblings were sublimated slowly, he identified with his age group and with himself. Moreover, from a blunt indicative statement, he expressed his wishes in the subjunctive mood.

Incestuous fantasies are fostered in reference to older women. Frequently they are acted out, since emotionally deprived children have great difficulty in delaying the fulfilment of their instinctual needs. Their unanswered needs are so great, insecurity and lack of faith in the future is so immense, their frustration tolerance so low, that delay could depreciate rather than raise their self-esteem. Though acting under the impact of great stress these boys are not devoid of guilt feelings. These may take the shape of "not ever wanting to get married" lest the wife "play with young fellows" while he would be at work. Guilt and sensitivity may take the shape of idolizing the woman in her maternal quality as well as providing for some legitimacy for the partnership with her, in being her children's playmate and protector. Thus, while the Oedipus complex is acted out, the youngster gratifies childlike dependency needs and uses rationalization to redeem the situation.

One of these mentally and emotionally underdeveloped boys was fourteen, but physically precocious. His present foster parents had adopted him out of pity. Now old and infirm, their home life was dreary and miserable despite their good will. The boy was pent up with frustration. He stuttered; he was a truant, slow of learning, and when sent on errands, likely to keep the foster parents' money without coming home.

Visits to a woman in his community gave him compensation for all that he had missed so far, the presence of an alluring woman, attractive living quarters, small children with whom he liked to play. He felt a need to justify his visits as "minding her children," thus assuming a paternal role which gave him an adequate status, at the same time, he gratified his unsatiated need to play. Time and again he would tell his psychotherapist that he had no space to play in at home, except for a board which he placed on his bed and upon which he had affixed the rails of his only toy, a small train that he moved back and forth along the rails. (See also the case history of Virginia, in Appendix.)

## The Death of Laius as a Symbol

In John (already mentioned in this chapter), we find another case of confusion involving incestuous desires. His father was a steady worker and though not without some guile, a most dignified person. The mother was hard of hearing, and made use of this infirmity in every possible way. She understood only what she desired to hear. She begged from agencies and privately from accessible benevolent people. She asked John for assistance because of his attractive personality, his splendid verbalism, and uninhibited fantasy.

There were six siblings; three boys and three girls in the family. The oldest and the youngest sisters were the objects of John's fantasies. The second sister was sexually promiscuous. The older brother had been engaged in numerous delinquencies.

John was referred to us at the age of barely thirteen, by the public school, for persistent truancy. At that time he used an identification with his father and a protective attitude toward the mother as motivation for staying at home. The mother, he felt, needed him. Away from school he helped her in her begging at agencies; he went fishing and supported the family in various ways. This he expressed with "I like to help my mama."

At a later date, due to our influence and due to skills acquired in the shop, he was intensely interested in restoring the dilapidated home to a respectable condition. He reasoned that his father was so old he might die soon. Of course, in order to appease his conscience he also had to save his father's life, thus becoming its creator. He feigned this role reversal by saying: "I wanted to be bigger than my father."

The resulting conflict, the self-punishment, the search for communion with the father, divinization and sublimation are revealed in the following story.

John repeatedly reported a number of accidents, each of which brought him to the threshold of death. "There is no place on my body where there is no wound and no place where there is no scar," an assertion which he could prove to be true. "I know," he would pursue sorrowfully, "I was bad and I dared God," but smilingly he would continue, "but though I was far gone, God must have been with me. He gave life again. You see, I cannot help thinking he must have wanted me after all." The boy repeatedly said that he was not sure whether we all knew what was "God-willed." John was well versed in the Scriptures and some of their profound interpretations. He asserted that it was his father who had taught him, though they never went to church. Their church was at home, they did not believe in those who expounded God's word for a salary. He implied that his father, and the son through him, had an immediate, not a mediate, relationship to God.

Because of the mother's complete inadequacy, John was placed in a foster home. He apparently did not have a chance in his own home to learn to work and to be reliable at any task. Though undoubtedly the boy profited by the placement, he was not far from the truth when he expressed his feeling that his own home was more humble, less self-righteous, and less sinful that the well-accepted and outwardly more acceptable foster home. He wanted to be allowed to be himself. In his usual, impressive way, he pleaded with a constancy derived from profound conviction. Because he had been so often near death, he was under the impression that a covenant was signed in his own blood. Any change, then, could only amount to making him lose this awesome, mysterious, and infinitely precarious and sacred tie.

His transference to his therapist was of a similar nature as to the parents, particularly to the mother, and his adjustment was partly due to his intense desire to assist her with the purposes of the Center. He thus displaced his concrete attachment to her to more general goals. The boy confessed, "To tell you the truth, you are the Center for me. I was born in the Center and I shall live in the Center until I shall die."

As John grew more and more independent of the mother, he would verbalize amply his relationship to an older sister who was murdered when he was about eleven years old. She had lived, according to him, a prodigal life, having acquired almost fabulous riches through gambling. Although married, she had a great number of "admirers," one of whom robbed and killed her. Substituting for his father, John accompanied his mother to the funeral, which took place in a distant city where this sister had resided. He pretended that this sister had willed him with a sum of money, that would be given to him when he became of age, for having once saved her life.

His relationship to this sister was very complex. He intensely and admiringly identified himself with her. He was her "life giver" and posthumous advisor, her son and lover, the one who, when he grew up, would enjoy the gifts of her devotion. It is remarkable that for him his sister's influence in this world had not stopped with her disappearance. He stated with profound conviction that her husband's death, three months after his sister's, was of her doing, although she was dead. "She killed him," he said, with deep conviction. Thus, apparently she substituted for his instinctive drives, relieving his conscience of responsibility for the consequences of his death wishes. This way, the sister's bequest gained symbolic significance as a surrogate for never silenced admiration, longing, and frustration.

At a later period, his little sister entered the picture. John wanted to save money; he wished to provide for her marriage. She was ten years old and was "going soon to come along in life." He was concerned about her morals and wanted to take her to church on Sunday, thus protecting and sanctifying their relationship. At this stage he pretended that he had many "girlfriends"; he identified in this manner with his oldest sister who was "killed for love or what you may call it," and in this manner he protected his youngest sister from his interest in her.

Furthermore he envisioned the time when she would be married. The man who was going to marry her was imagined as in need of John's economic assistance, of which, in John's mind, he would be assured in advance. John foresaw that he himself would be otherwise engaged. He thus found a legitimate or pseudo-legitimate way of consummating his eternal ownership of the sister, as well as a way to renounce her without loss, regret, and diminution of importance.

John's internal management of this emotional involvement with his younger sister points to the common origin of all human myth.

We find the very same relationships, as seen in the actual life of a destitute southern Negro child, in the Norse heroic legend of the Nibelungs, as well as in its recreated version by the nineteenth-century German author and composer, Richard Wagner. It is the story of Siegfried, the hero who makes himself invisible and conquers for the inadequate Gunther the invincible Walkyrie, Brunhilde, who becomes the wife of that weak and dependent man.

# VII

*Relation to Objects*

We have seen that these deprived children's relationship to objects is determined by material as well as emotional need. But being a conceptual and a suffering being even when most cruelly beset by circumstances, man barely ever reaches out for mere realities but for symbols of an altered status. We hope to give ample evidence for this conviction in this chapter. In discussing the transference to the house, for instance, we shall highlight the symbolism of the children's apparent vandalism. Due to problems of space we had to refrain from demonstrating by specific examples how vandalism may express, in opposition to what it seems, the child's violent bidding for being included and harbored.

This chapter will illustrate the child's relationship to objects as we can observe it in his spontaneous behavior in the therapeutic milieu and in therapy proper. We shall see the constant overlapping of real and symbolic needs, whether the child indulges in the comfort of undisturbed existence at the beginning of his recovery or whether he struggles with people dedicated to his welfare.

## The Helpless and the Helped Explorer

In the therapeutic home the child begins to turn to various objects which the Clinic has deliberately introduced for his benefit. He enters more and more into the inner recesses and enfolding coziness of the house, the friendly atmosphere produced by a seemingly infinite number of things, toys in particular, that are so precious to a child's imagination. To begin with, the milieu is surprising and fascinating. If the child were alone, left to his own curiosity, the object of his study as such would provide an answer to his inquiry. But it would stop there, either because the answer would have been gained at the expense of the object's remaining whole, or because at this stage of the child's development the object would yield only a limited, repetitive, monotonous response that does not stimulate motivation for further search. The child may not be able to make out even the purpose of the object, because he is not in sufficient contact with either reality or the surrounding culture. Stubborn attempts to force the "dumb" object, originally desired by the child as a promise of pleasurable gratification, into yielding more than reiterated responses to his quest for knowledge, can be extremely irritating. Instead of progressing, the frustrated child will return for exploration to each of his sensory tentacles finally resorting to the oral cavity as his last and predominant resource. A perverted or negative relationship to objects is an inevitable result.

Children left prematurely and almost exclusively to their own devices can be observed running vehicles back and forth or banging soldiers against each other. There are some who are no longer spontaneous enough to stop. There are others who let the movement gradually cease as if they were exhausted by their futile activity. Yet, in the mere presence of an adult, even without inspiring and properly timed guidance, the children will become more resourceful. Being watched fondly, and thus reassuringly, they become aware that they are accomplishing something, and their actions will tend to become more varied and reflective. These tendencies can be prompted by questions as soon as the child has gained self-confidence and trust.

This observation has practical implications. Emotionally disturbed children may not be able to do their homework by themselves. Usually their parents find it difficult to lend them the necessary support by their fond and interested presence and discourage rather than promote any tendency toward independent work. They show an irate resentment of the child's need of them and their assistance. They find as little enjoyment in the uplifting task of leading their child out of the darkness of ignorance and are no more inspired than the intimidated child in educating himself. Parents can be helped to recognize the fact that watching the child play or work provides as much comfort and reassurance as answering his call, "watch me do it." What he requires is silent approval for some daring act. He will feel safe in trying anything that the attentive or interested, protective or loving adult will not prevent him from doing.

Inside the shelter of the Clinic, where people gather, with weapons laid aside, children begin to trust the friendly animation that pervades the homelike atmosphere. They are at leisure to "recognize" their hidden wishes and take delight in their fulfilment. Motivated by the joys inherent in fulfilment, gradually they conceptualize what they have gained from play, and they retain what thoughts and language they discover. As time goes on they ask for more than help in dealing with the object at hand. They become explicit in the telling of their problems because they anticipate assistance. They will be more and more specific in the awareness, as well as in the communication of, their needs. Soon the child will be ready to project his own creative ideas onto his toys. To break the monotony of the object's sterile re-action, he will no longer have to run to the stores for promiscuous satisfaction. Whatever he has, he can endow with an endless variety of new answers which bring forth new questions, and real interplay of imagination between him and his now rewarding object ensues. Broken toys can now be cherished and preserved, for they seem animated and have their own history. They hold a promise for further developments. Penetration into the heart and hearth of things has occurred. The world, as a whole, begins to envelop the child protectively as does his own house seen from the inside and unified by his own way of being and of shaping things. He can lay away his weapons, he feels invited, legitimate, and ready to stay.

Whoever feels he can have his share in shaping the events at hand and in the world he is engaged in molding necessarily develops a sense of ownership and of belonging. Although still ambivalent or timid, the child has set his foot in the door.

## To Have as a Help in Being

*Ownership* is one way of becoming aware of existence and consciously aware of one's own existence and identity. When the mother has failed by unaccepting or wavering feelings to confirm her child's existence, the taking, the possession of objects and the, however vain, attempt to hold on to them may be one of the child's substitutional measures of testing the ever threatened reality of existence.

*To Be* means *to be somebody*, whether the child calls it so or its opposite "a nobody," "a bum." One of our boys once burst out in a group session with the joyous admission: "I feel like a big shot when I take something, but when I think of you [the therapist] I want to put it back." Because of "you," he needed no artificial aggrandizement, he now was someone, he was rewarded already, and the reward had constituted his conscious existence and made it legitimate.

Thus when a child has been invited and allowed to take hold of a place and make it his home, he has gained a first precarious hold of himself. No longer driven, shiftless, and overwhelmed by abysmal anxiety, he is already on firm ground, and advance is possible and likely. Though cautious, he will nevertheless be curious to discover a widening world. Confidence emboldens the youngster's steps; the direction and quality of the goal will be determined by the character of the loved object. Enhanced effort promotes enhanced self-esteem. The existing world will appear to him a vast vault which harbors all of his liberated moves. He no longer feels he has to fit himself into a confining and deceiving contraption. He soon will proudly add his own finishing touches as a fortunate co-owner who optimistically perceives the perfectibility of the world around him as well as his own inventiveness. Sitting inside, he is now entitled to contribute beneficial changes. Soon he will discover that the change in him benefits others, and he can know the pride of giving and the joy of sharing. But he will also become aware once more of obstacles and competition and of the pangs of adjustment to upsetting realities.

Ill-prepared for this struggle and exposed to his troubled pals inside the Clinic and to a cruel world outside, he will for some time to come falter in a number of ways. It would be most unusual, however, for him to revert to his old attitude of indifference to the wholeness of the world at hand, a world which, symbolically speaking, he once tore to bits in an effort to use these parts to build a whole of his own, a whole that contained only his yearning and angry solitary self.

Before the children come to us, a most frequent symptom is that of "finding" more or less fine bicycles, as the opportunity presents itself, which they dismantle with no other consideration than to build a new creation of their own. (We disregard here the issue of concealment of theft which in addition to its practical purpose may be carried out, as explained, for deeper motives.) Thus they assert their existence, their capacity for a Promethean achievement in defiance of the pitifully helpless "gods" who delude themselves in believing that they are the masters of the world order.

The child in treatment will soon change his method, building and rebuilding his own bike, desirous of making it perfect so he may be proud of his workmanship. To acquire the frame and its parts, he will now rely on the adults. Through loving trust in them, he is able to renounce his former Promethean arrogance, however impressive it might have seemed to him. Accepting help implies that he has begun to see his role and his abilities in perspective and to recognize the interdependence of men. In a new wave of more realistic independence, he engages in trading and exchanging, in finding pieces on the junk yard and storing them for anticipated use. Possible action in the future can now be recognized and foreseen. The suspense implied can be faced at this time, and the span of time is bridged by a creative play of imagination, planning, and action. None of this has to be taught specifically. These are the child's own discoveries. He uses his previously unknown fund of resources. Inspired by his observations, he ventures out, assured that he can return safely and confident that he will find another promising day rooted in the secure and friendly past.

The children's manifestations of loyalty are impressive. Those who used *to run away* from home, from family, and from school, chose *to run to* the Educational Therapy Center. Their coming ten to fifteen miles in the pouring rain or practically barefooted in the snow proved remarkable accomplishments, considering these children's usual disinclination to walk even a few blocks and their tendency to withdraw or their aggression in the streets. Some came to us from the country after covering as much as forty miles. Some habitually came to the Clinic when closed on week ends "just to be there and look at it."

## Objects as Means of Orientation to Self and the World

A house which is a refuge and a haven for deprived and disturbed children is necessarily a means for orientation and for finding one's self by more or less experimental procedures such as touching, throwing, making, breaking, or manipulating a number of things formerly unknown to the children. They were familiar with certain objects or toys, solely as advertisements in the newspapers or comic books. They obviously were struck by the fact that such things could be more than pictures to look at. To the first personal contact with that real toy they would react in an amorous way, approaching it as would a shy lover the first object of his longing. Some seemed to wonder that they could have lived to a day where dreams do become true. Others would stand puzzled in front of an unfamiliar object, looking at it before venturing to touch and manipulate it.

This observation is true not only of children raised in small communities devoid of the opportunity of seeing a profusion of toys exhibited in the stores. Certain children have lived so exclusively in their respected section of town that their experiences do not encompass what could normally be expected of a child. The anxiousness and helplessness of such intelligent children is truly striking. It may be used as a defense with resulting complete inertia. Proscriptions by an anxious or narrow family unit or intimidation resulting from its rejection or neglect of the child and the child's fear of a rejecting society initiate such a vicious development. Children who, on the contrary, have ventured out to those sections of town where they could see toys but could own them only at the price of an illegal act may be surprised and even suspicious when in the therapy session they have one of these fascinating objects so close at hand. They feel tempted and cruelly exposed to fear arising from their impulses to appropriate it. Sooner or later they become familiar with these objects and accept them as friends. Increasingly they find what suits them particularly and proceed from one object to the next. No longer reaching out greedily for just anything, they choose rather deliberately. They can explain or will demonstrate what prompts their selection. They gain a libidinal attitude toward the plaything to which they may return repeatedly. They now have a relationship of reciprocity, the toy is no longer wantonly destroyed, disregarded, or misplaced as a resisting outsider or the image of the rejected self.

The object now responds and has meaning. It rewards the child by stimulating sensory-motor activity and "let's pretend" games. The child is no longer under compulsion to rush from one delusive instant to the next. He can allow the present moment to linger. Fraught with unexhausted and inexhaustible promise, the object now is captivating, and because there is now so much fun in living, the child himself clings to it like all happy youngsters who do not want to bid farewell to the day. Provided that the objects to which the child is exposed are a proper match for his capacities, they are an opportunity for testing limits. Thus, dealing with objects becomes a lesson in realism, a measure of one's present potentials and a challenge to surpass them. The child has gained a goal; the object can be his fount of satisfaction. It can give him "all the answers" at least for the time being.

Dealing with an object in connection with its proper use or an achievement keeps its manipulation in suspense in a healthy tension and in anticipation of the outcome, and thus it keeps him interested in the future moment. The alternative of success and failure is recognized and means are evaluated to achieve a rewarding solution. Even children of borderline mentality will make sufficient progress to be eager and capable of explaining by what means they proceed and why. Concentration and more abstract attitudes are promoted. We observe that borderline children change from an existence on the level of the *homo faber*, the manipulating man, who performs by mere intuition to the state of a *homo sapiens*, the man who thinks. Though indeed the children do not turn into essentially abstract thinkers, they may, however, attain a stage where they establish principles about the manner in which a certain task must be attacked and certain jobs must be done. They have concepts sufficiently abstract to understand a simple engine and how its parts function together. They may offer to make a blueprint from memory and to explain it.

The adult no longer is feared because his superiority is intimidating; he now is needed as the child's aid for self-expression as well as for approval of his communication by performance and word. An accelerated pace on the road to knowledge, under the guidance of loved and trusted educators, is now desired. The toy has become the mediator between the child and the adult, between the child's present condition and his own womanhood or manhood. No wonder that a child becomes attached to the milieu which harbors so much promise and gratification.

But many a hurdle has to be cleared before the role of the toy as a mediator has been fulfilled. The sudden close contact with those objects which have been withheld and in the child's mind "taken away" from him "all the time" promotes anxiety. Therefore, the children show eagerness to be scheduled first for sessions. They are desperate if you cannot comply, as though thereafter all of your love would be spent and all coveted objects distributed. In their early psychotherapy sessions some children hesitate to touch a toy in awe of its inherent magic effect upon them. Most children, though rational, may, however, suspect the toy to be but an object of exposure. If they touch the toy, they might break it. Still others see in the toy a gift of an enemy across the track. Rather than compromise with him by acceptance of his gifts, one should resist him by independent means of one's own. We see here reasons why children angrily deny responsibility for illegal acts. They believe them to be justified. It is a matter of pride. The children might shout: "I don't want anybody to pity me!" They may cope with this feeling in being bad by defiance.

Difficulty in treatment may result, as evident from mute defiance which is a manifestation of utter distrust, the child's rejection of the helper and the position he represents for him. The youngster who challenges him by verbal impertinence actually senses dimly that some hope is left for thinking that the helper could be won over to "his side" or could convince the child that he is his friend after all. A mute child however, not infrequently, can be shocked out of his isolation by an interpretation which unfolds to him comprehension of his non-verbalized attitude. Stunned by an insight that seems miraculous to him and by the helper's detached, that is, non-resentful attitude, the child may give up some of his distrust and show a dawning of admiration and affection. These new feelings he may fear and suspect, however, and therefore he may resent that the therapist provoked them. He is suspicious again; he may avoid her. Day-care may help here. Encouraged by the trust showed by the other children to teachers and therapists, he may try them out again. Poor contact with his youthful companions is no obstacle. He simply reaches out for a thing which is obviously gratifying to others.

## Social Aspects of Ownership

When the child is confronted with a situation involving ownership, he will react incongruously precisely because he has to catch up with the lag in his condition and education. What inside the home could be a healthy tendency and an opportunity for development becomes delinquency in the streets, because there is nothing there that may be touched, that is free to be taken or a willing target. The whole world is pre-empted. The child is cast out on inhospitable shores. He is thrown into enemy territory, unwanted and unexpected. Nor is there any place where the child belongs to anyone but himself, where love and hate and the working out of problems in his own conscience may be achieved without interference. There is no domain that is not restricted by law, and this appears to be one of the reasons for the increase of juvenile delinquency, especially in the city.

What indeed should a little fellow do with an inquisitive mind, with his grasping hands, for the sake of a driving curiosity, when there are no frogs to tease, no more butterflies to tear apart or collect, no trees to climb, no sticks to carve, what is the child to do to subjugate his world? What is there to do in a city where there are no tree stumps to offer their cut surface for worlds of experience with a few pebbles, dry leaves, stalks, and dead wood? What is there to do in a city where a pocket knife has become a desired but frightening and suspicious weapon? What should he do when our economy, in creating specific and standardized desires, has blighted the fascination of things that from time immemorial have cast their spell over any child, inspired his discoveries and invested them with a thousand meanings; thus were stimulated first exploits in creative pursuits.

Social competition has poisoned the artless relation of the child to that world which may still preserve some charm for those who live closer to nature, a world which protects from the impact of a powerfully organized and all-pervading economy. Sensitive to inequality and excited by the display of technical toys, the children necessarily want what they see. The little fellow feels he must possess the material objects of his era, if there is any joy of living left to him. *It is his modern way of penetrating into the secrets of matter and the universe.* He needs to own these toys representative of our civilization in order to feel that he too belongs to it. Ownership has power to promote reciprocity between the owner and, through the owned object, society as a donor. At a certain age of maturing the desire to own a toy implies identification with the surrounding civilization to the extent that the child grasps its meaning.

In the child's interest in toys, we must read approval of those expressions of our civilization which are represented by these silent companions and teachers of childhood. Such approval is one of great momentum in the child's integration into this culture. The child does not understand but feels keenly what the exclusion from ownership means to his individual as well as social development and to his social integration. Necessarily he interprets it in terms of his subjective experience as an active rejection directed against him. Society, in withholding necessary ownership from the child, assumes the role of the ungratifying parent whom the child will want to coerce into granting that which for the sake of wholeness, or even survival, he needs. If he does feel he has to resort to destruction of his alleged enemies, as a rule he will strike at representative objects rather than people. Direct hits will use cold war methods rather than violence. But also for the sake of self-respect and a status of equality with his well-to-do brothers does the child feel he must partake in ownership. He must be allowed to manipulate, to study, to own, and to master these objects. Our economy is directed toward consumption; for the sake of its survival it must stimulate wants, while objects are surrounded by legal prohibitions. A child who is confronted with prohibitions at every step he takes, every gesture he makes, every thought he expresses, discovers that he is always wrong. He feels that evil surrounds him. He thus finds additional justification for resenting this world of obstacles, this world of prohibitions, this world that constantly says: "Don't."

When an ungratified pre-adolescent boy, arrested at the developmental stage of an infant, falls into the hands of the juvenile police or other potential helpers, the danger is almost inevitable that his size will misrepresent his actual stage of maturation. In his self-centered behavior and limited understanding, the neglected boy is capable of roving around and reaching up, symbolically speaking, to the fire alarm for an instinctive and confused outcry of anxiety. The child's leisure to manifest an anxiety which is derived from a history of neglect and inhibited maturation rather than being an opportunity for growth and self-help (if such a term can be justified) becomes also a source of new discomfort and increased anxiety. In the streets he is again neglected and deprived of guidance. His size and strength cause him to explore objects that he should have learned to leave alone. But in his disarmed condition he has, symbolically speaking, to explore the functions of his arms and hands to feel their existence. A fire alarm that he may instinctively have reached out for, to voice his state of emergency, calls out his "judges" rather than his Samaritans.

The child is as confused himself as he is perplexing to his observers. Certain objects he touches make him appear deliberate and thus responsible to his judges. But a minute exploration of what he was doing reveals that he was not reaching out for a specific answer to a specific need. Under its real shape the object was but a means for the child to escape a vaguely sensed state of discomfort and want. Reaching out for an object that means something to others the child may merely imitate them. It is a way of answering curiosity, a way of learning. Dimly aware that other people's condition is at variance with his own unrelieved state, he may, by imitation of theirs, try to overcome his own. But the thing that has meaning for others may have no answer for him. He may not be ready to appreciate it. It has no place and does not prosper in the child's emotional desert. To feel incapable of being gratified frightens the child, and the sense of being inadequate nurtures despondency. That he was wrong is impressed upon the child by his failure to achieve fulfilment. The object refuses to be his. The child would like to return his strange and unwilling companion. But its reluctance stands in the way even of the relief of getting rid of it. The object's return might betray him. A solution to the dilemma of holding an object that has no value and that it is painful and wrong to keep may be found by the child. A child who had been anxious to return stolen money may buy some minor gratification. But he displays it so obviously that immediately he will be caught. Thus is achieved momentary relief from want by a fulfilment the futility of which need no further be explored.

Simultaneously the adult is drafted for liberating the child from a complex anxiety involving a sense of being wrong. The adult who does not argue and further confuse the child, who does not punish and angrily chide a child already torn by contradictory needs, the adult who does not increase suffering by fettering a child who feels already the strain of his contended needs may actually offer relief. Supported by the adult who listens willingly, the child loses his sense of inadequacy. Relief is derived from clarification of thinking and orientation gained about himself, his relationship to people and to things. The child learns to foresee his acts and to prevent them. First he communicates with the helping adult, depending on concrete or moral support. Later the child relies on his own strength. The adult called upon to help the child has learned in his turn most specifically which is the child's present state of evolution and how the disharmony of its elements interferes with the child's behavioral controls.

When the child and his worker have learned to reach each other, the child need no longer speak by impulsive acts. These make him suffer for the love he longs for and cannot deserve and reward.

In such a case the helper will see with concern that no progress is made in aiding the child. He may be unaware of the fact that the child was thrown back. At this time the child is made to feel incapable to reward. An ambivalence toward the helper arises. The child cannot enjoy the love he does not deserve and tries to repress the resentment for the burdens of indebtedness. Usually depression results, sometimes a show of indifference or callousness to evade inner confusion. Such impediments to his improvement can be prevented when, due to a well atuned relationship, the therapist is protected from anticipating, by excessive expectation, a state of maturation which the child has not yet reached. He will not raise new desires which stimulate new tension, anxiety, and obsessions. He rather contributes to the fulfilment of residual needs of great urgency, in particular the legitimate exploration of the child's surroundings which is necessary for the build-up of his self. When the child's needs are still promiscuous, and his world is not articulated by the indentures of time, the worker will not stimulate an engagement with one object with which to be joined at the calendar date set by the adult. He will not set goals at a distance where they become imperceptible and escape the child with increasing rapidity as his tension from waiting mounts. Gifts must be as unconditional as the child's good behavior. Praise is in order as a reward. "You were so nice;" "you pleased me so much, I felt I wanted to please you too." This is a lesson in the reciprocity of love commitments and of deservedness. Rewards may be granted as the privilege to carry out a job or run an errand. The child is supported in his sense of adequacy and because he can be trusted. To help a child discover time and the future as an experience he must, in "working" on a project, learn to count the milestones he is in the process of passing.

Unless we fulfil these conditions, the children are tantalized outside the house by everything they are lacking; they are starved inside the home for the bare necessities of life. Forever misled and deceived, the children actually live in an inferno. André Gide says in *Thésée:* "Let it be known unto you that there is no other punishment in the shades below than the perennial beginning of life's unfinished motion."

Social exclusion as well as material deprivation will pervert the relationship to ownership and the object. The object being a relevant part of a social situation, its ownership can be accepted only ambivalently. It commits these children to an insecure status in society which they reject, thus making it a mutual rejection. Acceptance may be sensed as a loss of liberty to retaliate.

## The Tantalizing Quality of Ownership

At the very moment that the child appropriates an object in defiance and negation of the social contract, he paradoxically becomes an owner. This means that he has denied his own antisocial act by consummation of the very act, perpetrated to confirm an antisocial status. The responsibilities connected with the conservative status of ownership are brought to awareness immediately. The child's ambivalence between two opposite attitudes is one reason why the stolen goods have an astonishingly short span of survival. The child's changed status is brought to his awareness by the need to take care of his possession and defend it. As a caretaker and defender of owned goods, he finds himself caught in enemy ranks. Moreover, the fact that he cannot cope with the numerous tasks related to ownership impresses him anew with his inadequacy and lack of experience. The conflict between an antisocial mode of thinking and the positive attitude toward goods as an owner confuses him. In despair he may break up the stolen toy or smash it to pieces, angrily lifting up the bits, throwing them again to the floor, against the walls, through the windows, until they irk him no more. The vicious circle is closed, new desires will haunt him and new satisfaction will defy him. Exhausted and deprived, guilty and angry, his extreme needs may foster his dependency on an adult whom he might annoy with bad temper and angry demands.

Under such conditions, how could he be expected to be ready for school and its required regularity, its orderly object relations in ownership, its necessity for reliability and dependability—in brief, its trust in a mutually satisfying world!

When active tendencies still prevail, the child attempts to restore what he has destroyed. Restoration may not be aimed at restoring the object's obvious function. Rather it is a way of making the object his own by recreating and conquering it. It is a way of depriving it of its disturbing aspects. Breaking the thing down then is an attempt to assimilate it to overcome the indecision. But it is his indecision which stands in the way of any directed action. The deprived child who is exposed to using the one alley to ownership which is called wrong is more than likely to fail in his attempt to assimilate it. Its infiltrating growth will sap his well-being. To avoid such ambivalence and disarmament the child may withdraw. He refuses to connive with his enemy. Only the power to destroy remains and the need for it grows. Eternally ungratified, the child eternally reaches out again, slowly losing sight of why he does it. Finally, the adventurer in him, the little self-styled conqueror dies out. He cannot master and make his own the small foothold of territory which is represented by the thing he took.

In destroying, the lonely child finally deprives himself. In the beginning of treatment only this factor of his acting out must be stressed. As he discovers love, being wrong against himself remains as his last foothold on ambivalence. His last anchorage is thus set on the hostility of the world. With it he identifies when he hates and punishes himself. Only unalterable acceptance and painstaking attention can help him. The child sets sail with renewed confidence. Such an encouragement must not appear to be a reward for acting out, though it is by acting out that he shows most visibly his distress and that he reveals most clearly its specific nature and though it is then that he reaches out most ardently for comfort. It is by the consistency and permanence of solicitude that he must be shown that he is loved and worth loving. He must be convinced that he can reward and therefore he will feel rewarded.

## Exposure to Toys and Play Therapy

In the therapeutic home the child is at leisure to gratify in a legitimate way his wholesome urge to explore things by touch and manipulation. It is therefore in order to discuss at this time the technical problem of how to expose the children to playthings, play, and play therapy.

In the general group which could be called a "structured milieu with a permissive approach," the children have a schedule. Divided into subgroups they are exposed to a variety of beneficial occupations. These are atuned to their emotional maturity, their tendencies and interests and their mental age. Their schedule includes hours of learning and of physical relaxation, learning is through play and at pre-school level where indicated. Children with evident similar needs are grouped together. Few toys if any are used in class, unless a child has to have a specific single maternal object with a few elementary toys or materials, like blocks, clay, crayons, and paper. The children often create their own visual material by drawing and cutting. Collecting pictures by categories, provides for a central topic of interest around which to organize and classify simple knowledge. We described previously[1] how one or two pieces of string, a piece of cotton and a piece of hemp tied around a parcel challenged children to embark in fantasy on a dramatic imaginary journey. Pursuing their dramatic and dramatizing experience, they studied comprehensively the physical, sociological, and ethnological aspects of the places "visited." A program was outlined by which the children of a wide range of abilities engaged in a common endeavor of wide scope.

The children use toys displayed in the therapists' rooms. Our budget is limited in the area of therapeutic tools and we have to depend on gifts. Those coming from the stores, predominantly damaged, unsaleable things have proven useful in spite of obvious defects.

We mention this fact because of the surprising observation that these discarded toys did not necessarily elicit sensitive responses in these sensitized children. However, a number of diagnostically valid behavioral attitudes may occur. The children actually respond like any other children. Confronted for instance with an improperly functioning crane a youngster is struck by the fact that the pully does not accomplish the anticipated function. He attempts to produce this function either by a considered or a trial and error approach and finally recognizes the undeniable uselessness of the toy in that respect. The child may turn for help to the therapist who states that the toy is broken. The child then attempts to repair the toy or uses it on a lower level of functioning, that is, he may simply move it around, he may manipulate the pully by substituting his own motions for the mechanics of the toy, he may discard the toy altogether or finally use it in any capacity for a more structured game. In the latter case the obstacle obviously has become an asset. These observations are representative of the child's ability to make an asset of a liability, with accompanying gratification.

Defective dolls may be disregarded, discarded with emphasis, placed at a distant part of the room. The pre-adolescent girls were usually quite persistent, over longer periods of their treatment, in playing with large limbless dolls. They preferred them to the small flexible doll-house families. Their involvement with their own traumatization and helplessness motivated an identification with the infirmity of the dolls. The girls would nurse them, cloak their defects with wrappings fondly draped around them, or cover them up to make them cozy. The doll's injury was at times disregarded for the purpose of play. A serious attempt to make a doll whole was made by a boy. He was sufficiently preoccupied by the doll's amputated condition to provide materials and tools for repair which he brought into his next session. Failure to succeed has not to be feared in the therapeutic situation. With support the child can accept inevitable failure. It does not carry with it the connotation of personal inadequacy. The furthering of endurance, of a growing consideration of reality factors, reasoning about technical difficulties and thus anticipation of a negative outcome alleviate the child's irrationality and anxiety. Imagination and humour, implying the symbolism of the situation, may come to the rescue. Far from diminishing its therapeutic value the defective toy helps the child gather the curative potentials of the patient-therapist relationship.

Identified with the therapist's acceptance of the child as another self, the child is likely to learn not to lose herself in the doll, an attitude which implies a stagnating self-pity. Strengthened by the therapist's observant support, the child's interest shifts from nursing the injured to tending the "sound" dolls, having them move and relate in the doll house. Or, still concentrating her interest around her own person, she demonstrates by her desire to sew an apron or a skirt that she is striving for concrete tokens of her self-accomplishment.

A broken toy does not provoke so much anxiety as an unbroken one. It is not an invitation to conform. It leaves the child alone in the safety of his fancied pastures, no intrusion from a world of crude and harsh realities is even possible. No one can claim, "you broke the toy," since it was broken already. Broken as it was, it was all the child's. Its ties with ordinary values and meanings were severed. Broken playthings in the Clinic have a tendency to survive in spite of constant use. It may seem uneducational, not to discard them, since they do not point beyond the present condition of the child, but they are close to him, familiar to his status, representing him, approachable while he still feels profoundly inadequate and different. They are a means of introducing his world tentatively into our own.

The broken toy indicates where the child feels we have to search for the meaning of the one he is. Our acceptance of his incompleteness and his incapacity to function as expected motivates his creed and striving for enhancement.

Underneath the children's injured and injuring condition, we may discover an untrained, ill-trained, unskilled, or intimidated attempt to better themselves and their condition, or else a revolt against the handicap to aspired or longed-for betterment. We can see how it is done when children preserve in the Clinic the injured toys for the delight of play or in other words, when they feel comfortable being their genuine selves. But they greedily grasp the new ones wanted for self-completion, tending to hoard them anxiously, only to lose them inevitably in one way or another at short notice. The children "borrow" these perfect toys surreptitiously to play a part they cannot yet hold.

A similar attitude is manifested when they request to go to public school before they are ready. They are impatient to be as perfect and as accomplished as others and by means of "artificial limbs" they hobble toward their goal. If we pressure the children who are already too eager to compete too soon with borrowed strength, we expose them to strain and traumatic defenses. Symbolically speaking, they will never be able to discard their crutches.

## When the Object Cannot Be Reached

An experiment is suggested for solving the alternative of offering the usual or a reduced selection of toys to those children who are devoid of the capacity to select and concentrate on stimuli, impressions, and objects. At various chronological ages and various stages of their impeded evolution, we see the children wandering greedily and haphazardly from object to object. They will recognize and exhaust the possibilities of none of them. They will not benefit from the potential aid for orientation and growth inherent in an object which one takes hold of mentally.

Though they move around incessantly, some of these children show an early and unexpected tendency as well as capacity to relate. They may run in and out with an obvious, though merely impulsive, need for the helper. As time passes, they may cast a first furtive glance at him or her, smile, or attempt to tease. Thus, there is evidence of some form of apperceptive differentiation and social tendency, tenuous as it may be. These children must be gratified above all, not only because of the soothing effect of gratification but because gratification is able to arrest their errant attention; it can be a point of reference for choice.

In deciding whether or not to reduce the quantity of toys exposed to these children we move between two unsatisfactory alternatives. Place before the child too few toys and he will soon have ended his hunt; bored, detached, or tenuously related to the symbolic parent, he will leave the room to go on hunting elsewhere with aimless avidity for the forever evasive prize. Spent and irritated, he will finally find release in annoying others. If the equally exhausted and annoyed children react irritably, thus becoming a target for pursuit, he will finally learn to search for the thrill of annoying. Why should there be an end to the unrest at this time of release of tension? Though drained at that stage, the child is still driven to persevere, even more so. Anything can trigger a temper tantrum. Submerged by a volcanic emotional outburst, the child is at least for a moment unconscious of the misery that unleashed the outburst. Relief can come only from giving in to temporary death. When things do not develop to that extreme, the child satisfies his need to find an obstacle to his endless search and will tend to provoke it, as for instance a fight that arrests his attention.

What happens if we take the opposite course and attempt to expose the child to too large a number of toys kept in a room? Will he stray from toy to toy, from object to object until all or most stimuli have been haphazardly pursued? In our former experiment the number of objects was rapidly exhausted and the child continued to be driven by a dim and fruitless search for gratification. In our second experiment the child will also soon be exhausted by the profusion of tantalizing objects. To ward them off, he leaves the room. This is the most adequate defense as long as he has not discovered the way to his gratification.

The child was able in neither case to avail himself of the opportunities offered for experience. His reaction will be identical in both cases unless the toy objects for the child are properly and specifically adjusted in number and variety to his needs. If we prevent or are aware of the first signs of fatigue before the child's irritation runs its course, we can satisfy his need for rest and comfort and, symbolically speaking, rock him into relaxed forgetfulness.

At first such a random child will have to be gratified in a random way. He has to be "picked up," wherever he turns up. The special way in which the worker responds represents a particular lure to the child and determines in the long run his preferences. He gradually becomes selective and is no longer as driven; he now has a goal, a purpose. He stays where he likes to be. The wandering child finds his seat. He can now be "engaged" in an elementary pursuit; his motions and attention are further stabilized. With obvious serenity he takes hold of things by vision and touch; he notices and uses them. At this stage adult support is amply applied. Symbolically speaking, it is the stage where the child plays with his parents while sitting in comfort on their lap. From this posture he is going to rise to be more on his own. In turning to the adult, the hurt child tends to overcome the object's renewed defiance to his limited capacities. Results of his beginning efforts, though infinitesimal, give the child a sense of tremendous achievement. He has come from nothingness to life.

Successful manipulation of objects eventually widens the possibilities for finding relief. Having learned to shape and to explore, he now projects himself into the world by his performance. In his friendly surroundings, he discovers that he can contribute to the friendliness of the world. The child feels no longer totally helpless and disarmed.

Technically therefore, we may conclude that what matters is to help a child focus on the maternal object and the things that spring from her hands. Thus even the size of the room is shaped and made to close around the two of them. Any size room and any kind of toy or furnishings may offer the necessary start. Due to the quality of the relationship, stimuli of lesser importance are neglected. The child is helped "to forget about the threatening world," and to concentrate upon what is essential and gratifying. The capacity to concentrate on the edifying elements of experience is fundamental. The resulting optimism will prompt the child to an active attitude and in the long run to shaping his fate from wherever he stands. He will be saved from the danger of denigrating and censuring the world, unless there is a constructive purpose in mind.

The fortunate child who achieves self-realization by playing structured games, rather than by reducing the room to suit his purpose, widens it to encompass the entire world when, on his own scale, he experiments in conquering it. Both the one who needfully reduces the existing space and the other who opens it have begun to forge the metal of their existence.

## Interest in Models

Certain objects have a particular fascination for the youthful Clinic population. This fascination is derived from the joy of building, from the mastery of a step-by-step procedure that leads to a goal. Moreover the object is the child's own, unlike the building materials whose advantage of serving innumerable times has the disadvantage for the Clinic patient of being an object of collective ownership only. I refer to construction models which have an immense appeal for boys of a most varied range of endowment, whether this endowment is of an intellectual or mechanical nature. They are ideal media of communication between the isolated and withdrawn child and the world. These children first build their longing for comfort into the model. The most dependent ones show a first interest in boats which are their symbolic berths. They build their dreams of adequacy and potency into the planes, and the strivings for their own independent place in reality into cars—not jeeps or trucks, but *cars*. Finally aggressive or peaceful mastery of reality is tried when they no longer refuse to build jeeps or trucks for war or working purposes. They make enlightening remarks in reference to the ascending planes and their shapes; laughing significantly and slightly embarrassed, they tease a timid newcomer who needs to be "rocked in a cradle"; the boat is recognized as such.

Thus, though the child started with self-gratification and self-identification, his preoccupations open up further avenues toward the world, and new promises to follow. White children, we observed, went to the stores, searching for models not yet explored, new kinds and more difficult and complex ones to be mastered by an increasingly perfect achievement. Negro children, who sense that they would be less welcome in the stores because more readily sized up as insolvent, will pursue the same goal by traveling through catalogues. Both the white and Negro boy will try to find friends in the world to promote joy and growth. His appreciation is shown by fine and hard work. The boy considers his performance a monument or a document of his most representative self. He exposes his work for appreciation, he collects it for self-encouragement, as the token of an "improvement"; he gives it away as a means of vying for fond attention or as something overcome that is already irrelevant to his further maturing self. He begins to be interested in work rather than play.

In the early stages of the children's involvement with models, their attitude is greedy, passionate, irrational, and inconsiderate. Slowly a give-and-take relationship to the world develops. The model itself now begins to converse with the child and to stimulate curiosity. A bright boy who had acquired the model of a dinosaur skeleton read from one session to the next all the literature that he could find in the libraries about Sauria and the Mesozoic era. Almost any of these young, mechanically-minded boys will surprise you by knowledge of structure and function of the machinery he builds, whether cars or projectiles.

The majority of children are intensely attracted to playing with models. They are not the original, the creative minds who have to proceed on ways of their very own. The child who builds models searches, at least at that period of life, a prestructured situation to guide him to a pre-established, concretely perceivable goal, to a determination imposed from without. He thus manifests a longing for social conformity and social belonging. He is identified with the perceivable reality around him. He does not want to be excluded from the familiar landmarks of our culture representing society and its hierarchy to him. Nor does he wish to enter as an undesirable intruder, lacking education and proper experience; because he does not have the password.

Much emotion goes into these models because of their multiple meanings for the child, not least in importance being that as small scale models of a major object they also represent small scale tests that he can cope with. Therefore the model becomes "my baby"; it is talked to, caressed, and encouraged by words; the boy interrupts his work for a second, admiring "it," "her," or "him," letting it perform its anticipated function, and improvising the accompanying noise; or he "dresses" it up with paint and decals, overloving and overdressing it, compulsive in the urge to use all available decals. While usually the model is the baby, it may at times be the feminine object, proudly possessed, "the lady in a nightgown," in an "evening gown," or perhaps "it reminds me of my cousin," "my girl friend." Any of the vehicles may offer an imaginary ride to the boy's dreamland which he thus recognizes as an artificial one. "But it is beautiful while it lasts" remarked a young high school boy.

We should mention in passing the child's main attitudes to the therapist revealed through his play with models: he is extremely demanding and discloses intolerance of frustration when he can have no models. He sulks, blocks, withdraws, displays violent or insidious aggression, vindictiveness or incites other children to act out. Unwilling to accept substitution for the model, he shows inability to conquer his own obstinacy and to accept obtainable pleasures. Motives for yielding may be the fear of hurting the psychotherapist or anxiety of missing, by negative attitudes, too much of the precious time. Increasing realism is evident when he can see that costly toys cannot be available at all times, and he co-operates with the scheduling of certain model-building sessions.

Dependency is expressed not only by those who are in want of help for performance but by those who need attention and compete for it.

The children who show deep Oedipal involvement with their mother usually use their model as a means of self-enhancement. The mother's upsetting ambivalence is reflected in the child's hurried, sloppy, and messy performance, or, on the contrary, in the production of a perfect job for display of adequacy in view of acceptance.

One of our untidy "workers," eager to rush to "home, sweet home" always declared an unfinished job finished, pretending that by no means did he want to have certain parts built into his model. Actually he refused accessories that looked "funny" to him or reminded him of something "dirty." They were features that represented phallic or anal symbols to him. The same shape passed unnoticed when it was not part of a whole but the feature of the total object. Avoiding providing these planes or submarines with tanks, guns, or poles and categorically refusing to put in the pilot, he injected in them his "bumble bee" in the early stages of treatment. He said the bumble bee was he, his power that obeyed him and was capable of moving everything. Under treatment he completely forgot about it, but when he was angry against his mother, he remembered it and said laughingly, "I use it to annoy her." He tried to do the same with his therapist. But, while in reference to the mother it was predominantly a "spiritual," an airy, volatile, not a dirty means to possess her, in reference to the psychiatrist it was a means of making her inefficient, a hapless therapist who could not rid him of his symptom and to whom he refused to yield.

Children request models in excess of what can be granted or of so specific a quality that it cannot be provided. By means of such an attitude they impose upon the therapist the role of the ungratifying mother.

The children in the Clinic have never built their cars into racers, some of them stating that they will never race anyhow. They may thus realize the danger of racing. The car is for them a symbol of social respectability and the building of models a bridge to an ardently desired adjustment and social inclusion. Power is expressed by the quality of the car, but not always of a famous make. White children of another social milieu could often be observed playing the role of the radio or television announcer of races and racing accidents, preoccupied obsessively with dreams of owning cars and motorcycles and finally riding and racing them. They were driven by anxiety to be adequate males and the fear of being overtaken from behind or to be caught speeding toward a secret and non-admissible goal. The model is a symbol of too small a scale for a boy of "racing age" who needs powerful action to side-track an existent masculine drive, the gratification of which for more than one reason he tends to postpone.

The children at work with objects offer a wealth of information. They are operating with deliberation or by trial and error, leisurely or compulsively, following instructions by lecture or picture, working neatly or messily in reference to technique, performing at random or with an understanding of what they are doing, finicky in the use of the glue, pressing it out with force, making the solidity of the finished product unnecessarily safe in wasting the glue, smearing it or inviting the psychotherapist to take over this part of the operation which disgusts some of the children.

A most impressive stage has come when the child proceeds to the repair of old, broken models. This demonstrates that to shape form representing his own "broken" self, the child no longer needs the perfect opportunity. Anything can be made into a gratifying project. Sensitivity to not being given attention has yielded to trust, conquering the tendency to an excessive bid for attention and to contentment as well as to humility which is the prerequisite for "repair." Resourcefulness is now mustered and rewarded by a justified pride. The child is now far advanced from the stage where his barely started job on a new model was abandoned with discouragement and could not be taken up again. At that time failure used to be a seal to inadequacy.

At this time, however, a variety of new ventures are being attempted. Clay is no longer refused as messy or childish. Expressive artifacts of clay are dressed up with remnants of models, making these pieces worthy of others exhibited on the mantle. They intensify the builder's contentment with himself and the world.

### Use of the Doll House, Reduced and Different

Although we do not deny that the use of the doll house is a suitable device for clarifying the nature of a child's problems and their dynamics in terms of libido development, we must, however, maintain that its use should be subject to specific indications, as with any therapeutical tool. Suspicious and negativistic children sense it as being too obvious, too direct and directed an approach to painful experiences which they are bent on evading. The therapist who, in the mind of the child, lures him into playing with the doll house is not only an intruder into his secrets but, like everybody else he has known, has suspicious purpose in mind. The safest thing the child concludes, is therefore to be or do just the opposite of what is expected.

Those children at the Clinic who do take up doll house play are often observed to show the tendency to cope with the chaotic situation at home. The six-year-old son of an alcoholic mother lived with her in the home of an alcoholic aunt and her husband. He was exposed to these women's violent acting out and to the mother's sexual exhibitionism. Burning his home (the doll house) was dramatically staged in every session for a period of time. Furniture, bedding, and mattresses were thrown in the streets in an extreme display of anxious emotion.

Pre-adolescent boys make an extensive use of the doll house among other buildings which they erect from a variety of building games. In using the doll house for gangster and police games, *the boys transfer their problems from the family to the community level.* Confused fights and persecutions precede more structured games. Indecision between right and wrong, good and evil forces, official power and its opposite is clearly shown. The confusion originally displayed, and which in the early stages of treatment returns at the end of each session, obviously is a sign that the ambivalence can neither be faced nor revealed to the observer. Demonstrated ambivalence therefore can represent progress. It consists in a "changing luck." At one time the police, at another the gangsters win either by the child's "change of mind" during the game or by an undetermined outcome. To leave the playful events in suspense is a means of concealing with whom the child is taking sides. It might however represent a first incentive for structuring the game and for carrying it from session to session. One schizophrenic boy could never resolve the alternative. He was highly imaginative in keeping the story moving, but it became increasingly incoherent.

The doll house at times represents a more or less anonymous uninhabitable structure. It is one hide-out among many undesirable or censured places of concealment, and play is carried all over the room, as the image of home. The doll house represents the reality which the youngster beclouds. It is the original source of all his bitterness as well as the original target of his hostility. But most often he resurrects the "dead" ones who once populated the place of unrest and chaos. They were only taken for dead, the child declares. "This sounds crazy," one of them said, "but the bullets were dead ones and nobody got killed." The ambulance frequently is called into play as are the hospital, operations, and a cure. The burying of the dead with a respectable funeral service reveals that destructiveness is ambivalent or not devoid of elements of conflict. That the dead sometimes remain dead, in particular the crowd or the rank and file of the army or that at best

they are stuffed into a common sepulchre, testifies only to the greater
ease with which the world at large is condemned by him and sacrificed. To annihilate the whole world, even if you perish as well, seems
easier than to kill the father. The great majority of the children, however, wish he were a better man and would come home.

Expressing a thunderous elation, children treated in a group may
subject the world to chaotic annihilation. When their play becomes
more structured, they will argue that the enemy has invaded their
territory and has to be eliminated, cost what it may. If we remember
some children's deeply soul-searching confessions in individual therapy or their self-depreciating jokes in the group, we must wonder
whether "the enemy who invaded their territory" may not bespeak
their sense of being "possessed of the devil," the "stranger" who suddenly appears and "makes" them "do what" they "don't want to do."
Only total destruction can liberate the bad world within or without of
this invasive fiend. The children tend to leave the room in a mood of
elation derived from their symbolized omnipotence. An underlying
depression, covered by cynicism shows, however, that they realize
deeply it is by evil that they have conquered evil.

The therapist therefore suggests: "Would you clean up the rubble
so we might build up the city again"? By means of a new project for
the next session, expressed in the terms of the play, that is, by appealing to the children's imagination and to their buried inner motives,
relief and hope are achieved. We remember one session when one
of the four pre-adolescent boys of a group tried to prevent any constructive outcome of the session. Sensing that for him it would be
most meaningful to terminate it by symbolically reducing the world
to rubble, he left the room in an injured indifference. Thus he tried to
stimulate the other children's resistance to constructive compliance.
Their co-operative mood, however, caused him to re-enter the office
shortly and willy-nilly to "clear the rubble."

The further carry-over from this session was rewarding. The children returned next time as though animated by a purpose. They rebuilt the two enemy cities as usual, one boy more or less compulsively,
all with a sense of beauty, the two most alert ones with war strategy
in mind. Much more time was devoted that day to constructing, more
resources were mobilized, due as much to a tendency to delay the
destruction as to a need for an intense release in direct proportion to

the extent of the delay. In addition to the arsenal of airplanes and helicopters, space projectiles were used. Significant joking went on about one of the boys visiting his girl friend on Venus. The authority figures for the first time were endowed with individual traits though their part was only representative of their social role. They spoke in fatherly terms to the soldiers encouraging them to fight bravely for their country. Theodore, the illegitimate child of a feeble-minded prostitute, raised in a foster home, extemporized a remarkable speech, trying ardently to believe in his role and with conviction to identify with objectives that society presumably values. However, he could not hide his skepticism. In one of the following sessions Wilbur, about whom more will be said, took the lead, attributing negative and ridiculous traits to the generals and the colonels. They were drunk, caused accidents and were declared unworthy of driving a Cadillac. A mere jeep would suit them.

The children played in a similar fashion a few more times, holding authority figures responsible for the chaotic condition of the world. But quite spontaneously they recognized themselves with increasing clarity in the figures they ridiculed or censured. Having mockingly exposed the general, Wilbur suddenly exclaimed: "The general is I. I am a drunk driver like he is, riding around and hitting the curb." But, gradually, the soldiers became more civilized. Sent behind the front, they walked leisurely two by two through spots of interest and beauty in foreign countries.

A great deal of differentiation was displayed in building a complex city or city quarters, dramatizing events that had to do with the construction of life within a town and its buildings. Mishaps occurred on the scaffolds and roofs, or walls broke down, the children joking ambiguously about their symbolized ineptness as builders. The faulty structures were representative of their own "warped" make-up. This was Theodore's joking comment. He needed to be rebuilt "from scratch," he added. Real progress is achieved when the child no longer relies on the stability of his model for a symbolic support of the wholeness of his existence. He then shows enough self-assurance to manipulate the materials as they challenge his versatility and his capacity to be experimental. He can also be endlessly patient as he takes down and rebuilds time and again a structure that does not yet fully meet his increasingly demanding self-image.

## Reviewing the Function of Playing with Toys

Observing the relationship of the children, in particular the group of pre-adolescent boys we have had in mind, we registered the following attitude toward those special objects which are their toys. Intense and ever repeated appreciation of an ownership which, though scheduled, is sensed as total. The children give up the tendency of taking toys out of the room or the habit of asking to take them along. The familiarity with the objects and the closeness gained facilitate a fertility of the relationship. The child exhibits and reveals himself less timidly. A mutuality between the child and his toy develops. Because he had endowed the object with a rewarding quality, the object answers with new promises which entice the child to invest more imagination, endowing the object with further potentials for the release of emotions and relief from tension. Sooner or later, the toy's function as a catalyst will be submerged by its function as a partner in play. From inspiration to inspiration a series of more or less coherent performances will develop, revealing to the therapist a child's increasingly consistent preoccupation with solving his problems. The children's need to restage these problems many times, is increased by the attraction of the toy as a partner. They may keep the therapist wondering, "where are the children going and what is treatment doing to them"?

Suddenly they may widen the scope of their enterprise. Revealing that their imagery is growing richer and more complex, they grow "tired" of repeating what we might name their eternal refrain. They will begin to vary and modulate it and thus amplify it, as it were, into a symphony with a variety of movements, a vibrant *allegro con brio* coming usually at the end. A first step may be prompted by the intensity of the children's elation at play which calls for a more extensive instrumentation. The children begin to collect an ever widening range of instruments for self-expression which they succeed in applying for their purpose. Toys are borrowed in other offices; when the ones inside their therapist's office have all been made to serve, objects are brought in from outside the Clinic. Originally, collecting objects is an expression of anxiety, of oversecuring one's self in competition with other children. This motivates at times violent fights which interfere with the game. When the children learn that they can count on finding the desired objects for play in the impartial presence of the therapist, sooner or later such anxiety is alleviated. When the content of the child's project is remembered, anxious grabbing can be calmed through the meaning of the play. What the child has set outside himself by his performance usually returns as comfort. The child at play thus is the author of the peace of his mind. One example illustrates this.

Four boys were engaged in setting up their positions for a war game, building various encampments and placing the soldiers in their strategic places. Marvin Ronald, the least endowed and most compulsive of the little group, was trying to grab everything for his platoon. A fight was on the verge of erupting and of breaking up the game. That is when Wilbur, his play partner told him soothingly, "let them have the tents! Their camp is in the country. Ours is in town. We have the tall and strong buildings. We have no use for tents." Although the first child had been unimaginative and rigid, his pal's advice immediately was accepted. Marvin gave up the tents. Realism and fantasy overlapped.

Thus we are reminded of the fact that aside from its potentials of becoming a catalyst, the toy can become a solicitor of a child's imagination, inspiring the child to endow it with a wide variety of meanings. Anything can serve the purpose. Old leaves, pebbles, sand, pine needles, an old piece of wood, if the child, hearing its call for life, begins to see, like Gepetto, that the piece of wood can be more than appears on its surface. Once the child has animated it and cared for it with his loving attention, both the toy and the child become Gepetto and Pinocchio in one person. But Pinocchio forgets that he is also Gepetto, that it is also Gepetto's breath that moves him. In the play, as in the author's profound story, the unison with the animating father, alive but overtuned in the puppet's ear, becomes the result of an active reunion after experience in failure. Due to the author's infinite wisdom which is part of the poetical charm of the story, Pinocchio becomes a real boy only at the end of the book. This development was needed not only because a real boy is for educational purposes a kind and good boy, a status that one acquires by a long stage of failure in and struggle for overcoming opposite trends, but because a little wooden artifact is not mortal and his sad adventures throughout the story lose some of their deadly terror; also, for making so many unwise moves, a puppet can be excused; not so a real boy. When children stage and rehearse with toys the occurrences of a hostile world as they see it and when they release their own violent and destructive passion, the seriousness that all these feelings and events have in real life is lifted; it becomes a rehearsed, a playful experience and much of its terror is alleviated. As an artificial experience, not imposed upon the child by actual events but practiced at will, it can be faced. They can even ridicule it, make it a comedy or a farce and play the clown, attempting to reassure themselves fully.

As long as Marvin did not know how to play, he was so serious that any other child's teasing was answered by a dangerous retort. Reacting like a flash, he would throw heavy objects, anything he could lay hands on, aiming at the would-be assassin's head. His father had been killed while defending himself, having been in fights constantly.

The need to rehearse experiences most heavily fraught with anxiety, explains why we are made to be witnesses in therapy of periods of apparent stagnation "the eternal refrain." They are periods of practice, of getting into the habit of facing and dealing with tragic moments and their tragic effects.

The trying days when a child or a group of children reiterate the same performance again and again with barely noticeable variations or nuances are critical periods. Progress may be arrested or on the contrary promoted. Once the need for rehearsing had been overcome in the experience previously reported and the children had mustered courage to face their aggression against the "world" which so long they had reduced to rubble, the anonymous, amorphous "leaden" soldiers suddenly came to life. These soldiers immediately lived in a social hierarchy in which the children wished to believe or pretended they did believe, in an attempt to conform for the sake of belonging and for relief from anxiety and isolation. But after this new and bolder form of rehearsing, the play had to be "rewritten" and the prevailing skepticism had to be built in. The official authority figures of that new version of the play set rules and gave sound advice for a conduct which they themselves failed to follow. Their undesirable private life invaded even their area of duty; the authority figures themselves thus became the basic sources of chaos. The shiftless "general is I" implied the recognition that "we are so drunk, so confused, that neither you nor I can find our way." Unlike Pinocchio, who finds his way to reunion with the *model* father, our children discover their similarity with the "real" father, the elder as he *is*. Our children's insight must be deeper and maturer, and the resulting generosity with the united man, which is the elder and the younger combined, must be firmly rooted and potentially powerful. Will the stem of their growing selves become strong enough to withstand the storms of temptation?

## The Child as Author, Actor, and Audience

In child play, author, actor, and audience are identical. The children may start as acting authors, naïvely living and enjoying the "play." But sooner or later they become reflective and observant of the experience and their own audience for approval or self-esteem.

As authors, they are and represent the inmost core of themselves. Their suffering, their anxiety are greatest because yet "untold." Embodying as actors their painful experience and forlorn outlook on life and exposing them to others, they release the terror as it is shared, whether "the other," as the audience, is anonymous or not. A bridge is built, though haphazardly, to the shores of the other person.

That the child can become an actor and expose himself is evidence of the fact that he can share and potentially sympathize. He could not cast the bridge of exteriorization if he did not, in final analysis, anticipate a sympathizing audience in his companions at play or the therapist. That he is usually discriminating against outsiders to the group is at this stage a positive sign. It means he has chosen a core of trusted friends. The child who can play is therefore a patient hopeful of cure.

The third curative effect of child play that we here have in mind is derived from his role as the audience. As such he is the more or less reflective, detached element of the complex inner experience. He is the sympathizing observer of the villain he himself has created as author and interpreted as actor, in fulfilment of his two other functions in the play. He thus recognizes with less difficulty that he is what he exposes to the world.

The child, as we saw, will reveal that he recognizes himself in the *dramatis personae* and unfolds his awakening or awakened sympathy. That he has some realization of the way the play is functioning seems to be born out not only by the enthusiasm with which he plays and loves these sessions, but by the ardent interest in recording them on the dictaphone in order to play them all over again. The playing back of the recordings are usually occasions of great emotional display and comment about one's self and the others. Months later the child may remember what he considered most successful performances. He will request to play them back and take opportunity to compare, usually with generous condescension and often great hilarity, his former self with his present one. "That's my voice, that's me, that's the one I was."

In terminating this discourse on play therapy which aimed to explore the children's relationship to objects or toys, we should like to present the case of Wilbur Cecil. He needed no particular prearranged setting or other implied encouragements by his therapist to avail himself of the toys at hand, "marionettes," we might say, which he endowed with speech. Though thirteen years old at the time, while playing he talked to himself, only intermittently would he communicate with the therapist.

Wilbur was exposed to individual psychotherapy before joining the group previously described. He was the only and belated son of an elderly couple; the mother was a most unsightly limping woman, reminiscent of the witch in Hansel and Gretel. The father who suffered from diabetes was under insulin therapy. Whether or not the Clinic which treated him for this condition was aware of the fact that, due to poverty, improvidence, and total inadequacy, he could not obtain the necessary food to avoid hypoglycemia, we did not know. The fact was that he suffered from multiple small attacks of violence and agitation and, at rarer intervals, of paroxysms of violence and confusions. In such a state one day, he set on fire the old wooden garage where Wilbur lived alone with him at the time. The mother had taken refuge from her state of misery at a friend's home. Wilbur was quite preoccupied with the terror of that night as well as with the satisfaction derived from his act of saving his and his father's life. He ran to his mother as fast as he could in the middle of the night.

Wilbur was referred to us by the public schools for chronic truancy. His reasons for avoiding school were of a sensitive nature. The school children teased him and ridiculed his parents. Wilbur also was in the habit of staying out at night, frequently hiding under the porch of the home to which the parents had moved after the fire. He had a demanding as well as an Oedipal attachment to the mother, always inventing dreams of how to help her and always ending up by depriving her. But while about a year later he began his permanent stay in the foster home, he ran to her daily in the morning, secretly bringing her his good lunch. He wanted to justify his desire for and enjoyment of foster home placement by providing for his mother. Actually, this was a new version of an old family tradition, consisting of dependency upon agencies. Wilbur pretended the sick father had to consume all the available food and that none was left for his mother. His relationship to the father was one of extreme hostility which, due to intense guilt feelings, he tried to overcome. At one time he wanted to become a pastor.

At referral Wilbur was almost a skeleton, starved as he had been all through his lifetime. His parents had been dependent all of their lives. At an advanced stage of therapy Wilbur became fully aware of the fact that he had never seen the example of working parents. They were country people who for the sake of obtaining more substantial public support had moved to the city.

Our Clinic attempted everything to improve the economic, hygienic and emotional situation of the family, enrolling the assistance of other agencies. Foster home placement became necessary, desired by Wilbur and accepted with painful reluctance by the parents.

At various times, in therapy, Wilbur wondered why he was so playful and, on the contrary, so uninterested and incapable in every other area. Working and earning would be so important in his life, his needs being so great and some of them so specific. He would love so much to help his mother. He would explain all his good reasons for having a bicycle and why the one received from his foster mother would not do; he considered it a decrepit old thing. He needed a fine respectable new one. A low-priced English wheel would do. He would take good care of it and use it for work. Wilbur felt very uncomfortable, disloyal, and selfish for having deserted his parents for material advantages. The good new bicycle was representative of the foster mother, the real opportunity for survival as well as adjustment and as such the justification for leaving his parents. As it turned out, the material advantages in the foster home became in his mind a bait and adjustment a vice, a form of licentiousness. By surpassing his parents materially he felt he rejected them. In deep conflict, he destroyed the bicycle, surprising and hurting the foster mother who had bought it for him. Wilbur himself found a resolution of his indecision between his guilt-laden relationship to the parents and loyalty to them and the enthusiasm for a foster home that gratified all of his needs for "growth." He promoted a friendship between the mother and foster mother who spoke over the telephone daily "for a long time."

The child was remarkable for the quality of play, considering that he had had no previous experience in this area, no education, and, throughout his life, no stimulation whatsoever for his imagination. We should like to mention that when he had played his way into being sufficiently integrated and "able" and free to work, he had as much fun working.

He could captivate you by relating his efforts. At an early stage in therapy, he had sized up the potentialities of the toys as tools for self-expression. We recall that we had no typical playroom; the choice of our toys was imposed upon us partly by the poverty of our own situation: at that time our new venture devoted to children deserving help and chances for adjustment had to be demonstrated before the proper means for such demonstration were supplied. This liability we treasure as evidence that the material setting is incidental to the therapeutic relationship and the therapeutic proceedings.

For a few sessions, Wilbur used all the buildings which stood around to the exclusion of castles. A Western street and city blocks to build a town with an airport attracted particular interest. Fights between cowboys and Indians were staged. Wilbur reported that his father was of Indian descent and declared the Indians were utterly cruel. Wilbur then turned to the family scene. The day this happened planes bombarded the city. A large family group packed its belongings into a number of cars and fled to Texas with all of their belongings. The father was left in town with no means of escaping. It was an anxious and rapid flight, at the last stretch the cars were abandoned and airplanes were boarded. It took days to get to the family's destination in safety. The father later followed them and was accepted. His loneliness and his anxious endeavor to join them had made him an object of compassion, deprived of his menacing qualities. But it was the flight-play which was the most impressive to witness. After an exciting departure and a race through the major part of the first day, mother and son in a most imposing car at the head of the column arrived in a small town represented by the Western play town, its hotels and basic stores. After cars and people were settled, the family rested on the balcony of the hotel, admiring the landscape. "It is evening," Wilbur commented, "the shadows are lengthening."

## Relation to Objects Classified

Certain children's observed reaction to objects is of a threefold nature: autistic, antisocial or hostile, and realistic. Each of these conditions could be roughly characterized by a corresponding speech development or, in certain cases, linguistic pattern.

We should like to define the autistic behavioral attitudes as self-centered withdrawal. Lack of tendency to expand toward the object world is due to expectation of adverse responses to his own "utterances." As all other utterances, language is withheld.

At this stage, which may find more or less extreme expressions of withdrawal, objects, living or inert, are at best mere sources of gratification. Unless a totally negative attitude prevails, they are "imbibed," "ingested" or "grabbed" without any awareness of their objective meaning or accepted value. Speech at this stage is not a tool necessary for communication, and concept formation is at an extreme low. Objects turn up as answers to a momentary need. They have no objective, no general standard and therefore they need not, nor can they be stored nor disposed of for further use or reference. Problems of ownership, of administering them cannot arise. The child who speaks at all may dispose of a minimal vocabulary consisting of a few nouns and a scattering of verbs. When at ease, he may make up a name for the occasion which he may or may not drop thereafter according to the gratification or boost obtained through the object, thus whether "retaining" was stimulated by pleasure or well-being.

A shift from the autistic to antisocial or hostile behavior is to be expected when a "realistic" attitude begins to be in evidence. A dawning perception of the world around is initiated by a nascent sense of adequacy. Rather than deny reality, the child admits it; rather than withdraw from the world, he defends himself aggressively against it. This does not imply that he is aware of antisocial behavior when, from the point of view of society, he commits antisocial acts.

Felix, for instance, used to play with his stolen toys in bright daylight all forlorn in heavenly oblivion, in a state of innocent ignorance of the meaning of his antisocial behavior. In the early days of his delinquent actions the toys were the cure for his injuries. They restored his wholesomeness. The consequences of his behavior to himself or to those he deprived were neither registered nor comprehended. Real to him was but a state of want or of relief. At one time he collected old tin cans for the construction of airplanes propelled by motors. As soon as he became aware of intruders, he felt menaced, gave up this endeavor so important to him and never indulged in it again. Any human approach, with the exception of the therapeutic family, could discourage his appetite for living and for self-realization and incite him to recoil into himself.

Contact with reality is established, but the child doesn't care or refuses to listen. Consequences of his behavior are still not clearly understood or foreseen, since the outlook on the world he fights is reduced to an appalling degree and the immediate surroundings is sensed as the exclusive and responsible source of discomfort.

The majority of these children are challenged by obstacles and frustrations to leave their autistic island and to steer toward an encounter with the forbidding world they know.

Living unreflectively in a state of overwhelming discomfort, the children have no language with which to communicate how they feel and what they need. Unconsidered acts or interjectional language replace it with abuse that casts upon the incidental target the very qualities they object to in themselves. Though these children conjugate their small store of verbs which testifies to their capacity for discernment of an inner and outer experience, the border areas seem to overlap widely. Being not unperceptive of their human surroundings the children suffer from the awareness that their clamor by act or verbal injury is not understood. Only their vexations are registered, but these are vehicles rather than the aim of the children's behavior. The adult sought, though awkwardly, as a source of relief and a tie with the world has now become a target for newly nurtured hostility. The tie is severed and the object of potential gratification and love is removed to an indiscernible distance. Now the stage for antisocial behavior is set.

Loss of support from the parental adult has robbed the child of a state of mind conducive to thought and to the establishing of a socially acceptable value system. The child reaches out for material objects and, in need of a reciprocity denied him by the adult, for youthful

companions, as he is in need of them. In terms of language development it means that, in the case of his dealings with inert objects, he
needs no spoken language. In his dealings with his equals a "family"
jargon develops. A few phrases will be traded routinely with his
equals.

A new form of autism is in evidence. The self-centeredness has
yielded to the centering around the small group of compensatory
selves. The new aloofness and withdrawal is characterized by a particular loss of discernment of one's individuality. The young gang
member is at this time but an organ in a disturbed organism. Each of
two buddies or of a small group engaged in an antisocial act may be
confused about who wanted it and why. "I thought he wanted me to
do it." "I thought he needed the money and I gave it to him." A boy
may admit the other did not explicitly tell him to steal but had mentioned the whereabouts of the object wanted. However he can be
helped to see that he "listened" and did as he was told because he
welcomed a justification of his own intentions. Giving away the
object was also holding on to it and having it. The concomitant absence of social insight is illustrated by a boy's complaint that the police
took from him the flashlight he *bought* in the store and did *not take*.
He discounted the fact that the money was stolen.

In the Clinic a child is given opportunity to explore and explain the
ultimate and remote motives of his behavior and to learn about permissible sources of gratification appropriate to his needs. Immediate
gratification cannot be disregarded, but the child is helped to set goals
for himself that are attainable and thus realistic. The goals are not set
objectively according to the calendar of the adult but attuned to the
child's capacity to wait, to trust, and to comprehend realistic times set
into the future. Frustration span must be slowly extended, never over-
extended. In setting at too great a distance desirable goals of gratification we intensify the desire and weaken the resistance of children with
a history of chronic deprivation and a vague concept of time.

The non-intrusive and unprejudiced curiosity of the adult to learn
the meaning of the child's behavior encourages his trust. He stops
using defense by mute withdrawal, denial of facts, fabrications, and
evasions. In communicating with people the child learns to formulate
what he discovers about himself. He is relieved of the fetters of lacking insight and expression. He can speak up.

Since any syntactical language implies judgment, valid or not, some sense of realism is gained from a procedure which is in operation in the presence of guiding adults. Growth in the area of verbal expression is usually very noteworthy.

## The Emergence of Conscience

In discussing problems of behavior, the child learns to evaluate his attitudes and becomes his own judge. As his ear for the voice of conscience is sharpened, his need to listen to it grows. More and more he turns to the adult with a troubled conscience. The quality of his suffering changes. He has come a far way from the time where in undifferentiated unhappiness he threw rocks anywhere, not knowing how to eliminate his vague and ubiquitous misery.

Wilbur, whom we recently mentioned, became quite sensitive to his shortcomings to the point of feeling observed by any passer-by who, he felt, miraculously knew immediately that he had done something bad. Fortunately he was anxious and able to discuss in individual sessions his guilt and the sensitive nature through which it revealed itself.

In the group, children who feel censured by the judge inside or outside of themselves, like to stage trials before the forum of their own conscience or a censuring world they fear. The observing therapist represents an obvious support. One of these court meetings, suggested by the children as a means of airing problems that had arisen in the day-care group, is herewith reported.

Clarence was accused of undue aggressiveness against a girl in day-care. Theodore and Wilbur were also suspected but not caught. Clarence, now fourteen years old, had been referred by the Juvenile Court at the age of twelve for truancy and dishonesty. He had been a non-learner and incapable of getting along with either children or teachers in public school. He was the third child among his parents' nine boys and one girl. Clarence's sister was his deep love and his guiding star. He rejected all of his younger siblings but tried to emulate his elder brother's artistic skills and attributed great manual skill to the father.

The father, a skilled man in an unskilled job, was self-centered. He deprived the family increasingly and finally left. The mother, a youthful-looking woman in her early thirties, had wanted many children but was totally improvident and inadequate. The children felt loved but were insecure and slovenly to the extreme. Clarence's body care was inconceivably poor. Co-operation from Clarence's family was practically nil. His less backward relatives, though partially interested in Clarence, were discouraged. In the Educational Therapy Center Clarence's attendance was regular, but his behavior did not change. It reflected extreme dependency on the mother, extreme hostile aggressiveness against the younger brothers, a tendency to recruiting his peers for reinforcement and a slyness which tended to deceive the mother and retain her approval. Clarence's absolute refusal to work with any of the male teachers suggested his profound antagonism against his father.

But Clarence was in need of a better status. In the early stages of his small-group therapy sessions, he made skill, his father's only obvious merit, the measure of worthiness. He pretended that his father knew much better than the psychiatrist how to inspire good qualities at building. Model construction remained an obsession for a long period, his only capacity for self-expression and only means of gaining love and self-esteem. Having too much to hide about himself and his family, thinking was repressed for a long period of treatment, and language, though syntactic, was very laconic. With a Buddha-like detachment and smile he would withdraw upon his models. When the other boys' vivaciousness caught his attention, he would join them after having finished an accomplishment that had the meaning of self-accomplishment. His contribution then consisted in the painstaking efforts in building a bridge or another structure that fitted the game. He had great problems with identification. Due to dependency on the mother, he was unable to emulate the father's adequacy at work and had to reduce his endeavors to the scale of his toys. It never occurred to him spontaneously that he was fit to build models of increasing complexity. The father's ill treatment of the mother caused Clarence's identification with her and the desire to be the opposite of the father. Assuming the role of her protector and provider, he was ingenious in breaking into the Clinic, setting aside food and carrying it away over the week-ends. Employing "the goat as gardner," we invested him with responsibilities. Enhanced in his self-respect, he behaved well for months. A job in the kitchen was promised and the assurance that we were working to find the funds to pay him. Soon thereafter, he was caught carrying a bag of food. This setback coincided with the mother's developing interests in a man and his apparent competition with him as a provider. Clarence's acting out was a manifestation of his emergency and a devious means of letting us know that promises, though not disbelieved were no help for immediate needs. We assisted him in psychotherapy in co-ordination with the day-care program in a realistic attitude. His two friends, Wilbur and Theodore showed deep concern about him. For the first time Clarence expressed that he felt deeply ashamed of himself. He revealed appreciation of the help he received and willingness to deserve it in the future, a willingness that was carried into lasting action.

Sexual preoccupations were manifested by hostile aggressiveness against younger girls, an interest in pornographic magazines and a short period of homosexual activities. Soon after the father's departure Clarence was shifted for individual therapy to a male psychotherapist to counteract his tendency to depend upon maternal figures and reject paternal figures and the challenge to be active. He accepted the male therapist as a father figure and joined the sport activities under the leadership of the teacher he had most persistently rejected. The shift to a male therapist had been explained to him and was understood by him but through the months Clarence insisted that the female psychiatrist readmit him for treatment. Though his individual sessions with the male psychotherapist continued he was admitted to a mixed group of young adolescents. In this group, he struggled successfully for adequacy in his relationship to the girls and, accepting spontaneously social rules and standards, achieved a good standing among the boys.

The session to be recorded took place in the third year of treatment, before referral to a male therapist. The boys had appointed the court officials in the previous session and the jury had been sworn in. Clarence, the accused, had pleaded innocent and the hearing had been adjourned.

At the beginning of the second session, Theodore, the district attorney, immediately took matters in his own hands. To his right sat the one-man jury in the person of Marvin. Since he represented several people he was jokingly called several names, Mr. Ears, Mr. Eyes, Mr. Mouth, etc. (That he could assume this multiple role was evidence of much growth in symbolic thinking. His former concreteness was extreme. At intake his psychological rating showed him to be defective. At the time of this writing his I.Q. had risen 30 points, to an average level.)

Clarence, the accused, again denied being guilty. He was placid, composed, and matter of fact. A discussion followed between Theodore, the district attorney, and Wilbur, the judge. Theodore enjoyed playing his part despite the fact that he knew he was as guilty as the accused. But Wilbur became pensive. He was deeply affected by the discovery that it is difficult to be any man's judge. His troubled facial expression and the searching movements of his head showed how confused he was, how profoundly struck and groping for orientation. The psychiatrist remarked that he looked worried. This solicited his statement that he thought, "it is hard to be a judge." He said, "I cannot make up my mind about what is right and what is wrong." Theodore, who at that time still liked to escape responsibilities and laugh off problems, knew well that Wilbur would be incapable of indicting Clarence of a dereliction of which he felt guilty himself. Coming to everybody's rescue, he suggested that the case be dismissed for want of evidence. "We have no case because there are no witnesses to the crime," he proclaimed. The psychiatrist asked whether there existed any other means to establish the facts. The children answered in the affirmative, "the accused can admit his guilt." A witness however was found anyway in the person of a teacher. He played his role so adequately that Theodore, the district attorney, mixed up evidence of Clarence's case with evidences of his own and Wilbur's, all three boys having annoyed the girl that day. Very shamefully the two boys admitted that there could be no court, since Judge, accused, and district attorney were equally guilty. "Everybody is guilty," the two court officials said again in a duo.

Clarence had accepted his part as the sole criminal with so much stoicism because of group loyalty. But his impassivity also showed his refusal to accept the two "culprits" as judges. That the procedure revealed the truth and prevented that he suffer injustice protected him from becoming cynical. Wilbur, the most sensitive and the maturest of the three main actors, was in conflict. He doubted that group loyalty should prevail over truth. For Theodore there was no conflict. Group loyalty was uppermost. It protected all three of them from being exposed. To be fair to Clarence, he needed only to cover up. All three learned about the liberating function of truth.

Theodore wanted to prevent that guilt might be incurred again. He asked whether girls had to be admitted in day-care. It is bound to spell "trouble." He spoke about the girls' tendency to attract the boys and to be peeved when they give in to the lure, but he admitted, "it is mutual." "We also tempt them to get them in trouble."

Marvin reacted with a day's delay to the impact of this session. Information long withheld was released about his family situation. The awareness that even the judge can be accused relieved Marvin of a magic awe of the strict and punitive stepfather. It promoted a dawning awareness of a man's dual role, as a partner and fellow of a guilt-ridden mankind, as well as his incidental role as stepfather and "judge." Identifying anxiously and sorrowfully during the trial with Clarence, he was helped by the proceedings to discriminate between the guilty and the accuser. The former, not necessarily under accusation may have to be searched for among those who "judge you."

This dramatization is an example of the manner by which the children create a tangible forum before which they can "try their failures, expose their troubled conscience and find assistance in the 'process.' "

The children's chosen procedure showed them ready to acquire a realistic attitude. It is not by chance that they erected an exterior forum, symbolic of a social and legal authority not so much to be feared as to be understood and respected. Wilbur, as well as Clarence, requested individual sessions. They were serious in their search for more strength to master their problems dutifully.

Wilbur's father was in a mental hospital at the time and the mother lonely. He worried about her until after a long delay she was placed under the care of the Welfare Department. He and the mother had gratified mutual dependency needs. They deprived and weakened each other. But after having faced his problems in an overflowing need to communicate and when fate had come to his rescue, making unnecessary the sacrifice of all of his income, his vain search for a job and social inadequacy were overcome.

Language at this stage of realistic adjustment is adequate. Syntax is mastered. The children dispose of a variety of accepted idiomatic specifications of thought. For the clarification of an issue they are able to reformulate their statements in a variety of ways. Language has become a tool for inner, as well as outer, discourse. For Theodore, it remained a toy as well, a *fleuret* to wield or a musical instrument upon which to play with virtuosity the tunes of his new elated way of living. Enjoying his virtuosity, he constantly adds good phrases and expressions to his existing word treasure.

# VIII

## Identity in Relation to Objects

### The Seeking of Identity through Things

We mentioned that we had opportunity to observe the children's greed for objects. These are grasped for an answer to momentary needs and are dropped as soon as they have been reached. Apparently they represent no answer to the child's quest for gratification and are devoid of any lasting or generally accepted meaning for him. That for which the child reaches out escapes him over and over again. This reaching out is an impulsive self-healing attempt.

Even those children who have given up their insect-like aimless gathering and are purposeful, to the extent that they reveal by their behavior what self-centered goal they are pursuing, amaze the observer by the brief, wasteful, and unspecific use which they make of objects. Expensive watches may be stolen and trampled upon furiously minutes later. Impressing is the excessive need for dresses of antisocial girls. Barely owned, these are ignored and discarded. The dress for them means more than its apparent use—it is a "maker," a "director"[1] of its wearer, as the etymology of the word shows.[1] It is interesting to note that these young girls use defenses which coincide with such ancient attitudes in man which presided over language formation. As they covet the dress, they visualize an improved, a satisfying image of self, but the coveted dress fails to do what it was expected to achieve. Self-rejection is still intense and as soon as the owned dress becomes a part of the self, it shares the valuelessness of the self and thus loses its magic.

The girls at the industrial school appeared at almost every session in another outfit borrowed from other girls; some of them succeeded momentarily in gratifying their manifold self-love, delighted with the role assumed under such attractive disguise. They *were* at the moment the ones they appeared to be. One of the girls, not content to come to her interviews each time in different clothes, begged for them everywhere, to the extent of writing exacting form letters to all of her relatives. She was totally unrealistic in reference to her huge "consumption" of clothes as well as to her total neglect of them. She accepted all gifts with avidity, but like Goethe's Faust, at the moment of gratification, craved for desire. Some of the children are so haunted that a specific object which they pursue may be overlooked at the very moment it is at hand. The child may not recognize it. The object seems to have changed, due to the withdrawal of the illusion it represented. It is to the child but a translation into a meaningless idiom of the "real word" he is in need of.

We observed the need to touch and manipulate things that obviously represent a verification of the child's existence. Things are an anchorage to which the child in the street, unprotected and unsupervised, may cling long enough to violate the social order but too short a time to convey to it its purpose as an anchorage. During the earlier phases of his treatment, one of our boys would lose everything in the nearest alley. Some children were frightened of going out into the street. Although they needed the reassuring lure of objects, they were afraid of possessing what they should not have. In their driven state and indecision they might run headlong into a moving vehicle longing for relief by catastrophe, submitting themselves as it were to a final decision from without.

## Establishing One's Identity by Means of Touch in Crafts

"The balm of spring rises from the happy hand. The human being finds verification of his existence in exertion of effort."[2] Tactile perception and the manipulating of objects which are sensed as distinct and outside the body limits are instrumental in the discovery of one's own body image; this is a basic relation of man and matter.

## The Soft Matter

Herman Melville in his "Moby Dick" interprets our therapeutic intentions when we give the children, in the Educational Therapy Center, an opportunity for tactile experience which on the surface may seem quite ordinary. Melville describes the kneading of the spermaceti, a fatty substance contained in the head of the spermwhale. The liquid and more solid parts tend to separate but through kneading the lumps are squeezed back into the fluid. "A sweet and unctuous duty," the author calls it. "After having my hands in it for only a few minutes, my fingers felt like eels, and began, as it were, to serpentine and spiralize." Bachelard comments,

how could one better describe the lithe plenitude, the subtleness that saturates the hand and is reverberated constantly from matter to hand and from hand to matter. . . . This preciseness of the equilibrium between hand and matter is a fine example of cognition by kneading. How the fingers gain in length in the gentleness of the perfect dough, how they shape themselves into fingers, into the awareness of being fingers, the dream of fingers, infinite and free.[3]

Both Melville and Bachelard bring to our awareness how the synthesis of resistance and subtlety, a splendid balance between accepting and resisting forces is of rare value in staying the heat of anger. And indeed, if any man discovers through "the joy of the hand," the gentle touch of matter and his own appropriate response, his own capacity for gentleness, sensorial discrimination and nuanced motor adaptiveness, he has gained a mutual relationship with matter. In yielding to this relationship, he in turn makes matter yield more of its potentialities. Slowly knowledge of both the self and the non-self is gained, as well as a liberating awareness of mastery.

To give rise to any beginner's increasingly conscious awareness of his body limits and of his potentialities to alter things, sensed or situated outside these body limits, a sufficiently resisting substance must be offered. We must generate the awareness of being by means of prompting the need for opposing. But the substance must also be sufficiently yielding to bring to awareness the subject's potentialities for manipulating as well as the desire to alter what is at hand. Achievement brings a sense of adequacy and freedom. Therefore, the dignity of work overshadows its limitations; work is viewed not as man's curse but as his austere privilege.

The following observation illustrates a youngster's non-verbal communication revealing that to shape his world a child must be confronted with a "substance" susceptible to being moulded.

James Burting was a tall, physically precocious fourteen-year-old boy whose reaction to people or to any form of experience was a stubborn passive resistance. He spoke few words and those he pronounced could not be understood. Once he appeared to be in a positive mood to reveal himself. He took clay lying on the table and kneaded it persistently with an almost religious ardour until it had a creamy consistency. Repeatedly he looked at the therapist as though to verify that she was in communication with him and comprehended his important message. He shaped and reshaped a serpent, steadily improving the substance of the clay but also the shape of his object. Finally, the product was a piece of art. He had achieved the command of matter, the intensity of whose resistance to him only he could appraise. It revealed to his therapist, in terms of the highly qualified end result that he felt able to shape his world adequately and thus redeem it from its merely animalistic aspects. Circumstances had confronted him with an unsuperable resistance.

James lived alone with his mother. He shared room and bed with her to his pre-adolescent years and was an obstacle to the men interested in his mother's companionship. One of these "stepfathers" expressed his resentment of the boy's presence and his determination to get him out of the mother's bed by burning the soles of his feet with a cigarette while the boy was asleep. The boy was a chronic truant. He remained in bed late, thus laying siege to the house and opposing the mother's sex life. The mother stubbornly insisted on her way of life and the son concentrated all of his efforts on interfering with her mode of existence. This interference included his predominantly antisocial associations in the late afternoon when the mother had gone to work.

In his therapist's presence, James achieved his first harmonious interaction with a gently resisting matter of which he made himself the dedicated master. At that moment he was relieved of bitterness and anger.

Melville expresses with poetic emphasis that, through his molding and battering, participation of hand and matter may become so complete that dipping one's hand with sufficient devotion into the proper matter produces a sense of immersing one's whole being into it. The community of hand and matter sways into a relaxed, giving-in to the world: "I felt divinely free of all ill-will or petulance or malice of any sort whatsoever," we read in "Moby Dick." Yielding to yielding matter which has no object or provocation for rage therefore attenuates wrath. Through "the joy of the hand we reach the joy of the heart."

A minute element of a universe of matter by becoming an inmost part of its molder and shaper also becomes his active tie to the world. While he gives in to it, the part and specimen he handles miraculously represents the whole, and yields to him. This is, in symbolic terms, the meaning of work, man's conquest by dedication. The joy of being, of having, of generating, of actively yielding and gently conquering, all blended in one, engender optimism and hope. Fear of man then yields to a readiness, even a need for human partnership or, as Bachelard says, "the sympathy for the substance of things leads to the sympathy for the heart of men."

Events are newly interpreted in the light of the new outlook and as a result of the newly awakened need for human community.

Suspicious withdrawal from human glances sensed as criticising or destroying, yields to an increasing desire for eyes to behold one's creations, for ears to listen to the narrated revival of the rewarding experience. The child wants to please and to endow someone with his handiwork. He needs an ear to attend to the story of plans for future work and to hear him ask for more material which he will make to obey him and to be his messenger, his interpreter, and performer. Imbued with the process of being shapen, the product is full of the nuances of the imparted meaning. As the holder of the message built into its substance, it can speak to an audience and say that its molder too is in a state "of becoming." It is a tablet and the educator's or therapist's own opportunity to develop insight. It is from the educator's interpreting of such "documents" (objects) that the child can learn to understand the communicative value of printed matter and take interest in reading.

Play with flour and water helps the children associate the pleasures of the hand with the daily bread. Play naturally is connected with food and work, but the hand for making dough is rarely used nowadays. Therefore we substitute clay as an avenue for the child's developing relationship to the world of matter. Pottery clay that has to be mixed with water suitably replaces play with sand. It dries fast, can be preserved as a document of achievement and can be adorned by painting and glazing. It has advantages when the child has reached a stage of self-acceptance and sufficient self-assurance to expect and solicit praise. It is most suitable for initiation to culture; when a state of pure necessity has been overcome, man has leisure to adorn his surroundings.

The expanded self in the shape of the child's performance reduces a self-rejection in the child. A child's anxious inertia has given way to a hopeful expression when a child indulges in any kind of "output"— drawing, molding, cutting, or weaving.

The clay which hardens has disadvantages for the withdrawn and hostile child. It duplicates an inexorable petrified reality or world of feelings. The child may see in what he produces an odious counterpart of himself. While they shape "monsters," "ghosts," horrible animals or dejected people, those who talk may tell you that the product represents the self they hate. They will shape and reshape it to make it increasingly repulsive, finally mutilating it, for instance, cutting off the head. They seek to tell the therapist also that she is wasting her time, that they withdraw from her influence, that they are not an object for hope. Others wish to test whether they are worthy of concern and devotion and to prove that they can succeed despite their deformities. Children may throw their hardened product to get rid of the evil inside themselves or show that they harbor evil as a tool for retaliation, of destruction and self-destruction. Even when the clay product may represent the better side of themselves, as long as it has been made under the support of the adult and not yet out of an inner urge, it may seem untrue, a lie, imposed from without, a mere mockery of one's self.

In the early stages of rehabilitation the soft clay is a better choice. While they work it, the children destroy their begun or finished product which yields at all stages to their ambivalent manipulations. Destruction can be surreptitious. But equally surreptitious can be the slow insidious submission to a yielding matter which the child finds he can crush or construct. It is the alternation of sensations which conveys inevitably the comfort of knowing the matter one is shaping, and to which one can yield or command. *Ambivalence which held the child in indecision to do or undo has finally become an opportunity for a satisfying experience.* If he can overcome the fear of failure, he can also muster the fortitude of giving in to the joy of being in command of his work. He may still need support for overcoming the destructive impulses by which he manifests his refusal of self, but support will be acceptable if he has found people with whom to exchange trust. Trust will result in his readiness to share his product with the outside world and through it to reveal himself. New ventures will be started from where he stands. Penelope undid what she spun to keep unwanted suitors away because she *did* still have a motive for living—hoping that Ulysses would return. The child begins to recognize himself in the continuity of his performance, he senses that he has his history and is aware of a state of having been and of becoming. In treatment, he will be bent spontaneously on remembering and gathering the lost elements of experience for reconstructing the whole. Hope is born when things are not final and no longer deadly serious. The gateways to dreamland and fantasy may be open just enough at this time to evoke the child's curiosity for a new and more profound venture onto the promised shores of the future. Birth of the child's humanity now is at hand.

Children at this stage begin to ask for new materials that they discover and wish to use for self-expression. They make suggestions for improvement of our services; they gradually work for promotion either in their day-care classes or for an early return to the regular schools. They feel increasingly capable and willing to meet requirements and to deal with people. The children's requests reveal the development of their discerning ability and the resulting awareness of the specificity of their needs and interests. Accordingly, they are more capable of explaining the reasons for their past and present attitudes, their likings, wishes, and plans. In other words, they can now use language as an exchange for the future and the serious or whimsical play of their imagination.

The experience, that matter offers its gifts in return for one's attention to it, suggests that similar returns are to be expected from the human fellow by way of a tactful, persistent, and patient interaction. "Was not he the one who gave the clay in the first place?" (meaning the teacher or therapist) the child may now ask. The human fellow spans a bridge to the world and its inviting embankments. The child who now is hopefully and trustingly engaged in traveling toward the shores of a friendly mankind has in turn become fit to strengthen the creed of those who believed in him.

## The Hard Matter

These children now want to serve by the product of their hands and dare testing the metal they are made of on rigid and stubbornly resisting materials. Wood is such a material. It can be conquered.

It challenges and attracts the strengthened child; it causes his energies to converge on an "object" and his mind to concentrate on a purpose which integrates and enhances his mere existence. At times it is an appropriate means for strong masculine self-expression at an early state of treatment. It shows to the educator that the child may struggle with his anger, though vainly or by compulsive means. He may even hammer and saw slovenly and not achieve. But gentle guidance will help him produce an increasingly accomplished whole. This wooden creature of his, made in the image of his creative self, talks to him encouragingly and helps the little man love himself in his product, be proud of himself and love a world embellished by the work of his hand and ready to receive it. A new cause for anger and frustration is engendered when we allow the children to stand empty-handed, disarmed, and deprived of an "object."

Children of the lower-income bracket feel severely deprived when their clamor for materials to manipulate and shape remains unanswered. It is, as evident, an ever repeated experience of want and frustration, of an outcry that meets deaf ears and finally silences their outgoing tendencies. Some children retain enough strength to try to fight their way out of isolation. Usually their misguided efforts cause retaliation that isolates them further.

Materials to work with are not purely a matter for self-expression or a means for social and economic liberation, important as these functions obviously are or will become. For the deprived youngster, materials for manipulation are above all a vehicle and belated opportunity for proprioceptive experience, for the sizing up of one's strength and manipulative skill against and in comparison with the surroundings and its requirements. They are the necessary means of concentrating his energies and his thinking on a purposeful endeavor, patiently, persistently and with the aim of making a perfect and attractive object. To deprive a growing boy of the materials for such an exercise is to deny him the opportunity of welding his character for long hours of training and endurance.

The Educational Therapy Center has suffered chronically from the lack of materials for manipulation, play, and creative activities. Through many months of every year, due to budget limitations, materials have been scarce. With absolute regularity the children's hostile aggressiveness and destructiveness increased correspondingly.

Children ask for objects to manipulate "to keep them from stealing." One of the boys expressed it literally one day: "I am going to be destructive next week if I am not going to have the means of being constructive." Under the double impact of interminable traumatization and a self-defeating and self-rejecting contrition, these children have not learned to discover that guilt feelings may be a man's opportunity. Moreover, this "opportunity" has occurred at too early a period in their lives to be useful. Sound and constructive activity and the relief it affords is long overdue. Deprived of the means to produce, the children act angrily, not simply due to an annihilating frustration, but due to a deep realization of cruel neglect.

Gifts on the contrary are for them the most evident token of love and acceptance, the corollary of which is their deservedness, acquired or granted and sealed by the giver's loving kindness. That is why initially they insist so much on gifts that hurt you. These are creative of the new in these children. They sense that you have to be deprived of one of your ribs to gain a human companion. But when they feel elected, they are no longer in need of gifts to test you; they can be generous themselves. You may be surprised to find a few lollipops on your desk in the morning when you arrive. This gift by the child may not only represent a denial of the candy to himself and a loving offering to the therapist but the denial to himself of his infantile tendencies. It is the unfolding of a new trend to grow up, to be adequate, and to reciprocate. The child's loyalty may be to the therapist or any other worker, to the shop or the therapist's office. They adorn it and by means of their own work, they, as it were, "remain" in the room and retain attention even in their absence from it. The gift is evidently a means of competing with those who covet the same love object and with whom one has to share. It is most impressive that the objects the children make become a means of self-esteem, of self-improvement, of redeemed hostility. They ardently wish to take their work home "to show to my mama," "to give to my mama." When you encourage them to speak, you may find out that they were too ashamed to admit that in adorning their home with things that should have been there in the first place, they raise their standard and with it—so important to them for their own and "her" sake—the mother's status!

Much pathology is expressed in the children's autistic products which support our understanding of their inner experiences and their nascent expansion toward the physical world or people. They may not know what it means because they may not have discovered that things or words can have a meaning. They may artlessly begin to say what their creation "is for." This is placing it in the present with auspices in the future. "For" is mostly a purpose in the home and in reference to the mother, less frequently an immediately self-centered one. The product may obviously reveal a mind poorly integrated in reference to itself and the world around the author of the product. Proudly and smilingly the boy may convert all of his interest to a trinket shelf of his own design with a lamp affixed to the upper shelf. Some illustration in a magazine may cause an epidemic of production of an object that strikes a chord with the children, for instance, steps on a board, shaped like a *moon* crescent.

Hand and machine tools have been no problem with these extremely restless and destructive children whose main spontaneous occupation is fighting. Hostility is being absorbed by the wood. The hand tools represent support in gathering hostility in the direction of a suitable object.[4] The specific purpose built into each tool, the hammer, the pliers, the borer, conveys to it an individuality. With this individuality it invites the child to make a specific use of it in terms of its purpose. The necessary concentration and specialization of sensory-motor activity absorbs much of the diffuse hostile aggressiveness.

The machine is an object of love and pride and represents the dignity of big ownership. The young craftsman in the state of becoming will learn through the skilled use of wax or varnish to coax the wood to reveal its grain or compel it to hide it behind a coloring of his own choice. To use wood of different varieties is most instructive. The children have opportunity to become sensitive to the impression of the texture and natural color of the wood on the beholder. A communication between "consumer" and "tradesman" results. An inner speech develops when the worker anticipates the expectations and desires of the one interested in his product; he will anticipate his needs, the surroundings into which his product will fit. The way is paved for a mutual sponsorship of sensitivity and imagination and the stimulation of constructive goals by realistic anticipation. The child is led out of himself and his present state into interaction with the outside world. He can make a contribution in shaping its state of becoming and in molding the future he is investing with his faith and action.

Children who still want to indulge their hostility will use neither tools or wood. They induce other children's passive obstruction. Instead of accepting the instrument suited for converting and redeeming their aggression, they may insist on bringing knives.

### The Boy and the Motor

Introverted and dependent boys refrain from the outgoing conquest of the hard matter which the wood requires. Its "shrieking" resistance to being cut or coerced into shape is unbearable to them. They prefer the piecing together of pre-shaped materials into a structured whole. Work on bicycles and motor engines passionately engages their energies alone or in the company of a pal. The children's sole outgoing activity or verbal expression then concerns motors. In fantasy first and by more or less stealth later, they attempt to make an inroad on the world. They assemble their "motor" by searching for fitting pieces, collecting anything, with a tendency to be oversupplied. The junk yard is the source of their scavenging and represents the stuff "a bum like myself" is made of. They borrow and trade pieces and become discriminate in discarding parts unnecessary for the completion of their incapacitated engines. But the "bum's" ambivalence is expressed by its revelations that "I want it to run like a marvel." "I want it to be the most perfect motor you ever saw." "It has to be neat," "fast," a "jewel," a "dream." By means of his perfections, he conquers the state of being imperfect, thus conquering the ambivalence between despair and confidence. "I am a pessimistic optimist," said Jerry Stone at one time. For long months motors are being altered back and forth. You never knew there were so many parts to a motor until you have listened to these boys talk about it. The sense of inadequacy is overcome at last, temporarily, when the motor is "complete," or when "it runs" or "works like a clock." Again you may have to listen to innumerable details about how rapidly it can be cranked up, which is the engine's way of being under the boy's command. The youngsters will be sensitive to a host of sounds which are music to their ears, a music to which they want you to react. The unmuffled sound of a motor-cycle or a car in poor repair enchants them to direct proportion to the acoustic pains inflicted upon others. Contrary to the wood which resists the painful operation of being torn apart, the shouting motor expresses obedience to the boy and his power to command. The noise is not only a means of annoying others but a test that the assembler of the motor has greater strength and endurance than they. Nor does he "go to pieces so easily" anymore. A running motor is life itself; without the borrowed power of the motor or the illusion of its support the boys feel in poor command of themselves and of obstacles from without. The motor is the dream of escape to nowhere, to elsewhere or to varying goals as California, Florida, or to the birthplaces of the motorcycles, automobiles, and bicycles. Speed is their means of losing no time and effort between start and arrival and to skip the corresponding space. They are too anxious to notice, and much too anxious to enjoy, the green pastures on the side of the straight asphalt. Whipped in their fancy or in reality by the wind that they cause by their streamlined race, they stay untouched by the gentle courting of the breeze. Hence, neither time nor space can be filled with hopeful anticipations. It is anxiety itself which takes up time and space. This is the way some children described their feelings.

Jerry Stone whose story will be outlined below, was extremely tense due to such a condition. To cope with the abyss of his anxiety, he filled it with fantasies of accidents. Others may actually run into an accident or set an end to an endless distress. Anxiety may take shape in the form of real or sensed traumatization. Thus obtaining a character of familiarity the very traumatization carries an element of comfort and a boy may cling to it for relief, talking about it obsessively. Jerry discovered his mechanisms in the course of a long treatment. In a similar way a boy who had hallucinations and who was otherwise constricted to a robot-like motor and emotional stiffness began, when he improved, to *run* from his father.

Chester Clark, a fourteen-year-old boy of a respectable Negro home, had "never given any trouble." He studied with average success in high school and was, with an excessive zeal, interest, and investment of time, the father's companion in trucking all over the state. Within the space of one week or two the boy committed two irresponsible acts which he sensed as strange and inexplicable. He took a car—when he had his own as well as a truck for which he was paying with his own earnings. This stolen car he drove from the service station where it was parked to another parking place across the corner. The car was in his hands for about one minute. Explaining this behavior the boy said he wanted to get away with that car, but changed his mind, expressing thus the need to liberate himself of "his station," but also the need to keep close to it. He was not ready for the freedom and independence which he desired. He was prompted by the commands of his conscience, as well as held back by the social and material advantages which the condition of his family offered. The second act was to untie a boat and drift in it for half an hour, leaving it anchored at a different place on the owner's property. This was an act of longed-for leisure, a pause in his drive for earnings, overtime and during school vacation. The boy was less obviously exhausted than in a state of anxiety and confusion when referred by court after a third incident, an accident where he ran against a tree with his car, causing considerable material damage.

Chester's father had lost his own father at the age of nine and his mother had lost her father at the age of three. Both had worked very hard from an early age to achieve finally economic equality with a white man's upper-middle-class income. The father was kind, honest, very ambitious, but unaware that he drove himself and his son too fast. In need of relief because of his own long drawn-out competitive race with the dominant ethnic group, he relied too soon and too much on his son. He was inconsistent enough to deal with this son as with a grown-up partner, while simultaneously treating him as a young child who needed direction and strict supervision, and who had to give account of each of his moves. The mother had never been a solace to either of the two male persons in her family. Though devoid of excessive hostility, she was not endowed with much warmth and understanding. She was above all the husband's partner whom she supported by thrift and efficiency. Therefore, the boy had reasons to find her exacting and critical of him, never a support or comfort. In a session where this problem was discussed with the parents, the father remarked "this is true also in regard to the husband."

The boy reported that the accident occurred when he lost his way in the country, feeling persecuted by a white boy. He raced into a tree in an anxiety which rose to a panic when he saw he had reached a dead-end street. He could not clarify whether the police or anybody else was following him.

When treatment started, he was confused about who he actually was, a man or a child. He was as preoccupied with the trucking business and the large motors as by his secret love, a midget car he had bought with his savings and to which he slipped out when it could be done "to build it up without no intention of riding it." When the father discovered it, he was outraged that the boy could spend his money so foolishly. He had tried to help him become a provident man and that he would indulge in so "silly" a pursuit as "fooling" with a midget car horrified him. The father conceivably did not understand the deep meaning of play or the symbolism of Chester's toying with such a conveyance, the right-sized partner of an obedient child who still needs to "fool" with something after school rather than to assume major responsibilities.

Jerry Stone was extremely anxious when he drove with me leisurely through the countryside on a superb spring day. The roads were, as usual, free of traffic. Off and on, a car passed us with equal leisure; but the boy looked anxiously backward and tried to speed me on.

At the time of referral this thirteen-year-old boy with an at least average mental ability was intensely hostile and withdrawn. He was a serious behavior problem in school, insubordinate, provocative; he cursed and was pornographic in front of the class to shock the female teachers. He adamantly refused to study and had repeated one class four times. At a later phase of treatment he displayed a variety of phobic states, a condition which made it impossible for him to attend school, eat in restaurants, go to a movie or to a recreational center. At one period of treatment he could barely leave the very home he so hated.

Jerry was averbal for a long time; for years he had not broached a smile. He was extremely provocative and as in school he attempted to incite the other children to be insubordinate. In the Clinic, however, he assumed leadership by his obstructive, agitating, and shocking behavior. He was discouraged in such behavior by the day-care group, by its devotion to the staff and the psychiatrist, whom he wanted to hit. In the office of the psychiatrist Jerry would sit for an extended period of time in a most disrespectful attitude trying to shock and do all he could think of to provoke rebuttal. He wanted to play with firecrackers in the office, and at a later date, constantly played with matches which, he said, he "stole" from his mother, who smoked all day long. The heat they produced cracked the ashtray one day where he set ablast his mother's pyre symbolically. He would light the socks he had on his feet, hoping to provoke the psychiatrist's anxious outcries for his safety, a provocation which never failed to be rewarded by attention at home. His mother's predictable and anxious reaction irritated him intensely. Years later he said she was afraid of her own shadow. By eliciting more of this anxiety Jerry nurtured a hostility which otherwise was starved for expression. It gave him a sense of mastery he could not gain by any positive achievement. The psychiatrist would react to his lighting his socks, by asking calmly and kindly, why. He would usually respond by saying it didn't hurt him and let the blast die down. He then might light the other sock. When nothing more was said, he gave up playing with fire. He began to respect the psychiatrist when she consented to use the sessions for target shooting with real cartridges. The community between him and his psychiatrist began when he handed his gun to the psychiatrist, inviting her fondly to try a few shots of her own. She was to book the points. Now she was no longer as forbidding a desert as his mother seemed to be to him; moreover, the therapist had stood the test of valor. She was no longer identified with the mother, no longer afraid of her own shadow.

At a later date, he was racing on a motorcycle track, secretly at first. He felt protected by the secret. "I shall avoid the slightest scratch in order to prevent my father from knowing." When his father had found out, he was eager to prevent his father from worrying. I would feel it at a distance of ten miles, implying that the resulting guilt feeling may cause insecurity and accident.

This was very important to him because the mother's anxiety and indecision gave him no support. He thought very little of her; to be unlike her was one of his motivations for his overbearing behavior and spurious foolhardiness. The trust placed by the psychiatrist in his ability to deal responsibly and skilfully with a dangerous weapon, under conditions agreed upon, strengthened his weak self-esteem and gave him the experimentally supported proof that not only the mother figure, but he too could stand the test of adequacy and responsibility. In this function she compared favorably with the father. At the time, however, the boy considered him too paternalistic and anxious.

Jerry began to talk but needed the dictaphone as a mediator. He played the role of a television announcer for several weeks, reporting motorcycle races with great excitement, fatal accidents, and other less serious ones which proved to have little or no physical consequence for the victims. This talking would not last long and he would stretch himself out on the long table in the office, his hands folded behind his head and he would speak from the inmost recesses of his poor constricted self. Oases of experiences imbued with a poetical atmosphere, and filled with motors and their parts, emerged from an emotional desert. Dreams were revealed of climbing mountains with his motorcycle, racing, speeding, and challenging and outsmarting the police. All of his life and his personal associations centered on building and rebuilding motorcycles. But he was insatiable. Each time he reached his goal, he could enjoy it only mentally or because he tried to be appreciative (he had a desire to please and be kind); but, in fact, he remained ungratified and starved; the flower of love he wished to tend remained dry and puny.

A longed-for "perfect" gratification which he "had been dreaming of all of my life," "since I was four years of age" kept him speeding and "racing" madly, anxiously struggling for control. In sharing with increasing warmth his restricted domain of preoccupations, he became aware of the aridity of his emotional and mental territory.

He revolted against a self as reiterative and monotonous as his mother, whose tendency to repeat herself was the very thing that drove him to distraction. At the time he dared fate and kept open a wound incurred by falling from his motorcycle. For an extended period he bit his nails ravenously and picked his skin keeping it injured and infected. He pulled his hair and his eyebrows. His self-rejection became so intense that he could visualize himself only as a good-for-nothing, living from the mercy of institutions like the Salvation Army. His motorcycle for him was the image of his humble condition and the moving grounds supposed to carry him "to nowhere." His motorcycle was his morganatic companion to which he clung with utter faithfulness, until his father could be won over to approve of the liaison. His faith in his humble companion was his actual salvation. It helped him discern between genuine values as opposed to conventions and trivialities, which Jerry abhorred. Taking off in fantasy with his beloved one to new shores where he could "still see the sun rise when it has set," on our beaches; new light was seen and new plans surged in that fancied dawn. He wanted to become a skilled motor mechanic and stop tinkering with them, but he found that every school that met his standards of perfection, required a high school education.

One of the reasons invoked by Jerry for his opposition to school was that he had been coerced all of his life into doing what others expected him to do, school having been the most burdensome area of his coercive education and an actual serfdom.

The father who had been struggling desperately to "make him" go through school was helped to release his anxious grip and instead trust in the son's ability to discover what he needed for himself. Simultaneously the child was helped to see that he had failed to explore his own purposes, being distracted by his distrust of adult guidance and his determination to fight it without examining its merits. The emerging convergence of attitudes of father and son from there on replaced their former divergence. "I am just as stubborn as my daddy"—supported Jerry's new realism. For the sake of his very own purposes, the "service" to the long standing secret love of his life, the motorcycle, he was now stubbornly determined to finish high school. He felt assured that there must be a college for a bum like him, a connotation he now gave to himself humbly but smilingly. Not only did he study with determination, but he learned to endure patiently for the sake of his purpose some of the teachers he did not care for. But he learned to respect and admire others. As time went on he talked less and less of the teacher's attitude as obstacles for success and was more and more concerned about his own, thus deepening the insight in his human relations and tracing them to their traumatic sources. He learned to associate with boys and girls and the range of his interests widened to areas a young adolescent boy might be expected to turn to. He found to his surprise that it was easy to talk to girls nicely in good English and to speak distinctly in order to be understood. "With boys I speak indistinctly and use bad language." He read a great deal and took a particular interest in inspiring biographies. He was moved by the lives of men who, in their own way, had been disapproved of by their fathers but finally achieved an outstanding success which convinced their fathers. He felt that in his own modest way that could and would be his case.

The whole treatment had to be carried in opposition to a negativistic mother, who never could be enrolled for collaboration in spite of serious and repeated efforts. The mother's aloofness to the interests of her boy and her rigid and uncompromising insistence on her own approach, reflected the total lack of communication between the parents. The mother was an ambulant schizophrenic who had previously undergone treatment with no noticeable improvement. She blocked the son's treatment because it was undertaken, as she saw it, as the father's concern and project. Actually she had isolated her husband in the family by being unrewarding in every area where consideration or gratification should have been expected. When the husband's tolerance was periodically exhausted, he would "blow up," frightening the mother and the unsupported children, who were totally unprepared to understand the father's plight. The father therefore was anxious, authoritarian in his approach, considering his children's failures as his own. Consequently he was ardently involved in the success of Jerry's treatment. This success finally was brought about by the father's contribution. He relinquished his own immediate stake in the matter, which implied that the son of this father had to fulfil pre-established goals. As he learned to trust his son and let him find and fulfil his own "vocation," they could meet in a fond community and mutual understanding of goals. Both achieved a measure of tolerance for the mother's obvious weaknesses. The son discovered that he still loved the mother, and the father found comfort in knowing that neither son nor mother were totally deprived.

The motorcycles played an important "conveyance" role in Jerry's transference to the psychiatrist. In the earlier treatment period they beclouded inhibitions in his capacity to relate and concealed resistance. In a number of guises his talk about motorcycles, racing, trading, and building was his way of sharing what preoccupied him. He attributed to the therapist all the *dramatis personae* in the lived and fancied drama of his life. One of these, and not of the least importance, was the mother who in communication with the father—a condition he deeply longed for—he could use as a mediation for an independent and increasingly liberated relationship.

Covering distances, he had mastery over space that was measured by reduction and imagined annihilation of time, the telescoping of all his life enjoyment into a few exciting seconds. Life's fullness he refused to experience until later in treatment. He explained that he disliked the watch as a reminder of time and the enforced routine of existence. Routine represented the mother, her repetitiveness, her monotonous food, and her habit of showing him kindness by "stuffing down his throat" the few things he liked, until they too became repulsive.

## Preoccupation with Watches

When he went to a foster home, Henry Hawthorne gave away callously the watch received as a gift from his parents, breaking by this act his filiation with them. For some time he enjoyed the new watch received from his foster parents for Christmas. But when his attachment to the parents was revived, he confessed to what had happened to their watch. (He still was callous in the way he spoke about it, thereby hurting his parents, but at least he had come to the point where he no longer could live with the rejection of his progenitors without the need to confess.) We need to state specifically that Henry had discarded no other of his parents' gifts.

The "taking" of watches may be due to desired filiation to a respectable social milieu, a filiation which circumstances have led the "taker" to believe that he can achieve only by indiscretion and arbitrariness. Usually the children feel extremely uncomfortable with this prized object. They cannot deceive themselves about the real milieu under the circumstances. The symbol of a better condition does not fit; on the contrary, it highlights the discrepancy between dream and reality. These watches, then, are lost almost the very moment they are "taken" and in a gesture of hostility against what they really represent, as well as in utter and hopeless self-rejection, they are stamped to pieces as symbols.

In a desire to seal symbolically his filiation to his therapist, another boy, Leonard asked for a watch. He was extremely anxious not to lose it. Keeping the watch and being capable of preserving it in a workable condition was proof to him that he was living up to the standards this filiation stood for in his mind. With a mien of mutual understanding, he would point from time to time to his watch and, with triumphant staccato knocks, he would alert the psychotherapist to the praiseworthy achievement that the token was still preserved.

Once he had found an active and independent road to life, Leonard bought himself a new watch from his own earnings. Now he wanted to own his existence, as a man, to his own efforts. He significantly discarded the watch he once had requested from the psychotherapist as a symbol of the gift of life. However, then as well as through the years, he was most appreciative of the help received from her.

Preoccupation with a watch coincided, in Jerry's case, with a remarkable discussion with the therapist about life and death. At the same time he also chose to write, for school, two compositions on death. This all happened while he was loathe to own anything of his father's and even less of his mother's. In final analysis all this meant his denial of the gift of life. He refused to eat his mother's food, spent his allowance on meals in drugstores or went without food all day. His father could induce him to eat breakfast using all his diplomacy and psychology.

However, Jerry asked his father for a watch because his two older brothers had received one. He disliked his state as the youngest, which made him a strange "heir"—to handed-down clothes that his brothers bought in profusion. Jerry commented on their selfish exploitation of the father and their lack of desire to be independent. Nevertheless, he felt inadequate in reference to his eldest brother, an abhorred father figure who was close to the mother. But the father who had his reasons for feeling anxious about his authority with the sons, delayed, as usual, the granting of gifts that he had not thought of himself to give. When the watch was offered at the father's own time, Jerry felt like discarding it. He was troubled about being denied self-assertion in this matter, even when the father thought he had pleased him. At a later date, when Jerry called himself happy, he also reported he could not think of parting with the watch anymore. He accepted that he was *given* life but had found out that its conduct was in his own hands and that it could be attuned to the expectations from a world replete with opportunities to be embraced.

# IX

## The Problem of Language

### Speech as a Barrier or a Weapon

Due to the intellectual, emotional, and socioeconomic status of the parents, the children referred to us have known language not as a bridge between people but as a moat in a shooting war. Either the drawbridge is raised completely and the child is taciturn, or it is lowered only in order to send across a steady stream of words to attack the opposing forces. It is a means for coping with emergencies. These arise constantly, leaving no alternative other than to be incessantly in an attitude of assault, which precludes discursiveness.

This is reflected in their grammar. The imperative mood of the verb predominates, being used for the expression of wants. The present tense of the indicative mood is next in frequency. Past and future in the beginning appear most usually in the terms: "He hit me!" "I hit you!" The auxiliary is not used with the verb "kill" unless the child is talking to an adult about his alleged intentions. We see here a first indication of the result of discussions with the adult. The plural occurs with extreme rarity because of the children's utter isolation, their self-centeredness, and their unresolved primary relationship to their mothers. Similarly the children do not remember or inquire about people's names, and if asked to state their own will invariably mention their first name only. Not to know anyone's name may be a safeguard; it dimly means that you cannot be made to be a witness, and you do not actually know whom you know. When a child begins to speak of "a friend of mine," one can be assured that the treatment is having results. His relationships have become specific and represent a selection out of a plurality of choices which presupposes a sense of adequacy and some perceptive acuity.

Their limited vocabularies reflect a dearth of concepts which are due to lack of opportunity as well as to lack of desire for gaining new experience. Faulty articulation, suggesting a lack of communicative drive, reveals the child's despair: he cannot believe that anybody will "listen to what I have to say." Poor articulation may also be an expression of self-depreciation or a means of gaining and retaining prolonged attention. By poor articulation the child retaliates in kind for difficulties incurred in conveying messages or asking questions. Again, it may be a wish to appear helpless and in need. It is then a way to be deceptively alluring, as a dissimulation of distrust, shame, or hostility. Ambivalence in reference to the will to communicate, as well as doubts about the acceptability of the communication, may result in a very rapid speech tempo with slurred articulation. Low tone and monotony of voice are frequent signs of depression; alternatively, they may show that speech is used only reluctantly. The child wants to explain "nothing to nobody," not even to himself.

This reluctance impedes the development of syntactical expression. There is in particular no inner discourse or the eager questioning for the reasons "why" so characteristic of the healthy child who is almost flirtatious in his bid to retain attention, at times testing his auditor excessively. Reflection and the clarification of thought would serve no purpose with a child isolated by neglect or rejection; a limited verbal communication, however, satisfies immediate needs. These are best served by idiomatic phrases and slang, which represent communal bonds and a code for the initiates of a secret society. They are thus weapons used from an ambush. The use of idiomatic phrases may also express the children's desire to belong, to break through the language barrier without a serious and persistent effort. On the other hand, it can be language memorized or ingested and spit out with disgust. The positive relation to the psychotherapist can be expressed by the acquisition of syntax, discursive speech, and good choice of terminology; but *trust* may be manifested by the child's presentation of the key to the secret code, implicitly revealing that he is surrendering his weapons because he wants to be conquered. In terms of *syntax* the child's readiness to communicate is expressed in the replacement of the predominantly subjective, interjectional language which he uses during the early stages of therapy with proper discourse. He will correct his use of terms, and tenses, saying, for instance, "I used to . . . ," "I would . . . ," "I was in the habit of. . . ." The number of his prepositions increases and there is a slightly richer choice of adjectives, to convey specific questions or reflect a more discriminating experience.

*Discourse,* which in its simplest form implies a judgment, a statement about the identity of an object, also implies an element of suspense prior to the decisive acknowledgment that a thing is what it is. It is not surprising that the profoundly traumatized children, who no longer act impulsively, might however not yet be able to cope with suspense by making a definite statement concerning the identity of an object. Due to rashness, flightiness, anxiety, or frank ambivalence, they fail to distinguish between real or fancied perceptions, or in the sphere of volition and action they incessantly brood over or re-evaluate a situation, depending obsessively and vainly on the adult for a conclusion. The absence of gratification, via the grasp of reality then, may combine with an oral aggressive tendency to exhaust the adult by persistent and repetitive questioning. The gratification derived from inflicting annoyance may replace to a certain extent the ever evasive resolution of suspense and increase the incapacity to come to a decision.

### The Magic of Words

For these children words can be a terrifying magic, used for the transmission of wishes, good and bad.[1] This magic can bring relief or despair; it can punish or reward.

Without basis in fact a boy excused another boy's absence simply by stating: "He had an accident and is dead." An awful silence followed. To the other children, it was quite obvious that a death-wish had been uttered. Barely had he spoken his sentence, than the boy became concerned whether the other youngster would now *have* to die.

A schizophrenic child who never succeeded in expressing his thoughts, repeatedly insisted on a psychiatric interview. However, he could be counted upon to leave the Clinic the very moment he was to enter the office of the therapist. One day when he actually came to the interview he was asked in simple terms whether he was afraid of making a dreaded event come true by stating it. Surprised, he answered: "How do you know"?

The belief in the magic of words may cause a child to curse the other fellow's mother. Curses, the sharpest weapon of all, thus will be used as a means for offense directed against the other boy, or else to attack his mother, thus sparing his own mother. The target is fully aware of the danger threatening him through magic and nothing can prevent him from an irate retaliation. "One thing I cannot take," he says, "that's calling my mother names." The threat is deeply felt because almost invariably the retaliating victim, by exciting the original aggressor, will cause him to react more violently by cursing him *and* his mother, thus, so to speak, killing him from his roots up. "I beat you until you and your mother are blacker than mine," says an irate twelve-year-old girl profoundly rejected by an intelligent mother. However, the angry child cannot help fearing that evil will befall the mother, an evil which he himself has conjured up, and for which necessarily he will be punished. Nothing will prevent the child from fighting because he is really, as he says, protecting his mother. To protect her means to forestall the fulfilment of the curse. Until he can master his own hostile impulses against the mother, he will "hear" others, who have said nothing, curse her, or else he will stir them to curse her and in fighting them he will feel that he is her protector; he will redeem his hostility, annihilate the magic, and relieve his tensions.

The children distinguish spontaneously the *magic* of cursing from the *habit* of cursing or a need to curse which may be automatic or obsessive in character. Their reaction to these phenomena is different. They tolerate an excessive amount of all forms of cursing and take it for granted. It may be used as a pretext for a fight similar to the challenges preceding a tournament. However, cursing, having a magic significance, promotes awe. The children keep their emotions in abeyance as though in the anxiety of waiting for the effects of the magic. At times there may be no reaction but leaning on the therapist or teacher for comfort and protection and a return to rationality and reality.

## Verbalism Emerging from Treatment

It is striking to observe how practically all of the young wards of the Educational Therapy Center develop facility in speech. This gain obviously is of primary importance since the children's disturbed development is reversible and thus corrigible only symbolically and not in reality. The capacity for expressing their problems, their thoughts and feelings, which we recognize as a step achieved by the milieu, reflects the general growth needed to qualify them specifically for psychotherapy.

If we adopt a genetic concept of the evolution of personality, our share in "becoming" what we are cannot be disassociated from the influence of personal contacts and the general milieu to which we reacted and upon which we acted in the constant process of changing. Whenever the balance of this interaction with our milieu has turned out to be negative, temporarily or persistently, a particular effort is required to restore it, consisting of a reliving or a re-"vision" of the past with the result that we become, out of necessity, conscious observers of that bygone existence. Suffering is inevitably connected with this review and the attempted change of outlook, whether past misfortune is remembered, or the passing of happiness is deplored, whether we are pained or shocked by discovering our share in provoking, triggering or channeling behavior that we felt was inflicted upon us undeservedly. Deep regrets harass us when we realize what love and friendship might have been preserved, had we interacted with more wisdom; sadness may result from the futility of such belated thought and the doubt whether, considering the situation at that time and the actual state of all the people then involved, the tragedy could have been avoided or whether its outcome was actually inevitable.

When such insight has been gained, though confusedly and dimly, by the youngsters to whom we devote our attention, they may regard struggle with any aspect of life as futile. A profusion of bewildering problems may silence them completely, or else they may be reduced to only one tendency; to destroy the eternal obstacle, the world as they know it, because it is unendurable and not worthy of existing. When they do begin to communicate their feelings, they may reveal that it is a mistake to consider them ignorant. "People think I know nothing, but I know everything." With these cryptic words they give you to understand that laden with their kind of wisdom they have no use, no appetite, no strength for your brand of knowledge. In their experience the world you stand for is absurd.

But, incongruously, this simple sentence is also evidence that the world is beginning to make sense. The state of shock, of bewilderment, of hurt, fear, or shame that made them either speechless, or fearful or shy about using words, is in the process of being resolved. At the end of the evolution we shall find the child ardently interested in going to public school "to get me an education."

At the stage when he begins to speak, and in speaking to defend his position, even though he has begun to doubt its validity, he does not value the deep insight which he owes to his suffering and isolation. Actually, his total outlook is changing. He is no longer preoccupied with suffering, with the injustice or rigors of fate, or with the futility of all that is. He will have a goal toward which he moves. In order to live, he knows now, he has to make a place among his fellow men. That he can attain it he has found out in the experimental microcosm which is the Educational Therapy Center. He has found evidence that he is no more, but also no less, than "every man." As a tool for the social adjustment he now is eager to achieve, he is reaching out for valid knowledge which is his own. It is noteworthy that at this fairly advanced stage of treatment children become speech conscious in reference to their poor articulation and diction. They see that it represents a handicap for their newly awakened desire to communicate and the role they want to play in relation to their community. Therefore they will make active attempts to correct their weakness.

## "Listening" to the Silent Child

Basic to the encouragement of communication by speech is the necessity to "listen" to a child,[2] whether he speaks or not, whether he can at this time be stimulated to speak or not. When a child does not speak, one has to *be* with him in an individual rapport bent with all one's senses to receive the message which the child makes a tense effort to conceal by freezing up. This negative effort, which is transmitted via his closed mimicry, his motor rigidity, his frankly negativistic posture, gives the attentive observer, who is at best the merely tolerated partner of the child, the necessary clues for a behavior appropriate to his needs. Your understanding patience sets a child at ease. His strenuous effort to shut himself up and to shut the other person out will be relaxed with a resulting sense of comfort to which the child will become accustomed. A new state of existence results, a new habit which takes the place of the former constriction. A first communication may result from the child's first timid motion; grasping for, or helplessly glancing at an object, he might finally smile at you, proud of his daring and of the step made toward you by his outgoing venture.

When the child begins to touch a toy or even to look at the therapist questioning whether he may—proud that he dared, yet resourceless and in need of help—the stage is set for communication by language. If you feel that your noticing his behavior, and saying something about it will not cause him to fall silent again, you may call the name of the toy he has reached for, using the tone of voice most appropriate to the child's needs. Some definiteness in tone may give support to the deeply insecure child; a surprised tone may stir an emotion; a questioning tone may elicit, even though delayed, a repetition of the name. The child who has no speech, once he feels comfortable in the presence of your unobtrusive companionship, begins to utter sounds erratically when he plays. The child who *can* speak but withholds it can be caught napping if the observer enters his or her childlike or, where possible, autistic world.[3]

Charlotte Barden is an example of a nine-year-old whom we caught napping on the day of her initial interview by entering her world. Charlotte had allegedly lost her speech at the age of three, when the mother deserted her and her father, leaving no trace. The father was still deeply hurt and had not married again during the six intervening years. The original shock which caused the child's mutism and the loss of any motivation to relate by speech was continued indefinitely because the father's suffering laid stress on the state of deprivation. The child resented his depression which she sensed as rejection and to which she therefore responded by ignoring him. In play therapy, the child betrayed subsequently and inadvertently, both her volubility and the fact that speechlessness was for her a retaliatory device, a withholding of gratification from the other person, originally the mother.

On her first appointment she was asleep in the waiting room or feigning sleep. The aunt who had brought her was anxious that every second of Charlotte's session be used for her benefit. She shook the

child and talked insistently, telling her the psychiatrist was waiting
and that she must go right away. This caused the child to freeze
up. The psychiatrist spoke kindly to the aunt, reassuring her that
Charlotte need not be rushed; if she desired a little rest, she could
have it. The girl was reassured also and told that the dollies in the
office were anxious to see her as soon as she was ready to come and
visit with them. The psychiatrist then left the waiting room and
returned a few minutes later with a baby doll, assuming that the
need for identification with it would tempt Charlotte to play with
and nurse the doll. "Dolly wants to play with you," she said. The
child took the doll and laid her on her folded arms as one would a
baby, though without fondling her. Slowly Charlotte arose and, as if
accepting the doll's invitation, walked like a toddler to the office.

   There she nursed and tended the dolls, cooking for them, feeding
them, or serving dinner for the father and mother doll, while the
psychiatrist remained companionably silent. She was so involved in
her play that she forgot her need to withhold speech; in fact she
began to speak fluently, with perfect articulation and remarkable
speed. She not only spoke to the doll but commented on the meaning
of the play, engaging the psychiatrist in it. Without her commentary,
only the negativistic and destructive elements of her play would
have been evident. The strangeness of her play pattern was puzzling.
With the toy knives and forks she cut clay to pieces and immersed
it in water while manipulating it. She cut a hole in a rubber dog
and pushed the clay inside. Then she searched for something and,
finding the top of a box, laid the dog inside and bathed it with water.
Since Charlotte had been nursing and tending the dolls immediately
prior to this play, it looked on the surface as though she was now
bathing the dog, but elements of her activity did not fit into the
picture. Finally the psychiatrist asked whether the doggie was taking
a bath. "Hum, hum," she answered shaking her head. "This is a
turkey." And setting it on some toys as on a range, she added, "a
roast." It became evident then that the water was gravy; she was
basting the turkey. The clay pushed inside the dog was the stuffing
and the cut-up clay not used for stuffing, later on was served as
vegetables and potatoes. What seemed at the outset a hostile game
played in muteness and aloofness, with the destruction of a toy dog
and the ruining of the clay for others, was seen to be sublimated

and revealing. In this and the following sessions due to the purely expectant, observant, and "listening" attitude of the psychiatrist, Charlotte revealed her need of being a little woman, a housewife, someone who was adequate and acceptable. But she froze when we suggested, "Daddy might like to eat the turkey." We assumed in those early days of treatment that she did not want to grant what was not desired by the father. His mourning for the mother showed Charlotte in a cruel way that she could not fill the gap for the father and herself by *being* the little woman, replacing the one that deserted both of them. Charlotte's procedure, the accents of defiance and cruelty in cutting the clay and in cutting the "turkey," the violent way of stuffing it, justified the assumption that with this play she simultaneously gratified hostility of a multiple nature and indicated that someone more important than the animal had to be thus grated to be roasted. What interests us at this point is that the protracted shock and the muteness were overcome because someone "listened" to the child's behavior as it was manifested in the office and understood it in light of her case history. Her withdrawal was not interfered with. Instead of making her obey the requirements of the adults and their anticipation of her behavior, she was visited in her own world of fanciful play and thereby was caught off guard.

The children will frequently express appreciation for "listening" to them. "This is the best time I ever had. Nobody ever listened to me before. I love people." An intelligent boy said, "I feel inferior although I know I am not." In scrutinizing his situation, he mentioned repeatedly that his mother never listened. It tore him to pieces to listen constantly to her rambling thoughts. She "led him to dark woods and got lost with him." She did not know anything about him and built him up from pieces borrowed from other people and motivated by rejection, anxiety, and extreme ambition. No wonder the boy felt inferior because he "was nothing," and no wonder he resisted everything the mother needed and expected him to be. As for the boy previously quoted, he was dissociated by his parents' failure to listen from his own growth potentials and his own vocation.

In addition to being supportive of the integration of self, listening to the child is interpreted by him correctly as respect paid to his humanity. "You all treat us like human beings, you talk to us," are comments winding up the initial interview or reflections at some later stage of treatment. At such a time children wish that their loved ones could benefit from and be helped by the same privilege. "Let them sit around this table and quarrel in your presence, you might find out what bothers them and help them."

At the time of referral, most of the children have language which is not under control, unless by total suppression. This is evidently the reason for, as well as the effect of, their need to substitute acting out for verbal expression. The children have not learned to liberate themselves by the use of speech. A full scale of expression by movements, mimicry, crying, weeping, screaming, and, as we have seen, sporadic, irate outbursts of idiomatic phrases take the place of it. Even their most "elaborate" verbal expressions are simple in form and simple by the fact of their immediate relation to some proximate purpose. However, the most taciturn child may surprise the therapist by a monosyllabic expressiveness which throws light on a complex and consequential situation. Appropriate responses to the child's non-verbal and at times unfocused communication, the picking up as it were of the message sent out in space without any specific address, leads finally to mutuality in understanding and expressing. The child begins to feel very important because his messages are being received and answered. Importance is measured less and less in terms of delusive omnipotence and more in terms of intimacy and the human quality of the relationship. The child reaches a place of safety from which he can acknowledge his limitations and attempt to remedy them. He necessarily reaches out for help by means of the word.

Concomitant with the development of language into a tool of purposeful communication, a fundamental change of attitude occurs. The harmonizing of one's revealing words with the purpose of the communication at hand, presupposes a complex of behavioral adjustments, in the first place the postponement of these revelations to permit proper timing and formulation. In order to control timing and formulation, the child has to concentrate on recruiting for a single action all of his sensibility and mental energies and on holding them ready for release at the very instant that fleeting opportunity presents itself. This "sharpshooting of the mind" which is required for any form of purposeful discussion is assertive but not aggressive behavior and not necessarily hostile. Thus, in addition to self-assertion as manifested by discursive speech, self-control is required and through its practice it is acquired. Impulsiveness is conquered.

Delay of communication is inevitable in class and in the day-care group, where the children's impulsiveness must be regulated. The adult staff makes them aware that unless they can withhold their verbal explosions, they cannot be understood. The noise and the chaos resulting from simultaneous outcries make their words impossible to comprehend. The experience of gratification that would result from understanding them and the serious consideration of the manifested needs, encourages proper timing of the message a child might want to convey. Observing the staff who is trying to listen to at least two, if not several, children who want to talk, and in particular to those who are quarrelling and who take opposite views (and the necessity to help the children see both sides of an argument is an important preparation for verbal discourse), the children become aware that to satisfy their urgent needs and carry their messages they have to modulate their voices, articulate distinctly, and express their thoughts clearly. In this process of spontaneous learning, they are assisted by the example set by their adult surroundings. The obvious gain made possible by day-care can usually be noted in the therapy sessions, where the child begins to discuss alternatives clearly and, as time goes on, eloquently.

Moreover the repeated experience of waiting for the therapeutic session and the delaying of a gratification one has learned to rely upon is highly supportive of language development. The child has to think what he is going to say in anticipating the dialogues; he might think it over a few times or discuss it with a teacher, another staff member, or a child until the great moment comes which really counts: talking to his therapist.

## Communication in Time

When the child begins to speak, the use of syntactic speech slows down, though imperceptibly, the process of communication and defers the organized message into the future rather than the immediate instant. To verbalize in a syntactic form presupposes that the child anticipates both the future moment and the ultimate response to the message. This again calls for the discriminating and integrated control of one's thought and vocal expression as well as of one's mimicry, toward the achievement of the desired effect. Judgment as well as sensitivity has to be resorted to. Empathy and insight are promoted.

Acquiring the discriminative tool which is syntactic speech means translating undergone experience into concepts and symbols and miraculously storing them in mind in this abstract form. Using syntactic speech means resorting to previously stored-up experience and therefore extending the present instant back into the past as well as forecasting an anticipated period of time when the message will be heard. He who speaks thus resorts to the past and appeals to the future and expects it to respond. The continuity and integration of experience thereby are established, motivated by the factor of hope, however it might still and always will be mitigated by uncertainty. To reduce children constantly to silence, and refuse to hear what they think and have to say, discourages thinking and the integration of their experiences with a view to their purposeful use.

There is implied in verbalization the reduction of a long-endured suffering to an infinitesimal fraction of time by the symbol of the word. Translation into words necessarily objectifies suffering and thus, converted from individual to general terms, makes it fit for relating to others. These are equipped to understand, being familiar with the linguistic coding necessary for retranslation of the message and also willing to share it with compassion. Making experience objective or exterior, and the implied possibility of sharing it, contributes in itself to relief without regard to its specific content.

Each time a sentence or a proposition is advanced in correctly formulated language, it is the result of reasoning and as such represents an accrued growth. Every gain is accompanied by a pleasurable emotional state, stimulating the tendency to renew, amplify, and intensify the experience. Therefore, the children's growth will be encouraged not only by mental practice and speech processes, including their socializing function, but by the attendant emotional well-being.

By the same token the children's manipulative attitudes change. This is one aspect of a potentially unlimited development which G. Bachelard characterizes by the statement "ensemble, les choses et les mots prennent de la profondeur. On va en même temps au principe des choses et au principe du verbe." [4] (Things and words gain depth in common. Simultaneously one moves to the principle of things and to the principle of the word.) In its most elementary form this fact is observable when small children, sitting on the floor, look at objects or pictures which they attempt to identify, and as a result, will call the object's name out for themselves.

# PRINCIPLES OF THERAPY

# X

## *The Child and His Psychotherapist*

It seems proper that in an endeavor where closeness and community between the patient and the therapist are generated and assumed that we raise the question from which initial position the two move toward each other. Two different people, the adult and the child, the patient and the therapist, move toward a common goal but from different directions.

In the early days of the Clinic, when, symbolically speaking, we laid the cornerstone with our bare hands, the state wards were most urgent patients, fighting valiant battles for first place with their therapist. Felix, whom we know already and whom we are going to discuss repeatedly, would end up almost each time with a bleeding nose, not inflicted by any child in or outside the Clinic. Small in stature, a violent fighter, he seemed a battle-worn knight who came to his "lady" for the binding of his wounds. It was almost the only way he knew to be deserving of love, a man as well as a child, in need of nursing. He was an outstanding example of the children raised with neither the tender touch of love nor the gentle, but firm controls coming from a stimulating as well as challenging home.

In search of recognition and self-assertion, two complementary needs are displayed: the need for the parents' affection and for being opposed. Since the rejected children are deprived of love, and the neglected ones of both encouragement and the protection of controls, it is not surprising that the children in day-care pursue their goal of provoking opposition from parental figures by constantly fighting among each other. Then they return to these figures for sympathy and solace. With a sense of realism they usually challenge another child of their own age as a competitor for the prize in a violent strife. For the sake of this prize constant contact with these other children is needed which reaffirms a longed-for sense of being, some sort of acceptance and the proof that a threatened existence can be "healed" of the hurt incurred by exposure. Encouraged by the confidence that injury can be healed, children can then venture out for a new probing of the stuff they are made of and that of the one they oppose. The child, comforted by that same confidence, will not only seek to show bravery but will be protected from foolhardiness, because something has been added to the mere fact of existence. Each of the state wards used to struggle for the first place on the treatment schedule in order to feel first in love and acceptance. All of them were still infants, in that sense, with the claim of being a mother's little man. Sharing was still far away.

We were further impressed, more so than in any other absorbing therapeutic relationship, by the surprising fact that the therapists could become objects of love, passion, noble and great feelings or ideals, though these children had come from cultural and emotional deserts. Where did they muster those powerful potentials; how did they have affinities for their therapists whose interest, though compassionate, was, however, of a placid nature, gently expressed, deliberate in action and above all geared to all children alike? The very nature of the relationship and the therapist's way of expressing it, exposed differences in culture. Was the children's ardour to be loved first actually the burning desire to be relieved from a status which, for the sake of pride, they simultaneously defended by misbehavior? Was it the observed equanimity and apparent harmony for which they yearned from the depths of a volcanic upheaval?

The meeting of the helper and the one in need of help implies that both are different as well as alike. The helper gains closeness to the patient by empathy and understanding, which is the helper's guide to the bridges leading to the other "country," which any man is to his fellow (quoting a youngster's own words). But the therapist remains different and sufficiently outside the child's experience to be able to steer him toward a goal. The therapist himself is challenged to find his own optimal potentials, when the patient uses every means to oppose a betterment of his condition. As long as the therapist can fulfil the role assigned to him, he can become the chosen healer, the one who binds the wounds he allegedly inflicted. But he must not hurt in reality, or the illusion implied in transference is dissipated. If the emergency is weathered and the child calms down because his behavior provocations have remained unanswered, and thus, no new traumata were inflicted, the therapist will be loved and admired for his immunity to being provoked. The child will then first shoot forth his tendrils for support. With the passing of time, he will be identified first with the person who shows strength or resistance to what the child calls being bad, then, with the complex of attitudes which conquered the child's own resistance, to improvement. The children often dream of their future roles as professional helpers in the guise of the ones they have learned to appreciate in the Clinic. A few of them subsequently actually go to college with the intent of becoming psychologists, social workers, nurses, and teachers. Some want to help others and, while in treatment, bring them into the Clinic. In joining hands with the therapist, they want to save those who are in danger of sinking as they themselves were in the past. Usually, this is a period when the child is still greatly menaced and is reaching out for a significant experience of a longed-for ideal status. The child in need of assistance is seen outside as a replica of one's own past self. Finally, they seek to complement the therapist's efforts by working at their own improvement.

Their empathy with the therapeutic endeavor stirs them to help the helper and in so doing to know and help themselves. To quote Corine Landis' own statements: "In trying to please, I discover many sides of myself. With some very few people, I can be all of myself. I find that trying to please, I actually please myself."

What obstacles stand between people who cannot readily span bridges to each other's "countries?" Is the gap between these children and their therapist greater than usual? Is there an inevitable chasm?

## Language and Non-Verbal Expression

Between any two people who try to reach each other by the spoken word stands the history and experience of their whole lives. The imagery, the atmosphere, the meaning associated with each word is tinged with the reminiscences of the past. Every spoken word has a very different connotation for each partner to a conversation who can understand the other only by means of his own associations, thoughts, and feelings. This is the only way by which we can assimilate impressions coming from without and preserve the unity of our personality. The necessity to be self-defined and self-defining, indispensable for the continuity of our identity, limits us to our own boundaries— rich and vast as a man's territory might be. Understanding between two people can only succeed by way of translating the two languages spoken in the two "countries."

What is it that causes the feeling that through words there is a meeting of minds? All of us are familiar with the assistance to communication offered by the more general, the public conveyance of gestures and mimicry. But in language itself there are nuances of voice, of tone, of accent and tuning, acceleration or retardation of speed, scanning of rhythm, great varieties of articulation and their opposite, to mention but a few that help the listener catch the exact meaning conveyed by the speaker when he talks.

The richer the past experience, the more potentialities it holds for the attuning of the nuances and the meanings of the two "languages" spoken by two people, the more "conveyances" will be at hand for traveling back and forth between the two "countries." Actually the two people will share more than the mere "conveyance" of language, imposing as it may be, because both will travel together for some duration through the same "scenery," in the milieu that presently surrounds them and generates their responses to it.

When, therefore, a child in therapy speaks of his family and home concretely, or of the deep and meaningful recollections that arise from the vague and remote past, the therapist who has traveled with him for a while has gained some comprehension of the experiences that underlie the words. The miracle remains that an apparently satisfactory understanding results when none of the imagery girding the most fundamental words can be alike for both, though empathy and time may diminish their strangeness. That the child usually does not have a differentiated knowledge of the therapist with whom he communicates is not only of minor importance but a factor that favors the transference. It is less relevant that the child does not understand the psychotherapist's words in their specific vocabulary, since his understanding of the world is still gained more extensively by ultra-verbal channels, the more so, the younger he is or the younger he has remained in his morbid isolation. Properly timed silence, interruptions, or pauses may count much in the impact made on the child. The voice and the rhythm that chant to him or comfort him are what he responds to, rather than words and sentences as such.

## Child's Time and Adult's Time

Time does not mean the same thing to psychotherapist and child. To both as human beings time is comparable to a stretch upon which to move or to abide. What stimulates flight, or immobility, or on the contrary advance differs for an infinite number of reasons. Enjoyment of the creative moment, weariness, or fear cannot and must not be the same for the one as for the other, lest the psychotherapist obscure his role as a pilot to safety. Neither is time the same for patient and therapist in reference to knowledge about the patient. The psychiatrist has at the time of the first meeting a bird's-eye view of the child's life and personality. This view is entirely different from the self-image of the child. The child has lived his life, which implies experience of duration, of the stretching out, the storing up process of living in all its phases.

The psychiatrist who meets the child knows his chronological age in addition to a number of more or less rough facts and psychological data. The general concept of age is captured mentally within one moment that the child experiences as an extended continuum with sporadic highlights that stand out from the dimness. The predominantly intuitive experience of the child is in contrast to a predominantly conceptual knowledge of the psychiatrist. However, psychiatrist and child may not tread totally strange soil when they meet. The child also is able to and may translate the continuum of experienced life-time into an idea and call it by the number of years people have told him to count. The psychotherapist, moreover, knows the case history and has aligned, into a continuum, in his or her mind, the events lived by the child.

The tangible elements in the psychiatrist's grasp of the child's experience may still be at a minimum. What may be felt as a considerable duration by the child, might barely stretch out over a period longer than that needed for the psychiatrist to read the information and perceive more or less abstract facts, summed up quantitatively, though not totally devoid of quality. Indeed, what is needed for the psychiatrist's first approach, when the child is at the other extreme of the experience, overwhelmed by an infinite number of confusing events, is an organized whole or a tentative design.

Though the psychiatrist knows the element of time to be of paramount importance for the understanding of the child's problems, it is acknowledged only as a spotter of highlights to be situated early in his development. Neither the concepts of time and number, neither the intuitive element, nor the imaginative part of the experience are the same for psychiatrist and child. As time goes on, there will be a greater sameness in this respect, though achieved by infinitesimal steps. This implies that the road ahead will still be very long. Each station of insight conquered will still not bring into perfect agreement the psychiatrist's idea of the time past with the child's sense of his life's duration, or of the temporal extent of events under discussion.

In addition to his past experience of duration and living, an experience which is subject to constant change in relation to the child's development, a more conceptual discursive view of the past experiences is gained by the child through his work with the psychiatrist. This represents a qualitative change, from a predominantly intuitive experience to a conceptual grasp, by which relatively vast periods of time are telescoped into the thought of one moment.

A change in the course of treatment is brought about by the medium of identification. A child is active at this stage in trying to assimilate new concepts from without. But necessarily this is a transient stage. Once the child, as we see him in the Clinic, has set out to incorporate objects that move in and out of his orbit, human objects, offered for choice of identification as therapists and teachers, nevertheless are chosen for emulation and soon for formation of ideals. One can see children in class look at their teacher with adoration and others with intense warmth call him "my buddy," revealing the closeness but shyly concealing the veneration. The child may select a warm, understanding teacher for a mother figure. In psychotherapy to choose a conspicuous example, the children show an intense preoccupation with their therapist's profession and vocation. They want to be a doctor, a psychiatrist. Quite spontaneously they then remember their scholastic status, begin to ask what it takes to become a psychiatrist. Slowly the significant idea of service arises in their mind as they see it function around them. The time has come to help them discover that service is mutual. A general idea begins to benefit the child's individualization.

The psychiatrist proceeds in the opposite direction. Supported by ideas, he or she will share the child's inner life through participation in his concrete impressions and emotions, verbalized or acted out. The therapist will experiment with living through the child's experience rather than resort to observation exclusively from without. In this partnership of symbolic living together and in this community of discourse, enormous stretches of time are traveled together back and forth. The whole distance, a long period of the child's inner life, may seem identical to both. However, the complicated curve of the retraced steps of both participants in the endeavor, patient and physician, will be found to be quite unlike. The speed at which they travel from one differential of insight into the patient's problem to the next is variable. In other words, the time required for mutual understanding is very different. The nature of this understanding is never the same. Children termed "concrete" in psychological testing may be found to have a minimum sense of duration. Time may be but the inevitable location of thought in a nebulous, indefinite, and undeterminable past or future.

When treatment was started the child, through inner experience, preceded the psychiatrist in knowledge about himself. However, equipped with particular tools for understanding and not inhibited by such emotions and conflicts as are the causes of the child's specific condition, the rate of speed at which the psychiatrist gains knowledge about the patient and his emotional experience, exceeds by far the one the patient is able to travel. The psychiatrist's knowledge at this time, cannot be made available by interpretation, because the patient, left far behind is not yet likely to understand or to accept it. The element of time and travel rate apparently have placed patient and physician at a distance from each other. For the sake of the patient, the psychiatrist silently travels the road over and over, at his own pace, as well as at his patient's time and speed, without loss to himself and potentially at least, with gain to the patient.

What could be termed the traveling track also is different. Figuratively speaking, the patient moves by all sorts of means of locomotion: jumps, crawls, steps, and rides, and, proceeding by various speeds along the path of his memories, subjective association, traumatic events, and the vast deserts of loneliness or repression. The physician on the other hand may do no more than overlook the track, pulling the switches in order to establish his own abstract traveling tracks, his own associations, co-ordinating the branch lines of the child's utterances into a coherent communication system. While the child may offer only memories, the psychiatrist sees in them traumatic phenomena located at crucial life periods.

When treatment begins, the patient comes with an inner experience of himself which implies time in terms of many things: incidences, frequency and intensity of emotions endured, strains undergone, work accomplished, amount and scope of learning gained. Age may be envisioned in terms of distance covered or the remoteness of the child's previous "home" from his present one. Age may be envisioned in terms of imaginary travels through books, fairy tales, adventures and expeditions, discoveries and inventions. Those who have intense affinity with the poetic, musical or artistic genii of the past are imbued with an atmosphere that may add many years to their life. Childhood then may be extended to antiquity, the Renaissance, the Baroque, and life may seem extremely prolonged without a corresponding sense of being older. This kind of duration of life conveys a sensation of strength and wealth rather than of weakness. How constricted must be the lives of these children who never knew the blessings of an existence that extends itself into times immemorial!

The psychiatrist who meets the patient for the first time is totally ignorant of the patient's life time. What, at first glance, he has to resort to is either so objective as to be a mere framework into which everything can be fitted or so subjective as to open perplexing avenues in all directions; neither approach is of immediate help to him. He will, thus, have to hold in abeyance his own ideas about what years mean in terms of the patient's unique time lived.

## Happy Times and Anxious Times

To appraise what time means to children is not an easy task. At early stages of life the need for structuring and measuring experience seems small indeed. The child does not seem stymied by any road blocks which remind an adult of time passed or passing. Unaware of the time needed for development, the child will insist on the undelayed fulfilment of any of his justified desires or whims.

When Dayton was taken to the City Welfare Department, he became extremely suspicious and anxious because a home and a social worker were not immediately available to him. Another bright, unruly state ward called us liars when it took two weeks to organize his promised visit to his home at one hundred miles' distance. In both instances the procedure and exact reasons for the delay had been explained patiently in every detail. To force chronologically or emotionally young children into the adult's concept of time is extremely frustrating to them. In view of their dependency upon the adult and in view of the relative paucity of the experience to be measured and structured, the tool of time is barely needed. The child is yet unskilled in manipulating time or allowing the conventional tool of the adult to manipulate his childlike schedule.

Moreover, what is important to the child is not necessarily the same to the adult. The child is beginning from scratch, as becomes his creative mind. Lost in his "penetrating" exploration, he may be very slow and totally oblivious to the striking of the hour. The adult is anxious in reference to time and has long been resigned to a rapid glossing over the surface of experience. A revealing story to the youngster which he will need to relive an unending number of times has become an abstract code word for the adult who compresses it into a storable entity.

In brief, great discrepancies in time experience arise between the youngster and the adult and, unless handled with a deep understanding of children's "timeless" experiences, a chronic war may be the result. In reference to time, therefore, the adult and the child actually play on two different keyboards which are in need of synchronization. The adult cannot make the concession to break up the established scheduling of his timetable that in its turn is determined by cosmic, as well as compelling, social factors. On the other hand, account must be taken of the fact that the child's important developmental needs have to remain unscheduled in an overscheduled day. The schedule represents a coercive force, an infringement upon spontaneity and creativeness and, at best, a test of the child's social adaptability. Reluctance to obey the call of the adult's time may indeed be a symptom with a multitude of meanings. It may be the child's reaction to the educator's lack of awareness that the youngster has important business in process that serves the purpose of discovering and bringing forth the future man or woman in him or herself. The child is not aware of the nature of this importance but experiences it as a fact. He may feel vitally interfered with, extremely upset, and oppose interference by refusing to cooperate. Essentially creative people have greater difficulty fitting themselves into the coercive structure of a strict schedule. Children who do not conform immediately may be considered stubborn and arrogant when actually they deal with very important business.

Roland, a bright four-and-a-half-year old was asked to stop rolling his candy-filled dumping truck over his fine large book because he scratched its pages. Instead of complying Roland continued to roll the truck over the book. The observer assumed that he was stubborn and resistive, but, keeping her judgment in abeyance, she was rewarded by an impressive experience. "You see," said the little boy, "I roll it and I roll it and no new lines show on the paper." He then moved a few wrapped pieces of candy over the page and said, "these do not scratch the paper either; then I could not have made the scratches. They must have been there before." After having finished his experiment and demonstrated his thesis *per exclusionem*, this little Francis Bacon stopped playing on top of the book and both this child's and this observer's time rapidly coincided without a struggle or outbursts of hostility. Actually, the adult learned a lesson. Her judgment of the origin of the scratches had been precipitous and the child's judgment well considered.

At the age of five, he was unwilling one day to obey when told to go to bed. That day he was bent on finding a source of referral for a picture like one he had remembered seeing elsewhere. But though very much intrigued he could be induced finally to postpone the search until the next day. The next morning when the adult members of the family arose, he had accomplished his search and was happy to share his reference, found in one of a great number of the volumes of the *National Geographic magazine*.

In this instance obedience required self-denial. However, the carry-over to the next day and the successful performance promoted the child's realization that delay is not always a handicap. He learned the lesson that without detriment to his purpose a child can co-operate with the grown-up and make his and their time coincide.

The average man's maturity finds one of its basic expressions in his adjustment to a regular timetable. The growing child can be helped by a patient and generous approach that starts in infancy, bringing the definiteness of time and timing to the awareness of the child from the beginning. However, the need for freedom from the adult schedule or pauses from interference with creative moments must be foreseen.

Contrary to the views generally held, I hold the deep conviction that an infant should be fed according to a schedule, followed with leisurely self-evidence. The mother's accumulation of milk and the child's appetite coincide under such regime and mutual gratification is at an optimum. The "creative" pauses in between feeding hours are used by the infant at first for recuperation through sleep. If, on the contrary, he is allowed to be demanding at whim, he has less rest and comfort. His demands frustrate both the mother, who is fettered, and the child, against whom she reacts. Constantly deprived by his own attitude and frustrated by the mother's defenses, his need for gratification increases. Since gratification presupposes discontent, he has to foster the state of need simultaneously with the cries for relief. Dependency increases as well as the mother's need to defend herself and to frustrate the consuming terrorism of the child. To cope with the guilt feelings resulting from her own frustrations and the sense of failing the child, she may be inclined to resort to denial of her discontent. Her good-willed self-deceit and the need to maintain the illusion of happiness prompt her to indulge ambivalently the child's dependency and terrorism. Due to the hostile aspects inherent in the mother's servitude to the child, self-punishing and punitive motivations invade this mutual dependency.

The child's growth is doubly interfered with by the practice of silencing any of his utterances of discomfort by feeding him at any time. Even the nursing infant as man in the state of becoming has a wide variety of needs, each of which can be refracted in a spectrum of colorful nuances. Infants whose needs are answered with discriminate devotion will not readily resort to the oral cavity for every solace. Early resourcefulness protects mother and child from protracted dependency. To come to a child's rescue with the bottle or the breast indiscriminately at any time is denying him in final analysis development of and resort of his cultural potentials.

## Schedules of Child and Psychiatrist

It may be difficult to make the psychiatrist's and the child's schedules coincide too patly. How incoherent, unadjusted to reality, passive or withdrawn a child may seem! The child may have ideas of his own about what his day should be. Whether he seems incoherent, passive or withdrawn, he may be stirred not only by impulses of the moment. Being unco-operative with the school schedule may be due to a child's serious preoccupation with the mother's concomitant timetable of sexual behavior. Mother as well as son may have an interest in concealing what is going on. Therefore, a child's motives for truancy and his untold misery may remain hidden for a long time behind his uncommunicative and withdrawn behavior. Others may be driven by insecurity and the fear that younger siblings at home have uninterfered leisure to crowd them out of the mother's favors.

Sibling rivalry may tempt a child to interfere with another child's scheduled time, in particular when the little rival is very anxious for his sessions and has difficulty in sharing with others. "I want you now," the little intruder may say, "later I may not care for you any more," and "nothing might come out of it." A whole history of a child's anxiety and insecurity expressed in a small incidence of the transference interplay is condensed in such a three-way collision of time.

The children who are not enrolled in day-care have to be responsible for their arrival on time for their appointments. The mothers' sessions many times cannot be made to coincide with those of their children's, the mother's availability being limited as well as the overburdened staff's. The majority of the children are motivated by an intense desire to pursue the treatment. But some children are overanxious to let nothing interfere or they overcompensate their resistance; others again tend to cope with their ambivalence in reference to the treatment by arriving in the morning for an afternoon treatment session. They want to stay in the day-care group, they may express unwillingness to go to their session, give preference to a teacher's company or to some activity, or they give battle to the symbolic sibling. All these procedures are means of interfering with the other children's relationship to the therapist. Nurturing their own resistance and in search of finding motives for turning indecision into a frankly negative attitude, the most disturbed ones tend to disturb the program.

When there is no home to support the children, we enrol them for day-care only on the treatment day each week until they feel safe enough and enjoy the privilege of going to school. They may pass through a phase of bragging or making remarks about the "crazy school," most regularly without upsetting the one who knows why he is and wants to be in the Educational Therapy Center. In rare instances the little outsider may try to fit himself into the day-care rather than the public school schedule by acting out; when he is well enough he will request to be returned to public school.

When the child is to be home on time, his fear of reprimand and being punished may interfere with his treatment and while the sun stands at the zenith, he might ask whether it is time to go home. This attitude again may represent at three-way collision of time reflecting the child's anguish in reference to the transference and his guilt feelings toward the mother.

Time is the child's foreign oppressor, his tyrant, preventing him from living and from learning about its liberating aspects. Harassed and weary, he may want to forget about time altogether, because he cannot fight it. He will not get up in the morning; he will be late everywhere, stay out of school and away from home; fail his test under the pressure of time limitations or because he has no choice of the proper, the inspired moment. Time is synonymous with restricting "order," which is command and interference with the child's way of being rather than a beneficial structure, a means of orientation and comfort.

Anxious children tend to be hunting for the next moment, obsessed by some vague and evasive goal which in final analysis is evidently the mother's rewarding love. In the absence of experience in this basic satisfaction, the present moment is vapid. It holds no challenge, no promise, nothing to be explored. Educators and the psychiatrist are confronted with extreme difficulties in providing motivation for the child to linger for experience. Contrary to the child's anxious need for the next moment, the adult views the present moment as his opportunity.

Since unrest, the will-o'-the-wisp agitation, the eternal beelike gathering for an answer is the child's present need, preventing directly his moving around, as it seems, without a discernible goal, increases his anxiety and therefore diminishes his ability to abide for an instant and focus on an object. But the child's worker can abide by the child, thus becoming something specific and discernible. Since everything else shines up and disappears rapidly as the child passes it without rest, the child can be helped to mark time not by coercion but by his therapist's venture on to the unchartered ocean of the child's timeless wandering. Moving around with the child, he becomes the resting and arresting center in the panorama of fugitive apparitions.

In pursuing the treatment of these children in the Educational Therapy Center, we could not follow the ideal, the only logical and specific procedure just outlined. *We are however always available, always gratifying and offering lures of an emotional or otherwise promising nature for tomorrow, tomorrow morning, early tomorrow or as late as lunch time.* Thus, we become the children's goal, the object toward which they tend.

In some instances centrifugal tendencies which interfere with the treatment schedule are manifestations of negativism or challenges for the therapist to become the punitive or unrewarding mother. These fugues are attempts to hurt her and interfere with gratification and pleasure. At this time the child does not escape into the next moment. He is engaged in a present and familiar reality which he tends to transfer from his home to the therapeutic milieu.

The therapist who remains uninvolved, who is not bent on speeding into the future, anxious to accelerate the child's recovery but who accepts the child's retarding resistance, avails himself of an opportunity. The child, feeling no exasperating counterresistance, may be disengaged and relieved. Frustration may result from an unexpected response and from being deprived of a motive for hostile interaction. The child is likely to go on provoking, but soon his motivation will have changed. He wants to enjoy the fact that his provocations do not cause frustration and the danger of an enraged response. He begins to feel his freedom and that he is wanted. He attempts to abuse the power the loved one wields over the one who loves him. Love's labor, however, will not be lost if the dedicated therapist avails herself of the playful elements inherent in the child's new assuredness and the new meaning of his provocations. It is her way of showing her freedom which in turn liberates the child further. In any play situation there is charm. It ties together the playing partners. The child's isolation is lifted when he meets his therapist in an actual experience that is worth retaining. It therefore calls for renewal and thereby unfolds its auspices for a future in common. First the child "returns" to his experiences in common with his therapist. Spontaneously the child is alerted to the symbolic significance of their activity. Saying for instance, "nobody ever played with me before," he invites, as it were, the therapist to share with him past time and past pain and pleasure, and, by way of the joint recall, jointly they will build the future.

## Orientation and Adjustment to the Scheduled Session

The antisocial children treated at the Educational Therapy Center were extremely demanding; their needs were most urgent and they used desperate and destructive ways to express them. Critically in need of acceptance and the recognition of their rights to existence, they were, in the beginning of treatment, never able to wait for their scheduled time. When admitted to the office, however, they often did not know what to do with their opportunity, ran out with some loud accusation or curse or like Ray withdrew in a regressed posture under the table. It was impressive to see these children's eagerness between sessions being exhausted at the very moment when opportunity had come to pick the fruit of their longing. Had they been stunted, regressed, or were they precociously withered and unmanned?

The impulse toward life and living was preserved but at least partially distorted. Some of the children had to be fed the milk of gratification, incapable as they were for a long time to reach out for it. Others, afraid of accepting what was expected to be a false promise, refused it for long periods of time or attempted to provoke negative attitudes to prevent being offered a deceiving gift. A few were shrewd or took what they could get without feeling any commitment. Others were bound by commitment to a mother and were an inert instrument for the fulfilment of her needs, recognized as such or not. Others resented assistance and rebelled against it. The worst tragedy that befalls these children is the absence of an opportunity to become aware of their lovable traits. They know only of their "ugly" responses. Agreeing with those who reject them, they are unaware of their worth.

These youngsters were also extremely insistent and stubborn, irrationally demanding and impulsive in their attempts to deprive another child of "his time." They obviously acted under the impact of anxiety and the fear of grave loss. But there is in such behavior a struggle for orientation, for goal-directed behavior which will in final analysis result in the building up of controls, provided the goal is stable, reliable and rewarding. One of the manifestations of growing ego strength is the voluntary adjustment to a schedule, an expression of the child's increasing sense of security, of freedom from coercion and trust in genuine acceptance. It contributes to reliance on an orderly and consistent world. Orientation in time is furthered by a leisurely structured schedule and daily routine. This is anxiety relieving in itself. The schedule, however, may become an obsessive anchorage to a threatened child, a safety belt. When the "belt" is not thrown out in time, the child feels he is sinking or he may feel betrayed by the one supposed to rescue him. The acuteness of the need calls for so precise a response in time that unless gratified, access to the hour of treatment and the help it holds in promise is blocked. The child may not stay for his session or he may pout and be unco-operative. Repair is possible when his behavior is a means of retaliation. He may gratify his resentment and be satisfied with getting even. A child enrolled in day-care may "cool off" in the shop or with the supervisor and come back for his session spontaneously, glad that the door is open when he gets there tardily, having "paid you back" ten times. The *clarité* and *transparence* of scheduled time is a poor framework for delinquent acting out. It is a structure devoid of secret recesses. But it is true that children who deeply trust the therapist and feel profoundly secure also come to believe "that you cannot help it" when you are late.

There exists a correlation between dependency and poor sense of time, including the vagueness and subjectivity of concepts or the use of subjective word meanings in preference to general concepts.

Concomitant with poor orientation is a state of bewilderment, confusion, and anxiety. The child tends to lean strongly upon the adult. When the relationship is not satisfying, the dependency becomes obsessive; the child exposes himself time and again to new hurts in an attempt to verify the apprehended rejection, though never without hoping his experiment will fail. The hostile interplay is apparently his only opportunity to set in action a pendular or tidal motion, a to and fro between the two hostile parties. In the pacing back and forth, through the excitement which accompanies these motions and emotions, the child becomes more clearly aware of himself and his opponent as well as of distance and the passing of time.

This consideration illustrates one aspect of the fact that hostile and aggressive behavior is more promising than inertness or the motionless clinging to one's symbiotic complement. In the absence of motion, orientation in time and space cannot be experienced. If the relationship is satisfying, the child will not immediately want to give up his helpless state, one elemnt of which is his lack of orientation in time and space.

Without being actually ambivalent, Felix displayed both tendencies simultaneously. He was raised, as we know, without a specific maternal object upon which to focus his vital energies and from whom to let them radiate harmoniously. But due to a good intelligence and his responsiveness to his adoptive mother, he was at least selective to the point that he was never seen running around aimlessly. He knew what he wanted. It was self-complementation wherever and by whatever means he could find it. Raised without any training until he was almost four years old, he could resort to none of the usual road blocks of time, space, and social order by which the child, brought up with due dedication, is guided. He moved through space where he found objects to manipulate and to use within his autistic world. But he was not able to indicate properly where he was going or where he had been. He could return to the place and show it to you. Therefore we were confronted in treatment with the fact that when he was supposed to go to a determined place, not one to which he was driven, he was bewildered and expressed the fear, he might get lost. In the conventional world of the other people he was not oriented and reached out for support. On the street he wanted you to hold his hand.

His problem however was more complex. Your hand was not only needed to keep him safely in your space, it was needed also for what you and your space stood for. This meant growing up above all by identification and emulation and not by impulse gratification as within his own world. The outside things seemed unattainable. They seemed so much out of reach that he was fatigued even to think of moving along its tracks and was therefore unwilling to try. In his world there was no time and no distance. He would walk for miles and stay out over one or several nights without awareness of fatigue, hunger, and thirst. That he let himself become so helpless in our world, however, was not due solely to lack of orientation and need of support for finding his way around. Neither was it due solely to the need of putting himself totally into his rescuers' hands for alleviation of confusion and for the enjoyment of being nursed. He wanted to be held tight by the grasp of our hands, that he might learn to rely on us and might belong to us. Without that hand warmly and firmly tended to him, he could not help yielding to temptation. We were the ropes needed to protect that youthful Odysseus from his Circe, the enticing toys in the stores. Within his own world their role for him was entirely different. They were his accustomed companions and his protectors against an annihilating world. They were his only teachers and aids for his growing self and edification of his mind. In want of educators who were older than himself, he had to resort to taking refuge in "idols" smaller than himself. These he did not have to fear. They were his obedient servants and he their uncontested master, as long as he could remain within his own private world. To protect it he had above all to deny time. Therefore, he had to deny hunger, because its alleviation was connected with time, the destroyer of all that constituted him as a person.

Time was an enemy not only in reference to Felix's autistic territory, from which at least it could be shut out, it interfered also as a menace when Felix attempted to come over and explore the alluring pastures of human affection and loving care. It attacked him under many guises since he was unsure of everything. Time as a closed portal of entry aroused intense frustration and violence. The immediacy of Felix's needs, the inadmissability of anybody to the love to which he lay permanent claim would prompt murderous explosions—since his very life was at stake, he used to muster superhuman strength. One day he broke a standard typewriter and bent its strong metal frame. He would kick incessantly in such a condition.

He remained withdrawn from the children's group, but accepted one male and one female worker for comfort when not in the presence of his therapist. One was the shop teacher. He was a special bridge between Felix and his therapist. In the shop Felix could make rough little wooden boats, dreaming that one day he was going to float them in a pond which he fancied was in the yard of the psychiatrist's home. Boats were homes that carried him and the psychiatrist in isolation from others. In spite of such assistance it was for a long time a forbidding task for Felix to stay in the Center through the day. When not gratified by the presence of the psychiatrist he had to run for self-complementation to the stores. When he returned from his sprees with stolen toys, he would place them surreptitiously in the psychiatrist's desk drawers. They were in his eyes part of himself and therefore safest under her care. When he was told that certain toys were found and could not be accounted for, he would be embarrassed. Then he would be asked whether he happened to be the one who put them there. When we proceeded to the point that we found out how they got there, he would be greatly peeved and accuse the psychiatrist: "You never want me to have anything." The opposition he had solicited artlessly out of his autistic thinking he used as a motive for projection, the therapist being the one who denied him legitimate gratification. The explanation between Felix and his therapist was, however, a means for exploration of reality and orientation.

We tried to help him by concrete experience in window shopping or a lesson in the use of time as a tool of comfort and promise and as a medium for dreams that could come true if he found them to be persistent for some time and that their realization would be important. Soon he was capable of going window shopping on his own. At this time his therapist had become the center of orientation for him. The toys could no longer compete. But this was the time also when the relationship lost its demanding character. He had become sufficiently independent from her to occupy himself with observing, thinking, and planning by himself, nor was he any more in need of constant complementation by touch of the toys as objects of his desire for gratification.

For the sake of love, he was now able to offer his improvement and his growth as an adequate and worthy little man. In a splendid self-healing tendency, supported by our insight into the meaning of what he was doing and by our trust, he went to the stores daily. He now gratified his needs by an ever repeated, abstract experimental ownership. Hypothetical ownership of certain objects turned out to yield negative results and the original hypothesis that the object would yield gratification was now rejected. Felix became selective. He played with the idea of stealing and could discuss it. He exercised self-denial, reduced the amount of failure, and strengthened his will power and sense of realism. Slowly time became a framework and a supportive structure for an increasingly adequate self. Felix would return from his window shopping to a scheduled interview and on the appointed time for the much-enjoyed woodworking class. Conforming to his therapist's time, but not to rules, he would turn up as if from nowhere for a regular self-set "appointment" and a short ride with her to his home when the psychotherapist left the Center, after hours.

*Early Positive Stimuli: Their Relation to Developing a Sense of Time*

We could reconstruct the early lives of children like Felix by observation of the way very young psychotic and delinquent mothers treat their illegitimate offspring. We are further helped in gaining an understanding of some of the well-known symptoms, such as absence of sense of time and poor concept formation, by observation and psychotherapy of the neglected children whose early childhood frequently is completely obscured.

As infants these children are deposited with some woman who reluctantly consents to "keep the child for a few hours." The child remains unattended for a whole day or two or is nursed inadequately, possibly just to quiet him down; the mother may not return for days. Neglect of the baby is at times the women's defense against further exploitation by the child's mother. Next time the child will have to be deposited elsewhere and round and round it goes, sometimes for years.

"Adopting the child" by some motherly woman may finally stop the turning of the wheel on which the child is on the verge of being broken. By this time the child is apt to be traumatized so profoundly that he has become unmanageable and is "turned over to the city or the State." He may be lucky enough to produce serious physical symptoms in infancy. A neighbor's attention may be aroused, but only when the child is acutely ill may she act. The neglected child who suffers from a febrile disease becomes an immediate menace as a potential source of infection or epidemic, or seizures may arouse concern. Juvenile police interference, the public health nurse, or protective services of the city come to the rescue. The involuntary foster mother, chosen at random, may try to carry the child back to his mother or to a rejecting grandmother who categorically refuses to assume her daughter's duties. Rejection by the grandmother is rarely unmitigated. Mother and child are usually accepted in the home; hostility and rejection are acted out subtly. In one way or another the child, an object of contention will be affected by the rejection, the neglect, and the conflicts of the adults involved.

The most incompetent aged woman finally may be the one to "get stuck with the child." She is either unable to defend herself against the imposition or she pities the child. She may have ideals. "As long as I live no child will be without a home," she will say or indicate. Some women foster the unrealistic dream of raising the child as a future support and companion to helplessness and loneliness. The child may now belong somewhere, but his needs are not met. The woman may be totally incompetent, like one of the "ladies" who was known to have kept Felix in a dilapidated shack. She may be utterly improvident. These women may be only dimly remembered by the child later on. There were too many, and the impression was evanescent. They may be feared or hated; their memory may be repressed or the children may cling to them as to all they have, and the motive for pathological defenses.

In some instances the foster mother is actually the mother. She may have adhered to strict standards and prefer the role of the benefactress to the role of the fallen girl she cannot accept. She may want to be at liberty to give up the child. An employer called us one day, asking us to study the case of her maid's fifteen-year-old adoptive child, who was idiotic and apparently in need of commitment to a mental hospital.

Our study showed that this child was certainly not fifteen years old and not idiotic but emotionally neglected to an appalling degree. His birth certificate was invalid, borrowed from the alleged mother of the child whose trace allegedly had been lost. This child later reported to us that in the past he often knelt down in the country where he lived and ate the "dirt," that stilled his hunger. In the city such a child can at least steal food in the stores and use it as a pleasing substitute for school.

The rays of maternal graciousness never touched these children. They do not learn about the charm of a youthful mother who feels wanted herself and who, delighting in the joy of existence, motivates the child in every area of development. For the sake of this motivation a child will return home to the ever renewed source of life, instilled again and again with trust for venturing out and the desire to return replenished for replenishment.

Children like these do not pronounce the word mother in reference to any of the women who take care of them temporarily. The most fondly remembered of Felix's adoptive mothers was "the best woman I ever had."

A child under such conditions is devoid of the experience of the reciprocity of needs which begins when a child is fed from the mother's breast. The importance of fondling the infant and young child has been widely discussed in reference to the development of his body image, to the differentiation of sensibility and the responsiveness to stimulation as well as the atuning of interaction between mother and child. All of the child's life tendencies are elicited when the mother's fondling is accompanied by glances reflecting her delight and the awe inspired by the miracle of the child's being both parents conjoined in a new separate self in the state of becoming. The mother's eyes resting on the child protect her from losing either sight of or contact with him. Mothers' whose minds constantly wander from the child they hold automatically tap the little bundle. Imperceptive of the child's stirring and its solicitations, her tapping is no answer to these solicitations. The mother's motions irritate the child who expresses discomfort. He whimpers, whines, and attempts to withdraw into sleep. The imperceptive mother or the one who has to keep the child awake for fear of the magic consequences of her rejection will go on tapping until the irritated and irate child cries vehemently. The child's existence is interfered with. At times there is a tendency among these mothers to tap the baby on the arm or thigh rather than to pat it on the back, which is the infant's sole—the area of contact with his basic support. To pat the child on the back, therefore, is more comforting than to pat it on the extremities, main organs of motion which can have an inhibiting and menacing effect. Unlike the treasured child, such a child is not alerted to the pleasantness of intermittent stimulation, the play and promise of rhythmic sensations. The child senses no tension between stirring expectation of response and its rewarding occurrence. In other words there is no early paving of the way to enjoyment of time as a lived experience, ultimately to be conceptualized and remembered, nor is there stimulation for taking note of the structuring of the time continuum in discernible entities which in final analysis leads to counting and the conceiving of number concepts. When the child is fondly framed by an attention which expands his vital tendencies, everything becomes an opportunity to learn about the articulation of time. Language at the life period when it impresses the child predominantly by its melodic character and the rhythm of the short caressing sentences spoken to him, is one of the most obvious sources of such an opportunity. The humming of lullabies and later the reading of nursery rhymes, the singing of songs to accompany the children's bouncing on the lap of the adults, pat-a-cake playing, all are evident sources of learning about the continuum of time and its articulations. Schumann's "Kinderscenen" are a poet's and a musician's sensitive interpretation of the numerous measures, rhythms, phrasings that impress the child, rocking the cradle, riding, running. The duet of the mother's and the child's voices relieving one another "am Kamin" (at the fireside), the repetitions and alternations of desire, suspense "Bittendes Kind" (pleading child), and gratification "Glückesgenug" (perfectly contented), all of them speak of the oscillations and modulations of time forecast in the nursery where the child is treasured.

With negligible exceptions the children of the Educational Therapy Center were deprived of all of the blessings that mankind through the ages has lavished on its more privileged offspring. The few words spoken to them in the course of a day on purely practical matters may be too matter-of-fact or too irritated to be registered in their tonal and rhythmical character. That is one reason why poetry is seldom born in those dismal inharmonious homes. Under the impact of dissonance and rhythmical disorganization a child shrinks. He is not in a position to attend to and tend toward time, an experience so inherent to life and the idea of life that it has become one of the most outstanding symbols of life itself; the clock, the chimes, the dial, the calendar. Joyful and vivacious rhythms on the contrary are expressions of time and timing in all cultures.

The child who has not been fondled with affection seems poorly equipped to develop a well-defined and differentiated body image. Could it be true that he is also impeded in gaining a well-outlined and differentiated image of other bodies? Such a deficiency would imply that sources of spatial and chronological experiences are missed, that muscular co-ordination is at fault and movements awkward.

Under the circumstances, the identification of concepts can be impeded. We can observe these children to be completely erratic in word recognition. They read it one time, miss it in the next line, may or may not identify the word in the following rows. If we consider only these impediments to making experience and to forming concepts, we can well conceive the children's insecurity, bewilderment, their stymied, at times blocked or their frustrated and angry advance toward living and learning. The child's emotions conspire with those who deprived them and further cripple their development.

Not to try any more is a perfectly understandable defense, even were the child to feel it is worth trying. The children who try may experience the deception that the more they try, the less they succeed. They lack precision in reference to timing or directing the efforts to definite points in space inside or outside their body limits. Nor do they have a clear idea of what to do and how to do it. They may have no thoughts to express. Stuttering may be due to any of these factors, if the child does not refrain from speech altogether. We see children stutter because only after they start talking do they become aware of the fact that they have nothing to say. Similarly, children may start walking like tots with the drive to move but they have no goal, no sense of direction. They are unaware of the need for time, strength, and orientation for the return. Aimless scratching can be observed on furniture, upholstery or even on objects which offer more resistance as enamel which they puncture and scrape with their fingers or a sharp tool.

From the dawn of their days children like Felix are barred from the socializing effects of "time in common" with loving, guiding, and educating parental figures. Many of these children are referred with a history of having been deserted in their crib repeatedly at intervals for several days at a time. Their cries not having been answered, the urge to call or reaching out for gratification was silenced. Hunger may not be felt at the usual intervals, and the daily rhythm of waking and sleeping is disturbed, since the child remains unstimulated or understimulated in day as well as night time. The seeming indifference to food intake of some of our children is most impressing. They might quarrel, grab, steal, beg, or cry and scream for food when stolen from them, because of the trauma it represents or the defenses which are aroused. But they can forego food intake for a whole day or more without perceiving the discomfort.

The few stimuli that interrupt the monotony of such children's early days of existence happen at irregular, unpredictable intervals. They are too unfamiliar and irregular to create hopeful anticipation. They do not promote tidal sensations of discomfort, tension, and relief by appropriate gratification. These tidal waves of discomfort and relief, are as we see it, like the oscillations of a pendulum which pave the way for a future sense of the passing of time. Moreover, unless something happens regularly in response to the child's manifestation of tension or need, the early and later stages which lead to expectations, spontaneity, the setting of causes to subsequent effects cannot properly develop. Time as the medium of causes and effects, or a link of the present and the past as precursors and promoters of the future, cannot be clearly conceived.

Without expectation or anticipation of the promising familiarity of the mother's regular and loving appearance, the child does not have experience and is not stimulated, in his early days, to notice and to retain "experience" to the extent and in the manner possible at that age. Opportunity is wanting for conceiving in its time the idea of a consistent and predictable world. The world loses its logic. The child, bewildered in an unpredictable world, distrusts the guide of reasoning. Angrily he refuses to reason. You cannot reach him. "I am tired of that stuff," he will say. In fear of being deluded he runs from the sensed assault.

Concepts, deprived of the intuitive elements of time and space under such circumstances, remain vague. When stimuli have been predominantly unpleasant, receptivity to stimuli is inhibited and a state of alertness for threats is promoted against which defenses must be erected. The influence of early positive emotional stimuli upon life tendencies in general, and receptivity to learning in addition to learning readiness becomes once more evident.

One twelve-year-old girl complained she always lost her words. She wished that her schoolteacher, who at that time showed little understanding of the child's condition, would "lose her words" like herself, and have to stop in the middle of a sentence.

This child told her psychotherapist she would get to know her at Halloween where she would be disguised as a clown. She would wear no mask, her face would be painted like a clown's face. "When you rub the color off, their face is all sad."

When orientation, in the absence of regular and careful attention in infancy and the early years of childhood remains extremely poor, the usual divisions of time, e.g., weeks, days, months, seasons, may remain empty words, the meaning of which is not grasped and cannot be retained at a later stage.

The words are interchangeable, and only a general sense of past, present, and future exists. The past, we know, was vaguely perceived. It could be but poorly retained. Those memories which could be available for evocation may either not be worth the effort or even worth erasing. The past may be shrunk into an unvaried (in terms of time counts) moment of frustration and resentment.

The present we know cannot be captured because the child is unnerved when the moment has come to conquer and know it. When the child has learned to focus his energies on a center of security and trust, he has learned simultaneously to focus on the present moment. This means that he can begin to explore it. The future then loses its former character of an immediate and impending experience devoid of duration. So far the child was without ideas to populate this future time and endow it with the dimensions of space. Once more the mental capacity which was still preserved remained unused to glimpse the future with curiosity. The child in fear turns away from its gorgonic features.

Hansel and Gretel see an alluring gingerbread house from which the horrid witch emerges and tempts them with candy and goodies, only to make them more fit to be devoured. Like Hansel, these children prefer not to be tempted and to stay lean. Unlike the fairy tale character who retained composure, faith, and courage in spite of past famine, desertion, and neglect, these children remain aghast and suspicious in front of the deceptive gingerbread house, or in other words, in sight of the impending moment.

Improvement is evident when the future begins to be enticing, when it gains in extent. Hope and courage inspire action. Action is planned in view of desired results. The child struggles with undesirable tendencies and discusses inner threats rather than acts them out impulsively. Dates are set for the accomplishment of tasks and in anticipation of desired gratification.

### The Words We Work With

Felix was twelve years old when he tried to learn by rote and repetition the vocable "Friday" or the month of his birthday, upon which he might clamp the label "February" or "June" indifferently. What he knew was that his birthday would be soon. He may have been told it will be summer. But also for the latter concept he had no definite idea of meaning—it equally was "but a word." He knew that there was "such a thing as summer," but what kind of thing?

In his autistic play in the streets or haunted by his need to take toys, Felix would disregard the cold in winter. Clad in a thin cotton sweater, he explicitly denied that he was cold. He went out into the streets, leaving his coat in the psychiatrist's office. Felix was so vitally preoccupied for years with the pure problem of existence, that to take note of the seasons—to classify them—was a luxury he could not have afforded, even if somebody had talked to him about them. The cold season to these children may, thus, be many things, but not "winter" as we usually understand it. If there is any seasonal signpost, Christmas usually is the only one. This factor is an indication that some life tendencies persist. Christmas is not only a sad and lonely time for these unhappy children, but there is a great deal of excitement in the streets and many things can be carried out of the crowded stores.

The children are more prone to feel the heat. They try to escape it by going to the river to fish or swim disregarding dangerous spots, since they cannot afford the entrance fee to a swimming pool. The only free swimming pool for Negro children has been closed in this city for many years. Phobias may interfere with their swimming. The children cannot escape the torrid heat in the hot homes of congested slum areas. They may complain about sleeplessness until daybreak. They feel sluggish and giddy; they are irritable on a hot day, their anxiety undoubtedly is increased. That is why the heat is less liable to be disregarded even by children like Felix. But the change of seasons was barely noticed.

Some of the children bring flowers to the staff; children may pick flowers as a token of affection or a sign of the momentary serenity of their feelings, but they may not be aware of the seasonal appearance of flowers. Knowledge of the four seasons is remarkably delayed and for a long time remains an abstract word learned the hard way, by rote.

## The Missing Time

Misunderstandings between these children and other people necessarily are frequent.

One day we were intensely impressed by Felix's apparent insatiability. He had just managed to obtain the replacement of a transformer for his electric train which the other children had broken, when he insisted on a nickel for his monthly allowance. Several staff members had set out such monthly allowances as a means of stopping the children's habit of begging incessantly and to feel rejected when not gratified. Tearfully, Felix complained of the fact that one teacher had given a nickel to every child except him. He had been shopping around for days to find the cheapest transformer, but he did not associate the monetary value with the acquired object and thus failed to recognize his privileged rather than underprivileged condition. When it was explained to him that he had received a gift worth many, many nickels, he smiled happily saying: "I should have known." He gathered that it was a very large sum in comparison to a nickel.

About that time, he was baffled about why his foster mother pretended he was ten years old when he must be eleven. He explained shortly before his birthday he was nine; about two weeks later he felt that now a long time had passed since his birthday, thus, he must be eleven, he "knew it."

Dayton, trying to grow up and conquer number concepts, asked the psychotherapist to figure for him when he was born. He was then twelve years old. When his question was answered, he followed up with a new inquiry: "When was I born, when I was eleven?"

When Felix had to be returned to his home community, because of the policy of his welfare agency, before his treatment had been accomplished, he had to be prepared for the change. He was told that he could go home and stay at home all the time if he liked it. He was reassured that if he could not make it we would take him back. His attendance of school and other problems concerning his permanent return home were discussed.

He took an active part in the discussions. He remembered his old problems at home and aired them. It so happened that the psychotherapist had to take a vacation and had to mention to him that she would leave a few days before his departure. The child then cried out: "You go on a vacation before me! I thought you were going to leave when I leave and when I come back you will be here again."

I tried to find out where the discrepancy had arisen, between this statement and the plans discussed. Not ready to leave, he had not taken in the meaning of staying there "all the time." To him it meant he had to stay at home "overnight" or all the time of a day. That he seemed willing to try and discussed his apprehensions was due to his suggestibility. However, as so often, he expressed the fear of getting lost on his way home. That he made plans to go to school in his home community was due to his obvious bewilderment and to his belief that he had to attend school every day from the first to the last day of his vacation from the Center. He had not realized that it was vacation time for all schools. In this state of indecision Felix's emotions combined with induced deficiencies in mental maturation.

At an early stage of treatment, Felix gave as an exclusive reason for his withdrawal from and dislike of children the noise they were causing. Recalling his early experiences, he mentioned the noise of trains and the flashes of light at night which disturbed and frightened him and prevented him from sleeping. Under the stress of having to return home, he reported that his school, close to the railroad track, exposed him to the same traumatization then endured in the home. The frequent passage of rapid trains shook the whole school building to its foundation and, symbolically speaking, his whole precarious little world. This was given as the reason he could not learn. He was too scared. Only a few weeks ago he had insisted on being removed from his foster home because of the night noise, of passing trucks which made the house shake and cast flares of light upon his face. His age companion in the home, a happy, protected member of the foster family, slept under identical conditions in the same room without feeling disturbed in any way. Felix told his psychotherapist one day that he "loved the other children but it seems as though I cannot play with them." His profound anxiety isolated him. The more secure child and the anxious one did not find anything in common. Strangers, they shied away from each other.

This fear of noise seemed to point to an early traumatization in an area where the young child, in particular the infant, is especially sensitive. The persistence of this sensibility is due partly to the traumatization continued apparently for a long period of time. It is due also to the protracted state of helplessness which is a consequence of the child's stunted mental development. Dependency needs are not fostered solely by the frustrated emotional needs as such but by the detrimental effects on a poorly harmonized and integrated personality structure.

## The Neglected and the Rejected Child

Etiologically we must distinguish the predominantly neglected child from the predominantly rejected child. This distinction is therapeutically valid. It alerts the observer to a differentiation between similar symptoms which both the neglected and the rejected child display.

The predominantly neglected child, that is the child of improvident rather than frankly hostile parents, can be observed to move from extreme timidity, anxiousness, or beclouded aloofness to dependency. The vicissitudes of these children's lives are not correlated with annihilating parental hostility nor are they its immediate consequences. The cruelty of their condition as we could observe it was due to an appalling absence of care, to prolonged and repeated periods of maternal desertion to the extent that the children's survival seems almost inconceivable. It can only be assumed that charitable, anonymous neighbors or grandmothers took some minimal care of the children.

The problem of these children obviously is stunted or distorted growth due to want of fulfilment of their basic needs. In addition to persistent traumatization and their consequences, we deal also with inevitable auto-traumatization. In spite of this ballast of adversity, many of these children are still sufficiently alive to be capable of using their very needs as tentacles for replenishment. They are still sufficiently sound to yield at least passively, at times with delay, to being tended and "raised." Dependency, or, in terms of the observer, the children's indulgence of their helplessness, is usually the symptom that most obviously reveals its defense character and its usefulness for the forming of an intense relationship to a human object able and willing to answer with human compassion and insight.

A number of these neglected children may have preserved some strength and self-assurance. In an early display of selectiveness, sound affinities to the suitable objects upon whom to bestow their dependency may be in evidence. The hopeful prognosis for this child's responsiveness to treatment could be jeopardized by the unforeseeable, though frequent incidence that his therapist, whether he liked it himself or not, is an "itinerant" worker.

It is true that a fine therapist may leave behind him an endowment of trust that the child can bestow upon the next therapist. But not until some self-sufficiency is acquired can the child be expected to transfer his finally established roots and fail to be again bereaved. How he is able to deal with bereavement will depend on his own state and the actual state of the transference, on the child's resourcefulness and capacity for abstraction and the skill of the new therapist. The total therapeutic milieu preserves the continuity of the atmosphere in which the child is "at home." A satisfactory foster home may be equally supportive.

That the neglected children's needs and demands are also concrete when they begin their treatment and for some length of time thereafter has to be taken into account as the necessary consequence of both their concrete deprivation as well as their resulting mental and emotional deformation. The child's unabated insistence on fulfilment of his real needs, which formerly had remained persistently ungratified, paved the way for a deviation of attributes that otherwise might have become strongly positive traits of character. Obstinacy and lack of versatility ensue, crowding out potentialities for persistence and purposefulness. The child's resulting non-compliance usually is answered by the adult by rigid coercive and vindictive modes of approach which instead of subduing the child, as expected, cause reactions of utter despair. How self-centered is the adult who contributes to such a development or does not take interest in preventing it!

However, wanting to help and to understand what the child has to "say," the adult discovers further crippling effects of these children's cruel neglect. Usually excessive demanding is further stimulated by the unevenness of these children's development. Islands of hypertrophic adequacy, prematurely acquired by exposure to early struggle for existence, remain unsupported by areas of stagnated or deviated growth. Precocious adequacy under such conditions becomes growth in excess that draws heavily on the stunted areas of mental and emotional development and may assume malignant proportions. The child's positive potentials vie with his increasing deficiencies. In this stage of self-promoting disintegration the child feels helpless and lost. As long as he is still capable of suffering, he feels his discomfort physically. If he can still react he reaches out for closeness so desperately that he becomes extremely demanding.

Concreteness, however, may be only apparent. Despite their lack of concepts in those areas of development where man depends on direct training, these children have developed symbolic thinking and can use language in a figurative sense. Children who are no older than eleven years of age may converse among themselves in allegorical terms in group sessions with the intention of obscuring the social meanings of their discussions. What they say has an apparent and an underlying sense. At adolescence they are past masters of the art. It may be a *fleuret* they wield, a mutual testing of their mental skill and superiority. It may be a device for deception. In group sessions they enjoy their secrets and their alleged superiority. They tend to hold you in suspense, eager to divulge their secret but at their own time. This tendency and capacity for ambiguous expression is the sublimated tool of the Negro on all levels of their social hierarchy. On its higher levels it is mastered as a *repartee* of extreme alertness and swiftness. The children use their ambiguous talk for a display of distrust that actually is not serious and deep and which therefore they can use for pinpricking more or less playfully. It is a means of isolating the therapist, reversing the role of child and adult as they have experienced him, of child and society, against which they gang up by language understood only by the initiated, or as the Negro who is supposed to speak coarsely his incisive language but instead draws a rapier.

In less sublimated, less liberated, and less playful a condition, children ask for such concrete things as money but test your love, your consideration, your understanding of the reality of their situation, your tolerance of their demanding, your adequacy in coping with their testing of limits and their attempts to annoy. Certain toys stand for fulfilment of complex needs symbolic in character. For Felix, toys were means of achieving equality with his playmates, so that he would no longer be "Little Black Sambo" who "lost his mother." That is what he heard children in a group session whisper about him and what he pretended the white children living around him in his home community said about him formerly. In the therapy group nobody but Felix had heard it. The white children had wonderful toys, he reported, and let him play with them in their homes. But toys became a symbol of social privilege to him and for the sake of self-esteem he could not accept having no toys or discarded ones. Prior to his referral to our Clinic, his adoptive parents vainly tried to gratify his demanding in particular in reference to quality toys and were bewildered by his wanton handling of their gifts. The poor people bought him a second-hand bicycle on installments. The coveted bicycle was far too large. Felix preferred to steal one of his little neighbor's fitting bicycle, of a good make, and, as he had done so often, just ride off on it to escape to a neighboring city. In possession of this bicycle, he no longer feared comparison and could proudly park it in the policeman's stall near the White House (municipal building). Escaping his compelling fate, he felt like a policeman himself, to him the master of the street and the universe. Feeling like a ruler of the world of order himself, he would direct the traffic with his stolen tiny toy cars and vehicles, totally oblivious of the world around him.

In the midst of a modern city and its modern techniques and industrialism, this child created and recreated in fantasy a world of primeval happiness. He differed from other children by the degree of his sensitivity to interferences from without and by the intensity of his need for withdrawal, in total disregard of his physical well-being. The appeal of both the concrete reality of his foster home as well as its offerings of love, patience, and devotion were not sufficiently meaningful to keep him. Sensitive reactions which had been one cause of withdrawal were further fostered by avoiding contact.

These children are timid and aloof, essentially passive, and they barely speak spontaneously. Most of those whom we could observe had been in search of safety and comfort under the sheltering vault of the sky or under the more cozy cover of porches, bridges, cars or within them. At home they were exposed to the distress of being deserted repeatedly for several days on end or to the anguish of seeing the mother return drunk and in a shameful shape. These children may recover. One boy said, "I don't know whether I am more miserable alone at home or when my parents return to make me feel they don't want me." The parents are but insensitive obstacles.

Shyness is not simply an instinctive shrinking of a cornered and fearful child. He congeals not only because of the absence of love but in order to defend himself by means of the same stolidity that he observes in the rejecting or hostile adults. He thus obviates intrusions to which he is profoundly sensitized and to which he is for more than one reason ill-equipped to react. This is why these silent and cowed children "go to pieces" and break out in temper tantrums the severity of which is in proportion to both their emotional distress as well as their developmental distortion. In their presence one has to be unobtrusive and most sensitive to their needs. The child left to himself in one's presence can gain his composure and include you in his protective isolation which holds him together. He is now tied to a human being, the therapist, who has been so undisturbing that he gains familiarity and becomes a part of him. Once admitted, he can become protective and helpful.

Children may use the therapist's office as the street, a place for gratification by surprise. The various drawers are being explored as if they were trash cans or stores. We always saw to it that we gave motives to the child for continuing at the appropriate phase of treatment, to associate us with gratification searched for and found in the street, as if it were sought and found by his own efforts. Slow inhibited children become agile, busy, eager, and active. The leisure to stand on their own feet, to move by an incentive of their own, attenuates the pangs of dependency and its negative aspects. Dependency, nevertheless, continues for some time to come. The children store any of their belongings in the places which were the sources of their discoveries, thus these drawers, shelves, etc., change their character, they become the familiar nooks and corners, as in the home. The therapist becomes the keeper of the child's precious objects, a glow and promise that can be relied upon. Bachelard speaking of early imagery fostered in the dim and cozy corners of the house which attract the playing child says ". . . for our dreams we need a small house within a large one, where to find the primeval happiness of a life without problems. There we find shade, rest, peace, rejuvenation . . . all resorts are maternal."

To supervise these drawers and shelves is indeed a responsibility because of their significance felt by practically all the children alike. Therefore these sanctuaries may be threatened by sibling-like rivalry and the desire to show that the therapist cannot be relied upon. The promise for instance, with which the child invested the desk drawer, symbol of the protecting mother could be literally "broken." But as a rule, we manage to fulfil the expected role faithfully or to repair the damage when we don't quite succeed. A focal point toward which converge the child's tendencies now exists. Repetition of high geared experiences invite steadiness and the development of a meaningful routine which lessens the child's former restlessness and search for the thing he does not or cannot have. He begins to be content and may now be observed to appear serene and concentrating on his pursuits. He begins to care and take care of his little oasis which harbors his "properties" which symbolizes a co-ownership of his little world. For the security he needs, some basic order has become a necessity. As he reassures and pleases himself, he becomes aware that he pleases others and enjoys doing so. In a gesture of good will and pride, he straightens out the room before he leaves it. In a bundle he hands to you his beloved darts which formerly he may have placed in his own pocket and lost. Assured that his order is also your order, he may surprise you one morning. Alone or with his group, he has cleaned the room and readjusted the furniture to advantage. Gently smiling with pride, he watches your anticipated pleasant surprise. These surprises do not mean that the office needed adjusting or straightening out. They are gifts to the therapist given in appreciation. The improvement also symbolizes their own improvement, their capacity for a contribution to a world they are learning to accept and to shape.

Children who used to beg constantly offer to clean the room regularly to earn a weekly allowance. Whether adequately or helplessly, the job is carried out with devotion. They will offer to wash your car and you may hear an artless little fellow reassure you. "You know I am not going to charge you a penny for washing your car. I don't want to be hard on you."

The little bewildered and driven hunter has become a settler and hunting is at best only one of his interests. Necessarily he becomes more conservative and less destructive. The toy no longer is an object of displaced hostility or self-rejection but a tool. The child now needs to find it each time he wants to "work." He has become a little man. He will tell you by his drawings or his "brick laying," that he claims you for himself and that he has something to offer. Like Felix, who drew profusely and revealed his development also through this medium, they may tell the therapist for instance that her husband belongs in a boat by himself at the outer edge of the piece of world represented in the drawing. "I belong in the same boat with you and *I am rowing*." They build you houses like other children, their house in common with you. They use clay or the building blocks to make furniture. They want their products to stand when they are proud of them and their drawings to decorate your walls. These objects may be steppingstones but they may become monuments erected to the memory of a noteworthy event or period in their development.

One extremely timid motherless child of illegitimate birth could speak only through drawings and through them he tried to be permanently in the therapist's company. He drew profusely and left little space for others to stay in the therapist's room by hanging drawings from the walls. His drawings fascinated his peers and their predominance on the wall of the room was accepted.

The children play table games with the therapist. Some of them are still taciturn. The dialogue is not by verbal intercourse, it is performed. The game is comparable to a silent film, the child being his own commentator, uttering a few scarce words at long intervals. At first he competes with you with decreasing inadequacy, but then comes the time when he "can beat you." He gives you hints, advice, he comforts you that with three more strokes you would have won. Through the game, the dialogue at play, the child has learned to broach the dialogue by words.

## The Rejected and the Neglected Child: A Comparison

We are using the terms neglected and rejected as etiological categories. The treatment of the rejected child represents a totally different challenge from the treatment of the neglected one, whether the parents reject him subtly or overtly. Here we deal with primarily perverted emotions and perverted emotional relationships. Rejection is a much more complex and active attitude. The rejected child is not simply unwanted as is the neglected child with whom there is little or no interaction. Rejection, however, can have an infinity of aspects including their subtle modifications. It can be a cruel negation of the child's existence and quality of being with a concomitant urge to express the negation violently. The child therefore is not deserted. He is wanted as a catalyst of hostile attitudes, as a means of denigrating or eternally annihilating the individual or the type whom he, the artless victim, is made to represent. The child is wanted as a substitute or a duplicate for another object, another catalyst or as a representation for a hostile interaction that the mother in our one-parent families is obsessed to continue in her relation with the child. When the father is present and involved, the intricacy of relationships is necessarily more complex. Depending on the depth and intensity of the father's involvement, he may play into the rejecting mother's hands, he may make an inefficient display of his interest and his human and parental potentials or finally he may co-operate in the therapeutic endeavor for the benefit of the child. The child may see in the father another enemy, a pitiful and despicable nonentity or the father may slowly grow into a meaningful, friendly paternal figure.

Though the language and expressions of neglect and rejection differ fundamentally, both attitudes may shade over into each other. At this time we shall disregard nuances which are highlighted throughout the book and, for the sake of clarity and orientation we shall establish what could be called situational types. We proceeded in a similar fashion when we focused our interest on the neglected child specifically. In the case of Felix, neglect was actually an instance of complete and stubborn denial of his unforeseen and unaccepted existence. We felt justified in discussing him simply as a case of neglect because deprivation in its most cruel cloak was his early experience; very much in contrast is the experience of a child untiringly used in terms of aggression.

The symptoms developed by both etiological types may seem similar on the surface, but their quality differs. The withdrawal, for instance, a symptom observable in both groups of these unfortunate children is, as well known, of a more timid character with the neglected ones and expressed in terms of a contained aggressiveness by the rejected child. One child is hopeless, weary, and resourceless; the other, on the contrary, is at ambush, ready to break out indiscriminately, without obvious motivation or aroused by apparently innocuous motivation. He may be capable of attacking his target or its representation frankly, at times to face his would-be enemies with determination and not infrequently with arrogance. "I do not care," "I am not wanted anyway" is his way of expressing despair and indifference to injury that he may cause to himself or others. The obstinate self-exposure to risk or annihilation of a child trained in making interests clash contrasts with the withering of the worn and indifferent child destroyed by neglect. In his definite desire to perish the rejected child is animated by the hope to hurt. He dreams of getting even once and for all. This actually means finding peace once and for all. When he reaches a state of exhaustion, his last token of active life is his keen suspiciousness. Even though he is totally silenced, his watchfulness is still alert, alert to the venom that nurtures his distrust and justifies his defensive isolation. If he recovers, he will surprise you by the profusion and acuity of the perceptions he had at the time of apparent mental extinction; he will then permit you an insight into his erstwhile version of the panorama of events that apparently did not pass unnoticed before his eyes.

There is a difference between the neglected child's absence of trust in others and lack of confidence in himself and the rejected child's active distrust of others and overconfidence in himself. In his worst condition the neglected child shies away from the whole world, vaguely perceived as unfriendly; the rejected child in his worst condition still sees the world populated by enemies and frightening sights. The neglected child rarely has the resources to populate his vacuum. The neglected child, if offered assistance, tends, as mentioned, to become readily dependent. When his accepted condition emboldens him to discover the element of hostility in his timidity, he tends to react on the sly and find it difficult to explain why. As long as he is still in great need of attention and support, therefore, as long as he is still timid and very much afraid of losing love, he cannot admit that he reaches out deviously for more attention. He knows even less that he is beginning to test his metal or to react wilfully against his lessened freedom, and his obligations which result from the newly received care and training.

The rejected child is not as unaware of the world and its movement. He may have a realistic or a sensitive picture, he may use denial in reference to the importance of the danger which he wants to brave. He also tends to underestimate the supremacy of his adversaries that he may feel free to gratify his impulse to retaliate aggressively for injury and injustice. He senses the dangers of blindness to danger, but for the sake of needed aggression he does not care. When he tends to yield to the lure of love and to relax his alertness to assumed danger, he may be ashamed of his "weakness." He belies in his heart that he loves and enjoys it and mitigates the pleasures of relating.

When the child has exhausted his outgoing aggressiveness prior to treatment, his whole body is bent in a resistive defense. His withdrawal has an extroverted proclivity. The neglected child, though fearful, is folded up upon himself. When one approaches him he may be taken by surprise and duck. His apperception of what is outside is not keen. He perceives only the unexpected approach, not its connotation. His reaction is tinged by inner motivation, which is fear.

The neglected child was not exposed to influences from which emanated discomfort aimed at him directly. Discomfort arose from nowhere and was everywhere. Above all it was felt within the body limits. Therefore, the child was not stimulated to focus on the origin of a challenge. Confusion further paralyzed directed endeavors as well as purposeful and dynamic reactions. The rejected child had the advantage of being exposed to stimulation. He could become aware of outside events and the sources of his malaise. These, however, he may be inclined to displace elsewhere. To recognize the specific cause of his discomfort increases its pangs. Moreover, stimulation has been of such a nature that whether specifically intended or resulting from the parents' own discomfort, it produces only negative reactions, the invariable answer "no" or destructive defenses.

## Outline of Treatment and the Vicissitudes of the Rejected Child

When we are confronted with rejected children, we have usually a minimum of two hostile people to contend with, the mother and the child. The mother fights the child, the Clinic, and the world at large.

The father, as we know, is often absent, disarmed, and subservient; or he covers up his weakness and resourcelessness by a vain attempt to be a disciplinarian; or, the child is exposed as an anvil to the batterings of the father, a second instrument of hostility. His discipline is a means of rationalizing hostility, subservience, or ambush. In any of these cases paternal protection is absent and fails as a stimulant to growth, as an inspiration of ideals and motive for reflective action.

We alluded to the difficulty felt by the mothers in renouncing the child's role as a target or an object with which to achieve destruction. At the beginning of treatment mother and child seem like hammer and anvil in need of each other. The glow of a day's "good time" in the Educational Therapy Center will soon cause at least some immunity in the child to exposure when he returns home at night. As time goes on he learns not to offer himself as a target. He notices how those children in the Clinic do it whose position of seniority is envied and secretly admired. He has been helped to benefit by the unending series of his temptations and failures. His improved behavior in the home may be appreciated by the exhausted mother who in her turn senses the relief and not only the frustration of being deprived of a target. The child may improve and promote improvement in the home, backed by the mother herself who has received help in the Clinic.

Meanwhile, we shall have to contend with the child's negative expressions of fear of involvement, of fear because he is hurt, and fear of laying down weapons. Imbued with an inordinate sense of strength, he is not so much afraid of the outside world as he is in need to imagine that he is attacked. What he loves most is to fight and retaliate against any displaced target. But displacement may not be needed any more, when the child has created ubiquitous sources of hurt and hostile interaction.

In a few cases we shall have to cope with an arrogant display of an ardently desired yet spurious independence. Usually, however, these children are writhing in despair and give in to love, however, at first, only after each crisis. The aftermath lengthens, the crises become rarer, slowly the child feels secure and profits from his new advantages, finally he begins to live. Children try to enlist their parents in their experience of happiness. It may be their means of solving the conflict of allegiances by uniting the love objects at home with those in the Educational Therapy Center. Suffering may have changed its meaning and direction. If our love and endurance has caused the corresponding harmonics to sound in the child, he will be concerned less with the suffering inflicted upon him in the past but awakened to his part in inflicting suffering; as a result he tends to forget and forgive the enemy outside. He can deal with the enemy inside with tolerance and patience. All of us help him remain alert, help him cope with contrition without succumbing and accept some failure as inevitable. We attempt to offer a climate which keeps his hope alive and the goal of his recovery in sight.

A child who has not been able to promote in the home a similar mutation as he is in the process of achieving might lose what he gains if his love and endurance supersede his combative potentials at too early a stage of treatment. He may tend to condone what he once had the strength to revolt against. He will not live and die fighting but lying down. His hostility is unaltered, it only changed its sense. He has become ashamed not for what happened to him and around him, but of what he does and of the one he has become. His revolt died out. He has given into fatality. He no longer fights dangers outside.

The children may be imbued less with religious and more with heroic ideas and feel that as long as they are "mean," they can at least be proud of themselves. As subdued "sissies" they are no longer objects of their particular brand of self-esteem. Yielding involves them in the weaknesses of their homes. Giving in to one's surroundings, one is soon dissolved in them. The last vestiges of freedom are lost. Loss of hope, dependency, self-rejection, and desperate hate may be drowned in or expressed with the aid of alcohol or other addictions. Such solutions are extremely rare among our children, though not their parents. Some of these parents we meet too late to succeed in helping them not to despise themselves. Few of the adolescent boys may go on a single spree of drinking. One boy escaped to the mental hospital to evade his parents' aggressive temptations and their efforts to drag him down. Another indulged in a drinking spree when his girl friend, whom he had been reluctant to marry, deserted him.

The implications of this spree of drunkenness are worth mentioning. Because of the interference of the mother with the treatment, it could never be completed. She could not share her son's liberating investment in the therapeutic relationship. She could not be reached for collaboration and insight. She would not come. At the time we could not afford the home visits necessary to help her see the importance of her contribution. Moreover, she was practically deaf when she did not want to hear. Her deafness was a powerful weapon in the family and enabled her to gain services from its members. The father was subservient to her needs, her "ambassador" with definite assignments. When he came, it was in her name and to interfere "diplomatically" with treatment.

This boy loved the girl whom he refused to marry. He had not worked through his problem with his mother and could not shake off her impact on him. He was imbued with guilt feelings and feared marriage. He had not exposed other men's wives to extramarital relationships without identifying with them. He was sensitive to their being replaced by him because of the analogy of their situation with the one devised in fantasy to his father. The women he visited as a young man were much older than he was. He felt guilty and feared punishment. As a married man he might get it.

It was this complex of unresolved relationships and conflicts that caused him to stay drunk for six weeks after having been deserted by his girl. He was desperately hurt by the loss and by the humiliation which had caught up with him despite his attempt to escape from it by remaining unmarried. He had fought dependency by refusing to seal the marriage officially. What he had reaped was the partner's independence, not his. In his pseudo-suicidal condition he was a ready prey to another man who got him to participate in an attempt in breaking and entering. We knew of all of these events through the boy's numerous letters and through messages brought by his younger brother and sister to the therapist. He had a need to confess in the beginning of his confinement which started several years after termination of treatment. However, he had visited us from time to time. In confinement he wanted to be supported by his therapist's unshakeable faith and continued acceptance as revealed by his subsequent letters. He depended on this faith for the conviction that he was not lost and had not lost the source of "life." He believed that this faith could not fail to convince everybody that he deserved love and life.

*Thus when the revolt against the adversity or indignity of a child's fate is broken or undermined too soon, the child's strength is sapped by which he resisted the forces that are disastrous to his emotional well-being or soundness.* The symptoms may disappear but not their underlying and destructive causes. He has not been able to gain insight into the works of his own emotions and the weave of the family relationships which cause its faulty movement.

We are therefore increasingly aware of the persistence in the home of exterior and interior danger to the child's progress and the outcome of the therapeutic process. *The destructive influence of the family interaction cannot be overrated. We could trace to this source each case of delinquent acting out in our area of experience.*

In addition to the mothers' reluctance to give up their grip on the children as instruments of hostility, we are confronted with the problem of their attitude toward hostility itself.

They fear their own hostility and cannot stand up and deal with it. They are submerged or devoured or driven by it. This absorbs their strength and weakens further their resistance to animosity. They suffer from it but indulge in it. Through the use of hostility itself they attempt to be relieved of it. It is compensation for inflicted and self-inflicted hurt, companionship in loneliness and boredom and a tool of self-expression. Therefore they are inseparable from it and it is to hostility that they must say good-morrow. But there are also those who long to be relieved from their ordeal or the painful returns of the weapons sent out to strike. A mother may discover her own need for love, possibly in competing with her child. She may become dependent upon us and make a new and happier start. Whether the mother can help her child, whether the child can accept help at an early stage of treatment and permit therapy to be carried out while he still lives in the home or whether foster home placement is necessary, we shall have to contend with those tendencies which resist change.

*But whether or not we can conquer maternal resistance, we do not give up the child's concerns. If our united endeavor in therapy and day-care can help him localize his hostility, we can indirectly instil in him emotions that vigorously compete with his hostility.*

Increasingly compelling will be the need for the joy of being accepted and the relief that existence has a meaning. He may resist recognizing the merits of the help offered for fear that such recognition might change his whole outlook on everything and thus disarm him. Their interest in him is hard to believe and deception would be annihilating. The need for love and self-esteem and hostile impulses vie with each other for some time. The home goes on fostering hostility and the child goes on to use it. He transfers it to the Clinic in all of its negative accents or for relief, for testing us, to mention but a few.

Character formation by attitudes of educators and therapist is nevertheless promoted. It is most important to be consistent in one's unshakable acceptance, poised in manner but versatile in approach and constructive in one's decisions. Difficulties must find a satisfactory solution. Though the child's needs must be considered, his whims, as evident, must not be indulged in indiscriminately. There are times when he should simply be distracted, at other times discussion on the level of his emotional maturity is his opportunity to find acceptable or desirable solutions, and in its wake comfort as well as gain in self-esteem. If he is not amenable or refuses to reason, time must be given for thinking it over. He may pout, act up, try to get permission elsewhere, or complain. The whole scale of warm and kind responses will be such that he understands that irrational or coercive means are unsuitable to achieve his purpose. It is evident that a child's tendencies to rule and to have his way by dividing are not encouraged. If he has a valid cause, he may be referred back for better exposition of his point to the one he asked first or a session in common may be suggested where the various points of view can be expressed and integrated. A decision reached is final. It is a mutual commitment, a gentleman's agreement that some children like to seal by a handshake thus expressing joy and pride over a decision reached with them as partners on equal terms. It can be a carry-over of a Robin Hood attitude or of their gang habits. When decisions are definite, a road is paved toward a new goal. There is no lingering, begging, arguing. The child learns to enjoy the profound comfort derived from definiteness, fairness, loyalty, and clarity of relationships and the relief a decision can represent which is worth making. He finds out spontaneously or with assistance that for the sake of love, of pleasure, or because of demands of reality and necessity, adjustment is advisable and finally he takes such an adaptation for granted. Humor can help greatly or questions as: "Is it that you want to tease me?" "Would you like me to be so weak that you can't respect me?"

To keep their parental figures worthy of respect is intensely important to these children. It is basic for their self-respect and one of the first signs of recovery displayed by the negative, obstructionist, or resistively indifferent child.

Achieved progress encourages a child to gain further stature by comparing his past to his present behavior. This leads inevitably to his sharing memories with the therapist and an intense release of the complex of emotions connected with past mischief. The experience evidently is a sublimated form of enjoyment of mischief but simultaneously the child confesses and edifies his inner "court of justice." The child may express wonder that he formerly behaved as he did but spontaneously he will explain it himself. Aided by his "masters," the young "apprentice" learns not to condemn but pass sentences that bear the seed of new life. Therapy proper will have advanced to a stage where less or no support by play is needed. Recent events may or may not have to be used as a crutch to start the flow of communication or support it. The child may simply speak about problems, relationships, and conflicts. He may start his session by: "I have been thinking, wondering, worrying. I am confused about. . . ." This may lead to his revealing his attitudes and fantasies, and he may report about past, present, or repeated dreams that preoccupy him.

The child becomes very interested in himself and his sessions. Concomitant with a sizable growth which the child senses and enjoys, his world widens, and, to explore it in depth, the sounding line has to be lengthened. He begins to make plans for the future and solicits an evaluation of his personality or ability to realize his plans. His individual experiences are reflectively fitted with the events of the time and connected with recent learning. In short, *the growing youngster acquires an integrated view of life and himself.* The gained self-assurance encourages him further and further to verify his experience through association with his fellow men. He chooses the "nice" children and clubs which unite self-respecting young people. He follows the lead of those men and women who attempt to serve with dedication.

The development is not devoid of its element of pain and suffering. His own difficulties in "being good" may trouble the child in the early days when love has begun to compel the young wanderer to stay. He reaches out for assistance in his struggle, he becomes dependent and watches how you feel about him. He caters to your pity and exposes his home. He has yielded to the temptation of betraying it for his own benefit. He now is in conflict. He may resent it and resist the therapist. "You think you are so smart." But he can be helped as it were to cover lovingly the inebriate Noah at home and find how to give comfort to him or her whom he exposed. Through his aid and delicate attention he discovers both his former or present contribution to the turning of the Ixion wheel, the infernal punishment of family dissension as well as his capacity to slow down its disarticulating motion. It may be much more difficult to find a new way at home than in the Center, but what he is in the process of achieving here, he can at least attempt to do in the home. We can achieve the following positive results:

1. Due to our special endeavors with the mother, she changes to the point that a favorable interaction results with the improved child. The mother's or the parents' attitude to a very withdrawn or autistic child living in the home changes to the point of not promoting further impairment or admitting of small steps of amelioration. The parents' insight promotes an improvement of the whole family group.

2. No change is wrought in the home but the child can take the situation in stride. His treatment is necessarily prolonged. He is de-

pendent on us for all that the home is supposed to offer. In addition we are his school and his physician.

## Indications for Foster Home Placement

It is necessary to differentiate between the child who has the strength to cope with the situation at home and to defend himself by appropriate means and the one who tends to yield and succumb to his dependency needs. The latter we try to assist in his struggle for liberation and if necessary his desire to be supported by foster home placement. He can observe in day-care the obvious strides made by children living in foster homes at their own justified request. Our emphasis on the dangers of persistent mother-child or family interaction is increasingly taken into consideration by court and placement agencies. Every effort is made to prevent the mother's insistence on reaching out for her child with a view to absorbing him or sacrificing him to her needs. *A concerted effort by the Clinic, the placement agency, its workers and the foster parents is necessary to obviate the child's re-enactment of his pathological dependency and transfer its involvements to his new milieu.*

Berthy Vernelle, a twelve-year-old girl with a borderline intelligence rating, was committed to the Social Service Bureau for foster home placement at the time her mother was committed to the state farm for alcoholism and neglect of her four children. Berthy was referred to the Educational Therapy Center because she had a tendency to incite her brother's serious misbehavior as, for instance, his pouring detergents or rat poison in all vessels containing food in the icebox of the foster home.

We present her case as an instance where the family interaction had been transferred to the foster home. It was recognized as such due to our interpretation of the case history and the child's revelations in the initial interview.

It was the grandmother who had brought her daughter, the mother of these four children, to the attention of the authorities for alcoholism and neglect of her children of whom she requested custody. Her own drinking and stealing habits made her unsuitable for such custody. The mother was in the habit of disappearing at intervals and of returning home in an inebriate condition. Upon her return from the state farm her fourteen-year-old son was allowed to live with her. He had been returned from the industrial school to which he had been committed because of repeated breaking and entering. He was always in search of the mother, "hoping to bring her home." The eldest sister was allowed to live with the grandmother and at the age of sixteen was well along on her mother's track.

It was in talking of this sister that Berthy revealed her awareness of the grandmother's role in the family, and, unaware of it, she gave us a clue for her own behavior. She reported that her father could not stand alcohol. It made him sick. He had tried with some measure of success to wean her mother from drinking and make her go to church. But the grandmother told her not to listen and tempted her daughter, the child's mother, by bringing whiskey into the house. "Grandmother gives us everything we want. I love her but I am also mad at grandmother. She makes mother sick. She should not be allowed to keep my sister. She is drinking already," said Berthy.

The case history gave clues to the fact that the grandmother had fought unsuccessfully her oral dependency needs and was obsessed by the urge to let others act out for her. This was her way of not doing what she should avoid doing and by this means multiplying and perpetrating what she could not help wanting obsessively.

Berthy's mother and elder sister had succumbed to the "poisonous food," weakened by the grandmother's indulgence of them and by the grandmother's self-indulgence through identification with her "babies." In need of them as her tools only, their own vital needs necessarily were disregarded. When Berthy came to us she was repudiating incompletely her destructive needs by inciting her brother to act out for her and by assigning her tendencies in fantasy to other girls whom, however, she tended to stop by telling on them and thus relieving herself verbally of hostility. Thus fabricating, she had told the foster mother that two of her friends were coming with a knife intending to kill the foster mother whom they hated.

In struggling not to succumb like mother and sister, she had found no escape except to use the grandmother's defenses. In revealing the danger of the grandmother's attitude and revealing herself by behavior and fantasy, she seemed to reach out for help that she might conquer the danger. (Her oral dependency was also revealed in her psychological test.) In a concerted effort, our services, the protective service workers and the foster home, attempted to answer the child's call.

This example for a great many more variations on the theme of pathological family interaction is given to stress the impact and inner web of "temptation." Caught within its web the child has no chance for recovery. But our alertness to the extreme danger the child anxiously faces with open eyes can and must help him be relieved. Where we cannot carry alone all three generations, as it might happen in Berthy's case, we owe at least to the youngest generation aid for a healthy mental development.

An early severing of the concrete ties is of the essence. Whether the child's placement is temporary or permanent, the mother or the parents need to be enlisted in the treatment procedure with patience and persistence. At times they can be inhibited in their most deleterious impulses toward the child. At times they fight their impulses with increasing endurance assisted by a growing insight into their problem. Achievement of independence from the Clinic may be extremely slow.

# XI

*Principles and Techniques Characterizing the
Educational Therapy Center Approach*

## THE MILIEU AS A THERAPEUTIC TOOL

"La hutte est le centre d'un univers. On prend possession
de l'univers en se faisant maître de la maison." . . . "A ce
centre se concentrent les biens. Protéger une
valeur, c'est les protéger toutes."

("The hut is the center of a universe. You take possession
of the universe by making yourself the master of the
house." . . . "The good things in life converge on this center. To
protect one value amounts to protecting all of them").
Gaston Bachelard, La Terre et Les Reveries du Repos

Though the children treated in the day-care program are present only
from 8:30 to 3:30, we attempt to give the place the character of a
home. The children enrolled in the day-care group of the Educational
Therapy Center, with few if any exceptions, are underprivileged also
in the sense that they do not have a store of comforting memories
associated with the home. Nearly all of their homes have failed to
protect them from the anxieties that befall a child, nor have their
homes necessarily shut out the cold. They have not been stable dwell-
ings that foster "the sweet habit of existence," nor have they been
places where fundamental needs are met with a self-evident routine,
liberating their inhabitants for pursuits which give life its meaning
and its intangible enchantments.

Few of these children have a father to protect them and their
mother, a father who teaches them, a father to emulate and to be
proud of. The hearth is rarely tended by the mother and she seldom
produces the glow of comfort and the stimulation which open the
early buds of acculturation. The faces of many of the mothers are
turned outside when at dusk they sit at the window while their children, often hungry and forlorn, wonder what there is to see in the
dying day. When the mother turns back on the room, it is usually to

vent the bitterness of her own misery, her own frustration, and her loneliness. In the face of unrest, caused by parental indifference, overcrowding, strife, terrifying and humiliating sights, many of these children, rather than take shelter in the home, roam around the streets and are absent from school most of the time. They are outsiders, repulsed by forbidding surfaces of stone, looking for safety underneath porches or other places that cover and conceal them close to the ground where they seem to want to take root.

Therefore, the first step in treatment is to give the child a home. Aside from its evident and realistic significance, this step has a symbolic meaning of fundamental importance.

The child who is unwanted in the family or community or at best tolerated, whether inside or outside the house, cannot explore the inviting depth of a home and its accommodating atmosphere. Windows and doors are forbidding as are the "walls" of the street, the façades. But windows and doors at least offer lesser resistance and are spotted for an anxious and aggressive intrusion. The children come as explorers—they announce violently their rights and claims for acceptance. If any drive for survival is left in them, any tendency to associate with others, they need to penetrate the depths of things.

Penetration begins first with attempts at visual and tactile perception. The young child awkwardly attempts to bore his index finger into the sand or into any other matter that does not offer too much resistance. The curiosity to go beneath the surface is aroused intensely by the compactness of matter and its rigid resistance. The first reaction of the child, therefore, is an attempt to break the matter that usually confronts him in the shape of a resisting object and to explore it from within. His elementary desire to penetrate into the depths of matter for the sake of recognition and increasing differentiation becomes outspokenly "analytic." By tearing or breaking up a whole object, the child becomes aware of its parts and their relation to the whole, though not necessarily of its structural elements. Sooner or later, the child will try to understand how the parts hold together and how, if broken, they can be put together again. Some of the untrained children are skilful in rebuilding a whole from fragments.

The same energetic curiosity serves children who attend the Educational Therapy Center. Their curiosity had been discouraged as an intrusion, first by the family "that has no use for them" and later by the community, which they had invaded in search of activity that normally is permitted at home. They have no choice but to impose themselves as the very intruders they are, or are considered to be, whether they are sensitive about it or vindictive or whether they finally compensate the hurt by angry arrogance. Entering necessarily gains a hostile connotation for them, and the element of curiosity is either maintained or lost in the process. Belonging, when they are not wanted, is a vital need, a form of self-assertion, of proving "they can make it." Since self-esteem has been impaired by the reaction to their very existence, to be "able to make it," acquires the perverse connotation of "making it" as the undesirable, hence bad person, "the bum I am." Curiosity, until finally deadened, might be stirred by the children's exclusion. When children cannot satisfy their curiosity in matters sexual, they try to interfere with the observed relationship, or to find answers for this curiosity elsewhere, at times obsessively turning in the "forbidden" direction. They become perverted or attempt to withdraw from temptation altogether. Their forbidden preoccupations may encourage precociousness in this area of development to the detriment of the child's general curiosity and strivings.

In some instances, eager to become a provider and stirred by the drive to intrude, these children will resort to stealing, insisting on their share of the hidden riches that reveal themselves to them—thus they claim their share of the big "pie," as one boy avowed. Consumption is one means of exploration. It presupposes that the "pie" be cut or its wholeness be otherwise interfered with. With an innate sense for mathematics, not dependent on any systematic knowledge, the children insist on correct fractioning, inferring for those who understand, that sharing means participation as an equal, a "partner" in that great business enterprise—the world around them. They insist on breaking into the toy stores. This is a precursory move for attending, though belatedly, the early school of childhood and participating in child's play. They need to own toys, to share them with all children. The toy is coveted as a means of belonging to the community and to the culture of which the toy is representative. The children want to be spectators as well as actors on the toy bus. This conveyance, as all the others, in their way, permits the children's unsegregated inclusion in our society. The real buses spoke a language of explicit rejection, when Negroes were admitted to the rear sections only.

## Being Invited and Becoming Familiar

Inviting the child into the therapeutic home makes intrusion, whether by violence or slyness, unnecessary. Compared to the children's barren world, devoid of security and solace, the Clinic, circumscribed in space, is easy to survey. A warming vault of acceptance protects the child from anxiety. No therapeutic milieu must exceed the child-patient's capacity to encompass its physical structure and to organize in his mind what he can conceive as its meaning and function. It is the children who tell us so. The more purposeful children tend to run over the premises in the first days of treatment exploring, usually by combative means. The more verbal children will from the beginning tell you that they have to "understand that darn place." They may ask questions, usually implying criticism; they may bluntly express criticism or deviously, or excessively laud the Clinic. Orientation is sought as a basis for comfort and trust, as a means of integrating the world and integrating one's self into it. Compared to the confusing world outside, a concise clinical world is luxuriant in things one should and may have. There are sufficient things, however, which have to be denied to provide necessary opportunities to strengthen character and acquire a sense of realism. But no object or move which would be meaningful to the child is unnecessarily denied or withheld from him. Implied or stated prohibitions become measures of support and reassurance, as well as avenues of insight into the reasons for general restrictions and the manner by which they bind and commit all peacefully.

However, the physical entrance into the therapeutic house or home itself does not provide automatically a mutually intelligible means of language communication, familiar to all. Nor is to be inside the therapeutic home an automatic reassurance to the child that he is accepted. He cannot readily change the character of his defenses. Whatever else the child may want, his most important and recurrent urge is to fight. He readily finds good reasons for fighting those next to him. In view of the short radius of his experience and outlook, the child will hold those close to him totally responsible for the world as it appears to him and which, for his self-protection, the child continues to resist. His distrust will persist for some time, and though he will be within the house, close to the glowing hearth, his self-image will at first be that of an intolerant outsider. He may refuse to see the friendly blaze. He may not wish to give in to its warming embrace.

## Transference to the House

In the beginning of treatment the house is the preferred target of hostility, substituting for any relevant person in the children's lives or any of the staff members whom these children, almost without exception, are most hesitant to hurt. *Where they hit the house, and what situation triggered the outburst, are sources of information to the staff and an opportunity for the child to understand underlying motivations.* Of course, it is equally important to observe the children's reactions to their own violence, whether real or feigned, whether responsibility is denied or admitted, whether the child is profoundly confounded, whether willingness to make amends is shown spontaneously or can be encouraged, whether repairing the damage is offered, attempted, carried out, or whether the child forgets all about it.

The house can symbolize the defenseless child himself. He might find himself to be his own taskmaster, his own jailer—he and the outer world thus becoming confused. This is particularly true when the house reflects the child's helpless condition too clearly. It becomes the catalyst of an ever renewed panic. Aggression is actually invited. It is wielded against the menace represented by the object and against its sensed spontaneous dynamics which varies in intensity, being worse "when I am nervous." Aggression, therefore, more or less rapidly reduces this menace because of the resulting relaxation of inner tension and anxiety. The child may "feel good" afterwards or troubled because of guilt feelings. The aggression actually is carried out in blinding anxiety and despair[1] and in disregard of consequences, as a combined suicide and homicide. The displacement on an inanimate object, however, expresses a last hesitancy or a salutary fear to commit a final act. In striking the house, the child feels more or less realistically that the staff will be injured, though not irremediably. He can kill and resurrect living enemies like toy soldiers. Thus he wipes out the difference between binding realities and the freedom of mastering events which he has at play.

The children would interpret poor premises as proof of the staff's lack of power. They would then be regarded as "not real people" and thus unable to provide a haven in reality. In order to gain confidence in their contribution to the mastery of reality, the staff upon whom he is sensed to rely, must not be judged by housing that reminds the child of his disabled condition. Any diminished respectability of the staff offends and discourages the child who senses disregard of his worthiness, worthiness being gauged in terms of social success. Community responsibility is here obviously involved in the children's behavior.

The staff may even be included in the children's sensitive interpretations and considered as abetting community criticism and neglect by submitting to inacceptable working conditions. However, the children can be helped to see that they can meet the public half way, that they can gain and command sufficient respect for helping to improve the premises. They are made to feel assured of the unfaltering support of their educators and therapists. In a positive way, the importance of an adequate milieu was demonstrated in the simple and dignified quarters of the Rosa Bowser Library, augmented by the fond acceptance shown to them by all the librarians.

The new premises to which the Educational Therapy Center moved later did not keep pace with its growing needs and both space and upkeep remained inadequate for a number of years. The ever repeated traumatization of the sensitized children resulted in a negative transference to the house and a temporary carry-over to our third home. Competition for a maximum of attention was observed when the staff was still insufficient in number. However, we were not unsuccessful in creating redeeming circumstances which encouraged the children's eager co-operation with the therapist and made improvement or recovery possible. Paradoxically, the move from our dingy location to our new and better quarters was fraught with an extreme sense of deprivation. The children suddenly behaved as if they were deprived of a past and an inheritance. They knew that the old house was going to be torn down. "We shall have no house to point to any more and tell the people it is here that we went to school," was one of many expressions of proud association with a place of inner beauty.

Felix, seeing the house so desolate ran out of town or as it were out of his world, to nowhere, feeling for a moment he had lost all his roots and the continuity and heritage the old quarters represented to him. Others continued to return to the old place. Months later, when not a trace was left of its material existence, the children allegedly sighted its torn down windows and doors. Their wish that we should buy them was an indication that they still sought ways of re-entering the old home.

The children's sentimentality in holding on to the old house revealed that they had made it their own, a representative of their way and need of being. They took possession of the new house by trying to subdue it and cut it down to size. The house was explored from basement to roof for hide-outs and opportunities to be obstructive. Replacing the playroom, the house became, as it were, an experimental stage for a fight between "gangsters" and the "police," an ambivalently mischievous testing ground of their smartness and our endurance of provocations. But the home gradually became a harbor of love and care, which, out of their own need, they had to respect. The children in the group are each others' best helpers. Great encouragement was derived from the fact that even the liabilities of the Clinic's location could be overcome. Early acting out was a source of information.

## The Hearth of the Home

In the most difficult instances a child is at first intrigued by the appearance and behavior of many of the neighbors, but usually they remain totally unaffected after a relatively short time. The ambivalence of decision is given up. Rare exceptions were those children who interacted intensely with an annihilating mother whose problems coincided with those of the slum area. Extremely relevant material can be produced by the children and an insight into their antisocial behavior can be obtained, when their present experiences quicken specific memories from the more or less remote past. We shall illustrate this statement by the following observation.

Emanuel started a movement of extreme hostility against the puny little neighborhood grocery where the children bought candy. The previously friendly atmosphere between the store and the Clinic was disturbed. The owner finally requested that the children stay away from his place. Displaying a great deal of anxiety, Emanuel reported in his session that the storekeeper was selling "black whiskey" under the counter, the customers asking for "medicine," to conceal the nature of the beverage they were buying. Apparently more perceptive to the situation in the store than any other of our children, he spoke at first in general terms about the danger such stores represented. The whole neighborhood was strewn with stores engaged in the illegal sale of whiskey, he said. Deeply involved in what he was discussing, he finally forgot all caution and revealed his role as the mother's errand boy for buying illegal whiskey. He himself became the source of much of the insight into his own case history.

In giving the Clinic the character of a home, the role of the kitchen must be stressed.

For a time the Clinic supplemented liquid food, usually soup and dried milk, for the lunches brought from home. At the present time, the children benefit from the government school lunch program. Improvement in the nutritional condition of the children has resulted in raising their low threshold of excitability and in reducing their excessive acting out against the therapeutic milieu, the symbol of the unrewarding mother.

Before our new lunch program was instituted, the children rapaciously grabbed food from each other's plates. They begged from each other. Sensitive children were unable to eat for fear of being robbed or envied. Timid ones gave away their food to avoid being deprived by aggressive means. Children denigrated their food, whether justified or not, to make it disgusting for themselves and easy to give up or to deter the other fellow from wanting it. Comparison with feces were frequent, in particular when children had only monotonous meals of peanut butter to "enjoy."

To make a home, its kitchen has to be more than a place to gratify oral or nutritional needs. It is a hearth where the most anxious feels most at home, because most sheltered from the inclemencies elsewhere. But the kitchen, basing its function on the pleasure principle, can also contribute to the building of ego strength and the tendency to socialize. Bachelard, the eminent French philosopher, calls "work in common anticipation of the meal," "the festival at its morn." Pleasure starts and imagination is stirred when the child gets ready to contribute his share to the fulfilment of his own needs. The meal is then enjoyed also as a task well done. Those who share it, value one's effort. Their encouragement results in new efforts and generosity in sharing. The potential which apparently menial tasks have for being redeemed from their prosaic aspects, can be learned in the kitchen. Bachelard says: "To exclude a child from the kitchen is to banish him into an exile removed from dreams which will be forever withheld from him. The enjoyment of the meals is enhanced when we follow their preparation. . . . Happy the man who as a child has stayed around . . . the housewife."

The kitchen is an important therapeutic resource in treating adolescent boys who are traumatized on all levels of libidinal development. They are usually extremely dependent, listless, and restless. They do not study. They cannot be made to be interested in shopwork. They interfere with the other children's constructive pursuits by constant teasing or by "scaring them." They adamantly reject their male teachers. Having physical and emotional needs they cannot satisfy legitimately they are antisocial in their behavior. But they can be motivated to "help the housewife" who gratifies their dependency needs. Their achievement is tested with a tangible goal and the enhancement of their social status emphasized by the cook's white attire; the realization that they are capable of giving is illustrated by the privilege to serve food to the guests of the Clinic. Their white apron becomes an incentive to harmonize its cleanliness with the clothes and underwear underneath it. In one instance such an experience in the kitchen finally helped a chronic case of bodily neglect which had resisted therapy proper.

The case of Bruno is presented as an instance where the relation to the motherly housewife in the Clinic kitchen brought to a boy the awareness, by contrast with his previous actions, of his past motivations for antisocial behavior. The integration of the therapeutic endeavor is evident in the following case history, when the child remembers slowly more and more details which finally highlighted a coherent picture.

When Bruno was twelve years old, he was referred to us by the State Welfare Department for truancy and stealing. After a period of hostility, withdrawal, and an extended phase of resistance to communicating, one day, in a sudden upsurge of affectionate closeness, he remembered and revealed that he never stole anything unless he was hungry. He commented that he never was hungry because of a total lack of food. When his parents went to work, they always left food in the ice box for him, the five year old, and his younger sister and brother. But the food always had to be warmed up. This was too much work. In its unprepared state it made him feel even more hungry. Denying and overcompensating his need of being helped to food by maternal solicitude, he pretended feeling more capable of hunting for a sucker or other candy in the stores than of lighting the stove and "cooking." To be out in the stores was less dreary. Satisfaction was immediate. It apparently permitted the expression of revolt against parental neglect and the assumption of the precociously imposed parental role in his own terms as a little savage.

When Bruno was a little older, he went hunting pigeons and robins. One day he demonstrated his situation at home by asking for permission to take a mother robin out of her nest. When the nest and the eggs would be deserted and motherless, he would raise them himself with great care. Bruno explained how he would keep them warm and feed them, revealing his identification with the motherless and the fostered child, as well as the one identified with ideal motherhood.

Bruno came from a family of five children of whom he was the third. Both parents worked and were known to have a great deal of difficulties with their children, all of whom had court records. The welfare record described the father as cruel and the mother as "in need of a great deal of wearing apparel." This need was her apparent excuse for going to work and depriving the children of care, guidance, and protection. The father's earnings reportedly would have sufficed to keep the family budget in balance.

Sometimes the mother would prepare food for the children, Bruno explained, but often she could not arouse herself from sleep at 5:50 in the morning to do this. Bruno evaded facing the strange fact that the parents, returning home and finding the icebox untouched, did not wonder whether the children had eaten at all, and, if so, what kind of food and from what source. They did not care where the food came from or by what means.

Bruno's people lived at a distance of almost two hundred miles from Richmond. Therefore the welfare record and Bruno's remarks remained our only sources of information. According to these sources the parents tried to realize social ambitions against insuperable difficulties, at the expense of the children's physical and emotional well-being. His parents' lives reflected the obstacles Negro people often encounter in their pathetic strivings for advancement and acculturation.

Bruno, his brother, and sister had a number of accidents resulting from maternal neglect. At least in one instance, when they set fire to a closet, they desperately signaled their state of emergency. A second accident occurred when the mother had left food in the oven for the small children to turn off in her absence. The children had forgotten to do what they were told. Noticing the smoke coming from the oven, they opened the door. The blast of the burning food threw them against the opposite kitchen wall. They possessed enough presence of mind to extinguish the fire by pouring water on it, an act which might have been disastrous had the food contained a large amount of fat. The children did not report the incident and the parents did not recall the accident, but Bruno remembered being afraid to warm up food from then on.

Hours of unchecked shiftlessness through the whole day were followed by the forced yielding to the father's rigid controls when he returned home in the late afternoon. He considered his cruel methods of punishment appropriate and necessary. The mother returned at eight o'clock in the evening. She was at home only at night and on weekends.

At the time when Bruno was sent to school, he was completely unprepared for an understanding of the most elementary human inter-relations and social controls. Immediate urges had guided his actions during most of his lonely days. He could not be expected to fit into an organized and scheduled enterprise. School away from home deprived him of his unhampered hunt for food and his random sallies into the gratification of curiosity. Shifting from the playful or aimless pursuit of preschool freedom to the laborious and disciplined learning of the student requires acceptance of restrictions and purpose which children entering school cannot yet understand. But it is at the price of selectively restricted individual freedom that we constructively organize society. Properly motivated children, however, feel the importance of the transition from the leisures of preschool times to school discipline and conform either happily or with initial concern.

Bruno was no more tempted by knowledge offered in school than by the food he left untouched in the mother's kitchen. He needed, for his predatory pursuits, only a small vocabulary, no syntax, no reading or figuring and no other orientation than the one required by the limited area over which his legs could carry him. This territory included, of course, a food store, where, like Hansel without his Gretel, he would nibble day by day. Bruno's food of knowledge that was acquired by trial and error provided in return an intense adventurous release.

The Educational Therapy Center offered Bruno, though belatedly, the meal served in a protective home, which is the first and basic requirement for future acculturation in a sedentary society. *Lonely preying for food was supplanted by preparing food in common* and the intangible inspiration which thrives on a community of purpose, of feelings, and of action. He was weaned from a self-centered exploration of the world and the sense that his needs could be served only in opposition to guidance and controls. Our approach yielded evidence of his capacity to accept and give love, and to work with and care for others. His spirit was not broken. On the contrary, Bruno learned to assert himself in the presence of his father. First in individual therapy, later in group therapy, he vented his personal problems. But when his outlook broadened, hostility was transformed into a surprisingly mature and constructive criticism of the weaknesses of his community. He depicted its dreary and desert-like scene. There were only two decent houses in that rural area, one belonging to his parents. There were no nurseries and no recreational facilities. To find work the children had to thumb a ride to town, at times wasting half a day and losing the opportunity to work. But work was the only decent occupation available. He compared the disadvantages of his condition to the opportunities offered in privileged public recreation centers. He learned to understand his parents in light of their particular difficulties.

## PERMISSIVENESS

### Permissiveness and Conceptual Behavior

In the early years of our endeavor we were criticized in the community for the permissiveness of our approach. We found, however, that genuine acceptance, and the consistency of attitude and method that is implied in our concept of permissiveness, are not only necessary but highly effective tools, though not sufficient in all cases. We shall see how the children themselves identify with the method and general approach and win over the newcomers among them with a speed that the adult group alone could never achieve.

Having been the victim of parental impulsiveness as well as of their own, they usually respect, at a fairly early stage of treatment, the strength underlying an attitude which braves their challenges and which, instead of "tearing them to pieces," supports and builds them up despite these challenges.

Excessive or destructive acting out therefore is soon reduced in the case of the majority of the newcomers. Their interest in what is essential for triggering a destructive "explosion" is soon focused on those elements which are essential in holding their world and its parts together. Symbolically speaking, from the negating Mephistopheles in Goethe's *Faust*, the child has turned into the Dr. Faustus who discovers and experiences, in the anticipation of constructive action, the supreme moment of his existence. In changing his course, the child shows that he is developing a positive sense of values or, in other words, he begins to differentiate. Refinement and acculturation have begun to blossom when he starts to preserve what he selects and "treasures."

Development of a scale of values calls for communication and the need to establish relations with those who answer questions in reference to qualification and comparison. Once the child questions, he "recognizes" what exists and begins to make his contribution. He starts on a venture of infinite scope which he will encompass only by slow steps. At every stage of mental maturation, we have to explore established values before we can denigrate or criticize, improve or overcome them. Rather than acting blindly, we use discrimination, which inevitably calls for delay. In weighing the merit or validity of one approach or one solution against another, we discover new horizons. Unless the child has been assisted by trust to recognize and to explore an existing world, be does not stand on a solid basis. However correct and bold its superstructure may be, it will prove to be no more than a phantom.

Seeking knowledge from the parent who is the "ancestor" at

home, the conveyer of language, of knowledge and, in the widest sense, the transmitter of culture, or questioning of the teacher implies the confident turning toward the community of all men. It is the artless acknowledgment of a huge structure erected by mankind from time immemorial to continue to time immemorial. The child who trustingly interrogates his elders, joins the chain of architects and constructors of a common edifice erected by all men. In inquiring, he asks that the material be handed down to him with which to pursue what others before him have begun and carried on.

From the loving and attentive respect of the venerable ancestors of our human race we derive the inspiring awareness that we are of their kind. Understanding the great texts, the works of great art and music and being touched by them, we partake of the genius which created them and gain a profoundly lived and thankful experience of the privilege of being human.

Patient non-involvement and equanimity of mind offers the youngest generation, within its limited range of observation, the experience of a world which, through consistency, inspires a sense of security and confidence. It necessarily encourages curiosity and communication by word. It shows the immediate forerunner to be kind, composed, loving, and reliable within the limits of human capacity. Man is seen as gentle and dignified. The resulting self-acceptance by the child is based not only on identification with parental acceptance but by a convinced joining-in as a member of the human community not desecrated but dignified and noble. Words as "human being" will appear spontaneously when the twelve-year-old has begun to be proud of himself. When this state is revealed to him through the simple gestures of persistent love and patience, the child will not be intimidated. One of our earliest impressions of the kinship of our little street boys with the great men of mankind was gained at an evening club early in our endeavors. That evening an excellent church choir master, carrying a portable organ, had come with his choir; the musicians performed Bach, Handel, and other seventeenth- and eighteenth-century classics. The children's group used to be noisy, boisterous and refractory to any classical music. Here, they stood in awe, silent, their eyes and ears wide open. They listened and were impressed.

When thus challenged by a new and unexpectedly pleasant condition, a child begins to wonder, then to ponder, and finally to reflect.

A more conscious way of living means, as the fourteen-year-old Annette once told me, "living no longer day by day, repressing the past and refusing a look into the future." Beginning to reflect is the child's way of making happiness last beyond the phase of mere exposure to experience. It is a search for causes of events and a way of learning how to obtain desirable effects, or to further one's own contribution to the course of events. Thus a fortunate emotional condition is necessarily an *opportunity* to rise to a more abstract, conceptual attitude and the development of good judgment.

A group of four preadolescent boys, fairly advanced in their treatment was playing together with alacrity, taking the therapist's presence fondly for granted. They showed a sense of responsibility for the objects in the room because of this fondness and respect of her but also because of their own pride and dignity. One of them, however, fell into the glass door of a bookcase. Immediately the children began to argue whose fault it was. The psychiatrist intervened with the question whether the boy had hurt himself. He denied it. This is all that matters, she stated, since obviously no one had meant to do it. She suggested they take the debris out of the room to prevent any damage to any child. When this was accomplished one of the boys said: I still want to know how that accident could have happened. His disquietude now was not in terms of culpability, where actually there was none, but in terms of cause and effect. Another boy explained it shortly. All children were satisfied and went on playing.

This rise to a more *conceptual attitude* and the development of good judgment represents an *essential factor in making children amenable and responsive to treatment. The first step of the treatment procedure has been achieved by the total milieu.*

Trust we find to be the basic emotional condition for the child's achieving this first step in the treatment procedure. To invest himself with confidence in the world, he has to recognize it as consistent and a oneness despite the variety of its aspects. Without a basic and unifying certitude, mental as well as emotional, variety is confusing and for the sake of survival has to be ignored, totally, or at least widely. Hence, disregarding other motivations at this time, we see the child's withdrawal or constriction as protective.

When the child, however, begins to reflect or in other words to ask the questions why and how, he shows that a consistent world is acquired which he begins to analyze in reference to its parts, that is, the causal and the effective elements, the essential and the accidental ones.

Trust, then, is basic in helping the child to venture forth from an immobile, self-referred security position toward an outside which he curiously explores with newly discovered mental tools, unimpeded by and in disregard of its resisting or menacing aspects. The exploring self necessarily becomes in time one of the objects of curiosity, since it is one of the important causal factors that can be observed at any time. The child gets to know himself as an acting agent and, supported by benevolent but respected adults, he learns to look at himself with observant eyes, similar to those who view him either with approval or with doubt of the wisdom and advisability of his actions, or finally with the subjectively sensed disapproval of his behavior. Anticipating a rewarding session the patient will converse with his therapist or teacher, clarifying in his absence, some problems for himself and storing others for discussion. Thus conversing silently with them in their absence, the child develops an inner speech which is the precursor of a higher conversational language that he begins to develop. The affection for the therapist or the teacher and identification with a more refined condition than the one that has so far been familiar to the children help them aspire to a higher status and to develop verbal expression which is representative of it. *The acquired readiness for verbal communication, and the resulting reduction of impulsiveness, represents a second step of treatment achieved by the milieu.* Despite the persisting prevalence of intense emotionality, impulsiveness is reduced when the child has learned to confide in those of good will in his new milieu with whom, in their absence, he can engage in an inner discourse. Then he can adjust to the setting of limits and to a schedule. His confident awareness that love need not constantly be demonstrated in a tangible form, represents a further evidence of the known fact that the deep sense of being accepted is necessarily an opportunity for the development of a more conceptual attitude and of good judgment.

The house has served as a focus for the children's intense emotions and thus also as a suitable setting for observing their behavior. It is therefore in order to discuss shortly the role of observation in evaluating the children's behavior and its changes and to assess its value as a tool of therapy.

## Treatment by Observation

Observation may be defined as an active, yet not aggressive mental study of situations, events, or behavior. The setting should allow for a natural and not staged field of observation and interaction. Observation is intended to be unprejudiced and all inclusive, but our perception of the field and the proceedings within it are necessarily narrowed by our interpretive system. Experimentation on the contrary tends to provide a specific setting liable to promote responses in the specific terms of the system of inquiry; thus the orbit of observable material is reduced to fit a pre-established idea and method of quest. The answer can be expected to be specific and, due to the circumscribed focus of the inquiry, differentiated.

In the case of a psychological study, however, such a method is applicable only if the two partners, the subject and the object of the inquiry, are both sufficiently puposeful to stay within the confines of the setting. Such a framework is difficult to achieve with children, particularly with the youngest and the most emotionally disturbed. For observation we have to avail ourselves of life situations as they arise naturally, which is, in our special case, the interaction of the children with all persons living in the Clinic milieu. The material which thus becomes available for information is actually huge. An "experimenter" on the contrary reduces at the onset of his research the set of specific objects or facts under study. The observer in turn reduces the amount and variety of available information for understanding by classification. For this purpose he avails himself of his interpretive system. Such method of study keeps foremost in mind the total view and the general purpose of the observation whereas the "experimenter" subdivides the whole problem in elements and aspires to solve them step by step. This entails the danger that the whole is lost sight of in the face of an infinity of detail.

Both of these approaches, however, overlap. The office of a psychotherapist, we believe, should be considered an experimental setting. Patient and therapist meet under specifically determined conditions which isolate them for fifty minutes from exterior disturbing interference and which in the office of the psychoanalyst includes the couch as a special device. However, as in any experiment, observation remains a fundamental source of information. Contrarily, the organization of adjunct therapeutic services in the Educational Therapy Center, where we are particularly interested in observation of spontaneous behavior and the setting needed for individual or group therapy proper, implies that not only purely observational but more specifically experimental conditions are inevitably made use of also. The very fact that observation and treatment take place in a particular house with a specialized and emotionally stable staff, an inevitable scheduling of time, an organized and co-ordinated approach, represents a set-up which comprises experimental elements. Limits have to be set, as for instance the taboo of entering a therapist's office while another treatment is in process. These limits however are similar to certain prohibitions or fundamental dictates inevitable in any nonchaotic family. Though these basic rules are at the service of keeping the experimental aspects of the observational milieu safe from interruption, they cannot therefore be considered to be strange or in opposition to the real life situation which we attempt to produce and to maintain.

The staff, which represents the animate part of the "inner lining" of the house, allows the child to become and to be the person that he is. Though "permissive" they are not passive; though natural and relaxed, they are highly observant, that is, mentally active, notwithstanding the specific professional activities in which they are engaged with the children.

Observation is not simply a means of providing the observer with the information required for understanding and helping the child. It is a therapeutic tool. It has to be used initially with so much discretion that the most sensitive child can comfortably ignore it, thus permitting the first, most delicate, way of fondling without touching him. Observation can be used for protecting the child from himself and others, for giving him the comfort of not being alone, yet undisturbed, or the awareness that someone has time for him, enjoys his mere presence and thus that he means something to someone. Therefore observation may provide the observed object with a sense of being as well as of the quality of his being.

The hostile child may secretly enjoy and overtly tolerate observation sensing that it is a means of showing interest in him. Surreptitiously giving in to that interest, he may in turn watch the therapist shyly. He may out of suspicion hide his longing for love, attention and the bolstering of his self-acceptance. Struck by the evident benevolence of the therapist's attitude and the tactful withdrawal of a glance the desirability of which the child is not yet ready to acknowledge, he may broach a first smile or initiate a hide-and-seek game of catching and missing the other's glance. Incipient playfulness and laughter might follow. Observation thus becomes a token of love. Even the obstinately hostile adolescent youngster is not necessarily insensitive to patient, unobtrusive presence and discreet observant watchfulness of his needs. Observation may here obviously have to be "negative," impassively ignoring provocations. As time goes on, the therapist can burden the relationship with the test coming from interpretations. The fact that observation is a prerequisite for interpretation of motives of behavior is recognized by the child with increasing clarity. In other terms, the child becomes aware that he reveals himself through his behavior to the observant staff and the children in the group whose wits are whetted by experience and the acquired understanding of themselves and others. He relaxes under the observant eyes of his total surroundings and unguardedly unmasks himself. He is not exposed to any punitive or vindictive reaction. He will only be encouraged to explain what he had on his mind when he did what he did. As soon as he is able, he is helped to face underlying tendencies or to identify with the feelings of his opponent. The interest of the adult will support him in the difficult task of shifting from an impulsive to a reflective attitude and hence to assuming the responsibility for his behavior.

Necessarily, the cathartic effects of the unmasking behavior before the eyes of the ones who will not be shocked and who can accept him as the one he is and the one in whom we nevertheless believe will come to the awareness of the child. Therefore not only those who needed attention in the beginning, but those who feared or seemed to reject it, will soon desire and provoke it. They will react angrily when observation is lax. An intense concentration on the children, a genuine and unselfish interest are basic prerequisites for the reduction of excessive acting out, or a desperate display of destructive aggression within the therapeutic milieu. Observation should be relaxed, but never lax. Laxity of observation is sensed as withdrawal of love and support from the child. From the objective point of view, it fails to provide for the discriminate information which enables the observer to act and react specifically, that is, therapeutically according to indications.

We have discovered the therapeutic milieu as the abode of the child deprived of the benefits inherent to proper family living which are the loving guidance out of a state of physical, mental, and emotional helplessness and of want of orientation. Usually such a child is driven into the streets as a substitutional habitation and to its population as substitutional caretakers. Usually he meets the same fate as in his home, disregard until his unguided self-assertion, justifies a pre-existing rejection. We have further discovered observation in the therapeutic milieu as a means of responding specifically and helpfully to the human object and therefore as an expression of unprejudiced acceptance. The interest being permanent, acceptance necessarily is unfaltering.

## Principles of Permissiveness and Punishment

In indicating in the previous chapters that the behavior of these deeply hurt and isolated children is an awkward expression of despair and an appeal for help, we may have conveyed an understanding of the fact that we need to bind wounds whose infliction we have failed to prevent. Punishment is inappropriate and undeserved in view of the children's deprived and untrained condition, and is necessarily unsuccessful.

The permissive method, which is not the condoning of antisocial or otherwise undesirable behavior, takes account of the realities of the children's condition. It is therefore the only tolerable approach to their plight and the only fair and humanitarian one objectively.

Realistic acceptance of the child-patient as he is, and cannot help being, in view of the totality of his life circumstances does not exclude expectancy of change, as stimulated by the sum total of the therapeutic endeavor. Permissiveness includes that certain basic limits are set for the support and comfort of the anxious child, lovingly expounded, and impressed upon him with equanimity, definiteness, and persistence. Thus, he will learn to recognize limits as needed for his wholesome survival rather than a menace to his freedom of self-expression.

Supposing a new child comes to his initial interview well prepared by his parent or the referring agency. He will be given an opportunity to explain why he likes to come and what he expects. The child may already have learned, though possibly by rote only, that his contribution will be necessary for becoming a happy and successful child. To convey the idea that his daily attendance will be required, a variety of fundamentally similar attitudes can be taken by the interviewer. Assuming the child faces his problem and wants to help himself, he can be made to understand that a daily attendance is a prerequisite for success. A very immature child will require that one convey the fairy tale touch to the coming adventure. Something exciting will happen every day where we shall need him and could not possibly miss him.

One little seven-year-old who had been suspected previously of being a brain-injured and retarded child, a supposition not verified by neurological examination, proved himself to be quite adequate in his initial interview. A previous report invoked his playfulness as one of the evidences of his mentally and emotionally retarded development. The child probably had sensed that his playfulness gave him a minor status with his examiner despite the kind interest shown to him. He therefore was deprived of the only or main expression of adequacy he had. This interviewer, however, showed a pleasant surprise that he chose her for a playmate, thus accepting his way of being and giving him an initial encouragement. He was full of initiative and spontaneity and gave a much better show of himself than with his previous examiner. The child chose to play at the level of his brother, three years his elder. He remarked that his brother had a checker game; therefore, he wanted to play checkers with me. This was his way of placing himself in the privileged role of his brother in relation to the mother. That role was further characterized by the reported fact that his brother had a privileged position. In addition to checkers he also owned marbles. The little boy's lack of number concept mentioned in his previous assessment elsewhere, we found by our permissive way of interviewing, to be confined to the personal and family area about which he seemed confused since he did not know his age. He wanted to be as old as the brother, but being made to feel less adequate and acceptable he also felt the need to be only five years old and not ready to go to school. Nor did he know the number of his siblings, but he counted spontaneously and compared the number of checkers he had taken away to those the psychiatrist had taken from him, to cite but one example. When he left, he said, "I did not know I could be all right."

If the therapeutic milieu is capable of maintaining first the up-lifting shock and, persistently, the support of self-confidence and self-esteem, support inducing his school attendance will soon become unnecessary and we can count on the child's regular attendance. We shall have to enlist the parents' co-operation and assist them in stopping coercion to prevent a negative interference with the child's joy in his own adequacy, his freedom of action and his pleasure to please. One will necessarily fail when, interviewing a resistive child for the first time, one insists on obtaining information he is determined to withhold. It becomes a power struggle. If you tend to engage in it, you have already demonstrated to the child your inferiority to him in social strategy. You have exposed yourself to failure if you have shown that you have a stake in his consent or in his yielding. He will love and want your love only if he admires you and gains status by an alliance with you. But he also needs to trust you, and your whole effort, though without obviousness, must be bent in that direction. The child's yearning for a safe anchorage—whatever his apparent defiance—coincides with your interest in knowing the child, in order to be most specific about the kind of help you offer and the method by which it is given. It is in this meeting of needs that the child's first contribution to his recovery is made, because what you give relieves him. If he is suspicious or not yet willing to be kind to himself, you have at least drained off his opposition. You may at this time support his positive tendencies by taking for granted that you will see him again and may indeed be pleasantly surprised. A hostile, withdrawn, and sensitive boy might reward you for your trust by being present for his next session in his best apparel, broaching a smile.

Similarly, the new children in day-care may have been in the habit of being truants and their whereabouts may have been uncertain through the years. Success in the Clinic must be practically immediate lest these children associate it with all of their previous experiences. What they have had to face so far has been either coercion or the condoning of indifference. We shall offer neither. We are determined to see the children daily, but they will be aware only of the fact that in their absence we miss them. This conveys to the children the feeling that they are important enough to us to be noticed and that they are wanted for their own sake, unconditionally. The Clinic which has a high incidence of children with a history of chronic truancy has also a high attendance record.

Permissiveness in the day-care group does not mean that any kind of behavior is tolerated. Every attempt is made to keep the children interested and inside the classroom; the one who strays away will be met by the supervisor who gently attempts to have him return. If need be, she will have a discussion session. The child, alone or with others, is encouraged to express himself and to present his motives for leaving the room. He will be helped to face rationalizations, projection of failure, sensitive accusations, sibling rivalry, escape or withdrawal as a defense in the light of his own individual problems. His imperative needs for attention, for relief or release of emotions will be scrutinized and the child will be helped to return to his classroom in a co-operative mood. This way of dealing with the child's symptoms has the additional merit of providing a wealth of information about his concrete as well as lived experiences. In a natural and most satisfying way the child is guided to express his needs not by antisocial action or by hostile withdrawal but by communication.

Provocative behavior is met with calm and kindness. The only deprivation to which the children are exposed is the frequent denial to them of a target. However, they are helped to vent their hostility. They will be confronted and each of those engaged in strife given opportunity to tell his side of the story. Some control is inevitably imposed upon the children. If two or several children talk at a time, the child becomes aware of the fact that none can be heard. In order to encourage the children to take turns in talking, each of them will be assured of his fair chance. Moreover, a minimum of articulateness of speech will be a prerequisite for making one's self understood. Impulses will be mastered at the service of the child's own cause, and he will have to resort to civilized means of self-assertion. In cases of a serious nature, like dishonesty or violence against the house, matters are discussed individually with the child. It may happen that the misdemeanor has been discovered by the children and they call the children's court, an outstanding means of self-search and self-judgment, as well as generous identification with the failing child. The result is a charitable attitude and the desire to help him. Isolation is avoided, and the road to improvement is opened.

The need to express hostility by action is taken into account. The children themselves may cope with an incipient fight that threatens to get out of hand, by calling: let's get the boxing gloves. Thus they resort to rules and an orderly procedure for the control of hostility and for coping with their own anxiety; they make a convincing attempt to use play as a device for preventing "serious" violence. When violent attacks and fights flare up with rapidity and intensity, I have found it most helpful to venture into the thickness of the battlefield.[2]

When he was referred to us, Marvin was in the habit of throwing any enormous object, for instance a large metal telescope used for science experiments. In his first group therapy session he responded in his usual manner. He immediately interrupted his action when the psychiatrist walked between him and his target. Once or twice later he brandished heavy objects but needed only to be reminded soothingly and firmly, his therapist's hands lying around his shoulders, that he knew better. This approach is successful because it supports the child's trust in himself, in his dislike to be violent. It upholds his humanity. He loves the one who gives him an opportunity to prove his own human status to himself and thus, at a moment of extreme emotional upheaval to recover rather than to lose himself. In the case of Marvin it helped him to know that he was not condemned like his father to be uncontrollable, murderous, and doomed to die. It relieved his terrific anxiety. In the months to come, this boy developed, though not without divagations, into a self-respecting youngster who could discuss his problems calmly and present his arguments intelligently and comprehensively. He could consider all aspects of a problem and how all people involved in it would feel.

One day, he requested to be sent to a foster home. He was justified in asserting that he had no chance at home. He knew his mother understood his desire. He had discussed with her the obstacle he had to cope with in his home. He aired the matter of his mother's moving away from their present home together with him, but he felt the best solution was his own move, allowing the mother to continue living with the stepfather. In other terms, he did not want to force her out of her way of life, which she was too weak to give up.

When one supports the child in the disintegrative state of aggressive violence and restores him to himself, one must not forget that other children might be encouraged to solicit one's love by identical means. They are sufficiently weak in their own composure to be easily tempted. One way is to show attention to all children. But while such an attitude is comforting and gratifying, it is not the most important factor in preventing the children's misuse of the support to the failing child. Identification with the therapist is the usual response of the children. Just like the aggressor who stops his violence in the midst of an act already in process, they don't want her to be exposed to danger. Her interference was the best means of demonstrating the danger of violence and of conveying a deeply felt identification with its potential victim. That she knew how to alleviate danger and to provide emotional relief will intensify their sense of security with her and suggest identification not only with her as a potential victim, but as the one who could be relied upon to master an important problem without hurt to anyone. In preventing the undesirable act she confirmed its undesirability but showed that one can love and protect without censure or nagging the would-be aggressor from becoming an aggressor.

This does not mean that everything is terminated by the interruption of the impulsive act. The therapist will invite her little group to sit down and suggests: let's "think this thing over. This is serious; what happened?" The discussion will finally end in the children's understanding that Marvin's irrational anger was an outburst only triggered in the present situation. The children may report spontaneously that Marvin was mad already when he arrived this morning and Marvin will give the reasons why that was so and help us reveal the real motive and the real target. They will be deeply impressed by findings to which they contributed their surmises and solutions. Marvin will sit and go on pondering about his enormous discovery and its implications.

The reader might be interested in an instance where the permissive approach was applied to a case of dishonesty.

Spencer one day surprised his mother, Mrs. Sherwood, by coming home with a pair of sunglasses she had not bought him. We were duly informed of this fact by the mother. The child reported, and this information could be verified, that the mother had bought all children sunglasses with the exception of himself. Hurt and angry, he took gratification in his own hands and provided sunglasses without paying for them himself. This was his way, by defiance, of also having this gift. The mother was assisted in becoming aware of her unconscious tendency to trap and defeat Spencer. The child was encouraged to share his painful experience with us and explain what could be the mother's reasons for excluding him from privileges. A self-searching attitude was stimulated. At that time the child confessed that his case with the mother was hopeless, his good behavior was not even acceptable. We took the position that since he meant a great deal to us, we would not like for him to be slighted but on the contrary would like him to have what in all fairness he could expect. However, for his own sake and for the sake of the people who work for what they have, we would not like to see him keep what does not belong to him. He decided he was going to return the glasses. One of the workers went to the store with him, then to his infinite delight we gave him new glasses because mama could not afford them at the moment. We assured him she too wanted him to have glasses. By this time this had become true. We could not allow our act of comfort to the child to interfere with his relationship to the mother, our function being rather to become in the long run a bridge for their mutual love and understanding.

The most prevalent behavior in the day-care group is incessant mutual aggression. Whether the children have an early realization of what they are doing or not, they will learn step by step to attract needed attention from those they love by more appropriate means. They make sure that the therapist sits down right away as an assurance that she will stay with them, close to them. They make the therapist hand them objects, in an effort to prevent relaxation of concentration on them or their endeavors. They may begin to talk a great deal. Children who are not yet able to communicate directly may think aloud hoping faintly that they will be "heard." By such behavior they may stimulate themselves for action as a way to please. Children may visit staff members and make friends with them. They become alert to other people's needs and offer services to endear themselves. Now they are more spontaneous and resourceful. Realistic motives for contacts are found and worked for. Self-reliance is awakening.

The permissive method originally was used to free a patient from the rigors of a superego that caused him to repress his conflicts instead of admitting them to consciousness where they could be dealt with. In child psychotherapy, this approach seemed particularly appropriate since the released conflict revealed itself for observation in the acted out symptom, observation having to take the place of verbal communication such as between the adult patient and his therapist.

The permissive method, as we understand it and have learned to practice it, however, has a more general validity because it is essentially *ego supportive* and a basic tool of character formation.

## Fallacies of the Principle of Punishment

Justification of punitive attitudes and methods is usually superficial and serves purely practical ends. It is based on a narrow concept of right and wrong which takes account only of facts and acts in disregard of motivations. Judging a person on the basis of undesirable acts committed, we disqualify him socially and confirm the state of emotional or moral isolation which preceded the perpetration of the act and motivated it. Since the act belongs to the past, it is irrevocable and punishment is really the only means of re-establishing the equilibrium disturbed by the act. We have to step outside the legalistic order for "judging" and rehabilitating.

The confirmation through punishment, of a state of emotional isolation, which motivates asocial action leads in final analysis to a road of no return. Few "learn to think." Many derive from their emotional and social exclusion a deep sense of unworthiness or a deepening of their isolation. Instead of being stirred to overcome a feeling of unworthiness, they are convinced of it by its certification and submit to it, thus showing dependency on society and a form of recognition of its standards. But this recognition necessarily being self-annihilating, the disqualified person has to rally for survival. He feels weak and yielding when he submits and strong when he places himself outside society again, defending his status as an outcast and thereby overcoming his isolation. His character of an unacceptable member of the human community is turned into a weapon and unworthiness becomes his justification. Through censure and punitive exclusion, a state of permanent or at least of extended duration is attributed to the offender's subjective and real isolation. He is thereby disarmed to the point of having for his defense or his violently aggressive bidding for re-entering only himself as a suicidal weapon. In his state of despair, he no longer cares. In isolating himself fully, he overcomes isolation which is felt only as long as he cares for inclusion or acceptance and appreciation. Simultaneously, weakness and disarmament yield to an elated sense of omnipotence. For relief and elation, the isolated person has to resort time and again to suicidal aggressiveness, and he becomes addicted to it. Henceforth, he must entrench himself more vigorously against a society or a humanity, which denies him strength and elation and ordains the state of unworthiness.

Immune to punishment, invulnerable to threat, the offender has now become an explosive, uncontrollable force and society's disowner at the risk of his own physical or moral existence. Society reacts in legitimate self-defense. It disowns its constructive methods, its noble, uplifting spirit and with means similar to those of the aggressor uses force to fight back.

Only if we leave the cold world of facts and retrace the act to its motivations, that is, if we enter the experience of the human being who committed the act and only if we try to understand its meaning for him, can we hope to make an inroad into the vicious circle that we have just described. Only if we feel deeply the community and equality in principle with any of our fellow men can we join him fearlessly on his most isolated paths. Brave and bold issues may be then unveiled to the eyes of both, the one who suffers from isolation and the one who is afraid of involvement.

Once an act is accomplished, the tie between it and its author is largely severed. The severance may be so complete that the act may be felt as foreign, not understandable, unless recognized by the "recall" or re-collection of the motivating steps. A shift of interest from the perpetrated act itself to what motivated it implies that *emphasis shifts from the responsibility for our acts to the responsibility for being the way we are.* An act emanates, flashlike for seconds, from the whole of an individual's existence. It is *expressed* behavior in the sense of being exteriorized. Similar to the act itself, the consequences of an act gain independence from its author who started the chain of events. Our motivations, however, live with us. Changes of motivations are inseparable from the total of our existence. Not determinable objective entities, but psychic intangibles, of infinite complexity, motivations are in a permanent process of modification. They defy clear and so-called objective evaluations as being good or evil. These evaluations are too simple and totally inadequate.

"Good" or "evil," no longer isolates any man from any of his fellow men. *This alternative now lies within every man.* Man is constantly at work to maintain his state of becoming, to be self-restoring and self-edifying. This presupposes that his integrity and state of integrity are constantly challenged. This challenge is his real chance for a moral existence because it implies his capacity to struggle and his liberty to choose. The low points in our actions result from a real or subjectively felt isolation from ourselves or the other selves. Profound relatedness which "obligates" us particularly if it transcends the instinctive sphere of satisfactions, tends to inhibit digression. The crisis of isolation precedes and succeeds the state of disturbed equilibrium for which the digressor is not the sole responsible agent. We take due account of the general involvement in treating whole families, but to be complete, whole communities should be included and the cultural patterns of each society.[3]

The universality of responsibility redeems man's isolated condition and through equality of all men, which it implies, alleviates the anxiety inherent in the status of isolation. Punishment, in confirming and maintaining the sensed and enacted isolation by condemnation, stresses the inequality of the digressor. Inequality represents the most cruel exposure to danger and necessarily leads to extreme anxiety and an increased sense of isolation. To defend himself, the one who feels endangered resorts to shrewd or violent means. He has no other recourse since the legitimate ones are not at his disposal. At least that is how he feels with more or less justification. Children who suffer from such a profound feeling of isolation and inequality display their anxiety by carrying knives and attempting to own guns. Punishment then cannot be expected to prevent new digression.

As long as isolation and anxiety prevail, the defenses used for the establishment of illusory security promote a vicious circle of anxiety and defenses on both sides, that of the offender and that of society. The terrifying melee further prevents the return of the prodigal son. In order to combat his own anxiety and defend his endangered position and in order to gain ascendance over the prostrated sinner, the righteous prosecutor musters intensified indignation and goes to war with an expanded arsenal of steadily increasing armor.

Once we are convinced that punishment or isolation does not represent an answer to digression, more intelligent means of dealing with deviations from our culturally accepted ways will be devised. The first step necessarily is to alleviate rather than to intensify the anxiety which precedes and succeeds digression.

## Analysis of Temptation

Isolation and anxiety are also the inner experience of the "offender." The anxiety which precedes transgression springs from and exposes the core of man's tragic condition, his infinite distance from perfection. *It implies the longing or striving for a status that exceeds man's actual state. In his disturbed condition, however, man, the offender, is fascinated by what he should not do, for which he knows he will pay an excessive price. But the fascination holds him in its grip. The experience of failure, complicating the remorse or regret which follows the transgression, is in itself anxiety-provoking and develops new anxieties rooted in fear of the returning temptation. No longer is anxiety due solely to the fascination aroused by the coveted object but by temptation itself. Temptation becomes a second fascination and transgression an obsession. The original object of temptation may be lost in the process, even when it remains its symbol or representation.*

The transgressor's profound sense of iniquity and his contrition that succeed the transgression are equally ominous. Ambivalence may raise its Gorgon's head and the punitive aspects of the transgression, self-deprecation, shame, and anxiety take account not only of past but also of anticipated failure. Indulgence in anticipated failure is used as an enticement. The hazards of temptation become a stimulation, and danger inherent in the gamble begets anxiety which enters as punishment into the anticipated transgression. Anxiety now pervades every phase of the process. Rather than paralyzing the tendency toward transgression, it stirs it. An intense unrest is in process, a gratuitous motion devoid of a salutary aim. It further weakens the resistance. Thus punishment, here in the guise of self-punishment, rather than deterring transgression, sustains it. It provides a fraudulent toll for renewed failure by self-chosen and self-inflicted penitence.

A solution to the alternative of wanting intensely what also is not wanted can no longer be reached and is no longer sought. Indecision and obsession have become a way of life. Choosing one's own punishment as an acceptable substitute for the consequences of one's actions also expresses anxiety. It is promoted by the sensed inability to endure an incurred fate, the anticipated blow of which is dreaded.

## Rigidity and Permissiveness

The use of punishment in education represents an approach which imposes by coercion values which the child is not yet ready to make his own. Children may well be indoctrinated by such methods, but by so doing a number of grave risks have to be faced.

When children thus raised are not yet able to understand why they are punished, they are not likely to focus their attention on what meaning the educator intended to impress. Instead of being exposed to the privilege of learning by insight and that kind of obedience which is to "listen closely," the children are prompted to avoid danger by submissiveness. This represents a fundamental lack for the individual and the culture in which one grows up and which one will be called upon to represent. Lack of resourcefulness and creativity result, as well as lack of conviction in reference to knowledge and ideals, which the child will be ill equipped to defend. In view of insecurity and lack of well-founded convictions, the adult himself has to resort to coercive methods of education which, history has shown, lead to the decaying of culture by power struggles and chaotic succession, over more or less extended periods of short-lived authoritarian regimes.

Education supported by means of coercion does not take into account man's inherent tendency and right to doubt, nor does it acknowledge his fundamental need to search for truth, independently and individually. Resentment cannot fail to be the result of such educational shortcomings. The eagerness and rigidity used in impressing, by punitive methods, one's own mind or conviction upon a child is liable to convey special connotation. The child will feel that he is not respected as potentially equal and may fail to reap the benefit derived from example which, due to resentment, he refuses to emulate. "They try to bombard me into manhood" said a bright and sensitive boy, and "I am all confused," said his sister. "I want to go to the creek alone where I can collect myself and can find out who I really am." Less privileged than the child favored by edifying example and the opportunity for developing and defending his convictions, the child coerced by fear of punishment is inclined to feel he is a mouthpiece, used for the educator's purpose rather than for expressing his own convictions. This leads to revolt. Principles forcefully induced upon the child today may not at all be defended by the man tomorrow. Insecurity on the part of the educator is sensed with increasing clarity by the child. Why should his teacher be so eager and harsh if he defends a position that would necessarily carry conviction when its validity speaks for itself?

The need for surveillance and *steering* does not imply, however, that these measures have to be supported by an eagerness to punish nor that at all stages of education proper guidance could not be effective if it takes into account a child's own need for testing reality. It is the psychiatrist's daily experience to hear thoughtful youngsters complain of their teacher's or parents' anxiousness which tends to prevent growth, through "testing" and self-experience. Anxiousness begets the fear of exploring.

## Appeals and Responses

Appeals can be made to the *human* person as early as he stands erect, for then he finds his upper extremity freed for action and his eyes able to capture a widening horizon. He feels the need to act. He is constantly at work making discoveries and finding out things to do by himself. Prohibiting this trend does not easily inhibit it unless education is sufficiently faulty to have a stunting effect on the child's initiative. The child who will wait for the second that the mother has turned her back to pull off the table cloth or turn over the ink may be prompted by improper training, by too many unwarranted prohibitions, or by an improper tone that indicates irritation rather than assistance. The mother may forbid for the sake of her comfort rather than the child's guidance and welfare. Instead of obeying, which is to listen willingly, the child may be frustrated. He may have picked up mother's irritation and responded to it. His mischievous attempt to do exactly what is forbidden necessarily leads to new irritation, to a good spanking. Now the state of war is on between mother and child.

But experience cannot be transferred, it must be acquired. Borrowed experience, unless verified by one's own observations, does not carry conviction; it leaves an uneasy condition of uncertainty. How intrigued a two-year-old child must be to remain in suspense long enough for the auspicious moment when he can reach out for the forbidden fruit? The mother of the young child has no other choice than to eliminate dangerous temptations from the child's sight or reach or to warn by a sweet but definite "no, no" or other expressions commensurate with the child's growing vocabulary and capacity. Understanding inspires trust. The mother at first gives an explanation in jargon or in the child's current language. With the child's advancing level of understanding, she shows him with delicate prick that a needle can hurt him. Where it is possible, she allows the child to experience an experiment. The educator's role should be one of the unseen guardian angel who protects the child in his searching inquiries. The educator allows evolution and maturation to take their courses, aware of the fact that the child's failure to "mind" is not solely due to wanton impulses, but to his admirable search for knowledge and the discovery of the universe by experience. To forbid and to punish requires less dedication than to be abreast of the child's mental and emotional development and thus to know when to encourage or discourage his boldness. Children who grow up in an accepting yet understanding educational climate feel free to discuss their problems, hopes, and desires with their parents and educators and, should it seem important, to ask them for greater margin to have their own experiences and to insist that advice at this time cannot substitute for a brave venture of their own. Where trust rather than fear mediates between the child and his educator, the need to test the contrary to what is advised is greatly reduced. Children who have parents who discuss problems with them tell the therapist how the parents' real or assumed disapproval effects their decisions. Mutuality between parents and children in the conduct of life inhibits impulsiveness and limits excesses. Usually, permissive parents who allow their children to venture out within the limit of safety or acceptability are likely to have demonstrated throughout the years thought and the acceptance of responsibility, the corollary of which is caution. When the time comes, the child claims his share of responsibility for which he has long been prepared by example and encouragement. He usually anticipates results and takes account of them unless he is under the impact of intense emotions.

Mutuality of trust and love between parent and child is likely to protect the child from succumbing to devastating emotions at the expense of self-realization or the higher purposes of his existence. The fact that parents treasure him and respect him for himself and not as a tool for their own purposes is bound to promote self-respect. Having become self-contained by such trust and love he can yield with total abandon to emotions without fear of sacrifice of the purpose of self-realization. If he is in opposition to his parents but believes in their integrity, and has learned the permissive and patient approach, he can postpone decisions until, with the passing of time, they are convinced of the validity of the younger person's judgment in reference to living his own life. The offspring of a family who did not use the deterring approach, however, still is heir to the human frailty and some failure is inevitable.

But his companions, raised under menace, will not be equally able to do so. Education has not equipped them with sufficient self-assurance and the conviction that it is worth overcoming impulses which are unacceptable in view of one's essential goals. Cowed or hostile and aggressive, they tend to act out rather than master undesirable impulses. Their behavior can be expected to be dependent and reactive, not self-determined.

## The Child's Own World

By the very laws of evolution and by the fact that the child is an entity at every stage of development, he lives in a world of his own. He fulfils purposes of his own in the present, though the various phases of completeness in adulthood are anticipated. Once the state of self-awareness is reached, the future man or woman grasps the meaning of educational advice in terms of his present stage of understanding. He buries the seed that the adult passes on to him for fruition in its proper time. This seed is rejected if the child is in a state of overt or covert antagonism against the adult. He cannot accept the future which is represented by the world of the adult under these circumstances.

By the fact of his rapid growth the child lives in a realm of transitory meanings and values. At all stages preceding adolescence, these are sensed rather than consciously appraised. This is one reason why he lacks the time, the concepts, and documentary media for developing a positive method of explaining and defending his own world.[4]

Only the artist and the poet, by means of the documentary media of the adult can capture some of the indefinable fragrance of childhood dreams. They "carry us away" by conveying the indescribable and reviving those great moments of serenity when a child ponders, muses, and plays within his own unconfined universe in total oblivion of the adult and his world.

Happy the child whose habitat and whose parents' moderation were favorable to such fruitful and irreplacable extraterritoriality! Resorting to temporary oblivion of the world around is of immeasurable value for finding one's self and for the recovery of self-affirmation and pride. In his unequal struggle, like a Lilliputian in a giant's world, the child may be compelled to compromise and to conform at times, whatever the magnanimity of the adult. That a child will come to resent his own lack of valor as well as the educator's power to defeat and deprive him of his pride is an almost inevitable consequence.

Adult appreciation and praise, coming at such a moment may tend to promote awareness and intensification of sensed vexation. The child will possibly feel that he does not deserve recognition because of his resentment and guilt feelings. The rift may gain an unnecessary momentum if a vicious circle develops between inappropriate and sensitive responses by the child and reproaches by the adult for the child's refusal to accept kindness. Praise for yielding will have to be dispensed with particular tact, lest a sensitive child misinterpret it as a vindictive or at least ungenerous stress laid upon the adult's victory.

## David and Goliath

An educational program which needs support by punishment, particularly corporal punishment, does not stress the fundamental human equality of child and adult; thus it underscores differences of age and experience in an ungenerous way.

Nature has outfitted the child with grace and attractiveness, suggesting, it seems, that adults conform educational methods to the size, shape, and stage of maturation of the youthful denizen. Self-centered adults, disregarding the child's physical frailty, may cause him to become violently defensive about his status. This status becomes a total liability if credit is not given to its assets in childlike charm, assets of which the child remains totally unaware unless it is gleaned from the approving glances of the adult.

Nor is the juvenile lightweight fully aware of the discrepancies in physical vigor. When physically attacked by the heavyweight adult or otherwise punished by steamroller procedures originating from the arsenal of the giant adult, he may bravely, unwisely, and disrespectfully take the challenge. Although he will soon learn to understand and do better, two opposite warring camps may become well established, the one owning all the powerful and forged weapons, the other able only to become a constant nuisance with his guerrilla tactics and the fight from ambush with weapons of chance. Who will incur the more serious defeat depends on the individual case, in particular on the resourcefulness of the child which the adult may not have taken into consideration. But one factor seems undeniable: The adult fighting with weapons which are not good or equal will lose face and he is bound to be embarrassed by it. Nor will he have impressed upon the child a mature and dignified image of man. The grown-up usually knows this, hard as he may try to repress his awareness of it or to rationalize his behavior. Moreover, the adult has not shown a great deal of foresight. He is more likely to find himself lost in turmoil which he did not intend to create. He assumed that he was dealing with a malleable substance and foresaw falsely that it would become increasingly manageable by his imposing educational procedure. He did not anticipate a defiant fighter or even less an obdurate enemy from a far-off camp. Nor would such a development have been the child's choice had he been free to decide.

### Permissiveness Used by a Child

The child needs guidance and basically desires it. When used with patience, availing itself of the child's own resources which increase by infinitesimal steps, guidance represents comfort and support and offers optimal opportunities for the unfolding of the child's potentialities. Any child appreciates leisure for self-realization. The adult who uses with discretion his superior position to provide moments of relief from pressure, can usually count on the child's joyful co-operation. First the child learns that he can lean on the understanding adult, then rely on him and later consult him, particularly if the adult, tactfully adjusts to the changing needs of the growing youngster.

Children thus raised by the peaceful method of *permissive guidance,* not only identify themselves with the adult and try to emulate him but at a surprisingly early age, they try to verify the validity of the principle of positive permissiveness by discussing it.

Ray was not privileged to have any education but had spent a few months in day-care in the Educational Therapy Center. He was a tough, rough, and sturdy thirteen-year-old boy, referred by the State Welfare Department for treatment. In spite of his borderline mental capacity and in spite of total illiteracy, Ray had leadership ability; however, because of his antisocial record of long standing one could look upon his future role in society only with serious concern.

Ray was one of twelve children of chance born to his mother. She was utterly improvident. Her children had to find their own food as soon as they stood on their feet. Ray felt extremely privileged because he knew his father and he spun an unending series of happy illusions around him. Actually the father was a rag picker who recognized his paternity, but did not provide for the boy. In Ray's mind his father was an independent businessman with two employees. His sense of dimensions was so poorly developed that, to demonstrate the importance of the father's business, he sized it up as twice as large as a box of playing blocks.

Actually, the standards of both parents were such that he was ashamed to have anybody see them. In individual therapy, he always spoke well of his mother and of his genuine fondness for her. However, Ray could be observed to confess his concern about his mother to another child whom he knew to have lived under a similar pressure. In the group, he might remind the children of their privilege as a ward of the Center. If they knew, as he did, what it meant to be one of the many children born to his mother from her "thirty-six husbands," thirty-six being his word for innumerable, and to be hungry all the time, they would not cause trouble.

When we first met Ray, he was an extremely unkempt child who had a panicky fright of taking a bath. He constantly had all fingers in his mouth. His behavior was furtive. When he was supposed to come to the psychiatrist's office, he would stay for a moment near the door and suddenly be gone or else sit astride the window sill and, in sudden anxiety, try to escape to another window, looking longingly over the wall for escape. Then came a period when he would settle down in the psychiatrist's office. But he needed a particular shelter. Withdrawn under a table, cuddled up in an embryonic position, he would have all five fingers in his mouth, the other hand around his genitals, relying upon his own body for every comfort, protection and libido satisfaction. Regression was total, but it revealed the beginning of a relationship. Though still most insecure, he knew he could find his particular shelter in the psychiatrist's room. He could relax in comfort and let her know, though mutely, how he felt. The communication was then still negativistic. (This term is not meant to imply that Ray was schizophrenic.) For his own benefit and comfort and in order to put the psychiatrist in her place, it disclosed his self-sufficiency and his total reliance on himself.

Other children were afraid of Ray because of his touchiness and constant readiness to fight violently. It was not long, however, before the boy began to identify with the Center and to assume positive leadership, displaying tact and mannerliness as well as self-denial in a most surprising way. One day Sammy Boone, a new child who was as "savage" as Ray had once been, and even more irrational, began his treatment. In his anxiety Sammy ran to the porch roof outside the psychiatrist's office. Within seconds Ray, climbing up on the porch columns, was at his side. The psychiatrist, who was not unmindful of Ray's rough ways only weeks ago, was wavering in what attitude she should take to prevent a fight on the roof top, when she heard Ray talking sweetly to the boy. "You are going to hurt yourself" he said, putting his arm around him and gently carrying him inside the room. Then he knelt down before him, the younger and smaller boy, and told him: "Now, you stay here, you'll find out she's a sweet lady." Following this recommendation, he left the room.

Ray spontaneously and resourcefully adopted the permissive method which apparently had convinced the once bewildered child who but recently had thought of an adult only as one who pursued him as necessary prey. His new insight he used most effectively on his symbolic younger sibling and on his younger actual siblings at home. Ray's behavior was deeply impressive. It was a complete reversal from all of his former primitive attitudes. His old stock of experience in climbing to escape from the "cop" was suddenly at the service of a positive and social purpose. He gave the first evidence that a development which long ago was arrested at the level of mere interjectional language now was advanced to the extent that it was under control of syntax, so that even in a compelling situation and under pressure of a bewildering density of thought and feeling, he could capture his thought in one short sentence highly expressive in its simplicity. Ray understood the newcomer, he knew how he felt and how unwarranted was his anxiety. He felt comfortable enough to remember and to encompass in his experience the terrors of the past and the relief of the present day. Therefore, he could speak to his likeness of yesterday, implying from his own present vantage point that Sam would not want to hurt himself. He could convince him by a dramatic performance why life is worth being saved and being lived. By a gentle and embracing gesture he restored the composure of the distressed, the torn-asunder little man. He invited and fondly welcomed him. He showed a brotherly concern, generously helping him to avoid unnecessary suffering, which Ray himself had endured. He displayed the willingness to share what he loved and trusted most. His trust was most obviously demonstrated when he left the source of replenishment and comfort unafraid of rivalry. He also showed that a little male hero can grow up under gentle training and stand on his own feet in proper time. Moreover, Ray told us by his behavior: "you can take care of this small helpless kid. I am brave now; you need not worry about me at this time. I learned the world is full of people like you, if I know where and how to find them. Some of them are right here in this house." At a later date the staunchness of his faith was put to trial: he lost his foster home and had to be returned to the study unit of the industrial school where all placements are decided. The welfare worker informed the psychiatrist with apparent good faith that they expected a better home to be found. In spite of intense despair over the loss of the foster mother's commitment to him, Ray consented to return to the study unit and trust the psychiatrist. No home was made available, but Ray still continued to confide in the therapist and came for treatment regularly. The promised but not actual placement was repeatedly discussed but that it was the therapist who had deceived him never occurred to him. He trusted her and he was realistic enough to take into account the limitations of her realm of action.

Ray repeatedly expressed interest in helping his younger siblings. There is every reason to assume that rather than gang leadership, he will show leadership of the fraternal or paternal kind and within his radius of action.

## The Punitive Needs of the Child

All children suffer from guilt feelings. Whatever their problem and whatever their overt behavior, they elaborate their inner conflict and their specific defenses.

Hostile defenses often do not represent sheer defiance but, in addition to being a manifestation of anxiety, they are awkward ways in which the child deals with the sense of unworthiness. Callousness, flightiness, cynicism, or stubborn aggressiveness may mask his despondency and shame. Acting out is only a specific dynamic form of expressing despair. As long as the child has not recovered, we may assume that he is but contrite and not yet ready to gain relief by reform. He may want relief as a grant to him, or he may be more sensitive and feel that he should not expect help in his undeserving condition. This may be expressed ambivalently by new undoing or by provoking a rejecting attitude from the adult.

The need for punishment is great when regrets or repentance are incomplete, and the subject wants to keep the door open for new motives for digression. This places the educator or therapist in the dilemma, either to satisfy the child's needs for punishment or to ignore his asking for it.

When we punish the disturbed child, we allow ourselves to become involved with an unending struggle between the child and his conscience. Punishing him, we may confirm the guilt feelings he is fostering or contrariwise help him to appease his conscience.

Punishment, in his eyes, may equalize the scales of justice, but it dulls his sense of responsibility. Inasmuch as punishment is a need, it is longed for. Its painful aspects, however, may upset the desired solace and the scales again will be unbalanced, but in the opposite direction. New resentment is likely to have been aroused. At this stage, the child is not yet beyond bargaining. He wants to get it over with at low cost. Punishment, being no pure comfort, is resented and the child attacks not to solicit punishment but to inflict it. This ever renewed challenge by the child enslaves the adult who is at the mercy of the child's wantonness or his obsession and thus the child is deprived of adult leadership and support. The effects are grave. Deep-seated anger and the barriers of hatred tower between the grown and the growing person.

If, however, the adult can take the challenge in his stride, the child is bound to register the fact that these defensive mechanisms fail to provoke the desired reactions. More adequate behavioral attitudes then are likely to develop. With such an educational policy the adult is the one who holds the reins in guiding the youngster who in turn loses his false sense of power.

When the provoking behavior is aimed at obtaining some form of attention, ignoring undesirable behavior discourages it. Punishment, on the contrary, may encourage it. Frustration of the specific need for punishment and resulting anxiety may be prevented, if needed attention precedes provocations.

It is of fundamental importance to forestall wooing for attention, or in other words love, by perverted means. The danger is very real indeed since punishment has a double connotation, relief through incurred pain and love-hate for inflicted discomfort.

## Child and Adult Community

The ways of the child and the adult will meet when the youngster learns the complexity of things, when he learns that partial inadequacy is the inevitable condition of all men. Their ways will also meet when the adult on the other hand remembers that whatever distance he may have covered, he too remains in the condition of the child unable to penetrate the intricacies of a world which forever exceeds him and forever evades his grasp.

If those terms of equality are the basis for the child's confidence, the adult might say to him, "Come along, I burned my fingers at this stove, you better watch it. If you believe me, you will forego the anticipated pleasure of touching it and avoid pain. If you have to try, you will experience what you do not anticipate. You will have to decide later if the price paid for concrete experience was worth it. Whichever way you choose, you will find out that experience and maturation are at the price of pain or denial." This attitude of the adult bears testimony that he has learned to acknowledge the limitations of his effectiveness, and has lost the undue anxiousness to intervene. He will be resigned, without sensing defeat, that the younger one must learn himself about the boundaries that confine him. The adult's fears of letting the child pay the painful price of certain experience may cause the child to doubt the infallibility of the adult's convictions and thus dare to question the value of maturation.

Obvious and excessive pity for the child shows that the adult is still sorry for past and painful experience of his own and that the fruit that grows from the seed of sorrow is not worth its price. It shows that the adult is still greatly in fear of adversity and struggle.

Allen once told us that the intense trouble he gave his mother may be to her advantage rather than to her detriment. His own suffering was intense and his insight profound. He was the gifted son of an intellectual family. There was a fifteen-year discrepancy in age between the parents who were, according to all evidence, very congenial. They had fallen in love at first sight, but courtship was extended for two years. Allen, their only child, was born after three years of marriage.

Both parents had been subjected to strict educational principles and the first years of Allen's education were spent under an equally strict regime. The father actually fell victim to his education which was authoritarian to the point of preventing him from choosing his vocation. This, in the father's mind, excluded him forever from equality with the privileged and austere status of his father, Allen's grandfather, to which he had gained access only through the back door, by business associations with his father's professional colleagues. When the father's advancement, at the turn of the fifth decade of life, finally disrupted these contacts, Allen's father suffered from repeated depressive stages and subjected himself to shock therapy. His twelfth shock treatment resulted in his death.

The father's disease and treatment had diverted much of his mother's attention from Allen from his sixth to his ninth year. He competed with the father by means of his own symptoms and his own depression. Although of bright normal ability, he was a poor learner and poor reader from the onset and resisted school attendance. However, his problem of non–co-operation began in nursery school; there is every reason to believe that stern educational controls determined the negativistic and obsessional elements of his pathological responses.

We met Allen and his mother after "ten years of trouble and concentrated difficulties" following the father's death. Allen was sixteen years of age. After the father's death strict methods were first continued. The son was sent to a military school, later to a religious school of high standing but extremely austere in its approach. From nursery school on, because of an obstinate refusal to co-operate, Allen had been expelled more or less diplomatically.

The mother was a gracious, most articulate woman of great refinement of feeling, deeply religious in a generous and broad-minded way. At the time she approached us for assistance she had become anguished and cornered to the extreme, and was totally at a loss to control her son. He held her tied by an alternating course of defiant lack of cooperation and short stages of sweetnesss.

Before summarizing briefly the dynamics of Allen's case we should mention some emotional traumata he had incurred. The suicide of his roommate Allen Johns, by hanging, he witnessed from a distance; forewarned by his absence, he suspected some ominous happening. The boy had threatened repeatedly to end his life. Allen ran to open the sling, but the emergency squad's attempt to bring Johns back to life failed. Allen suffered from serious guilt feelings. He had participated in the mockery, with which the students of the religious institution had covered up their own anxiety, aroused by the suicidal threats of Johns. The fact that they shared the same first name increased Allen's anxiety.

Another close friend and daily companion of Allen's died suddenly in a car accident on an evening which, by chance, our patient had failed to spend in his company. The three sudden deaths had imbued him with a sense of life's utter futility and at least two of them, Johns' and the father's, left him with profound guilt feelings.

Allen was extremely ambivalent toward his parents. He identified himself intensely with the father as his way of reaching as well as escaping the mother, who herself seemed to have an adoration for her departed husband. This made Allen's task of living difficult and abstract. The glorified man could not be emulated, and there was no human ideal image with its encouraging and heartwarming influence to impose limitations, no one for closeness and enjoyment. Nor was there opportunity to dissolve the resentment of the father who had deprived him of his mother. Allen, at the age of sixteen, therefore insisted on retaining the father and clung to the period when he was alive. He refused, as obstinately as he could, to be more than a nine-year-old. The father though dead for years, still was sensed as present, similar to a phantom-limb unchanged in its former condition and function. This was death within life. But death was also sought beyond life.

Allen's relationship to the mother was equally complex. He still used to join her in her bed at the age of fourteen and up to almost sixteen years of age, symbolically in her absence. The mother's continued adoration for the father was resented. It imposed upon Allen an inordinate competition as well as a task for emulation which absolutely exceeded his strength. The mother's devotion to the father had taken too much of her attention from Allen during the father's illness, and it continued to do so after his death.

Competition with the idealized father was impossible; but Allen *was able* to compete with him and emulate him as he recalled him—depressed, obsessive, imbued with a sense of futility and irrational in his morbid preoccupations. By these means he could retain his mother's attention and cause her at least as much concern as had the father. It was a means of reminding her of the father as he actually was and whose real traits she denied to herself.

Allen also had to be convinced that the mother herself did not meet the requirements she established. It would have meant to him that she exposed him to the exaction of emulating an ideal, the father, that exceeded her own strength. But this strength of hers was all he had for support in the reality of life. To test her qualifications as the representative and the ideal image of the parent, which in his terms meant to bear one's fate whether by enduring life or death, she had to excel her son in the capacity for endurance. This was possibly his meaning of doing his mother a favor by worrying her.

As long as she was anguished she could not be the master of a son who identified himself with the dead father. If she were elected to be truly his mother, she had to consent to going through any test imposed and not dread it. Thus, to use the poet's words with a modified meaning:

> And to irrigate my desert
> I shall cause oceans of suffering
> To spring from your lids
> I am the wound and the knife
> I am the blow and the cheek
> I am the limbs and the wheel
> And the victim and the henchman.

Whether we deplore the painful way in which Allen attempted to extricate himself from the unacceptability of his condition or whether we share his view that most painful experiences might be optimal opportunities, the fact seems incontestable that, at the period we are referring to, he had no choice but to be his own and his mother's henchman and thus to continue the revolt against the father. Though his behavior seeking to educate his mother was not acceptable, his mother seemed to understand his condition and to accept the lesson when she said: "If Allen comes out of this, he will have made me a woman."

That is what actually occurred due to her profound understanding, her redeeming availability and her unshakable consistency in applying the permissive method. Her apparent immunity relieved excessive guilt feelings, which had they been held, would have made approach and return prohibitive.

Of course, Allen himself was inflicting punishment and not without success. However punishment as inflicted by him does not coincide with the terms as used in the preceding discussion. Rather, the punishment inflicted by Allen was his only way of surviving. Death, as the father, had to be included as the protector in his dangerous community with the mother and the identification with his father's pathology as the only way he knew of the painful way to be loved and tended to exclusively. The mother as a component part of his pathology could not be excluded from suffering.

As the awareness of universal inadequacy resolves the child's problem of isolation from the adult group, it tends to solve his problem with his own age group. No longer does he need to gang up with them for fear of the conceited adult's regimen, nor has he to deny it and depreciate it in self-defense. In a world of universal limitation, jealousy of his contemporaries is out of place because he loses his wrong conception that he alone fails to live up to the expectations of the adults and thereby loses their love.

Thus the whole idea of punishment is obsolete in a truly contemporary society. Not that the community has not to protect itself, but to use retributive punishment is merely entering into a vicious circle. It is a negative procedure whereas true, purposeful permissiveness, as it shall be understood here, represents a positive progressive procedure in favor of human equality.

## The Essence of Permissiveness

Permissiveness is understood here to be an educational and therapeutic avoiding of immediate and impulsive responses to hostile challenges. It delays reaction to the symptom and insists on a persistent, motivated and versatile attitude, based on four main pillars: (*a*) human empathy, (*b*) skilful observation and understanding of the disturbed behavior, in particular of the dynamics of emotional pathology, (*c*) respect of the rhythm of the patient's development, and (*d*) his tendencies of recovery in view of anticipated goals (self-realization).

To an uninitiated observer this may appear to be a passive and condoning attitude. However, the apparent passivity or delay of immediate responses to individual manifestations is motivated by the educator's appraisal of these momentary manifestations in light of a longitudinal life perspective. He therefore adjusts his responses to the underlying meaning of the overt behavior and relates his expectations to the child's actual capacity to fulfil them. A permissive educator, were he at all tempted to threaten or punish, for the sake of the child and the educational pursuit, would not want to expose himself to the defeat resulting from a vain threat. The educator who uses the permissive method should be well grounded in its general principles. He does not then lose his own direction, when, in order to find where the child actually is, he has to find his way through childhood's green pastures as well as its dismal swamps, and keep off the rigid highway which the more conventional are prone to use. When the adult can brave the child's unchartered routes, his gain of strength and experience thereby is realized by the child. The child will admire such an educator and feel supported by the certainty that, with fortitude and understanding, he will steer him to security. It will not be long before the adult's chartered waters will also be the child's, who will find on their surfaces as well as in their depths, vast opportunities for exploring the world without and within.

In view of his convictions, the permissive educator does not lose sight of the ultimate goal of education, which is the self-realization of the person. Far from insisting on the here-and-now solutions in preconceived terms, the educator or therapist envisions a multitude of ways, and is willing to let the child feel free to explore and discover rewarding paths of his own. The enchantment connected with adventure and at times with its success, is likely to stimulate new positive endeavors and ever increasing enjoyment of and devotion to the adult who is close enough to the child's world not to discourage it. The child's investment of trust in the adult is an abstract attitude which promotes other positive abstract attitudes. The child who questions the adult and talks to him learns to evaluate alternative solutions which in turn implies delay of action, the testing and anticipating of reality factors by inner control rather than by impulsive action or random trial and error.

Education by intimidation and punishment, on the contrary, is characterized by too much concreteness and therefore narrowness. The educator is intrigued by and responds to the symptoms at hand. The total situation of the child as well as the educational design is ignored, or the impulsive means employed are used belatedly as a justification of method. Such an educator has no patience to delay impulsive responses and work on long-term gratification derived from a completed task. Indoctrinating rather than education of a bewildered child results. The child fearfully shrouds the fact that he does not understand what is going on, and he conceals his anger while losing his path to security and orientation.

Similarly, education that uses threat as a deterrent is not based on well-conceived principles. The educator's inability to cope by himself with the deeper educational tasks or problems at hand is revealed when he summons Daddy, the police, or the court. Anxiety-provoking phantoms or obscure forces have to be invoked to frighten the small offender, in that way increasing irrational behavior. The mother who regrets her impulsive behavior shortly afterwards usually does not carry out the threat except to bring forth an irate Daddy at the end of a day's struggle for existence. Lasting anxiety has been brought about for the child. He finds support neither from a helpless and vindictive mother, nor from an upset father, be he punishing, indifferent and condoning, or resentful of his role as a punitive agent. The child then feels tension between two frustrated parents. He senses that he caused it and withdraws, deeply troubled and guilty, into himself, only to find with bitterness that there is peace nowhere.

The parents themselves are distressed by a sense of inadequacy and guilt. All too frequently they project themselves and pour over the child an interminable stream of criticism and reproach. The resulting chronic discomfort interferes with the proper conditions for growth, and repeated sessions of scolding are thus needed to shift blame to the child for the parents' failure.

Certain educational approaches may find the educator unprepared. Failure, however, need not lead to guilt feelings, nor should sound principles be sacrificed just because their application does not succeed in all cases. The very essence of the human condition is its imperfection, the corollary of which is man's admirable and perennial striving for perfection. Satisfaction is achieved in pursuit and anticipation of a perfect action which, however, eludes man. We need not particularly incriminate either ourselves or the child or the well-considered method. With such an attitude, error as well as success are opportunities for ever renewed and modified attempts which are assisted by the rewarding or disappointing experience. This is productive. It braces one to meet constructively the challenge that life holds in store. It is a firmament of infinite radii whose ultimate extents can never be reached, but which can be approximated only step by step. Such a view of the human condition is affirmative despite a full awareness of human limitations. It remains optimistic and confident.

Neither success nor failure is wholly attributable to us as individuals. At best we are allowed to make a contribution. This is our limited area of influence to which we humbly refer our responsibility. It must compete with a universe of concurrent and adverse influences which no approach, penetrating as it might be, can completely overcome. Similarly, our own contributions are influenced by such innumerable, intricate, and complex forces as are represented by our present state of knowledge and experience, sufferings and maturation. Awareness of the limitations inherent to human nature is likely to cure the educator's excessive zeal to punish. It rather suggests an observant and studious attitude co-existent with a tender watchfulness that encourages the child's natural growth. Such an attitude is essentially preventive and usually precludes the need for corrective measures.

## The Working of Permissiveness

A child who has not been coerced into submission, but who is convinced by example and valid arguments properly presented at his level of maturation, enjoys at an early age the liberating experience of freely consenting and co-operating, with a corresponding sense of worthiness. As a result of the permissive approach in the Educational Therapy Center, manifestations such as permanent pouting, nagging, attacking and accusing other children and adults, yield to more pleasant and co-operative attitudes. Good spirits and laughter, unheard previously, reveal to the therapeutic team that the effects of the child's past suffering and frustration are being overcome. He is able at this time to "pick the day which is in bloom." He newly rejoices to be a human on equal terms with his fellow men. A "virtuous" circle, to replace a "vicious" one, develops from delight in contributing to the sense of achievement and merit. Some children overflow with love and good will. In others, firmness of attitude and wholesome self-assuredness contrast with former apathy and inertia.

We attribute to the permissiveness in our initial interviews the high percentage of co-operation, from the beginning, by children from whom one would expect it least. Their apparent hostility, their withdrawal, and their depression are eased as soon as the children feel that their humanity is recognized, and many a child will feel encouraged to the point that he or she will then shoulder his responsibility for the venture into treatment.

Education by intimidation expects both too little and too much. It fails to promote growth and maturation of the personality or the quest for autonomous principles of conduct as well as the courage to stand for one's convictions. It expects too much on the other hand where sufficient knowledge and experience must precede the ability to account for one's actions. Punishment is so often administered before the child understands its significance and at an age when even explanations of the reasons for punishment are premature. Bewildering shame and embarrassment are then the consequences. The child takes for granted that he is in the wrong without a real understanding of the reasons for it.

To be safe, a threatened child feels that he has to bow to force. Reasoning and insight are stunted by this paralyzing menace. In order to alleviate the resulting insecurity the child automatically tends to lean on others. Under the imminent impact of the cudgel, the educator's human traits seem to him remote and likely to disappear altogether. Having no ideal image with which to compare him, untrained in judging him and in penetrating beyond his menacing exterior, and longing for help and closeness, the child will follow anyone. Since he is cowed, frustrated, and resentful, he is apt to search membership in the hostile camp.

The educator who trains by threat and force is himself under the scourge. As the basis of every threat there is anxiety and fear of isolation. Children raised under the scourge of menace, whatever shape it assumes, sense the educator's uncertainty. Not able to understand, they in turn react by anxiety and isolation. Thus the very action which the threat is supposed to enforce yields doubtful results. The complex of painful and ungratifying emotions, as well as the anxiety in dealing with the rationalized rather than with the understood needs of the child are manifested by excessive supervision, rules and threats, carried out in anger and exasperation. Violent punishment will alternate with bribes and threats. Confusion hurries the child on to the dark woods of emotional disturbance where he loses his way altogether.

The story of Eli may serve as an example. He was referred by the State Welfare Department for staying out late and being "incorrigible." The slender and refined appearance of this thirteen-year-old boy was matched by bashfulness and soft-spoken manners. Conspicuously expressive eyes dominated the otherwise immobile face. With these he wooed for love. He could be observed using his innate charm to entice people regardless of their sex or age. His mood was depressed and only rarely did a mischievous smile flash over his face when he glanced at other boys.

Eli was the adopted son of an elderly couple, the man in his seventies and the woman in her sixties. He had been wanted as the comfort of his adoptive parents and was to be the beneficiary of their savings. The child was constantly "whipped" into providing the expected gratitude. The mother's observed anxiousness was similar to that of an investor who is uncertain whether his capital is well placed. The child was coerced into saving the "titles" by a threat held constantly over his head that his misbehavior might contribute to the father's death and thereby lose him all the economic and material glamour of his present position.

The mother was extremely thin and withered under carefully applied rejuvenating make-up. A retired professional woman, she was intensely aggressive, agitated, and domineering. The couple lived in comfortable circumstances due mainly to her efficiency. They provided the child amply with what money could buy. The mother, intelligent but narrow, was proud of her standing in the church and the community, and when she came to the Clinic, she tried to impress us by dressy clothes and an overwhelming quantity of costume jewelry.

Our impression of her corroborated all previous reports that she was anxious to shape Eli into a perfect child and thereby to achieve improved standing in the community. She talked and directed Eli incessantly and corrected him about trivial points of behavior. She mentioned in his presence that she probably had spoiled him and had been too generous with gifts. Almost in the same breath she explained how much the parents needed him, and she encouraged him to make every effort toward being a good boy to hasten his early return home.

Disregard of Eli's deeper needs was noticeable during her personal interview. From home she wrote regularly, laying emphasis persistently on the father's old age and weak condition and his constant longing for and worries about the child. Our contact from the child's home community denied the alleged seriousness of the father's condition of health. The mother visited Eli too often, constantly interfering with the successful transference of emotions to his foster mother. By reminding him incessantly of his obligations, thereby creating guilt feelings and a sense of inadequacy, she held him bridled to his original adoptive home.

Eli soon entered into a mutually dependent relationship with another of our wards, Bobby, an extremely aggressive and voluble boy. Bobby was at that time on the verge of recovery, but was still struggling with an urge to steal. He too was refined looking and well-mannered. He needed a friend to follow and support him on stealing sprees. In a transitional stage he would exclaim, "I wish someone would break me of stealing." His stealing was compensatory. He took weapons—guns and "BB" rifles. Eli needed and admired Bob for his daring and for prowess in which he could participate as an observer. Eli's need was to know only that the other possessed them. Since the meaning of Eli's apparent indifference in ownership was not understood by Bob, he did not feel encouraged to steal by the decent and gentle fellow and was assisted in giving up a habit which seemed a liability rather than an asset in their important new relationship. In scrutinizing his relationship to Bob, Eli gave us important clues from his own previous associations, regarding the problems of his upbringing and his "incorrigibility."

Uninformed about his status as an adopted child, Eli had nevertheless begun to doubt that he was his parents' natural offspring, sensing his instrumental and conditional role. He mentioned this role in reference to house cleaning. Comfortably seated in armchairs his parents would observe him, remonstrating constantly. He felt that he had to perform the role of a daughter and a "maid." At times, each parent wanted him for a different purpose at the same time. His own needs were mainly discounted except for material things like clothes. What the parents considered failure was punished by a strictly imposed denial of privileges. Everything was strictly organized and timed. Relaxation was allowed only after fulfilment of the tasks of the daily schedule.

Trying to escape the rigors of his perfectionistic home and to assert himself elsewhere as an independent person and a young boy, he joined a group of youngsters who played at calling distance from his home. Too timid to select his friends, he moved, groping from one group to the next. At first he would return home when called, but soon he ignored his mother's summons. What held him, however, was not pleasure, but an obsession to be liberated and to gain a sense of adequacy. Eli would start out from home perfectly dressed, with his timid, girlish manner totally ignorant of the other boys' ways and devoid of resources for coping with them.

Eli's princely clothes proved a liability. The boys' playground was improvised and unsupervised, a vast, impenetrable area of brambles and thistles. He went there in quest of community, disinterested exchange, and in hopes of an intense self-expression. He was shockingly initiated. The boys threw him on the prickly ground, sat on him, tramped and beat him, ruining and soiling the fancy clothes. But the struggle released his constriction. It represented a violent, emotional outlet and relief from pent-up hostility. The relation became more rewarding than the one at his monotonous home where he felt himself to be an inert tool of narrow people with shallow feelings. Inadequacy with the boys seemed not total. They too used him, inciting him to be "nice" and then assailing him again. But he also sensed that he could be a source of pleasure and he in turn had become dependent on the release of tension which their attack unleashed. The admission of being loser and victim coincided with battle weariness and exhaustion and was therefore not altogether unsatisfying. The punishment was desired, because he had persisted in being bad and resentful at home. The need for punishment outlasted, however, the wearing away of the emotional exacerbation and was manifested by a chronically depressed mood. Actually, his acting out with the boys gradually became an unredeeming and unrelieving obsession, intensifying his sense of inadequacy in reference to his parents as well as the juvenile group.

Eli's story reveals how the use of coercion and threat as an educational tool leads to unwholesome dependent relationships. Intimidation resulting from constant pressure and the sense of impending menace inhibit reasoning. The urgent need for safe harbor causes a tendency to cling to any object, without choice. However, the hostility inherent in any dependent condition kindles a tendency for associations antagonistic to the traumatic source and the acting out of the impulses which have been interfered with by that source. Emotional stress and the absence of spontaneity provide attitudes fraught with delinquent potentials.

## The Heart of the Matter

The negative consequences of punishing attitudes are even more profound than the preceding illustrations make them appear. A very young child begins to walk and move around. At this wonderful stage of man's arising, immense horizons suddenly unfold before him, grasped primarily by eyesight. He is stimulated to extend the radius of his new world further and further, advancing toward objects or reaching out to them with his liberated upper extremity. The discoverer is born and the experimenter verifies by touch observations made by sight. Not so long ago, he may have tried to attain by touch the sounds that emanated from the mother's mouth. The young explorer discovers a universe of pleasant experiences because his sensory and cognitive curiosity is gratified. But he also meets with unpleasant experiences and on his level of maturation he becomes acquainted with the nature of obstacles and with his own limitations. He begins to be cautious and more and more circumspect in exploring a world of which he feels he is no longer an omnipotent agent. The world has become divided into pleasant and unpleasant experiences which call for orientation and choice. The sense of failure or inadequacy derived from slightly unpleasant encounters with obstacles embarrass him, but he tends to conceal embarrassment and to deal with them by himself. Thus he restores his sense of competence, which again liberates him for new ventures in exploration. Only when badly hurt will he scream or run for support. Comforted, he will again proceed with exploring and manipulating the world. If by anxious and stringent methods, the mother interferes with this natural and, on the whole, peaceful process of humanization of the child, the result will be fundamentally different.

The child, let us imagine, reaches out for something unsuitable and harmful to him. The mother, rather than eliminate it from his view and gently distracting him, that is, instead of providing a substitution, angrily slaps him and tries to tell him that the thing is not for him. This should be conveyed to him in a pleasant tone, whether seriously or playfully, depending on the importance of the taboo. The friendly mother is more likely to inspire trust. Opposition and obstinacy of a child at ease is not likely to be aroused. His peaceful world is full of challenges. He need not cling to the one at hand. He can allow himself to be distracted. The irritable mother, on the other hand, unless she atrophies the child's curiosity altogether, may have promoted rather than deterred the child's desire to touch what he should leave alone. The mother's excessively irritated interference emphasizes the thing formerly devoid of any specific significance to the child. It was just one more object for exploration and enjoyment. It could easily have been forgotten and substitution would have been acceptable. The child would have remained in paradise, protected from a precocious "knowledge" that in its very "midst" harbors the viper of temptation.

In describing the three basic principles of our therapeutic attitude we have seen that it rests on the creation of an atmosphere of *acceptance, attention,* and *respect.* The therapeutic home and the permissive atmosphere that pervades this home enable the child to live and find himself in reference to human and material objects, that is, to become conscious of his existence and enjoy his title to being human. This joyful awareness of his human condition is gained in an experimental workshop within the confines of which he manifests his self in relation to its adult and youthful population. Acting out as a form of self-expression and self-assertion, is a first step in the making and strengthening of the child's personality. Acting out in the presence of respected love objects, and either feared or admired sibling figures, tends to promote an increasingly conscious form of existence which is supported by the discursive use of language within the therapeutic and educational milieu. A growing acculturation is manifested by a mounting volume and quality of verbal communication which diminishes impulsive acting. In other terms, a move is in process from impulsive to thinking manhood.

The element of observation represents loving attention, care, and protection. Knowing that he as well as his peers are watched benevolently, the child learns to watch himself. He gradually becomes the judge of his feelings. He observes and controls them. He becomes a responsible master over his behavior and is no longer merely reacting to stimuli from without which he no longer holds responsible for unconsidered attitudes. To help the child accept his educators as regulators of his conduct, the educator must seem lovable and his behavior must deserve the child's reverent attitude toward him. Tolerant of the child's inevitable weaknesses the adult educator must not expose weaknesses of his own. It follows that the therapeutic home and the child's refuge must not unfold to the child discord among those he is supposed to emulate and who should implant in him the belief in human values.

# XII

## Therapeutic Education

### Essential Aspects

Two fundamental aspects should be considered for education integrated with therapy.

First, due to the rigidity of the sick child who is able and willing to function only under reduced conditions, teachers must at first be in a position to adjust themselves to the restricted needs of their students and to ward off disturbing intrusions upon them by the outside world. The teacher's knowledge of the child's inner experience has to keep pace with the understanding, reached by the therapist, in order to shape the teacher's approach to the highest possible refinement, specificity, and precision and thus to prevent interference with therapy. Teachers and therapeutic staff have to be in constant touch. Observations of both have to be exchanged as need arises and in regularly scheduled sessions. These observations must be tied in with communications received or gained from home, foster home, or agency. In understanding the child's typical, improving or relapsed condition in terms either of the treatment process or new traumatizations, the workers will be enabled to determine whether a more expectant and permissive, a more encouraging, stimulating, or a more structured educational attitude should be taken. Change of teacher or student group may be advisable because of transference problems that cannot be worked through at this time. These will slowly take care of themselves or need to be faced again at a later period; otherwise resistance to improvement may become too intense and may also involve other children. As evident, the schedule must be flexible.

Second, the general educational approach should be based on the awareness that the neglected child did not have anyone to "listen" to him at the pre-verbal and the verbal stages of development and nobody to question at his age of the incessant "whys." He therefore must be helped to wonder again on that level and his silenced appetite for life and learning must be revived. The class atmosphere should vary, depending on whether we group together a few dependent children, who have to conquer contact with reality close to the mother figure, by scribbling, drawing, and manipulating simple materials and objects, or whether we are dealing with restless and boisterous preteen boys. In the latter case, it is of utmost importance to create an uplifting, inspiring group spirit and to promote competitive sportsmanship. Positive competitiveness is valuable for two reasons. Threat coming from siblings and anxiety create so intense an aggressive drive that it evidently cannot be and should not be suppressed; but it should be channeled as a source of productive energy. However, children, in particular immature ones, cannot be expected to strive disinterestedly for a super-personal and absolute goal. The object of their exertion at first is self-centered and relative to comparable achievement. Once the joy of accomplishment has been experienced, the way is paved for doing well for the sake of it. Achievement may not have to be supported necessarily by praise. This might stress dependency and be resented, making the child prematurely aware of the fact that he is yielding to requirements. Praise thus may promote conflict of allegiance in reference to the child's "friends." Above all, success may then be a means of gaining advantage when it might otherwise be a pillar of self-esteem to the child's growing dignity. The enjoyment of achievement should rather fit in a general atmosphere in the classroom, one of enthusiasm that comes from the adventure of a mental exploration and conquest. The child must be so challenged that life in class competes successfully with outlets for which he used to search in the street with the gang. Action and movement, physical as well as mental, are needed. Therefore learning has to be staged and dramatized. Simultaneously it makes learning and its subject a lived experience. It channels unrest into the enjoyment of expression and thought.

Under restrictive circumstances, as the ones experienced when I was the only worker of the Clinic, in its first five years of existence, when no noise could be made since our quarters were above the Public Library reading room where readers wanting quiet might be disturbed, resourcefulness was essential. Some readers took offense even of our unobtrusive presence. Motion then had to be experienced by emotions. The children then traveled with me vicariously over continents and countries represented on maps. Identification with explorers was stressed. We were always wondering what was going to happen, what was going to be found; there was excitement, danger, escape from danger, the solace of a subsiding storm, the relief of the stars' guidance or the inviting vegetation on shore. Things were offered slowly, tension mounting from suspense. The "angry sailors" were distracted by questions about the immense horizon and by some astonishing facts such as, about light traveling at miraculous speed reaching us today after a long journey from some stars, continuing since the time of the birth of Christ. A wonderful awe gleamed in the children's eyes. They were so close to the narrator that in none of them was there fear.

Early education should appeal to the romantic imagination in the child, father of the man. Nothing in our lives has real living charm that is not resonant with tunes from the playland of early childhood. The educational-therapist gives the child the opportunity to feel the experience of tactile closeness missed in his earliest days when no loving mother, moved by the miracle of his existence, hugged his little body, patted, and rocked him.

Teachers and therapist have access to the literary and musical heritage that almost any child delights in and is attuned to and for which he will be eager to abandon his former self upon his emotional liberation. That which is deeply satisfying the child will want to take with him. He will sing and recite and sense the beauty of a dream in the beat of the rain against the windowpane while he is sheltered indoors, or the enchanting silence of the falling snow as it blankets the street, in the soft gleam of the sun. All of these experiences will be tinged by a fairy tale atmosphere and the lightness of nursery rhymes. Enveloped in the gossamer cloak of poetry and dream, the child's whole outlook, even when at home, changes and not only in his most intimate and precious hours of privacy. He may find a partner in one of his siblings, or his feelings may become attuned to those human elements in the mother's existence and those "joyful hours" in her life that "have passed away." When on the other hand, the contrast has become too great between the child's new innermost experiences and his home surroundings, he will begin to talk freely and revealingly in the Clinic and he will thus help us intensify our endeavors in assisting the mother more specifically to realize his needs, or in planning for both him and her.

## The Spell of Learning

As evident, none of the children referred to the Educational Therapy Center are ready for learning, but they are at different levels of preparedness. By sheer necessity a child is invited to function at his own level. We have children who just sit or who participate erratically. As a rule they are placed in a small group, preferably with a woman teacher, and are offered an opportunity to play in a way that provides the pleasure of self-expression and achievement. The child who expresses himself by doing communicates increasingly with the one who is going to behold and appreciate his product, thus confirming the child's existence as a value. Dependency on attention, help, and praise, when wanted, is lived out. Self-assertion grows as skills in performing or "reading" the secrets of objects and shapes grow. *Four* little sticks may come together to make a house. The house becomes also a *square* with four sides and the square becomes meaningful as the sides of a house. The child may be invited to name those who carry each wall to the house, *four* children in the room or elsewhere, thus making the *four* sticks or walls come alive. If the child is very immature or regressed, his fingers may go "marching" one by one to the house, supporting body mastery by the conscious awareness of the singularity of each finger which may be named specifically in reference to the house. Subtracting might be learned by using an additional stick, giving him jokingly the name of a peer with whom the child does not get along, and by suggesting that we don't need it and by "taking it away." Playing angry with some humorous obviousness, a first form of sublimation of aggression, is promoted.

If idiosyncrasies are being revealed, the teacher must be sensitive to them and she will attempt to understand their meaning. She is being equipped for it by the sharing of all relevant therapeutic information. She should be, and usually is, prepared to avoid improper playful suggestions, those that could solicit sensitive reactions and be associated with areas of traumatic experiences. She may make observations which lead to further understanding of the child's condition. While a world of approaches are being used implying a world of meanings at the child's level, interest is motivated and evoked and the child is made to feel his growth and its further potential rather than his limitations. Hopelessness is diminished and on the way to being eliminated.

At all steps of the educational effort an integrated attempt is made to stimulate simultaneously the infantile personality in the areas of (1) body mastery, (2) mastery of perception, (3) mastery of social relations, (4) mastery of learning and memory, (5) manipulation of things, and (6) intelligence.[1] To stimulate curiosity and wonderment at any level of development or maturation is a prerequisite for helping the child question the world again.[2] The teacher must not know all the answers before the child has gained or is helped in discovering an appetite for knowledge. The teacher herself must be and appear to be inquisitive and intrigued. Thus whetting the child's appetite in an imaginative way, she must play hide and seek in the area of mental curiosity or, in other terms, help the child enjoy mental give and take. *It is in both the willingness to accept and the willingness to release knowledge that the child needs to be stimulated.* In playing a game, for instance, tinged with cheerfulness and joyful surprise the teacher helps the child relax his reluctance to taste the bitter, less pleasantly offered, food of learning, whether by experience, or directly fed to him at the adult's time and bidding and in the adult's kind of pattern, as in academic teaching.

A playful competition between teacher and child is not only acceptable to the child and permissible educationally but definitely indicated with disturbed children. The teacher asks questions in a wondering and enticing way, questioning also more or less playfully —depending on the child's mood—who is going to know. The child thus is tempted to release as it were, at his own whim, and not by coercion the important information he has to convey. There is no more reason now to withhold it.

Generosity rather than niggardliness becomes his means of self-assertion, and knowledge becomes its tool. All tools are demanding of perfection and promote it. Knowledge representing a tool promotes more sublimated goals and the means to implement their achievement. Generosity depends on an increase in quality and quantity for maintaining the flow and value of its gifts. These are representative of the child himself who tends to create them in profusion as measures of growth and supports of self-esteem. Becoming more and more independent of a source of nurture and of the need to hoard what he is at liberty to produce, the child's interest in the adult as a provider has changed. He questions as one eager to learn and be free, notwithstanding other motives. The child will look for guiding models and for objects as resource material. He will want to measure up to the persons who inspire his new life tendencies and interests. Not to discourage him, and not to cause a sense of inadequacy and the futility of trying, the teacher must be understanding enough to value the enormity of a gift which is negligible by superficial appraisal and to help the child enjoy the distance covered from which he had set out to accomplish it. She must be alert to its inherent beauty and value. If the child is alone with the teacher, standing on the podium of his first good answer, he can be stimulated pleasurably to draw on further simple resources of his own, thus learning to recall stored memory material at the time when it is needed. He thus realizes that he knows things worth telling and that he is not so "dumb" or deprived of means after all.

The child may at first refuse to make the effort or to recognize abilities which obligate him to prove himself further. He still feels too inadequate. By a friendly play with the vicissitudes in relating, childish silliness, as "my little boy is hiding that big piece of information, I'll have to look for it," making gestures of searching in space, the emotional climate may be created for the child's release of his "spasm" and of his mental hoard. It is due to his sense of utter deprivation that he has to cling to it, constricting further all of his being. Soon the borderline of knowledge is reached and the child needs help not with willingness or pleasure in recall but in clarification of dim, distant, and poorly registered perception. "I wonder if you have ever seen a tree that stayed green even in wintertime?" the teacher may ask. Perception of stored experience then is stimulated by the suggestion of something distinctive which arouses or arrests interest by the element of wonder and surprise. In a small classroom an element of speed, a tending of sinews, as it were, for a little race with answers, will keep the ball rolling, and a reluctant child may be induced to become a co-operative part of the group. The child feels the integration of his whole personality in making a joyful effort at the high level of his capacity. He feels strengthened and longs for more of this comfort.

At all stages of educational maturation the child must be approached from the center of his preoccupation or obsessions; thus a community of interest with the child is established and the teachers become acceptable and an integrative part of the child's life. Not feeling censured for his bizarre preoccupations, the child will give up undue wariness and in his desire to hold on to his "buddy" he will make inroads into that buddy's mode of thinking and feeling. Through the joy of relating, widening the range of his interests will become enjoyable and knowledge itself can fulfil the kind of gratification which whets the appetite for more. Like a wreath we shall lay around the core of the child's natural quests and enterprises academic pursuits which are regarded at first as at the sole service of these pursuits; scoring, adding, measuring, reading catalogues, figuring costs of what the child desires.

The infinity of ways by which interest in geography and history can be stimulated cannot be explored here.[3] At the time when the children were learning through dramatic adventures, discovering countries on the trails and in the wakes of the original explorers, the geographic scene became the stage of historical and social events; historical events were dramatized within their time and geographic setting.

As Columbus we set out to ask the king and queen for money in order to implement what seemed a dream. We were ardent, angry, bitter, enthusiastic. Before we set out, our means of transportation were explored. The children found out whether we needed to travel by water or land; provisions were discussed and "provided." We revolted and suffered, we yielded to the visionary who led us. We were increasingly tense with hope and exalted when we reached the clement beaches of solid land. Vegetation as a friend greeted the sailors who were tired of the unrelieved company of an arid ocean, which, however, had surprised and distracted us with its curious dolphins and flying fish.

Motivation by emotional and inspirational means, however, is never allowed to supersede fully the realistic and objective validity of knowledge. As time goes on, the exalted, inspirational motivation of knowledge will yield to a more reverent approach with an increasing appreciation of its dignity—a dignity which the child wants to respect. That he partakes of this dignity enhances him. He now wants to reach out for its offerings in the public schools which to him have now become its austere temples. They are the very schools the entrance to which he formerly shunned and forfeited. He is now eager to enter "because I have changed" and so has his view and tolerance of the world. Nurtured by the therapeutic sources of the child's change of attitude and his trust in the perfectibility of the world, knowledge itself is recognized for its realistic values. The child has explored it in his young way as a two-way bridge of communication and thus as an instrument and a help for mastering abysmal obstacles. Knowledge becomes a means of extending the self to distant shores and, for the adolescent, a promise of socioeconomic security and social expression. Children will treasure books, borrow them and one of our most deprived and disturbed patients was finally seen to embrace his books fondly with his arms, saying "I have learned to treasure them, they will help me rehabilitate all my past disgrace." At this time he was extremely ambitious in school and his behavioral adjustment was fine. He subsequently took a college entrance examination and planned to become a "dedicated" clinical psychologist. Psychology was an "outstanding" field.

The tendencies in children to satisfy their curiosity about facts and function of living and inorganic nature, as well as things of man's making, is most successfully stimulated by use of the inductive method. Since the child is devoid of experience that would stimulate his need to question why, to identify an object with itself, to compare it with others, to count, etc., it is the method he pursues spontaneously.

Unfortunately, only little use is made of this method even in the biological disciplines. At the Clinic, it is the method of choice. But our location and transportation difficulties represent a handicap. Children who have no contact with nature and who are confined to their uninspiring city homes and their environs and whose sole possible inspirations are church, movies, and television respond enthusiastically. When their only source of inductive research is the trash can or the few objects proper for manipulation which they take in the stores, teaching by induction becomes a delinquency-preventing device.

It is an inspiration to see the method work and with remarkable results. Walking or sitting in natural surroundings, the teacher can arouse curiosity by appearing curious herself. When intrigued by a plant, a flower, a crawling insect in the palm of the hand or a spider at work, when a snake or a snail in its natural habitat is *discovered*, the teacher does not have a hard time gathering the children around, and if he or she has a gift for narrative the children will delight in listening. Those who have strayed away on their own exploratory pursuits or in need of exercise will soon be told by the other children what they missed. The lively report of those who stayed around the teacher benefits both groups. The former listeners become the narrators who rehearse and lecture about their new knowledge to those whose curiosity is stimulated and to those independent explorers who on returning are prone to bring new materials for "research." In this connection, it is worth mentioning the approach of a German teacher who had met the fatherless children of war prostitutes in the rubble and taught them on the spot, using any object of their interest as the sole point of departure. Examining an old engine, for instance, as if intrigued to know whether all the pieces were at hand, he would talk *sotto voce* to himself, calling the parts by name, and manipulating them he would talk to himself as though verifying their function. All the boys around him would watch, and it was not long before they followed him, ending up in the classroom.

## Learning through Crafts

Crafts essentially link mankind in time and space. Their divisive national aspects are overcome when we are recipients of the friendly gifts of each specific culture and are capable and unafraid of integrating them without loss of our own cultural identity. All crafts were initiated in the home as true servants and representatives of civilization in its timeless as well as its changing aspects. They are most suitable teachers for children unfamiliar with a home having cultural aspects of living. They have missed the home where both sexes together adorn the cherished dwelling—the women putting to use the nimbleness of their hands, the men bringing in their "trophies" and the products that yielded to their strength and ingenuity.

In the Clinic, through their own strivings to make a contribution, the children take their place in the home and the community of all men. They sense that they are partaking in a meritorious and meaningful pursuit. Isolation is miraculously overcome. Whether serious, anxious, or smiling, whether performing with religious ardor, the child yields to the world. He may relinquish his product passively at first, too incredulous about his worthiness, the value he has to offer and the honesty of the receiver's appreciation. Later he will offer his product and through it offer himself with all the joy and will of abandon.

Initiating the children to the age-old craft of weaving, we gather them serenely around a table and give them an incentive to work in common in a purposeful activity thus learning to "collect" themselves; or, sitting on the floor, the children enjoy a timeless posture of comfort, and in this sitting for communal leisurely endeavors there is storytelling, rhyming, and singing. In general terms this is a frame for the early beginnings in the enjoyment and creation of literature, art, and music. What the children create can and should represent in principle an integral part of our sedentary culture.

Such an integrated pursuit of leisure-learning draws on perception, sensibility and sensory-motor skill. This integrated result cannot readily be accomplished by children as restless and aloof as those whom we attempt to interest in this kind of activity. Motivation might be derived initially from their compulsive needs, though tenseness, excessive seriousness, irritability, and fatigue may interfere with a concentrated effort and the completion of any project.

However, the small and awkward products which at first the child has such difficulty in "accomplishing"—in the double acceptance of the term—may serve tangible purposes in the home. Even the child who is raised under the stress of sheer necessity can conceive these. The useful object is a product of leisure activity and automatically partakes of play and luxury. The child's joy in shaping it as best he can, the choice of colors, his very effort at a self-chosen task, one not dictated by necessity, contribute to an inevitable meeting of the practical with the aesthetic purpose. Thus by love of beauty here too is conquered man's bondage to necessity. In the area of fancy and play man is royally free and his position in the universe appears to be unique. Each of his products and their arrangement in space from where it may "look back" upon its creator, reminds him of his freedom to influence the order of things.

Only with a resourceful and whimsical mind will we be really equipped to quicken the desert of the stunted young lives that surround us in the Clinic. Even the prosaic looking puny potholders the children make will be animated by poetry and liberated from the narrow utilitarian limitations and the heavy texture of cotton. The child is his own master in choosing color. It will not take too long and he can vary the pattern at will. With redeeming lightness and "kidding," once the child's responsiveness is aroused, the teacher can give the child a first inkling of the potentials of imagination inherent in a human mind and inspire a wish to explore its depth. It can be symbolized by attempts to find a new pattern for the modest little potholder. The performance fascinates without presenting excessive demands. In working on this humble product, the child fills space with what formerly failed to stimulate his own creative imagination. Only his forbidding and bleak anxiety used to be there to occupy the space from which now his product speaks to him. It also reaches those who devotedly guide him, those who behold it and those he will specifically endow with the product.

Our unassuming weaving loom can also take on the potentials of a calculating machine. In weaving up and down a great number of times, a sense of repetitive continuity is experienced and the feeling that one action is added to another of its kind. Up and down can be followed by "one, two" as the initial steps that lead to counting up to higher units. Soon the children will know how many cotton bands they need for their total product; they prepare them, planning their work before they begin it. When the children use a variety of colors for an organized pattern, they can learn to add, multiply and divide the skeins needed and learn their tables up to 36 or 72 at least. When the child is not yet ready to study systematically, he may spontaneously use his product for barter and sale. With the little potholders or rugs, hats, pocketbooks or whatever combination product they have achieved, they take their first steps on the long road to financial self-support and independence.

Their first relay is their learning readiness. They also trail ingenuously, though with equal devotion and intent on perfection, the endeavor of those great intuitive minds who create the geometry and art of an oriental rug.

Identification of the weaving children with women and men of other cultures and other periods may be achieved by the accompanying words of the teacher, spoken leisurely in a fairy tale manner, while she assists the individuals of her group with their work. Their own or the teacher's reading may be geared to coincide with the current occupation of the children and visual material is a useful resource. In an over-all review of a complex therapeutic and educational endeavor these few highlights must suffice.

## Teaching Children To Read

In the course of my observations, during the first five years of the Clinic's existence, I became increasingly aware that insight into reading difficulties presupposes a basic knowledge of some principles of spoken and written language. Mankind has devised two fundamentally different types of written language: (1) picture writing, as by the ancient Egyptians and the Chinese, and (2) sound representation, as by the Semites and the Indo-Germanic peoples.

In picture writing an individual word is represented as a whole. The present symbols are schematic simplifications of pictures of objects. Every individual word has its individual sign, and the number of signs and their complexity grows indefinitely with increasing experience and thus increasing vocabulary.[4] Each of these signs has to be taught individually and retained by pure memory. Consequently, only a privileged few can devote sufficient time to gain mastery of a sufficient number of symbols to be able to read any text. This method has proven to be a fundamental hindrance to the vitality and the dynamism of the historic Chinese culture. If the written language succeeded at all in keeping pace with the increasing knowledge, the average reader could not read the increasing number of symbols.

The alphabet writing method is an abstract procedure based on the combination and permutation of a given number of visual symbols, each of which, representing a sound, can be an element in the whole word.

Western culture is unthinkable without our writing system by permutation of characters. Gutenberg's method of printing, by means of movable type, is as it were a concrete performance inspired by the principle underlying our phonetic writing system. *Democratization and internationalization of learning is based on this ingenious principle.* With a few relatively simple rules any foreign language based on this writing system can be learned and easily read.

Every spoken word is a sequence of sounds. Thus, as an audible entity, it takes place in time. Through an instantaneous mental act it is perceived as a whole; only then do we understand what is heard. The inventors of alphabet writing of necessity have provided symbols for every sound element and thus reproduced the heard word visually. The reader has only to be familiar with the visual code of the definite and limited number of alphabetical sounds and the principles of their combination and permutation. Nothing else is needed, in particular, no further memorizing. He simply revocalizes in his mind the silent visual representation of the spoken word. Reading *skill* is achieved by habit formation, i.e., by a repetitive performance of an act which is *in principle* always the same.

In fact, writing and reading is an ever repeated re-creation of the original idea of sound writing and reading. Gutenberg simply liberated the letters and restored them to their individual mobility of which they had been deprived when cut into solid blocks of book pages up to that time.

It is true that the swift reader no longer is aware of the process of gathering or gleaning the sound from its visual code, a procedure indicated by the word *lesen* in German, *legere* in Latin, "to pick." Nor is the swift reader aware of the sequence of the collected elements in his text and the synthetic act can be brought back to consciousness only by a new analytical process as in writing and spelling. Analysis and synthesis are correlated in translating the sound into its written code and in reading and thinking or pronouncing the text. It is most noteworthy therefore that reading and writing are closely correlated. Spelling is not a parrotlike memorization but a well-understood calling out of those visual code signs of a word which represent its sounds. It does not have to be constantly practiced as a special subject, if the child is taught to express his thought and knowledge in writing from the day he begins to read.

The Gestalt Psychology[5] discovered that we read whole words and even longer units at a time. This discovery caused modern educators to introduce the word reading method by which a word is read as a whole. They unwittingly applied picture reading to our sound symbol system, depriving our flexible and scientific reading method of its superior characteristics. We regressed from Gutenberg's method to imprison again the single movable letter in an image unit.

The theory in short is that an intuitive whole is sized up back and forth against its background. Its characteristic shape is thus brought to clarity. But for taking apart these wholes, structured according to principles of discursive, not intuitive thought, we need symbols in the shape of the letters, the constructive elements of the written language. These symbols are taught, indeed, but too late. The children then use the alphabet only for analysis of the read word and not for synthesis because these educators do not take advantage of the discursive element in the thinking process and concentrate on its intuitive aspects. The analysis then loses its incentive for reconstruction of a discursive whole, and we see the children's reluctance to learn belatedly how to analyze and *comprehend* the written word by reconstruction of its letter elements.

The rules which presided over the construction of the marvelous edifice of our phonetic writing and reading system must be used also for its application. Unable to understand, the child guesses at random at times offering sounds which are not even in the words. Guessing, a trial and error procedure, is unscientific and useless. Many possible words might fit into the context. For many a word, its opposite or contradictory term might be reasonably guessed.

Not knowing how the words are rebuilt out of their sound elements and unaware of their motion in time and space, the children do not understand the importance of letter sequence. We do not have to appeal to the discrepancy in eye-hand dominance, nor should we. If the incapacity to read letters in proper sequence were inherent to mixed brain dominance, this incapacity would bespeak a serious deficiency in the child's mental integration. This is contradicted by his tendency to maintain the sequence and direction in his sentence and page reading, to quote but one relevant factor. Reading disturbances not based on improper training, like speech disturbances of the aphasic type, according to H. Head, are disturbances of symbolic thought and expression.[6] He justly declared it hopeless to explain these disorders of the higher intellectual functions by disturbances at lower physiological levels, as are the motor and sensory ones.

Appraisal of the correspondence in length of the read and spoken word is lacking when the correlation of sound and its representative written symbol are not understood. Prefixes and endings cannot be isolated from the word root unless the child learns it belatedly by special training. Most crippling is the incapacity to isolate letters which the child has improperly combined. A child who happened to read *gray* or *brown* before *gold* or *blue* might have a hard time isolating the *g* and *b* from the *r*. A child may be unable to drop the *r* in the word *thought* because he happened to read *through* before. He persists in reading *throught*. The examples could be multiplied indefinitely. *They illustrate that through the picture approach to a phonetic reading and writing system a rigidity is promoted which is a serious handicap not only to the handicapped.* The child is deprived of the versatility of the letter writing system itself as well as of the versatility promoting effect upon the reader. In not associating the sound of the spoken word with its written symbol, the child learns neither to discern consciously the sound elements and nuances of the spoken word nor to develop a discriminative articulation. Reading the whole word, children identify its visible picture with the audible Gestalt they have in mind, a child pronouncing *fireman*—"fiman," *Florida*—"Fioda," *penalty*—"penaty," *Atlantic*—"Atlanting" will not correct his pronounciation. The advantages of literacy are lost and its communicative merits on an individual and supraindividual level. Language based on a phonetic writing system tends to even out dialect differences that stand in the way of a mutual understanding between people of the same linguistic stock. The child with poor auditive language discrimination and poor articulation is in the throes of a vicious circle when not taught by the phonetic method. Anxiety enters the picture. The child feels driven to try again and again, losing control instead of gaining it. He has no clues to redirect him.

The letter gleaning method is based on a *minimum* of *memory* material. The Gestalt method resorts to a complicated and slowing process of evocation, recall, and recognition for word identification. Spelling is taught by mere rote, unsupported by any kind or degree of understanding. To assist memory, a number of sensory devices are used to promote helpful associations as tracing the letters, looking at pictures. Associations, however, are not logically necessary relations. They are non-essential to our phonetic writing system. Pictures offered in the books for regular associations are not compelling and not a reliable aid. Associations being subjective and depending on memory may be quite erratic. A playful, creative child might make his own unexpected associations and drop them again. The dull child fails to make any at all.

Prepositions, conjunctions, pronouns and even adjectives and adverbs abstracted from their nouns and verbs, as well as abstract
nouns cannot be properly pictured. But prepositions, conjunctions,
pronouns and certain adverbs are essential for the syntactical structure
of language. These are the very words over which children will stum-
ble, they will wildly guess anything: and, said, then, they, when, why,
who, there, for, from, in, on. These are the words which make
children despair of reading by themselves. They represent road blocks
at every step. They are the words without which an understanding
of any text is utterly impossible. The child therefore is completely
discouraged from reading and practicing reading.

If the child cannot build up new words, what he does not recognize
he does not read. "I have not learned that word yet." Consequently
reading does not increase his vocabulary, unless he is very active
and intelligent. For example, a child might come across the word
*rickshaw*, with which he is unfamiliar. He cannot "get" it at all. This
is one of the reasons for the widespread reading difficulties up to college level.

When the child has learned to associate the visible word, the Gestalt
with its meaning, he will have difficulties with synonyms and with
those words which are synonyms in his mind. Look and see, house
and home, iron and steel, wolf and fox will be confused. Such a confusion will interfere further with the making of rules for phonetic
grouping and the establishing of a system of classification. Such a
system of classification, however, is a necessity because we have to
reduce the task of memorizing an endless number of words into a
restricted number of word classes.

Familiarity with the sound character of the alphabet is inevitable
and belatedly introduced as it were by the back door.

But what happens now that the child is not used to letter reading?
He will take the letter for a word: *d* will be duck; *m* will be mother;
*c* will be car. These are three examples of failures by three children of
different ages, intelligence, sex, and race, out of a multitude of such
failures: *bread* was read "bearduck"; *once* was read "on-car"; *man* was
read "mother an."

The reading text has to be adjusted to the necessary support of rote
memory by innumerable repetitions of the words the child is in the
process of learning. Learning to read and the acquisition of knowledge

is pathetically retarded. The child and his growth, whether mental, emotional, or in reference to ideal formation, are not promoted beyond their existing status, nor is the enjoyment, as time goes on, of advanced cultural pursuits. These finally are resented and its core of devotees may be ostracized. In countries where the phonetic method is generally used, children are seen satisfying their curiosity by reading the printed word anywhere. This behavior is evidence that the phonetic method is a fit tool for an early independence in learning to read, contrary to the claims of the word reading method. The children taught by that method depend for a prolonged time on the adult for "giving" them individually the new words to be learned. A certain ratio of them is acquired per chapter and book. In reading as it were "instinctively" the sound reader gains by constant practice, great speed, and proficiency at an early age. The word reader here is whipped into speed and subjected to "drilling."

Since this method depends on pleasurable associations the schoolbooks are full of colorful pictures. This charming attraction however has disadvantages when, as is frequently the case, the pictures, used as clues for words and the meaning of the text, become a vain promise. When the picture is consulted rather than the text, the first influence is exercised over the present generation to become "skimmers" of illustrated magazines rather than readers of books.

## Principles and Illustration of Our Procedure

The method favored at the Center is based on an understanding that the spoken language destined to reach the human companion through the auditory sense has been translated for use *by vision*. Symbols had to be created which, when seen, would evoke sound.

Twenty-six symbols were found to be sufficient to represent all the sounds of language if shifted around in certain definite ways.

Of these twenty-six symbols or letters, five and sometimes a sixth are the real sounding, musical ones, the really voiced ones. The rest cannot sound without them and in fact stop the sound. This is demonstrated as well as the function of the consonant to shorten the vowels which, as called in the alphabet, are long and explained, with words as "in, an, am, at, as." A funny rhyme then is made up and read line by line as it is produced. Curiosity is aroused about what is going to happen. The first rhyme consists almost exclusively of short words containing *an* and *at*.

This method has the following purposes:

1. It makes the combination of this vowel with these consonants *automatic* by repeated practice in a meaningful and humorous little text. These and other combinations acquired subsequently will be read as units in the future, regardless of their position in a word.

2. The child will learn to *classify* by the discovery of similarities without having to learn dull and meaningless word series. Classification is suggested by the rhyme and quite naturally out of the reading material and with double emphasis on sound and visual feature. If word series are established, it is done, so to say, by induction from the text already read, as a means of recognizing the words in their similarities and dissimilarities and to be assured that they are read also outside the rhymed context and not memorized. The child is encouraged to make short sentences with these words.

3. In further rhymes or self-made texts the child will learn new words where consonants precede and follow these units. Each consonant is learned when it is needed; it is called by its name and by the sound function *be* or *b*, etc. The child is not overburdened. Familiarity can be established with each consonant. It is endowed with specific qualities and the road to discriminative capacity is paved. This is a great help to the schizophrenic child, more so than to the mentally slow one. The schizophrenic child is not necessarily devoid of discriminative ability but rather overwhelmed by the problem of selection. Although the child will not be taught to build up words letter by letter in their sequence, the definite feeling for the importance of letter sequence is established by emphasis on prefixing or suffixing letters to the core of the word.

4. The child is not overwhelmed by an increasing number of words, none of which seems to have any phonetic relation with the other. A secure basis is created by the establishment of simple sound combinations which are gradually enlarged by new rhymes related to the established ones. We worked on cats, rats, bats in all sorts of funny contexts that permitted the natural association with other words of that class. It followed a lad and his dad and situations that permitted the use of bad and sad and mad meaningfully in a quick rhyme of two beats. A little man with a watering can followed and

so on. By a geometric progression the sound combinations and words thus mastered will increase very rapidly. Rapid progress can be achieved because it is built on understanding, careful grading of difficulties, and on the establishment of automatic responses through repetition of sensory-motor action which is in principle always the same.

5. The diphthongs which are supposed to make reading of the English language so difficult and unpredictable for the child reader are brought down to a common denominator: the children know that short objects are lengthened by addition of another similar object to the first one. Consonants having shortened all our vowels in words, we are in need of lengthening some of them again. The first vowel is lengthened by a second vowel. For all vowels it can be the silent *e* placed behind the consonant that shortened that main vowel or a vowel placed right behind this main vowel. It is explained that certain vowels associate (keep company, marry) with others as *a* with *i*, *e* with *e*, and *e* with *a*; the apparent contradiction of read (pres.) and read (past and past participle) is explained etymologically and well understood even by the slow child. Other apparent inconsistencies are explained similarly as they occur and only relatively few words remain which the child has to take for granted. These are but a sampling of the clues that help the child understand what he is doing and that he is not exposed to a disconcerting randomness with which he cannot cope.

Furthermore the children were made to understand why man, since the dawn of history, had felt the need to write. Reading and writing became a necessary attribute to any man whether primitive or not. Picturesque stories were told of primitive men in the mountains who wanted to warn their brethren of dangers and means of circumventing them. After letting the children find out by questioning to which senses we appeal in using the spoken word and to which when we write, the miracle of man's ingenuity was depicted in finding ways to speak to vision. The need for such communication then was explored at the level of the children's understanding. Once the principle of talking to vision was understood, thus the object of translating sounds, we set out to sound out and depict sounds and found out that there were but a few which we sang to emphasize their vocal quality. All others were noises made to stop the sound. There again

I illustrated vividly why stopping the sound was necessary for the shaping of words and the holding of attention and how shortened sounds needed to be lengthened. Reading then was taught by rhyming, writing down the rhymes, and reading them.

The children read their own as well as the "foreign" text and were asked what goes on in the story. In discussing the children's interpretation encouragingly or in questioning them for further elaboration, understanding was deepened but not explored to excess. Thus the light touch of the approach was maintained. The children learned to express themselves increasingly by writing. They wrote down their own experiences, their own adventures, their wishes, feelings, and fictional stories. Then they read them to the adult or the group. The merit and mutuality of communication were fully explored. Spelling was not memorized but treated as a process of unfolding in slow motion each sound element of a word and, in writing it down, pinning it to the page for review or for "speaking to the eye." When printed books were used, they were chosen for their inspirational and literary value on the child's level of mental, emotional development and capacity for achievement. Serious lags such as their unfamiliarity with nursery rhymes, fairy tales, classic heroic adventures and explorations were caught up with to the profound delight of the children. "Oh, I love that!"

The children may unfold to life, asking to be read to with eyes on the book, spontaneous dramatizations may be inspired by it, they may write poetry, recite some of it, use phrases inspired by such knowledge. They learn to give by reading spontaneously in return for the beautiful gift of being read to. Certain children will reverse the roles, simultaneously revealing family interaction. Assuming the part of a domineering parent, a child may bid you harshly to sit down and declare: "*I* am reading now, not you." The child may simply want to becloud shamefully a romantic note in his relationship to the teacher. Soon we shall meet the child on his very own newly discovered grounds when we ask about the woundrous stars and the marvel of the traveling light or miracles close by that have intrigued him in his lonely observations and destructive experimentations. These highlights illustrate shortly the method in education upheld through the years at the Educational Therapy Center.

### The Ideal Education of Teachers

A few short remarks about the education of teachers seem in order here. We believe that it is not sufficient to have the future teacher travel on the straight and narrow path of teacher training in the skills of education and subject matter. For no one can find within himself all those subtle qualities that give meaning to the world. Unless touched by certain intangibles of experience, they will not inspire the well child, and even less the sick one. Teachers have not really been initiated in their vocation unless in their own childhood they have tried reverently to become familiar with the legacy of mankind's great geniuses. They must have been uplifted by their inciting vision, a vision that they then carried as the guarded and sacred flame into their court of innermost reverence. The most "unnecessary," the least "useful" preoccupations, those least determined by goals of "efficiency" and the crowding of an undifferentiated quantity of work or knowledge into a set number of college years will prove to be and remain the most valid experience.

Fortunate is the teacher who listens to the accents of the poets not only in his mother tongue and its familiar spirit, but who has also adopted in mind and heart other tongues and has become familiar with their literary heritage. (We must not refrain from alluding to the role of music and the arts in contributing to an elevation of spirit and to an inspired outlook on every sight, humble or squalid as it might seem to a naked eye.) A colorful spectrum of experience may shine for the imaginative teacher at the end of a dark and isolating passage from which she may kindle the child's emotional life. Teachers who have developed their sensitivity and intuition by uplifting intercourse with the geniuses of mankind are prone indeed to approach a frozen, repetitive, and monotonous child with more versatility and resourcefulness than the ones who have learned to classify or categorize behavior. Those privileged by a professional training that permits a deeper insight into the child's individual problems and the subjective uniqueness of his experience may be less likely merely to observe him, disarmed, from a distance.

A mute child who communicates to the extent of pulling blocks from a container and handing them to you with a coarse gesture until fatigued, and out of the little control that he has, might be thanked with varying intonations as fitting as an identical refrain to the changing moods of the verses of a poem. The back and forth motion between the child and his worker, the vocal emphasis on repetition which implies an increase of the number of acts, the diversification and intensification promoted by the concomitant modulation of voice and movement encourage a living relationship with its surprises and thrills. Thus is achieved a fundamental change in quality of the formerly automatic and monotonous repetitive behavior of the child. While improvement may not be obvious, in view of the absence of emotional display, it can be registered by the child's willingness to come to his sessions and his tendency to pick up where he and his worker left off in his last sessions. His memory has been supported by positive, though unexpressed feelings, since his interest has been sustained for a whole week. Mothers who co-operate with the treatment report that their children pursue similar play activities with them and on the whole show more spontaneity.

The nascent emotions not yet expressed by a smile, laughter, or jubilation or even by the acceptance of physical closeness are, however, intense enough for the child, not used to feeling, for him to become fatigued. In one case of such a child smiling, jubilation, and dancing actually occurred under similar circumstances, and an ever growing, spontaneous and amazed exploration of objects, their motion and functions. Indulgence in purposeful action which engages the child's dormant mental capacity contributes to the exhaustion. The child may give up his serious pursuit and his striving for adequacy manifested in the handling of the blocks or trying to empty or fill a container; he may instead run to the door, banging against it or playing helplessly with the doorknob. He may be ambivalent about the tendency to stay for play or leave for relaxation and rest. He still strives for adequacy, however, on a qualitatively lower level by the achievement of noise and the display of the power to be mischievous. The teacher may support the tiring and slightly excited child's tendency to carry on his elementary struggle for existence and survival by a tuneful rhythmic "bing, bang, bong." This can have a soothing effect and due to the rhythm, a definiteness which structures a situation which may tend to become dissociated because of the child's fatigue. The child may be helped to set the door ajar for relief from any sense of constraint while each time the refrain "bing, bang, bong," is repeated and the word "o-pen" is scanned with emphasis on the tuneful vowel. Thus the child is helped to associate liberation from constraint with words and the pleasant and civilized "bing, bang, bong" with the opening of the door. By this procedure repetition has become relaxing, pleasurable, and educational, in other words, meaningful.

The example, viewed superficially, may not seem very convincing. Any mother may proceed likewise without previous training. But this would not disprove our thesis. Everyone knows that love may be enough to guide the maternal instinct in the proper direction and arouse the mother's sensitivity to a child's needs. When maternal love and "tact" are associated with an innate, though untrained intelligence, we see outstanding educational results. But there remains an essential difference between the average person who "plays the piano" and the one who has been trained in music and masters the instrument of his choice—let us only mention the number of overtones the master can elicit from the keyboard. Of two teachers who have chosen their profession because of vocation, the one who has undergone the influence of great literature and music will be more prone to touch the unresponsive keyboard of the disturbed child's dormant sensibility and to elicit its "harmonics."

To be and become attuned to a susceptible and withdrawn child, we believe an education in the humanities to be a prerequisite. While the great masters differ by their command of the form which they lend to their medium, the sick and the genius have in common contact with origins to which we have to return in order to find the common ground that belongs to all men.

Moreover, teachers who have not been misled by their own education to stop wondering will continue to live in awe and admiration of the mysteries of the cosmos like Archimedes or Newton, like the great thinkers, like Milton or the Psalmist. They will not allow the deadly dust of routine to collect on their teaching. With them the children proceed to knowledge as though responding to the wisdom of a fable from which they derive their own moral.

In treatment it may become apparent that in their contact with the teachers the children have been stimulated to wonder and meditate, to draw conclusions of their own and begin to fuse the islands of knowledge to an increasingly coherent terrain from which the mist begins to rise.

Through beauty and the arts the child is associated by admiration with great models. The distance at which they live creates awe and admiration, longing, not fear. Admiration raises the youngster's self-concept. The capacity to admire must be stimulated, as it were, from the fringes by heroic models whose real or legendary uniqueness are brought forth down through the literary heritage of mankind. Through and with admiration the child gives in to the master and imbues himself with the spirit and quality of his work. Due to the enjoyment of the work through responsiveness to its charm and the understanding of its meaning—whatever the degree of consummation of such an enjoyment—the artist and his audience belong together and are complementary parts of one whole. Being therefore of the noblest stock, because a human being, the child senses his dignity as an audience and feels justified in his existence, a fact that does not escape his observer. As a self-respecting human being he necessarily respects in the other person the image of man. Disappointment in everyday reality cannot alter this image in principle. What is true in the adult's contact with youth can and must also be reversed. The strength remains behind in the primal sympathy which, having been, must ever be. The self-concept that underlies this attitude is promoted by teachers who understand the importance of their task because they are imbued with the respect for the fiery thornbush that burns or can be kindled to flame in any man.

At the frequent staff meetings at the Center the children's pathological dynamics are discussed and teaching techniques are explored. Our methodology is by no means confined to a rigidly set pattern. We hold the conviction that within the limits of the spirit of the place each teacher's individual resourcefulness should be respected because only in his autonomous way can he genuinely express himself and be of greatest help to the hurt child.

A fine example of a joint effort of teachers and psychologists is our sports program. The children play competitive games with other schools and institutions in and out of town. They derive pride from it, a sense of belonging, and a great deal of joy that carries over to more demanding pursuits. From the teachers' initiative has sprung our most recent endeavor "the father-son days." Most enhancing is the success they obtained from a community endeavor with parents and foster parents in our parent-teachers group. The parents' and foster-parents' identification with the Clinic and their proud work with and for it has been happily stirred and is being enjoyed by them as well as by the staff.

# XIII

*General Introduction to Therapy*

*Preparing the "Untreatable" Child for Therapy*

Because the main purpose of the Eduactional Therapy Center is the psychiatric treatment of very deprived children (previously considered untreatable as ambulatory patients in child guidance clinics), we use an approach that is particularly geared to assist such children. They are isolated not only in the family but also in the community, whether because they belong to a minority or subculture or because they belong to an underprivileged and ostracized socioeconomic group, within the predominant (in numbers) population, within a given geographic area.[1] *One of the advantages of the method to be expounded is that it shelters the child at the height of his emotional, socioeconomic and cultural solitude, but does not isolate him completely, in an institution. He remains in the community.* Thus, while he still feels he is in "enemy territory," he is free to withdraw or make tentative sallies for liberation, in accordance with his actual and changing needs, his growing confidence in himself or in his community environment. In other words, he can continue to function socially.

Although theoretically any emotionally disturbed child of school age qualifies for our services, in actuality, and partially because of imposed segregation, we have dedicated our efforts, particularly in day-care, to those children most in need of them—the socioeconomically most underprivileged Negro children. It is in this group that our method has been tested and it is this group which has kept alive and enhanced our faith in the human potential of all mankind.

Necessarily the method of treatment had to be adapted to those elements in the situation and behavior of the child-patient which had originally disqualified him for ambulatory therapy as practiced in the classic child guidance clinic. This meant that a concrete approach had to be added to the usual symbolic relationship in which the child accepts the therapeutic framework of a room representing the child's world and a therapist who represents all of his loved ones as well as the objects of his troubled human relationships.

*To children who are as deprived as the ones with whom we are concerned, psychotherapy proper is a necessary but not a sufficient measure.* Equally necessary is a milieu that at least reduces actual traumatization, especially those traumata that recurred constantly in their lives. To make a proper way of living possible and inappropriate reactions unnecessary, however, does not constitute a therapeutic milieu. An emotionally disturbed child obviously does not only react to actual stress but is disturbed in his development by chronic traumatization with which he has interacted all of his life. A therapeutic milieu then, in our definition is *a substitutional home* that responds to the child's actual and legitimate needs in addition to offering him an opportunity for the repair or correction of damage caused by past omission or active destruction. In other words, a therapeutic milieu has to be more than a shelter, a hearth, the source of adequate food or the presence of a family-sized number of accepting people displaying a fundamentally harmonious way of dealing with each other. The mutuality of relationships of the Clinic population as well as the child's present gratification, cannot make up for basic gratification missed in the past or the pangs of physical and emotional starvation, of vexation and punishment—all of these will have left disfiguring scars which hinder the acceptance of the gratification offered. Because these scars are so deep these children were formerly called "incorrigible" by other agencies and deprived of proper psychological assistance. They remained unresponsive to the "care" provided for them, whether with naïve devotion or resentful cruelty. We have demonstrated, through our method of educational therapy in a symbolic milieu, that such "incorrigibles" can be successfully treated.

Previously, the most forbidding hindrances to the usual approach in the child guidance clinic were considered to be: poor symbolic function (i.e., the inability to think abstractly) and the tendency to project. Indeed if a child clings stubbornly to his natural mother as the only one expected and permitted to reward him or to repair the damage done to him, past or present, he may display a complex of attitudes by which he prevents or resists relief. If his attitude is not altogether negativistic, he may at least reveal in its most elementary manifestations a profound ambivalence between an unquenchable thirst for life and the fear of unbearable new deceptions, which paralyze any advance toward a truly rewarding source of restoration. In other words, for the sake of life and gratification, the child turns to his mother's suffocating embrace. An irreconcilable and deadly resentment for what he has not received is simultaneously expressed by an unalterable expectancy that the deceptive and necessarily elusive past be belatedly restored. He stubbornly demands to remain the nurturing mother's helpless child, thus penalizing both. Trying to satisfy his hunger from a source that is spent and incapable of or obstinately refusing to make a contribution of his own toward accepting other gratifications, he vainly overlooks the vanity of his attitude and the inevitability of further frustration. At the same time not one of his least needs is to use his mother as a source and motivation for projection. Insisting, against all hope, upon her alone as a wellspring of positive gratification, he is sure to lay open her obvious failure and thus have justification in accusing her of a world of misery in which he has become actively involved and for which he hates and despises himself.

It is interesting to note that the defense which produces this complex of attitudes is a premature "specialization" which, in extreme cases, narrows down the child's radius of perception to the focus of a special obsessive interest—the mother.

The mere acceptance of rewarding and liberating maternal functions of a substitutional or symbolic nature and even more the reaching out for them on his own is thus prevented. Since normal maternal functions include training and education, it is evident that such a child is unable to perceive their merits, never having experienced these functions through his mother. Fascinated by the gorgonic features of the one who gave him life, the child actually is paralyzed. Clearly he is not able to test maternal potentials elsewhere or explore promise for the future. In less desperate cases, he may tend to consider what causes might obtain for him a desirable effect. In extreme cases, fear keeps the child grafted to what causes fear. We are here dealing with the child who, whatever the case may be, is too weary to talk, too involved to reason, too tied up with the past to perceive or desire a foothold in the present from which to rise to a future which, because of his condition, he is unable even to imagine.

Since these children are prepared neither for psychotherapy nor for immediate acceptance of answers to their well-understood needs in milieu therapy, we are faced with the necessity of searching for preparatory steps to lead us out of the dilemma.

How can we achieve *the goal of treatment* which, in general terms, means providing motivations for a new and uplifting relationship with the world? We need to replace the child's deadlocked and stifling interaction with the mother and his confinement behind the inflexible bars of the narrow and thwarted world of his thwarting experience with liberation to enjoy love and life. The basic attainment must be the overcoming by the child of his compulsive desire for ubiquitous rejection and the resulting motive for retaliation by punitive (of the mother) withdrawal or aggression. Unreserved dedication to each child individually must, therefore, characterize our endeavor. Each staff member must remain personally unaffected by the children's provocations which are solicitations for rejection, particularly in the early phases of treatment when these solicitations are intense. These are the usual manifestations of frustration resulting from unanswered hostile aggression, the main form of human communication that the children have hitherto experienced. Insight into the motives and the meaning of the overt behavior will foster and support the staff member's patience and equanimity.

Since every aggression is necessarily temporarily exhausted when physical and emotional resources are spent, the child is susceptible, at the ebb tide of his aggressiveness, to a discreet and gentle expression of affection, care, and understanding. There is danger, however, during early treatment, that the child will bring about these orgies of violence in order to arrive at these moments of exhaustion that will lead to the soothing closeness of the therapist or teacher. But the soothing closeness also begets the child's love. He wants the comfort extended and benefits by its intensification and differentiation which results, as by now he has experienced, in an interchange of words. He soon has pleasant memories to which he wants to return and for which he will not need the dramatic overture of a temper tantrum or an aggressive explosion. The intensive and steady flame of the hearth will take the place of the devastating flare of hatred. Those who are not ready for words, even though they are approaching adolescence, may communicate by rocking or putting their fingers in their mouths, conveying the meaning of how incessant the frustration had been and how comforting it is to have their wants met.

At this time the child no longer clings stubbornly to the hope that the damage done him will be repaired by his blood kin or the ones who inflicted it, but accepts another person as the representative fulfilment of a previously denied function. He shows that he consents —by the apparent regression (which is his tool for maturation)—to a symbolic re-enactment of what should or could have taken place in the past. Such an acceptance implies at least an instinctive feeling and intuitive insight into the concrete fact that the clock cannot be set back. This form of implied "realism" usually comes at the beginning of treatment proper. It bespeaks the child's acceptance of treatment or even his consent to it, using the stranger as an object for ungratified love and longing. One source of the child's instinctive or intuitive appraisal of the fact that the clock cannot be set back is the number of sensations connected with the chronology of his development. If, for example, on account of his regressive trends, a child feels unable to walk, or if he resists doing so, in a great number of instances he will still be aware of his locomotor ability. His paralysis, which is a "crying" means of communicating objections to the vicissitudes of his condition, may not be a persistent symptom; its appearance or disappearance will depend on the circumstance and the presence or absence of relevant people or therapeutic figures.

Serious as his suffering and his general emotional condition might be, grave as might be their manifestations, they do not necessarily mean that he is resigned to them. On the contrary, they might indicate that he has preserved the capacity to appeal for love, charity, and care. An ultimate trust in a favorable response may be expressed by regression rather than by aggression. Whatever else the meaning of his symptoms, they are an alarm rung to awaken the conscience of those whom he wants to touch because he is not unfamiliar with pangs of remorse and is longing for relief.

The child who obviously disarms himself by regression appeals for help. To arouse the "rescuer" in his educator and with it renewed awareness of the absence in the child's past of the adults' responsibility and loving kindness, the child senses he has to incur the vital risk of extreme exposure by a lurid regression.

In a do-or-die behavior, he forces himself either upon the specific object of his longing or upon the world as a whole. By bold exhibition of suffering he is able to explore elements of dedication in those to whom he now appeals for help.

Such behavior reveals that not all hope is lost and that time does not stand still. "Frozen" into the refusal to live and let live are elements in the past that remain a wellspring, however sparse, for dreams of restoration in the future. These small sentiments may be detached pieces of remembered devotion, perhaps single moments in the child-mother relationship where, in an emergency, compassion was aroused. Children will keep concealed such reminiscences like embers under the ashes, and such moments of a mother-child closeness, experienced by both or as the child's solitary secret, may encourage him to fall back on the "past," so there may be "recovery" and thus a "future." Because of the rare and precious moments of the past and the alluring dreams of the future, there is fear of separation and a reluctance to desert the love object. Here, to avoid both isolation and desertion, the child needs help. He reveals it by his symptoms which tie him to life and to people. If the child's dramatic appeal (his regression) for help is heard and answered, the need for the symptom, as the child's means of revealing himself is overcome. The self-inflicted "disarmament" represents a painful limitation. It inhibits the child's outpouring of joy that springs from a gratified condition. The happy child jumps, he does not cripple himself by a regression to helpless infancy.

The hurt child's *chronic* symptom is fostered to induce a permanent solicitude. The ever repeated deprivation and the chronic self-limitation create a state of suffering which results in the loss of faith in parental love. The symptom remains, but its function is gradually altered. No longer an appeal for love, no longer a tie with life and the future, it becomes, when not heeded, a weapon to punish and drag into paralysis and annihilation the ones who mutilated his existence. (It is thus that the patient becomes the ruler of the family.[2])

In therapy the anxious child who is not yet devoid of hope can and will grasp any suitable or, at times, unsuitable life belt with which to be pulled back or, with support, swim back to shore. The hopeless, the withdrawn or angrily, isolated child will at first not be or want to be aware of the helper's hand.

For him, therefore, to be therapeutic the obvious *milieu* has to be endowed with intangibles, to be discussed later.³ They are, to the damaged child, appropriate pretexts for an investment in a milieu of unique complexity, as well as simplicity, which makes it for him a home. While equipped to offer the discernible elements needed for growth, these elements must be fitted into an embracing whole for him which constitutes and thus precedes the existence of its parts, as will be explained in the following chapters. Originally, the day-care milieu represents an atmosphere for the mere existence of the most timorous, withdrawn, and imperceptive child to which he can yield and awake at his own pace.

Slowly parental figures emerge from the situation, which, in a few serious cases, is holding the child in a state of suspension between mere existence and an increasingly discerning engagement with life. Sensitively responsive as well as intelligently perceptive to the child's changing needs and to his awareness of the milieu and its population, the therapist slowly pervades his existence. Through rising levels of interaction a form of kinship is established which, we have very good reason to believe, can never be fully uprooted, whatever decision at the crossroads of later developments the patient will make. Even his so-called failure may prove to have elements of success.

Those in need of protection from stimulation and those most defenseless in the face of aggression, may be harbored with one teacher in the most sheltered place which will become living room, dining room,⁴ and kitchen progressively, and the days go by. The one-room abode allows the highly vulnerable child to feel more secure. He can overlook the world around and espie dangers he still fears might assail him. The place soon becomes most familiar and doubly safe as a place of habitual security appropriate for the discovery of the self and the outside world. Other children love to be in the group, though withdrawn, sensing only that there are people beside themselves although they barely seem actually to perceive them.

Attention is constantly required to absorb constructively the restlessness of the newcomers in order to give opportunity for an attachment to a first object and to the milieu. Aggression by a number of other children usually is chronic and insidious. For a long time this will best be coped with in terms of these children's anxieties, frustrations, and insecurity in reference to their primary object relations and the resulting sibling rivalry. Thereby we protect the aggressor as well as the "attacked" child, who may possibly promote aggression, to prove the world hostile and "mean."

In blocking off emotional growth, or in tending to promote regression or restore the past; a child cannot ever attain or reproduce an exact replica of parental responses and attitudes. Above all the child cannot remember early frustrations as such and what troubles him is registered as a more or less vague discomfort and later as condensations and elaborations of actual memories confused with other people's stories. If this child is to be helped, whether by foster home placement or by treatment or both, he has to accept something completely new and unique of its kind, something that is only similar to his old and painful relationship in that it is a model of what the relationship should be or should have been, namely an answer to needs, the opposite of what was painfully experienced or else rewards he knows or believes others are having. Even the most deeply withdrawn schizophrenic child will have to learn a "new" organismic preverbal language, translating the sensory-motor communication which is going on between him and the "new" nurse into a new and positive object relationship. The new relationship must be started at a level below the child's present state. Change requires arousal of stimulation and growth but also calls for the relinquishing of experience no longer relevant. The "new" mother is not only providing what can be expected from any good mother, but she should be able to accomplish the whole act of curative nursing through an extended period of time. The foster child who remembers his own mother, will go through a period of ambivalent and taciturn tolerance. Later on, he may declare "I *call her* my mama," implicitly saying what she is not, and can never be, his mother. Though his original home may have reduced him to a mere existence, he may pine for it poutingly for some time. He will carry a long while the sense of being intolerable to others which he gained in his original abode. We may see for instance such a child moving rigidly, lending his body passively to the surrounding world, noncommittal in his verbal responses, unsmiling, obviously a stranger to the world, hampered in shaping a gift that he feels will not be well received and intimidated in his ardor to give obviously in a state of indecision whether to yield or resist.

The child who can free himself from paralyzing bitterness toward what *is* and can test what *could be* is ready for the usual therapeutic approach. When reasonable safeguards are given, this child will venture to experiment with the parent-child relationship in all of its aspects. This is an indication of his potentialities, of his own spontaneous and even creative abilities in shaping and mastering his life and his world, whether by imaginative action or thought. The Educational Therapy Center has only a few children enrolled in its day-care program who are in such a relatively favorable condition. The complex therapeutic endeavor must attempt literally to lift the forbidding block of resentment that discourages and paralyzes the children's surviving vital tendencies. Unprejudiced observation of the child's spontaneous behavior in children's groups has to be made in an attempt to understand the meaning concealed or revealed by overt behavior.

Through the years we have been struck by the difference between the children's behavior in individual therapy, in group psychotherapy, and in the general day-care group. In the latter two circumstances, the children feel more exposed, therefore they live and react more impulsively, acting out violently. In the presence of the therapist, however, self-awareness is awakened, springing from the child's intense need for acceptance. At the time of initial contact and at the earliest stages of treatment, so basic for a child's acceptance of therapy, the difference of behavior necessarily is most obvious, but it may persist through an extended period of time.

## Choosing a Therapist

In the *initial interview*, the child reveals almost invariably his ambivalent relationship to the mother, that is, his dependency upon her and longing for gratification as well as his simultaneous violent hostility and urge to promote her rejection. Initial interviews represent as many variations on the basic theme of ambivalence in reference to the mother as there are children. They are played on the reduced scale of a few fundamental behavioral elements; sullenness, weary aloofness, or covert hostility held in check in order not to lose control of an unfamiliar and feared situation which the interview represents to this child. Distrust is evidenced by near-muteness, lack of spontaneity, the reducing of answers to a minimum, at times impatience when confronted with questions. Usually, however, the interview moves on to some apparent warmth and closeness. With the exception of some recalcitrant adolescent boys and girls, the children gradually show a readiness to reveal, in confidence, what troubles them, making either a peripheral or central approach to their problems. Adolescent boys may burst out with bitter and sarcastic accusations. They may shout at you as though holding, not without good reason, the whole world responsible for their plight. Others show their need for power over an actually unconquerable world by being shrewd and deceptive in their communications and thus enjoying their triumph.

However, when the children leave the session a great number of them show a desire to return. The wish to return to the interviewing therapist may persist for a long time, despite a satisfactory and progressively successful therapeutic relationship to another Clinic worker. The persistence in holding on to and wishing to repeat the first satisfactory experience finally recedes. In the meantime, protecting the child from feeling that alluring people are unresponsive to him, we must find ways of gratifying his desire that do not affect his therapeutic relationship to another worker.

Usually co-operation is requested of and obtained from the children in the choice of their therapist. The children may have been deeply impressed by the first person they encountered in the Clinic, that is, the psychologist who tested them, or they may express the capacity to relate more readily to a person of their own or the opposite sex, their own or another race. Others show indifference to the choice of their therapist, because of general aloofness, submissiveness, or indiscriminate acceptance of anybody. Children who impress us as incapable of deciding between alternatives or who cannot remain in suspense for a few days do not have the opportunity of choosing a therapist.

We may usually assume that those children whose co-operation is appealed to vainly fail to co-operate not so much because they are confused or blocked, but because they feel hurt. This is true in particular of those who show indifference to the suggested choice. Having invested so much in the initial interview, to the point of confiding and yielding secrets, they are sensitive to the awareness that they have prompted so relevant a commitment on the part of the interviewer who does not choose to be their therapist. Such painful traumatization of a sensitive child must be anticipated. The need for assigning such a child to another staff member must either be avoided in particular cases or explained convincingly as an expression of a common and concerned endeavor of the *family of workers*, one of a variety of ways to impart the feeling of being fully accepted.

The engagement of the child's co-operation in the choice of his therapist is as much an exploratory measure as an initial therapeutic step. One can only appeal to children who would not be overburdened and confused by making decisions, assuming or sharing responsibilities, or in a state of such emergencies that an appraisal by the child of his situation is out of the question.

However, asking the child to make the choice of a therapist is indicated in all those cases where an emotional response can be obtained although it is a minimal and cautious one. Soliciting the child's help in making a choice that from his point of view would be the most desirable is a first test of his willingness to consent to treatment rather than yield to it passively. It is the first step in a positive co-operation, the first constructive use made by his minimal surviving social potentials. It is an indication of his interviewer's respect for him as an individual, of his recognition as an equal: this involves also the recognition of his legitimate needs. Few, if any, of the children treated in our day-care program have ever experienced such consideration. Thus the acceptance of them as human beings, expressed by the engagement of their collaboration in the choice of their therapist, immediately may spell to them acceptance and inclusion. In spite of being stunned or possibly because of it, some children give in to the charm, sustained subsequently by their experience of an essentially co-operative attitude in the whole therapeutic milieu. Others struggle with their doubts and the incapacity to believe in the "miracle." The interviewer, in his subsequent role as the child's therapist, or as the Clinic director, may have to be put to the test. Instead of being encouraged by the tokens of respect of their human equality, certain children become cautious or suspicious. Feeling hopelessly unworthy, they may suspect that the interviewer's attitude represents a trap, a bribe to "keep" them "from misbehaving" or, in other words, acting out. They may suspect a trap that commits them not to be or to remain who they are. They may consider the therapist naïve and in total error about their actual characters. However, since this specific matter, the choice of a therapist, comes at the end of the initial interview, the error of burdening an unsuitable child with the responsibility of contributing to the choice of his therapist can practically be discounted. Sufficient basic knowledge about him is known at that time and success depends largely on the emotional atmosphere that can be built through the session. Even the youngster's suspicion may be a matter for scrutiny. It may relieve him of the fear that antagonistic feelings, prone to silence their relationship, have to stand between him and his interviewer.

We may have a good opportunity at this time for clarifying the youngster's human status in therapy and, in an approach accessible to him, emphasize the fact that none of the persons concerned with his problems and their attempted solution are incidental: they are all important, he, his family, the therapist, the Clinic population, and the people who referred him to us.

## Sharing Responsibility with the Child

All of us feel and should feel actively responsible, not only at the present moment in helping him help himself, but in view of the future. Responsibility has to be borne also in reference to the lack of help in the past. Failure is tactfully shared. It is not laid exclusively at the door of the child who feels both disarmed and objectionable. With such an approach we may relieve him of an undue responsibility that in all fairness is not his and which, exceeding his capacity, causes him to repudiate it altogether. We may simultaneously succeed in making a first inroad into his compensatory resorting to evil. This attitude is forced upon him when he is considered by his defensive parents or a defensive society to be solely responsible for his shortcomings.

The resorting to evil is an almost inevitable result. It is the enjoyment of existence, perverse though it is, that the child can experience. From this is generated further energy and the pleasure of retaliating or joining a gang which will keep him aware of his importance. Interfering with the order of things and with the emotions of people, he can thus hold the attention even of those in high places. In no other way than by maintenance of anger and the assertion of anger in a variety of ways can the child discover his own self as a separate existence. As long as failure is due to involvement in an inextricable mutual dependency between mother and child and as long as the mother penalizes the child for his behavior, despite the fact that he is primarily the executive organ of her own destructive needs, the child can never experience himself as a self-determining agent. Necessarily he remains confused by his inability to know what prompted his actions. He is weakened by compulsion, its power of insistence, and the intensity of the lure. To be thus fettered and incapacitated represents a self-replenishing source for an ocean of anger which engulfs the child itself within its all-embracing waves. Therefore, the mother's negative stimulation is resented in spite and because of the inescapable and enticing dependency. The child who enters treatment cannot turn away from what fetters him; his resentment holds him in the bonds of bitterness. He deplores the absence of ties which in actuality are not absent but perverted, turned in the negative direction of love. He is fascinated by the maternal rejection, her cruelty and the annoyance coming from her habit of egging him on by constant nagging, "making him nervous," "preventing him from forgetting." The child may be reminded deviously of whatever forbidden things he allegedly should not do: "now don't you go again in those stores and bring mama. . . ."

When the child has fulfilled the mission outlined for him in negative terms, he is censured. The mother denies responsibility for the child's intentions, which she induces, and for the actions she has prompted. Some mothers are not content with this form of persecution but for fear of loss of their weapon are driven to accuse the child everywhere. Thus defending themselves, they simultaneously deprive the exposed child of any chance to escape his assigned role. It is not the child's conflict of loyalty and the shame of having "reported" the mother as she has reported him that causes his recalcitrant reaction but the fear of disarming the mother, who is for better or for worse, for life and for death, linked with him. What appears to be fear of disloyalty on the surface may be mere self-defense, his eternal subjugation to the problem of conquering the mother's rejection. This attitude is not unlike the loyalty of his gang by one of its partners, an apparent loyalty that actually is the self-defense of a member of an interdependent organism. None of its organs can survive on its own.

The real or token sharing of responsibility in the initiation of treatment usually represents these children's first experience in dividing responsibility with a supporting helper. Because in school, for good reasons, individual responsibility is taken for granted, the children are expected to assume it voluntarily and generally, a maturity for which these children have not been prepared. The psychiatrist, on the other hand, approaches the child in his initial interview with regard to a vital problem of his own.

The idea that *each* of the partners, the child and the interviewing psychiatrist, carries his share in the present and the future endeavor is more or less vaguely understood by the child as trying to do something "together," playing together, being heard and not forced into something he does not want, that we will explain what is going to happen and let him have his say so. Though the child is unprepared by positive experience to make decisions and be the originator of his spontaneous *acts*, the longing for a wanted fulfilment could cause a child to be silently prepared for such a freedom. Others, living as though in an ambush for revolt or warfare, accept the relief of liberation. The appeal to co-operation might therefore be answered by some form of positive response. A first realization is experienced that the power of hostile action is unnecessary in a relationship in which the child is being consulted as a person. The tendency to exercise such power, as the child understands it, may be checked, because already he has learned that he might have something to lose, a trust, the community, an incipient affection. However, the child may fear a new dependency and try to invalidate the new commitment and the mood of the first encounter. We shall have to reassure the child by repeated attempts to stimulate his interest in himself and his relief from his dependent and frustrating condition.

If a child regresses in the course of treatment, the movement of events will differ widely, as evident from his former stagnation and the passivity of his involvement. Dependency will become only a stepping stone toward final emancipation. A powerful dynamic struggle with himself and the outside world will be in process through which he learns to outline the boundaries of his personal existence.

It need not be stressed that in our initial interview we appeal to those vital and sound tendencies in the child which can most readily be aroused and that we do not call indiscriminately upon the exercise of responsibilities and performances which the child cannot yet master and which should they be appealed to would of necessity arouse a host of negative defenses.

If in the process of treatment both the child and his mother gain a sense of individual responsibility, their responsibility will slowly have to be defined, in view of necessary reciprocation and mutual understanding. An active rapprochement by mutual identification will be necessary and resulting empathy will lead to a new closeness based on choice. The fetters of the original dependencies are broken and the child is free to seek the mother as an object distinct from himself, becoming aware, to some extent of how mama feels when "she comes home nervous," from work. This does not alleviate his burden; it might increase it and he may revolt; but he thoroughly becomes the child of a person *like* himself who is acting out and should be loved and helped "to be good" rather than "punished." This means that mother and child promote each other's self-realization as human beings with a resulting gain in emotional well-being and enjoyment of living. Finally, by identification with the mother, the child gains a clearer awareness of his own condition and how his needs are met in treatment.

## The Beginnings of Self-Confidence and Self-Esteem

This process is sponsored by the general group experience where self-confidence and self-esteem are developed. Whatever a child's roots may be, once he has learned to stand his ground, he has lost the sense that he is condemned to "rot" because of these roots, nor is there any need for condemning or cursing these roots for the pain they cause. Once he has gained the pride of standing upright, he will not need to hide but want to cover with loving generosity what no longer causes his blight. Thus, the child can become the healer of the child-mother, when corresponding help in understanding herself and her mothering is gained by the mother in her interviews with the psychiatric social worker. Mother and child become closer to each other and to themselves. A more objective view results, and projection upon each other becomes less likely.

New therapeutic impediments may arise, however, from an awakening conscience and a tendency to cover up lovingly and shamefully parental failure. Setbacks, due to the flaring-up of hostility or regression and above all the resistance to change, because of involvement and the need to foster resentment rather than love, may have to be dealt with.

In the initial interview, we are, at times, able to shock or move the child out of the interdependence with the mother upon which he stubbornly insists and to which he clings obstinately. When the pathological process is not yet frozen, it has been maintained by the chronically frustrated longing for maternal love. Therefore, some children may tend to respond, though with more or less reluctance, to the lure of maternal love coming from other sources and give in to life. Simultaneously, a first explosively sensed belief in himself has to be sustained in the child. Since almost any child can have charm for him who has senses to perceive it, encouragement can be offered by an obvious, though discreet, response to it. Even though the child may reject an accepting glance, the comfort was felt before it was refused and the longing remains, though it may be feared for a long time to come. Moreover, relief will be derived from the child's sensing that the interviewer is not deluded about him and his environment.

The child senses, though dimly and incredulously, the redeeming potentials of his home and of his condition. When he has not yet reached adolescence, his opposition to society and its representatives has not reached such proportions that approval from these quarters is meaningless. In the interviewer's lack of criticism, the child may find the license to love and to hope for the recovery of his pride in reference to his family status. Evidently such an understanding cannot be expressed discursively. It must unfold as a design out of the proceedings of this individual interview. It becomes the hour of birth for the child as a self and a first transfer of his loving potential. Therefore, when the interviewer cannot also take over the treatment and accompany the child through the vicissitudes which hopefully will lead the bewildered youngster out of his calamity, responsibility has to be assumed by the therapist to preserve the validity and permanence of a decisive experience. Every staff member must be animated by a profound sense of reponsibility, dedication, and awe of the minor universe with unlimited potential in every man. Equally necessary is the realistic appraisal that, in spite of a first step in the right direction, the child will for a long time to come not be ready to fill even his small size shoes and that therefore he will be awkward and terrifically afraid of stumbling.

Most children have serious difficulties in accepting the mother's co-operation with their treatment, fearing that she will impart to the Clinic and thus to their therapist her conviction that he is the sole cause of his troubles, thus widening the encirclement by rejection. Many a child finds comfort, slim as it might initially be, when he is reassured that his mother's co-operation with the Clinic is testimony to the fact that from now on she assumes, with conviction, her share of responsibility. Another might venture to express doubts that she is sincere in this and a third one might declare her incorrigible anyway. The distrustful child will be reassured that in treatment he will not be incriminated. He will be accepted as he is and can be. We will share responsibility with him on his way to mastery of his problems. This entails a process of learning in common. Emphasis is laid on the willingness of the therapist to listen to whatever the child may want to say or convey. While those who are not able to overcome their suspiciousness will sullenly bear with promises that in their mind no doubt will be broken, others will foresee relief from a needed and long delayed emotional communication. Many children feel and mention resentfully that the grown people think they know everything, meaning among many other serious complaints that they fail to listen and fail to give the children an opportunity to explain their version of their story.

To be listened to relieves a number of these children of the feeling that they are insignificant. In an initial positive encounter between child and therapist, the child gains a dim awareness that he is not necessarily a nobody and that at least for once he has been considered worthy of notice. Certain children thus reach a state of mind which can be exploited in an unending number of ways, not only in reference to the information to be elicited but the atmosphere which develops further during the interview. This depends on the child's age, his capacity to understand, the susceptibility to humor and the readiness to be emotionally playful, his responsiveness to friendliness, warmth, and insight, or his serious need for ego boost. On the *leitmotif* of a child's mournful mood might rise the first tentative notes of an expanding melody of cheer.

An important impediment to acceptance of therapy is the fear of being molded into something one is not, one cannot be, and therefore refuses to become. The child may be extremely fearful of being torn to pieces and cut to size. It is therefore important to impart to the child the confidence that the therapist will not want to "alter" him in view of a preconceived idea but help him find out who he is and learn to be himself and true to himself.

More deeply affected children may be made to feel at ease by a mere existence in common where time does not seem to count; the interviewer enters as it were the child's isolation, sharing his "shelter" which protects him from all the menaces, including noises and movement. Comfort and tranquillity might be sensed and revealed in a number of ways by rocking, thumb-sucking, an approach by a searching glance or motion. Only the most profoundly withdrawn and negativistic children will fail to show some sign of life and reaction susceptible to guiding the interviewer in the successful management of the interview.

There are children who will be able now or later to find comfort in the awareness that their suffering was not only a liability but a source of early wisdom and that they had received an endowment from which they might allow others to benefit. Such aspects of interviewing confer to children who can take a more generous view of life the status of a potential giver; they are aids in motivating the proud one to accept adult help. Isolated by a complete impoverishment in all areas, having conceivably been impressed only by what was denied them, they necessarily have at all times had the feeling that from their empty hands could spring no life. But more or less dimly many are conscious of their burden as well as the morbid wealth of their experience. This may serve hostile purposes. To be shown, however, that it can have appreciated constructive value represents an ephemeral ego boost which can be revived as time goes on.

Interesting the children from the beginning in taking a responsible attitude in reference to their treatment is a goal that must be sought. Children have to be accepted in their dependent condition as they are, passively or ambivalently yielding to treatment or bent on using the Clinic as an opportunity for acting out hostility.

A great deal is learned, by this means of approach, at the initial stage of our contacts with the children about their capacity to deal with responsibility and about the way they fail. Most significant are those who co-operate apparently but do not show up for their therapy sessions or who refuse to come up to the therapist's office from the day-care quarters.

Overt "consent" and subsequent withdrawal may have been but a hostile act, a retort in kind for having been deluded in the past. It may have been just an easy way to decline without having to face refusal to co-operate. The child may also have meant what he said, but in the absence of his interviewer, and thus deprived of her support, he was unable to carry through his intent. Contrary influence brought to bear by the family or other children inside or outside the Clinic or their disapproval just taken for granted may be enough to deter him.

The day-care group will, for a long time to come, remain the catalyst of the children's negative attitudes and help them manifest what directly they are incapable of expressing toward parental figures. As you would expect, they are not yet in possession of the civilized and acceptable way of presenting an argument, i.e., verbal discussion. Therefore, the children's group becomes also an ubiquitous target upon which violent manifestations are displaced, in an attempt to spare the real or the Clinic parents. These are needed for love, hate, care, and self-respect. The child lives in awe of parental status. It is a remarkable fact that impulsive and violent as these children can be, they do not venture to attack any grown person physically. One exception is conceivable. Parental status is denied by the child to a person whose anxiety or aggressive hostility is felt. Such a person must be ruled out as a potential source of support and may promote a panic reaction.

A tendency may prevail to avoid an early affiliation with adults in order to maintain the character of the group as an ever present target for the sake of relief from tension. Under the stress of utter insecurity and anxiety, the additional anxiety of reciprocal commitments and the resulting pangs of conscience cannot be endured. Chaos and confusion can be a safeguard with which the child surrounds himself to forestall intrusion or assault upon himself. In a chaotic situation you are at leisure to prompt motivation for aggression through the behavior of others. In view of his own needs the other fellow readily consents to being provoked.

The growing boy obviously avoids a face-to-face meeting with parental figures which carries the burden of its relevance and confronts him squarely with his fundamental problem—the child-parent relationship and all its "vicissitudes." Only by intense hostility and a violent revolt can the resourceless and untrained boy attempt to tear the ties which hold him in a deadly grip. He has, as it is, more to cope with than he feels capable of handling, and it is not only because of a prejudice against parental figures that he defends himself against new and complex attachments. Those youngsters who felt the need to borrow strength from antisocial gangs will bring into their individual treatment a particular ambivalence or conflict of allegiance. In certain of these cases, group therapy will have to precede individual treatment.

## The "Transparency" of the Clinic

Though each child has his own individual or (small) group therapist, each of the professional workers accepts any child that wishes to see him or her, so long as the youngster does not intrude during sessions with other persons. Some of the workers have a scheduled "open house" hour. These techniques serve the purpose of letting the children know that they are excluded nowhere. To be one child's therapist does not mean rejection of another. Such care is not only dictated by the children's problems but by the "transparency" of the whole Clinic. This "transparency" is of great therapeutic and prophylactic value for suspicious children. Their distrust has been nurtured by exclusion from parental acceptance.

The children's impromptu visits with any staff members who appeal to them are an important opportunity for unguarded emotional expression, and a source of information for the staff. In running from therapist to therapist some children may manifest an aimless randomness in the first weeks or months of treatment. They are obviously in search of an answer to a question which they are not equipped to formulate. Above all, they are in search of themselves. The visits may represent belated choice, motivated by an intense affinity to the person or predilection for the person's sex or race. Since the response to the child is genuine and therefore potentially meaningful, these improvised encounters may promote the child's tendencies toward deeper attachment and thus to the exploration of life and living through the experience of relating. Important material may be disclosed in these impromptu sessions. It is attempted, however, not to let them interfere with the already chosen therapist and the work in process, unless there is good reason to expect that the new therapeutic relationship would be particularly promising and that the child's behavior is indicative of its appropriateness to his needs. For instance, when a growing boy feels he has outgrown the need for a maternal therapist and cannot alter the meaning of the relationship in transference, and when, by persistent visits to a male therapist, he displays his emancipating tendency and needed male identification as well as his choice of an ideal figure, a change of therapist according to his choice seems in order. Unnecessary changes of therapist, however, work against a child's improved capacity to work through his problems in transference and deprive him of an opportunity to invest his human relations with depth and intensity. At times children express a desire for treatment by both parental figures as well as an ardor to join both. This may represent the need for reassurance and the wish to see put to the test in reality parental figures who co-operate on his behalf; this co-operation has never been shown in his own family. The child may not only display such a need, but he may communicate it verbally. In such cases both therapists thus elected join their efforts.

The child's need for parental unity and harmony must be answered, and the edification of such an ideal must emanate from the spirit of the Clinic and the Community of all its workers.

# XIV

## Main Aspects of Therapy

### Steps in Therapy

A. *The diagnostic procedure:*

1. The first contact with the patient, as elsewhere, is indirect. The study of his preceding life history and his background made at "intake," is established by interviewing the child's parents or guardians. It is based further on written information concerning the child and his family obtainable from physicians, hospitals, schools, courts, and welfare workers. The initial interview, however, could not fulfil its diagnostic function if it were not also therapeutic. It must include the promotion of a trusting relationship to the Clinic, the need to gain insight and the desire to obtain help for the child, or better, for the family as a whole. The latter insight in particular may have to be obtained by subsequent contacts.

2. The psychological study including intelligence and personality testing of the child, at times of one or both parents or several siblings.

3. The initial interview with the child which again includes the establishment of a relevant relationship not only for best diagnostic results but it holds the promise of future gratification due to the interviewer's insight and acceptance.

B. *Planning:*

1. Day-care—advisability of day-care enrolment or eligibility for it. The therapeutic *planning* is made by the total therapeutic staff. In case a child is considered for day-care, the teachers' supervisor and co-ordinator assists in the deliberations.

The therapeutic staff first establishes need or desirability for day-care. The co-ordinator, an inviting and most accepting person, then discusses whether services can be made available, what the suggested procedure in day-care under available provisions could be, what difficulties will have to be taken in strides. The balance between certain children's tendency to act out and others to be sensitive to it has to be considered, and how much isolation of the one from the other must and can be provided.

We accept all those children whose symptoms reveal that for emotional reasons they cannot cope with school requirements and children who need a protective environment through the day but can live in a home or are expected to stand the trials of their own home with support of treatment to child and family.

Not eligible are larger, aggressive boys who would cause constant disquietude to the smaller and weaker ones, whether the latter are provocative and acting out or sensitive and tending to withdraw.

Regretfully we are no longer equipped at this time to take girls, though the need for these services has increased. Our luncheon program absorbs the space and the teachers. Children eligible for day-care must be toilet trained.

We have been bold in that we accept children with a doubtful prognosis and have been encouraged by good results. We had all to gain for the benefit of the child and the community and very little to lose in the absence of more appropriate means of assistance. If we fail to achieve a full success, some improvement of the child's symptomatology usually had been achieved; at worst they had to be referred for institutional care, in the majority of cases in a state of readiness or preparedness for co-operation with their treatment. In all events we benefited by the experience, and the child had gained a place of safe anchorage and motivation for his return to the community.

2. The assignment of a therapist for the child and one for the mother or foster mother or both parents or foster parents.

3. The decision whether group therapy or individual therapy is to be given, in the former case whether the parents are assigned to a mixed group or not. This decision may depend also on sociological factors (working hours, etc.).

4. The planning of the specific approach and treatment is dictated by the dynamics of the symptomatology and of parent-child or child-family interaction.[1] The diagnosis plays its part only insofar as it is implied in the psycho-dynamics.

C. *Treatment:*

Every treatment or planning session is recorded and information correlated between the child's and the family's therapists, as well as with the observations of the teaching staff. Recording is obviously important for documentation of procedures and results—it promotes the thinking through of the meaning of the observed phenomena and the verification of thought. In the light of the process and progress of the treatment itself and of the knowledge about current child-family interaction or parental emotional or socioeconomic crises, treatment either takes its course or has to be modified in Clinic staff or teachers' staff sessions or both. Modifications concern, for instance, intensification of treatment, regrouping, return to individual therapy, or, on the other hand, readiness for group therapy, need for foster home placement, return home, or dismissal as improved. The learning schedule or approach may be modified. A child not in day-care may be admitted to the shop or recreation activities.

Information in conference is regularly exchanged with, and interpretations are given to, welfare workers or school psychologists, guidance teachers, and probation officers. In addition progress reports are given regularly; reports for further disposition of the child's case in court or for adoption procedures are made on request.

The first step in actual therapy is the establishment of a relevant relationship in addition to the initiation of the action motive: letting the child find sources of gratification and implement them. This is his opportunity to build up his self-esteem under the auspices of the permissive approach in the protective surroundings of the therapeutic milieu. The therapist is usually the main object of the child's affection. Though the milieu tends to be ideally accepting and a model unit for the promotion of a positive "transference" of emotions and emulative tendencies, it is not devoid of opportunities for differentiation and choice. The reality aspects of the milieu as well as the symbolic aspects which are attributed to it by the child and to which it lends itself, again stimulate spontaneity and the strength needed for asserting one's affinities as well as for learning to inquire into their motivations.

In order to help the child achieve a positive transference to the total milieu, the one presently favored by the child and the main recipient of confidences and complaints must, to remain the confidant and love object, be gratifying. Thus he becomes a suitable mediator for rewarding and trustful relationships elsewhere and a deterrent to meddling, manipulating, nagging, and projecting. The mediator tends to be a moderator and to stimulate the weighing of one's own position and arguments providing the child has gained a base stable enough to admit the reasons and arguments of the opponent.

Thus each worker and any child identified with the Clinic as a whole can be of help in dissolving, minimizing, attenuating negative attitudes to people and resistance to progress. Wherever possible the child is also given an opportunity to find gratification in the area of learning.

Negative transferences are likely to be manifested in reference to those adults who are in the children's permanent presence and therefore widely absorbed by those adults. Though permissive, they must not allow the orchestration of the whole program to be interfered with. Though the mode of dealing with problems is gentle and by intention, certain limits are set by safety and fairness.

Negative transferences have been increasingly manageable, due to the function of the maternal supervisor and her high skill of dealing with acute emotional exacerbations. A contribution towards this end has also been made by the increasing conviction, dedication, and skill of the staff which includes a constant attention which edifies the child and gives him the certitude that the world has a place for him as a person. The teachers' dedicated attention alerts them to the children's needs and in promoting the teachers' empathy generates their insight and resourcefulness.

More frequent and more resistant are transferences of sibling rivalries. It takes time to help children traumatized in the home or in foster homes, struggling with transference symptoms. We try to avoid a renewed exposure of the child to traumatizations as formerly incurred and to promotion of negative transferences. Love and security, as well as interpretations, finally prevail in the great majority of cases as well as identification with the adult model of behavior. In cases where several or all children living in a foster home were referred to us we treated them in a group, if indicated, in addition to assisting social worker and foster home.

The children's resistance to treatment or to improvement can be expected to be in terms of their usual defenses. When these symptoms are due to resistance, whatever the stage of treatment, we shall have to consider influences coming from outside the therapeutic endeavor as well as motivations derived from the treatment process. In the former case the outer obstacles have to be taken care of as well. As evi-

dent, if these resistances occur at a time when a transference relationship is established, the child at times can be made aware of what he is
doing by a simple question which hits with marksmanship and thus
takes care of an interpretation.

Excessive demandingness of every possible description, and in many
an instance it will be of a sadistic nature in reference to the therapist,
or, deviously, in reference to rivals, can be expected at the beginning
of treatment. Deceptiveness may be used. Exceptional children will
resist by non–co-operation, non-attendance or mute and noncommittal behavior, unconstructive and unedifying use of time for extended
periods. Some will be late coming and leaving. On the whole, defenses
and resistance in treatment are treated similarly. Only the references
differ when interpretations are given.

We deal with demandingness by first gratifying it. Since the milieu
as a whole is gratifying, the child who is guided also by the desires of
his peers will become aware of multiple desires and sources for satisfaction. Thus he is distracted from becoming excessively and unrea-
sonably demanding in reference to a single love object. The other children, as guides toward pleasure, lose their character as competitors or
can be tolerated before they are accepted. (It is evident that by means
of this same process the mother at home is liberated from the punishment of excessive demands provided she does not counteract the liberating movement.)

When the child has a need for hurting, the aggression may have to
be ignored; next the child can be helped to explain his need for hurting and later he can be assisted in empathizing, in accepting the pangs
of regret and in not expressing despair by aggressive or sly hostility.
At this time the child, fearing loss of love, will summon his own
newly discovered potentials for sympathy. In the moments of distress
about himself, when he tends to isolate himself from himself or the one
he has hurt, there is always some youngster or adult at hand who is
sensitive to his condition and can help him find his way back to the
fold.

The totally passive child must first be left alone, exposed to the lure
of participation in day-care. In therapy he might be shocked out of
his isolation, for instance, by a play that in apparent artlessness performs his situation and problem in the dollhouse, a puppet show or
with toy figures or inert objects on the floor. Depending on the mo-

tives for passivity the child will be more or less alert to the guile and resist it, especially when he is under his mother's commitment. Much time has to be invested to overcome his passivity. A sound and co-operative father who is considerate of his sick wife but who cannot be disarmed may represent an invaluable assistance in this effort.

The obstinate child may have to indulge dependency needs before he can yield to the lure of love and invest in it generously.

Children traumatized on the Oedipal level of development frequently need treatment in day-care because of a symptomatology that reveals traumatization on almost every previous developmental stage.

On the whole we are guided in treatment by the person the child is at each special time when we are called upon by the treatment procedure to react to him therapeutically. We tend to obtain an insight into his relationships to men and the world and his way of dealing with them. Any appropriate therapy is also an artistic, strictly individualized endeavor "proceeding by flair and intuition."[2] Theory is a measure for sifting the necessary intuitive perception and a *design* for orientation, that is, the gaining of an interpretive system for therapeutic action.

We quote Glover, who discusses the therapist's compulsion for making developmental reviews as a tendency, similar to his patient's who is obsessed in "making things clear, rounding them out," etc. "Overanxiously clinging to a structural point of view . . . the analyst may find that instead of analyzing his patient at some given moment, he has simply been engaged in a process of scientific description. "The fact that his unconscious processes have been attuned to the processes going on in his patient's unconsciousness enables him to keep tally without conscious efforts."[3]

Therefore, to develop steps in the therapy of these children further we feel the need to bring the story of their lives in the form of a usually extended observation.

## Choice of the Mode of Therapy

Strained by those human groups which succumb or struggle not to succumb under the pressures of an inadequate and dense society, clinics have found their own devices not to be submerged. One method has been to set criteria in child guidance which have eliminated from treatment patients and their parents as unsuited, unresponsive, or not ready for a specific approach. Principles or intake procedures have served as measures for separating promising from unpromising cases.[4]

Even group therapy is not meeting all needs; hence the attempts of group therapists to sift out early in treatment doubtful cases who would be liable to cause waste of professional time.[5] On the other hand tendencies have arisen to widen the therapeutic embrace even further and by a community therapy[6] and its complex approach, reach not only more patients but the "untreatable" ones.

Originally we gave individual treatment to all our patients, using the day-care group as a dramatic scene representative of the child's life and needs, the natural as well as transferred pathological needs. In making each child a dramatic actor, the stage drew in the withdrawn observer and lured him to play his part on the scene, or to interact from afar with its protagonists. But day-care being also life and a minor world, realism as well as adequacy could be explored and developed. The presence of the staff was and is offering an ever present sympathetic audience ready to become the "God out of the Machine," when the drama otherwise might have come to a tragic end. Day-care having a core of a long-term population which however is open to a steady trickling in of newcomers, the children previously enrolled are guides to the newcomers, supporting identification with ideal parents and, as time goes on, with desirable goals.

Strength is tested continuously in coping with one's impulses, in following the dictates of insight and reason as well as in withstanding temptations under many guises. The adult handling of antisocial tendencies, supported by the children identified with acceptable standards, is of such a nature that the child feels included, however not supported, by a soft-peddling of improper attitudes of his. Thus is avoided that the child holds on to his hateful self-image as an excuse for remaining hateful, excluded, and justifiably antisocial. Antisocial tendencies of the child who is made to feel he belongs "inside" are weakened in a slow process by the lure of the milieu and its adult and young population. In addition to genuine acceptance the child is exposed to demonstrations of fortitude in danger, the danger to yield to temptation, to react impulsively to challenges, etc. He is exposed to seeing impartiality. To be "smart," he has to give up antisocial behavior because the

Clinic population makes him find out "that it does not pay" and "he cannot get away with it."

Most helpful in coping with the children's problem of ambivalence in reference to the mother has been the exposure to group living alternating with the privacy with the therapist where the child can fall back upon his inner experience. The children's dependency needs can be expressed in greater intimacy and closeness. Responses to the child are most specific in that tête-à-tête community. The children in the initial stages, when they are most reluctant and most ashamed to uncover their dependence, are rewarded by the group, a forum for faked public abdication of love and a testing ground for independence. But its "counterdelusional"[7] function being necessarily more obvious, expectations and stress needed to meet them are greater, and resort is longed for and received again in the tête-à-tête of individual therapy. There you can love in secret, mute or pouting, turn your back because you are ashamed of your love and resent it. You can listen to silence and suddenly hear "the kettle begin it." Then you can invite into the room a population of increasingly threatening phantoms of the past. The support felt in facing those ancient phantoms and the resulting strength intensify the relationship and the positive aspects prevail over the negative ones, helping the child to overcome inhibitions, anxiety, and resistance. The tentative practice of courage thus achieved and the greater elation of mood experienced cause the child to face actual challenges in the group with more confidence and insight. Dependence on the therapist will diminish; now he will be sought for purposes of maturation. In the group the child will no longer make a pretense of reneging his love, but affirm and emulate it.

Thus we find the role of day-care and individual psychotherapy to be complementary. Together they are particularly well suited to ambivalent emotions of the hostile pre-adolescent and adolescent boy.

But exposed to increasing pressures for admittance and determined, by being flexible, to keep our doors open to the children who need us, we explored psychotherapy by small groups first, as an adjunct or substitute for certain cases of individual psychotherapy. Larger groups were also formed for growing children and adolescents who have undergone individual therapy. These youngsters may have passed through a small therapeutic group that widened its circle, usually by their attraction to other children.

In our experience then we found the therapeutic group to be a catalyst for social tendencies in withdrawn children and adolescents. We also found it to be a catalyst for social manifestations of a positive or negative nature and for verbal expression. But, due to the artlessness of young children, it proved itself to be a valid therapeutic means where expression of intense dependency needs was necessary. Under certain stress or under intragroup pressures, and at times precipitated from without, adolescent boys and girls will express their dependency needs aggressively and without control. At times they feel the urge to request to be seen individually. Individual therapy as the method of choice had to be omitted in certain cases, but valid results in terms of the children's attitudes were obtained due to the intensity of their relationship to the therapist and the interaction with their peers. Insight was gained at the level of the children's optimum capacity.

Discoveries of unexpected possibilities were sponsored by the children themselves. Spontaneous encounters between children in a children's world may reveal affinities which can be exploited therapeutically. Marilyn Burus, the intensely rejected, only child of an intelligent and efficient unmarried mother, was referred at the age of thirteen by another mental hygiene clinic, for a severe learning difficulty. She could be pleasantly shocked out of her extreme, timid withdrawal which was coupled with a tendency to burst out with "smart" verbal aggression and to deny the vicissitudes of her condition. But she remained anxious, inhibited, and unproductive as well as surprised at the miracle of her acceptability. Her mother had engaged an old woman to "watch" her constantly to prevent her from playing with children lest she get into trouble or be impregnated, as it had happened to her. Marilyn asked that I let other girls play with her and refused categorically to play with boys. I did not readily yield to her desire, convinced that it would be more helpful, if she could work through her predominantly hostile dependency needs. One day she saw a new girl, eight years of age, who had preceded her in my office. She asked me whether she could invite her into her session. Lilly Morrison, the new little girl, was in the Clinic for an initial interview. Her welfare worker had not yet returned for her. She too was extremely timid. She was under the impact of protracted emotional shock due to the sudden desertion of her and her two half-sisters by her unmarried mother. Marilyn immediately began to gratify Lilly's dependency needs and by identification gratified her own. She was timid but gentle. She revealed she wanted a little sister. However, she also showed competitive impulses and in this and the next session, subtle cruelty. Despite these negative aspects, Lilly seemed to enjoy the attention of the "elder sister" and the games which gave her an opportunity to prove her adequacy. She knew how to defend herself. At the end of the session, she requested "doll play" for next time, thus showing that she had already some business to attend to. She showed identification with Marilyn's role. We can expect that in conferring to the dolls the treatment she received, she will let us know which aspects of Marilyn's attitudes she appreciates and which she dislikes. A promising start was made. We enlarged the double sessions to the formation of a group of four children, built up around the potentials for dynamic interaction of their problems.

Two nine-year-old girls, Ada, autistic and speechless, and Charlotte, obstinately refusing to use her fluent speech, met because the former had arrived too soon. Neither of them were in good contact with reality. Ada ran into the session of the other and began to interact awkwardly, surprised at the other's presence. Since both played with each other and Ada talked occasionally, the following experiment was carried out. Each of them remained in individual psychotherapy where both could act out their earliest dependency needs. Ada, the autistic child, began to speak in an articulate way, reiterating, for instance, "make Dr. Riese mad," or expressing in similar short terms her oral requests. Between their two individual sessions we inserted a small group session consisting of these two girls and a seven-year-old boy, deserted by his mother, who was enrolled in our day-care program. A mentally adequate boy with well-developed speech, he was in individual therapy with a male therapist. Though his treatment proceeded most satisfactorily, he had persistently looked for a pretext to see his first interviewer regularly. He met Charlotte in the general office, and she enjoyed the contact with him. She brought him into the session. Ever since then he remembered the day and hour of this group session and appeared for it on schedule. He tried to endear himself to the girl although he noticed her condition. In his presence Charlotte behaved more adequately. In individual therapy she was mute, but the group stimulated her social tendencies and she spoke. Between the two girls a slight sado-masochistic interaction developed. Charlotte and the boy played constructively together. Charlotte, for instance, was the house-wife who cooked, cutting clay and soaking it in water; he set the table, they fed the children, had picnics, and played ball. She had the ideas and mutely realized them. He fit himself into the play in a manly and gentlemanly way. Mutely Ada encouraged him to speak into the dictaphone and attempted speaking into it herself; but so far no more than the tendency has been in evidence. In front of the apparatus she can utter no words, though it helps her proffer sounds. It gives her joy to hear them. This was and continues to be a spontaneous endeavor of hers. That both girls benefited from the accepted contact with the boy seemed obvious. But the boy also benefited. At a time when he was in an emotional crisis because of a change of foster homes, at a time when he was moody, unpredictable and had violent temper tantrums, he drew support from these little girls and the role of the dignified little man he could play with them. He showed the one how to speak and gave the other a play husband. As a husband or as himself he could also pursue his own goals; he would go hunting which was shooting his darts, truck-driving as the provider or he could be the therapist's big boy, who drew or wrote and asked for assistance for his "superior endeavors." One day, he was asked what he was drawing. His answer was: "I don't know yet what it will be." He thought by drawing one turns out an incidental result which thereafter is "read" like a text. He was aware of his effort but not of a design of his own for it.

A most interesting contribution to a successful therapeutic group-ing was made by Theodore. At that time he was seen alone with his brother, a new patient of ours. The object of this endeavor was the working through of their problem in light of the family interaction.

The foster parents had raised them practically from infancy. Due to the increasingly serious marital problems of these foster parents and the foster mother's closeness to these two boys, they had taken refuge in a female identification. This had lead to an incestuous homosexual relationship and to a homosexual relationship to Clarence another pa-tient who had visited them in their foster home. The fact had been brought to our attention and was therapeutically dealt with. The brothers finally became unproductive in their sessions. The younger one was quite dependent on his therapist. One day they asked for permission to join the group of the four sisters described later. The tendency was to venture out into healthy and pleasurable heterosexuality for which at the time of inception the therapist's support was needed. The girls were asked whether the boys were welcome. After an initial timidity on the part of both boys and girls and the separation of the sexes in two groups, they began to tease each other, the girls being at first extremely hostile. But after a while the boys began to exhibit skill at dart and ball playing, the girls grew into an enthusiastic audience and finally the "teen agers" played together jubilantly. Theodore hesitated to throw back to the girl the ball she had caught and thrown to him. Turning to his brother as though to aim the ball at him, he artlessly and significantly said to the girl: "I am afraid to throw the ball to you. I'll try it out on my brother first." But he threw the ball in her direction. After a few sessions which moved on the same pattern, Theodore and his brother asked me for permission to introduce Clarence into the group. Clarence told me he knew the girls would be hard on him first. But contrary to expectation they welcomed him into their club which, in an artless self-irony they called the Savages Club, from then on. The sessions were opportunities for an intense exhilarating release of tension between the hostile girls and the timid boys. Each time there was a crescendo of emotions, relief, fatigue. Then the curve had a descending branch. Both sexes sat down in two friendly, yet slightly apprehensive camps, still uncertain of their capacity for control. Significantly dependency on the therapist and display of affection to her by both boys and girls increased. Both groups vied with each other spontaneously in "cleaning up the mess." They left separately, though this had not been requested. As time went on the boys conveyed the girls home fondly and respectfully.

One of the sessions was noteworthy. The battle of words had gone out of control and the children reacted by qualms of conscience. One girl became sleepy and talked of church, one of the boys pretended the therapist looked sad, another one said, "there are no ladies in this room but one." The children from then on set their own limits of behavior and the girls who came well groomed and charmingly dressed preferred to be recognized by the boys as "ladies," gay and young.

We may be confronted with the problem of children who do not qualify for group therapy because they are too menaced by the children as competitors or catalysts of an ill-contained hostility, whether their behavior is constrictive or quick-tempered. By the same token they may be too menacing to the group. We may be confronted with the problem of availability of only a female psychotherapist for a young adolescent boy traumatized in his relationship to the mother on all levels of libidinal development. These children, depending on the relationship to the father or a substitute father figure, may well work through their problem with the female therapist.

Thus the child who feels immediately deprived of strength in the immediate presence of the adult, the one who is resourceless and so dried out that he has lost his appetite for play, or the child who feels self-conscious in the presence of a female psychotherapist can nevertheless be treated in individual therapy, and his problem can be overcome without excessive anxiety whatever the therapist's sex.

Jerry would brave his anxiety in the early days of his treatment by sitting arrogantly in a comfortable chair, his feet sprawled and placed on the table. When he found out he could not create anxiety, he lost his own. Another boy would engage the assistance of an evil ghost for annoying the therapist in her dreams. He played the ghost and the therapist was supposed to be harassed in her sleep. This was performed in stages. First she was only frightened, then she was massacred by the menaces of the ghost, exposed to the eternal fire for refusal to be evil, finally her bed was set afire, she was asked whether it was not getting hot already, and how it felt to be burned up. He would always wake up the therapist with the words; "all right wake up. It was only a dream." One day, he said, "I almost called you Hertha, but a little boy like me cannot do that. I don't want to do it."

At the beginning of the session, he had asked that the door remain ajar to the next room "where daddy could hear us." The therapist, attempting to comfort him by her ignoring any "danger," expressed doubt that this would be a good idea. Therefore he introduced the door into the play. It had to make a squeaking noise to announce the frightening approach of the ghost. Then it was closed.

When he started his treatment, the boy was constricted by fear and moved like a robot. He spoke in a crackling voice and an abrupt rhythm as though taking away the few words he ventured to speak. He coped with his anxiety by filling the extended conversational vacuum that would have arisen by pointing in the direction of the sun dial and telling what cities lay there, always calling the same cities. He withdrew upon drawing. All his drawings were empty pages crossed by one main street or a street crossed by another, seen in bird's eye view. The compulsive order was expressed by two or three regularly lined up street lights or signals saying: "Do not enter," "No parking," "One way only," "Stop ahead," "Yield the right of way." As so many children he used as an avenue to verbal communication the talk through the dictaphone. Deadly anxious and utterly resourceless, he preferred noises and animal sounds as though intent on revealing his abhorred animality to himself and the protecting and accepting therapist. To encourage himself and deny the nonsensical character of the dictation, he played back almost each word and commented joyfully, "that's me; I am saying that," pointing to his chest.

To the children's group may be attributed the part of the protective male and to the therapist the role of the non-threatening mother. Her rewarding function on all levels of the child's emotional development must be gained through the interaction of the total group. It is often helpful to introduce a threatened child into a group which is already feeling comfortable in reference to the maternal group leader. The interaction in process between the children in such a group has lost its potentials for excessive expression. The children may be ready and willing to open their ranks to a newcomer. They may identify with him and manifest acceptance or the desire to help him. They may on the contrary want to keep their ranks closed and bluntly call out, "we don't want him." Attuning your response to the children's feelings, you usually can win over their co-operation. The other children's confident and easy way of expressing their feelings considerably attenuates the newcomer's anxiety in most cases. A similar influence is exercised by the children in the day-care group whose attitudes have improved. With few exceptions, their anxiety and resistance against the therapist is greatly diminished. The newcomer may feel supported by the children in his barely contended need for hostile manifestations and understand that he is safe in releasing what "bothers him" and what to us may explain his symptoms.

In contrast to the child who uses the children's group as the supportive male, there is the child who sees in any other child or group of children a threatening agent or a competitor. By his anxiety he creates anxiety and exposes himself to the very danger he fears. These dangers he also ardently needs as a means for a strong and explosive release of tension.

This was the way Daniel Miller frequently used his session in the group and the way he tended to relate to the children in day-care. This boy was his mother's sixth child, born out of wedlock, after the desertion of her husband, the father of her other children, much older than Daniel. He was conceived at an age when his mother did not believe conception was still a possibility. A sullen, unhappy woman, devoid of warmth and of a mature interest in Daniel, she had been distraught with anxiety and anger while expecting the child. He was bottle fed and was a very poor eater all of his life. In the first six months there was reason for great concern because he refused the food offered. After that period "he began to eat sometimes." No other problems were reported except his subjective feeling that he had a heart condition. He kept "pounding his chest as though he wanted to cough up something." We could observe that Daniel, who had had to prepare his own food, never ate a balanced meal. He complained of being constipated. The mother denied that he suffered from rectal bleeding as Daniel claimed he did. She believed it was simply an excuse for staying at home.

Daniel's father lived a hundred miles from this city. He still showed some interest in his son. He saw him extremely rarely but expressed willingness to raise him. He did not take responsibility for his upbringing but provided for gifts that impressed the boy. The mother had lived with him for years in a common-law marriage, then she returned to her first husband in a northern town. The first husband was thirty-four years of age when she had married him at the age of sixteen. The reunion occurred after a separation of sixteen years. When we met Mrs. Miller she was separated from her husband for the second time, but still predominantly preoccupied with him, his unfaithfulness and desertion. She had refused to sleep with him and shared room and bed with Daniel instead.

Mother and son, living alone together have moved not only from family unit to family unit, from city to city, but frequently within the city. Due to her dependent and deprived condition only unsatisfactory houses and quarters were available to them. Almost no contacts were mentioned with the children from her first marriage. They, too, had been shifted around constantly. One son was said to have made a very poor adjustment in life, he appeared from time to time to take shelter in the maternal home. Until recently Daniel slept in the same room and bed with the mother and still does so when the mother's "boy friend" is absent. She takes Daniel, dressed like a young man, to strictly adult entertainments.

Daniel, a slender boy, was thirteen years old when referred by the public school for his irregular attendance and his unpredictable behavior. The report mentioned that he alternated between docility and rebelliousness. The mother was described as condoning any of her son's behavior. Until recently, she considered him a model child, but finally began to worry "because he does nothing in school and at times stays out all night. He plays exclusively with very young children. He is untruthful and he steals. He has destructive outbursts followed by threats, self-pity and a sense of 'persecution.'" It was reported by a visiting teacher that he once ran out into the streets in extreme anger, sat down in front of the school and even approaching cars could not make him move. Another time, he sat in the classroom window and it was feared that he might jump. Because of his failure to do class-room assignments and his pretending never to understand how to do them, he was placed in a special class for a limited period. His school problem had begun only eighteen months earlier, when the family moved and Daniel was transferred to still another school. He loved his old teacher and rejected the new one.

To prevent Daniel from staying away from home and returning in the early morning hours, the mother bought him a television set. While reducing to some extent the problem of staying out, it promoted the intensification of his truancy problem. He was glued to the television set all hours of the day. At the time of referral he had been excluded from school attendance because it was feared he could be harmful to himself.

The period of referral coincided with Daniel's and the mother's move to a two-room apartment. Our following contact with Daniel was an opportunity to observe how enhanced he felt by this improvement of his living quarters. As typical of him, he ignored all of its overwhelmingly negative aspects. The mother had then given him an additional television set of his own to secure privacy for herself for visits with a boy friend who came at regular intervals and who was a stabilizing element. He had helped her find a job, the first she ever held. Daniel denied any hurt resulting from the mother's new emotional ties which isolated him. In the children's presence he emphasized loudly how good his mother was and bragged about the gifts he received. He was so much in need of attaching himself to the tokens of her kindness that despite his usual good-naturedness he was indifferent to the great distress these boasts caused those children around him who had no mother to attend to their needs. He also fostered the illusion of good social standing. But when he heard the other children express discontent with their home or foster home situation, he invited them in child-like artlessness to live with him. His mother would love them too and give them a television set. No child in the group was as artless as he was. They just looked at him with silent surprise. This soon brought him down to earth. Silently and thoughtfully he gave up the dream that he and his mother could grant privileges and that their love had a value to others.

The mother, as we know already, was absent from home from seven in the morning to seven in the evening. The center of gravity of her existence then was her work as a maid in a hospital for chronically disabled white children whom she served food. The children showed her great love. The mother seemed interested enough to come regularly to see our psychiatric social worker. She unfolded a picture of a long life of dependency and socioeconomic misery. But it remains to be seen at this writing whether the mother has a genuine desire for assistance in reference to her own as well as her son's problems. At the time of this writing she tends to delegate all responsibility for his unpredictable behavior to him and declare herself disarmed in controlling it. She seems incapable of making an effort on his behalf. She is inconsistent and bribes him to co-operate.

The initial interview was made in view of an emergency admittance at the request of the visiting teacher of the public schools. Only her report and a resumé of the test made by the school psychologist was available.

Daniel spoke fluently in a nasal tone. His mouth was held open when he did not speak and he produced much saliva, although he did not slobber. He willingly gave information, obviously tried to please in a slightly unctuous manner and to display adequacy. He immediately assumed a status of familiarity. He unfolded his whole family history, his and the mother's relationships to the father, the stepfather and the stepsiblings. He emphasized his appreciation of the mother's maternal virtues by expounding the other son's maladjustment as a proof of his want of gratitude.

It was obvious that Daniel used identification with the mother to defend himself against the temptation of failure. He affirmed a dissimilarity between the stepbrother and himself to convince himself that he really was different, that he legitimately belonged to the mother. As her adequate and faithful son, he had a permanent place with her, contrary to the brother for whom the mother's and his home was a temporary shelter. As we know, however, he tended already to use his home as a foothold that he would desert for part of the night.

On the other hand identification was revealed in this session with the helpless white children whom his mother assisted in the hospital. Immediately after reporting what kept his mother away from home and at work during the day, he acquainted us with the fact that he loved to play with small children and to put diapers on them. He added that he enjoyed the company of those white children in his neighborhood who want to go to school with him. It was immediately obvious that he had a complex problem in reference to his mother's devotion to other children, in particular of the white group whose fight for segregated education at the time was sensed inevitably and painfully as rejection. It also showed that indulgence in regressive tendencies would find a limit in his pride. It also was apparent that he had a sense for basic responsibilities.

He spoke elaborately about his school problem in terms of personal relationships. He was extremely happy in school until he moved to another school district and was separated from a teacher he loved and who loved him. The teacher with whom he could not get along he said, "in strictest confidence" between him and me, "never stayed in class for five minutes." She was depicted as violent and threatening. She broke up a fight in the cafeteria by raising a chair to throw at a child. He asserted that the teacher had made a similar threat against him one day. He said he felt so cornered that he wanted to escape through the window. But "you know," he added, "I was not going to do something desperate." He finally stated: "The children pick after me and the teacher does too." His self-criticism was identical with the mother's statement that his main problem was "hard-headedness."

Daniel was assigned to a male therapist and enrolled in day-care. The teachers' supervisor assumed successfully the role of the ever-present rewarding mother. She made him feel that in his absence he was missed, that he was wanted, awaited, and needed. She knew when to give him an opportunity to reveal his distress and when to distract him from it. His male therapist was his first opportunity to be a real boy in the company of a father figure. To cope with the problems of controlling him, the mother had kept him home with table games, before buying the television set. All male teachers had been rejected by Daniel. At the time of the observation that we shall report, acceptance of Daniel's male therapist had not prevailed over the boy's indiscriminate dependency on all female staff members, though his relationship to each varied to some extent. In fact, Daniel was not altogether lacking in awareness of specific compensations he could expect from his numerous love objects.

Daniel's multiple attachments were not a bee-like gathering of a child who cannot focus long enough to hold on to what he has. He knew how to obtain partial gratification from all of the female staff members. With no detriment to the good rapport with his therapist, Daniel became interested as time went on in the male social worker, his mediator between the mother and himself, and therefore an element of growing comfort and support. He knew also to establish a hierarchy of importance in his female relationships and to nuance them. His "promiscuity" was attention-getting; it was a means of being acceptable and recognized and above all, a means of escaping the children and the class situation.

Daniel chose to come to the Clinic with a stylish hat, a necktie and his Sunday clothes. This necessarily exposed and isolated him. He aggravated his situation by stressing his vulnerability to damage done to his clothes. Those children who had a problem similar to his could not resist teasing him. They fought in him the outside representation of problems with which they were struggling inside themselves. One boy expressed it saying: "I don't want you here. You are a sissy," adding, "I at least am fighting it, why can't you?"

Daniel's self-exposure tended to make him more dependent on the protection by the maternal figures in the Clinic. Their failure then became justification for withdrawal behind television at home. We attempted to channel his needs to his therapist and the supervisor, but in the beginning he needed not to feel rejected and worthless, he needed to be acceptable everywhere and always. He was swept away in a torrent of tears and attempted to drown his environment in a stream of self-pitying and accusatory words. Each of us had to contribute to the security he derived from a token or symbolic admission to our presence. For the sake of love and fear of loss, he co-operated. He used to steal and nothing was safe with him around. The first symptom he gave up was stealing, knowing he could attach himself more safely by mutual affection. Gradual support came from the father figure. Daniel's regressive tendencies were increasingly absorbed by the supervisor.

He continued to remain competitive with the children who underwent group therapy with the psychiatrist. He always found ways to be in the room before it was noticed, either secretly conniving with a child or being officially introduced by a child who, for one reason or another, begged for his admission. A compromise solution was found to avoid hurt and he was enrolled in one of the groups. Before this was done, Daniel's adjustment tendencies upward and downward were explored. In a mixed group of children of his ability and his age, he played the entertainer, sang, danced, and let the children see that he was a young man with the necessary experience. But in a group of boys of which he was the oldest he could not hold his own. He could, however, isolate himself at a dart game or at checkers with a reassuring, relatively mature youngster.

This latter group we met when we acquainted ourselves with Nathaniel. In one of the sessions the children put up a radio program which they recorded. It was flighty talk fraught with sexual ambiguities. Daniel's part in it revealed a man's exposure without a hat. He addressed a "bald headed guy" that was going to get "a lick on the head." But the stick immediately became a sex symbol and the sign of superiority.

Another day the children were boxing in an orderly fashion. Daniel made an excellent showing of himself as he did so often later on at boxing and at dart-throwing. Accidentally, a button was torn off his shirt, a factor which would have remained unnoticed but for his sudden desperate cry, "If you want to have my shirt you can have all of it," he screamed, weeping and enjoying his tears and his running nose. He had thrown the boxing gloves into the room and it seemed he was trying to tear his shirt to bits. In a powerful crescendo of excitement and suffering he stripped himself of almost all of his clothes, including his shoes and socks. The scene seemed to be staged deliberately and dramatically—the audience was in suspense. The children looked at him in amazement, sensing also his general accusation of their evil intent. It looked as though he was going to strip completely. The children were worried and embarrassed because of the presence of their female therapist. But as unexpectedly as the tempest had mounted, he brought himself under control to the point of leaving at least his underpants on. He sacrificed his passionate self-expression for decency. The writhing creature seemed to turn into a martyr.

The clothes were no longer simply "cover" and protection for his body nor were they representative of his social status. The drama was changed into a passion play. He recovered himself due to an unshakable feeling of decency, the respect of the mother and the sensitivity to the other children's fear that he might overstep the limits. He was no longer afraid primarily for himself. In spite of Daniel's anxious expectation of the contrary, and the obvious hostility of the aroused group, his tantrum did not hurt his physical and personal integrity. On the contrary, it restored both by an attitude which alerted him to his behavior as seen through the eyes and in the judgment of a beholder. The group had assumed the function of the healer, not the destroyer. In so doing it had experienced its own purifying catharsis. As involved observers of the dramatic performance they had partaken of Daniel's sufferings and were terrified by its manifestations; they were so deeply touched that through the weeks and months they brought up the subject repeatedly and obviously were struggling with their own responsibility. The profoundly impressive drama had also its epilogue on the day of its occurrence. Daniel called back to the fold by the other children's silent astonishment began to talk to them with the therapist as an audience and, still deeply stirred up, he shared his experience and justified his behavior. He felt no longer singled out and superior by suffering. He was no longer arrogant. He realized he could not regain his infantile innocence and was no longer an innocent child. He accepted being covered by his "figleaf" as a little man, driven out of the paradise of infancy to struggle in the sweat of his brow.

For weeks Daniel behaved perfectly adequately until, two weeks after the previously reported episode, the following observation was made.

The children were as frequently anxious, aggressive, and dependent at the beginning of a session. Daniel had appeared in his Sunday apparel and kept his hat on. When the children had calmed down, Marvin triggered a new unrest. He took Daniel's hat off with the result that he screamed as though someone had cut off a part of his body. Marvin, who usually pinpointed a person's vulnerable spot, sensed that Daniel felt exposed without his hat—uncovered or even naked, as once before. Avid for an intense excitement at Daniel's expense, Marvin suggested with irony that he strip himself of his clothes. Marvin, who was intensely jealous and hostile in his jealousy, knew well that he exposed the therapist to the predicament of taking sides in view of the possible imminent divestment. The therapist, however, simply assumed an attitude which could represent support to Daniel in order to attenuate the sensed danger and give him strength to defend himself. It was hoped also that the children themselves would take care of the situation. Daniel anticipated more partiality than could reasonably be expected. Holding his genitals as though to protect them, he shouted at the psychiatrist that she had deserted him. All the children saw his gesture and took it for granted. He also started coughing intensely for a few moments and to feel like vomiting.

While he was crying and shouting, he complained about the social worker, saying he had counted on him for changing everything but nothing had happened. When he noticed that he had inadvertently given away the deeper reasons for his agitation, he added, "nothing has changed in the Center." At home everything was fine and he is going to tell his mother. Then he sat down and indulged himself in a good cry and peeved pose.

Marvin considered Daniel's crying as an incontinence and explicitly stating it in his own terms, he brought up the subject of enuresis. This had been, in the past, one of his own problems. The therapist had been sitting opposite Daniel and near him. The children now closed a circle around us. Johnny Samuels who had also a problem of enuresis joined last, but did not reveal in any way that his own problem was under discussion. Marvin appeared to feel sorry for having hurt Daniel so severely and seemed to be identifying with his painful embarrassment. But he was not capable of exposing himself overtly. He spoke about experiences in our summer camp last year and about those children's embarrassment who wet their bed. He spoke at great length about their various futile attempts to hide their weakness. He was anticipating this summer's experiences and trying to give the once painful problem a humoristic note. The children could not figure out any reasons for a child's habit to wet the bed. Marvin was the great talker. He first mentioned drinking too much. Quite spontaneously this lead them back to the subject of childishness and childishness was associated with feeding. The children spoke about Theodore and his brother who were big candy eaters and at night raided the ice-box at camp. Marvin's jealousy blew up again and he wondered why I gave Theodore's brother the privilege to attend camp in summer. Because he was not enrolled in day-care, Marvin was not aware of the fact that he, too, was a patient of the Center.

To recuperate their manhood, the children began to box, with the exception of Daniel. Nathaniel caused the table to fall over, trying to shirk a blow and the children called him a sissy like Daniel. But they corrected themselves immediately calling Daniel a baby. Nathaniel commented, "at least I can take a defeat without crying like Daniel." He then took a drawing out of his pockets, his storehouses for surprises and treasure troves. He handed it to me. It showed a girl behind whom a boy was kneeling. He said he drew it and defied everybody to draw as well as he could. Johnny laughed, trying to raise his status from the enuretic, motherless child he was, to the one of an independent young man. He commented dryly, that he would never kneel before a girl. Nathaniel was intimidated and denied that he had drawn the picture but felt bad about a retreat which he knew was useless anyway. He commented, "at least I can take a flop without crying like Daniel."

When the children left, Daniel was not ready to go and had to get even with the group therapist. He was mad and accepted no comfort. But talking angrily and with violent profusion he revealed how many ties to the mother the fine clothes represented to him, the hat being the most prominent token of his mature community with her and of those hours when he made her boy friend's company unnecessary.

Coming with these clothes to the Educational Therapy Center, it appeared then that he aimed at a position of similar importance and complexity with the symbolic mother. Therefore being deprived by the group, his assumed competitors, of the hat, pre-eminent symbol of the desired foremost position with the symbolic mother, represented a terrific blow.

To be the mother's companion was indeed confusing. It tore him in a number of directions. Precocious growth was the lure as well as the price to pay for the community with her. It was the condition which made him less dependent on her and was an anticipation of her dependency on him. It lead into conflict and flight from her. His dependency upon her, however, was fostered despite her desires. It simply made her a lure on all levels of his desires, with a solution for none. His flights were a means of not being bad by being bad, his way of repaying her by disquietude, his refusal to be docile "for nothing." Return was possible only if he accepted helplessness and could justify it inside himself by showing her what she is going to get.

Next day, a sashless window fell on Daniel in his home. Two staff members went to see him and to assist the disarmed mother get him to the hospital for the minor surgery that was necessary to close a superficial gap under his chin. The intensity of regressive defenses used by Daniel and the mother's way of coping with her son's behavior was noted. She either bribed or threatened him. When our workers arrived, he sat on a stool, squeezed in between the range and the washing machine. There was no evidence that this behavior was due to shock resulting from the accident. In the hospital he acted up violently and soiled his pants. He ran away to the Educational Therapy Center where he was calm and slightly dependent. As a rule, however, the mother could be trusted sufficiently to care for him in his dependent condition which she fostered as a more manageable one. This condition made him the stronger of the two and made her dependent on his feeling "better."

We learned from the sessions that Daniel was not devoid of ego strength. When he broke out and exploded, he showed, it is true, violence of emotion. But he had spoken the truth about himself when, in his initial interview he said: "You know I would not do anything desperate." But his strength did not consist only in the capacity to bring about necessary release without actual dissolution or destruction.

Throughout the outburst he kept an exactly circumscribed control of himself and of the situation. He showed violence of expression, as it were an artistic power to communicate by dramatization. But this very mastery which was clearly observable gave to his outburst an element of wantonness. Doubt was aroused whether his performance was unavoidable. His use of the group seemed due less to an obsession than an indulgence in temptation, a self-propelled gratification by acting out in transference the despair against the mother. It had been nurtured on all levels of development finally to reach towering heights. But he also had learned to love and to respect. It is his transferred respect and love of the mother and his respect of his little audience consisting of his other selves that set a limit to what he dared. It tied him to the reverence for intangible values. *It is reverence for what exceeds us which refers us back again to our own status.* Daniel also protected the future man from a dangerous sense of grandeur when he did not claim an invulnerability which was not his condition.

Though we could not overlook the creative elements inherent in Daniel's behavior, we could evidently not permit it to go on. In final analysis it was a stagnant procedure and possibly depleting. Each time Daniel felt "better," he was aware not only of the limits inherent in his existence but in his actions and the procedure used in defending himself. But the lesson had eternally to be learned anew from start. He never gained a higher platform for a wider outlook and a newly consolidated insight. His distress was constantly nurtured at home, it is true, but also fostered by himself. At the climax of his suffering which was also the climax of gratification, he was not amenable to help. Suffering, however, became also a self-chosen road to redemption. It enhanced him to a point where he could grant comfort to his parental figures. He was master of the situation at the period of upheaval and for the duration of truce.

Thus he became his own redeemer and his elders' comforter at will. Daniel was in great danger of aiming at an arrogant solution and in psychiatric terms of developing paranoid traits. That he used the group as a means to his ends was most understandable, but it also pointed to further danger of usurpation and presumption. We could see but disadvantage to the other children in this kind of test of the metal they were made of.

We felt assured that it was untherapeutical to let Daniel "die" again and again for "rebirth." Instead we saw the need for support of permanent survival. We intensified his therapy with a reassuring fatherly therapist who could not be exploited for the triggering of a pseudo-suicide in view of an ever repeated real or transferred lashing out at a traumatic mother. As evident, the mother at home had to be assisted not to go on hurting and exposing herself to hurt.

At this time Daniel is learning to renounce the concrete and absorbing "possession" of people indiscriminately. He is learning to trust tokens of a less immediate and tangible nature or in other terms to consummate symbolic relationships. Renunciation and the implied liberation from the obsessive fascination of a single unobtainable object, result in the freedom to choose among the rich offerings of life that beckon to him; as the seasons advance, he can harvest the fruit he chose to sow. Renunciation could be achieved in this case due pre-eminently through the help of his male therapist and the supervisor as mother figure.

That the phasic elements of these relationships could be accepted by the boy was due to the fact that each real contact was fully gratifying and edifying. It is evident that the boy's dependency needs had to be met. But the quality of the indulgence eliminated the need for it, thus fostering spontaneous maturation. Insight necessarily is based on great sensibility. The resulting accuracy of the marking as well as the delicacy of the application elicit satisfaction, in other words, fulfilment. The mutuality of the experience of both child and therapist is therefore completed and temporarily overcome. Separation of both partners to the experience is not only possible but necessary. The completed experience is in the process of being integrated separately by each individual partner. Until full independence is reached, the child moves phasically toward the gratifying object for replenishment and releases it when replenishment is completed. We attribute importance to the fact that Daniel was given assistance by a couple of parental figures. This was fitting to his emotional condition in disharmony with his state of chronological development. We admit that such a therapeutical constellation may not be an absolute prerequisite for success. It is certainly an opportunity for its promotion. Daniel thus was not weaned abruptly from dependency on a maternal figure nor from his need to reach out for immediate reassurance here and there. At this state of development, a renewed and exclusive dependency on a primary love object would have seemed an unnecessary and therefore harmful indulgence. What he needed was support of existing strength and the tendency to grow, that is, help was necessary in recognizing and developing his more sublimated needs and in learning to distribute selectively his tendency to relate. The therapeutic parents were complementary by gender and qualities; this contributed to the differentiation of his needs, to the anticipation of specific responses and to the determining of whom to turn to and how to proceed. Such a choice implied delay and the use of time as a means to implement his purpose "wisely."

We understand why prior to treatment Daniel could not reach the same liberating phasic relationship with the mother and why he had to sit at home waiting and pouting to fill the hours of boredom. The mother was simply fulfilling an eternally uncompleted duty. She was trapped with the child. As a by-product of her existence he was tended to from its fringes and not as a constituting element of her life, inherent to its whole. The non-specificity of her casual attention, which fettered her, kept him "wanting." Moreover, she was his only love object. There was no one else to reach out for in the home.

Enabled to renounce the mother's constant material presence, Daniel is freed to reach out for answers to needs that are no longer silenced by his constricting possessiveness. Natural growth can now take its course as well as healthy experience in relating. Life in its reality aspects can now be discovered, understood, accepted, and enjoyed. "Pain says: pass away. But all delight yearns deep deep eternity." Satisfying experience for the sake of its survival must be detached from the fetters of concreteness, and the mere fact and time of its birth. It is permeated by conceptualization and codified by language. It is available to recall and lends itself to being endowed with "deep deep eternity." Thus joy becomes a main vehicle of experience, of the deepening of experience, and of differentiation and individualization of experience. With joy as a conveyance of experience, challenges can be met and mastered, self-assurance and self-confidence can be gained. No more sampling of support ubiquitously will be required or as it were reliance on statistics which is relative and conveys no certitude. No experience can be final. Collecting and counting goes on.

Daniel overcame his promiscuity at an early stage of treatment and soon related with intensity. Very different is the child who relates through the detour of role-playing and promiscuous narcissistic exhibitionism on an imaginary stage. The children talk to one person and seem to ignore everybody else, but they speak as though for a big audience. In our experience, this is the case of neglected motherless girls before their teens. They imitate, almost ape their foster mothers and make the pathetic impression of wizened, precocious little women. An exaggerated display of importance overcompensates their sense of being negligible. In the initial stage of therapy, they tend to reverse the patient-therapist relationship. A deep dependency relationship in therapy is necessary, intensely gratifying and not easily given up. Other children need guidance lest they carry the burden of the past in a confusing way into the new outlook. The tendency must be overcome to interpret unrealistic dreams not come true as disappointments inflicted specifically upon them by a mischievous fate. It is their fruitless way of displacing an appetite for hurting and being hurt.

We need to return for a few moments to the other children of this group. They, too, needed help in understanding, to the extent that they were capable, the meaning of the dramatic events of the last session as well as their particular role on the stage of events.

The children, however, were not yet sufficiently united as a group to discuss it together in the next session. But, as mentioned, they were preoccupied with the implications of the events and repeatedly brought them up later. At this time Johnnie Richard was moving and playing in the group, brave and successful at surviving. He related mainly to the mother figure, who was felt as gratifying. She knew how to draw him into the group by a casual appeal to his self-centered interests. Thus, introverted preoccupation was shared with others. For survival he still had to ward off disturbances of almost any kind and therefore he tended to withdraw. But shyly and slyly he would stand in a corner sending darts into a doll's body lying close at his feet.

Charles Lofton and Johnny Samuels were actively testing real interaction but were still cautious. Charles was not ready to review the situation and tended to escape. He was beginning to act out and had no use at the moment for reasoning and collecting new inhibitions when he was barely shedding the old ones. Johnny was on guard lest anybody intrude upon the sacred altar he had erected for his mother in the most secret recesses of his being. He alone had been at her deathbed to alleviate her agony and to be with her to the very last. But he was already sending out first tendrils of affection and stepping toward exploring life. Interest in learning by experience was awakening; he was no longer intensely menaced. His mind could be seen silently at work.

Marvin, the catalyst of Daniel's outbursts, felt guilty and was ubiquitously projective. This was his usual defense or rather his way of living. He would open the box which held the boat model on which he was still working. Without even looking at it, he would accuse someone of having taken a part of the model and, as usual, the accusation proved unwarranted. The therapist would come over to him, lay her arm around his shoulders to give him a feeling of wholeness and security and talk very softly to him, asking him in simple terms why he felt so exposed and why he feared the children who loved him as well as did the grown people. He once gave as an answer an instance where another child had accused him wrongly. He looked impressed when the therapist simply responded: "Now, then you know how it feels." Without being able to help it, Marvin repeated his unwarranted accusations on several occasions in this session. Nobody paid any attention to him. But Marvin became aware of his behavior simply because he sensed the therapist's awareness of it. He tried to bring the impulse under control. When he thus had exposed repeatedly his irrational sense of being deprived of part of what belonged to him, the therapist wondered out loud whether this was how Daniel felt when his precious hat was taken from him. Marvin looked sad and uneasy. "Maybe we better protect him from hurt in the future," she said affectionately, encouragingly, and with a certain lightness, indicating that between the two of them they would not find it too hard to do.

The situation was discussed singly, with Nathaniel and Johnny Samuels as observers. Nathaniel had felt attacked and wanted to coin, at least for a short moment, this alleged attack into the advantage of getting pity and attention. But spontaneously he stopped, too gratified by what he had already to test the situation in a greedy way and by excess of demands risk loss rather than gain. He knew that he had made a contribution to Daniel's distress.

Marvin's own mutilation anxiety stemmed from his insecure position with his mother who could not sever her ties to a brutal, alcoholic stepfather. His behavior in day-care and observations in group therapy showed his urge to expose children with problems similar to his own and to observe serenely their explosion as well as their relief; and he revealed to us that he gained temporary relief as an audience to a dramatic event. As a spectator he was interested, happily fascinated, felt comfortable and superior. He commented on his observations or interpreted them. Deprived of such an opportunity he suffered from a kind of abstinence symptom. This discomfort, sensed for instance by Marvin as the stage director in the absence of Daniel, his main tragic actor, was further stimulated by guilt feelings. These in turn had thrived more readily on the soil of want. He felt bad because he missed Daniel for interaction as well as for having excluded him. His sense of loss was displaced on the objects of his playful activities which were part of him. For these delusional losses, he needed causes in the objective sphere where they were located. Thus, he accused children anonymously. Marvin also still needed to project his guilt feelings. But at least he could benefit by help on which, however, at the time of this writing he was still dependent.

Daniel's case was produced to give an account of why, in a special instance, a child might fail to benefit from group therapy at a certain period of his development. It also shows the resources of a day-care program. The child could go on fostering his nascent relationship with the Clinic as a whole and be relieved through acting out how he felt. He could be helped to renounce for his benefit an element of the total milieu and accept, though at first with hesitation, the profusion of all of its other offerings. For the whole remained constant and rewarding. There was no devastating loss of love, nor loss of qualification for inclusion in the small community he began to cherish. As time went on, the boy's male therapist became more and more desirable and the relationship more enhancing of his self-esteem. It helped Daniel find his soundings within himself. Meanwhile he received warmhearted and understanding support as well as guidance from a purposeful maternal woman. Due to her permanent availability, the breaking down of frustration tolerance could be obviated as long as waiting for the absent love object was a serious problem. Though going through numerous circuitous paths, the child finally loses interest in a sadomasochistic interplay in his relationship with an unshakably poised, reassuring and edifying parental figure. The comforting relationship was not allowed to become so deep that survival would depend on it and competition with the other children in the day-care group would become intolerable. Daniel could be allowed to "float" within the day-care group until he found himself sufficiently involved with its program, the children and the teachers and to ease into it with an increasingly strong and confident investment.

At the time of this writing the child's mother has made great strides in her own purposefulness and the consistency of her line of conduct. She has moved again but with the difference that she has found adequate quarters that will give her enough time to search for a home she is on the verge of purchasing. She has in mind particularly to endow Daniel with a place for him to root and from which to expand.

## Indications for and against Group Therapy

Children referred back to us, after a stage in the mental hospital or the industrial school, who had been subjected to group therapy successfully, will be treated in the group in the Clinic as well. The treatment is preceded by an initial interview for exploration of the youngster's acceptance of this treatment device and the change of approach, if formerly he had been in individual therapy. He may yearn to return to it, attributing all of his progress or of his potential progress to the therapeutic relationship. He may have outgrown it. If not, evaluation is made if a temporary indulgence in the regression, which may be expressed by the desire for individual therapy, or valid needs of a mature order for a return to individual therapy shall be met. Equipped with the information on the children's previous traumatizations and behavioral attitudes, on the test results, and a child's attitude and communication during the initial interview, we are usually ready to evaluate which mode of therapy to choose, individual or group therapy. We can determine at this point with whom the child feels safer, that is, with whom does he feel protected from his own hostility or from outside menace; is it the adult male or female, is it the peer group? Are the menaces sensed as forbidding or can the child be exposed to one or the other method for his benefit, when the method of first choice is not available and immediate help is essential? If the child's inclination is toward the group, what are his motives? Only the avoidance of the adult and the seeking of refuge with similarly minded or complementary peers? Is it the need to seek for catalysts of aggressive behavior? Is it the impulsive or obsessive urge for displacement of hostility on sibling figures? What is the intensity of the need? Are the hostile tendencies, violent as they might be, attention-getting and bids for love?

We must be ready for surprises at all times. Though we may be aware of the fact that a withdrawn child uses the group as a release of his pressing pent-up emotions, he might suddenly break down the wall that loomed between him and the world with unexpected violence. Rather than sensitized as we may have feared, the children in the group may be extremely tolerant and forgiving. They may defend themselves adequately; they may empathize. The immunity in the face of the upheaval may not be due to lack of feeling but was built up as a *potential* strength stimulated in a menacing environment. Due to lack of support, however, it could not come to fruition and be used. Sometimes such adequacy is the child's positive reaction to the consistency of acceptance and the poised reactions to all of the children's modes of expression, a consistency and a poise which were lacking in a home not devoid of its positive aspects. The latent potential then is brought to life when the circumstances demand it and when the resorting to one's resources is promising. Like all real heroes the children perceive the danger and show their anxiousness when the outburst occurs.

They may be guarded in the next session, but in the third session they may be fully reassured by the support to all children alike of the strengthening of their positive defenses by which they braved the outburst and the resulting sense of adequacy. At times the upset child needs however to be eliminated from the group. At other times the child is simply seen by himself, a varying number of times before the next group psychotherapy session. Additional individual psychotherapy may be taken up again for an extended period along with the continued group psychotherapy.

Contrary to what one would expect, the children may show acceptance of the child that discharged his pent-up hostility in so violent a manner. Neither do they necessarily ostracize nor display anxious submissiveness. When Marilyn thus exploded one time in the little group of four in which she was treated, she insisted upon being returned to the group. She must, she said spontaneously, and would prove herself in the future. Lilly tended her a hand silently like an affectionate miniature mother. It was evident she had a positive transference to Marilyn. She wanted Marilyn back, the image of her own mother. Harsh or loving she was still longed for. At that time Lilly felt closer to Marilyn than to the therapist. She could be made to verbalize her feelings. Marilyn seemed more real to her and therefore could be trusted more. Marilyn was less menaced by fear of failure and of loss of love in her relationship to Lilly than in the relationship to the therapist.

Small agencies such as child guidance clinics, because of the great demands made on them, are not always able to offer the most suitable answer at the very moment it should be available. At times, children are not very promising therapeutic material. They may not be able to relate to either a paternal or maternal figure in individual therapy nor be able to endure the pressures coming from a therapeutic group.

This was actually the case with Marilyn. But in offering her the group at her ardent request, the individual therapist was sensed as understanding and rewarding, which produced a positive carry-over to the individual sessions. The privilege of individual attention which she kept as a hoarded secret alleviated her hostile competitiveness in the group and therapy could be carried on. She slowly stopped holding on by her teeth and biting the therapist and became loving.

As mentioned, we may be confronted with the necessity to decide between refusal to treat or the offering of a female psychiatrist to children who have a deep-seated problem with the mother on all developmental levels and do not qualify for group psychotherapy because they are too menaced or too menacing. In attempting a treatment rather than refusing it, we found that excessive anxiety could be overcome in the case of children who had never had the slightest foothold on adult support and therefore by anxious anticipation of further rejection had caused their peers to react rejectingly in school. The decision concerning the approach has to be dictated by discriminate and sensitive evaluation of the family interaction and an equally sensitive and versatile correlation of the work of the Clinic. The day-care milieu may be of invaluable help. Exposed in day-care are not the withdrawn children predominantly, but those who passively solicit or actively provoke angry reactions. By appropriate reactions anxiety will be attenuated. What remains is the need to be angry. The child that was taken into day-care as an emergency, usually at the request of the public schools, normally calms down in the Clinic within days. By then he knows all staff members. The initial interview is made wherever possible as a prerequisite to entrance, but tentative acceptance of an emotionally disturbed child who would be unguarded in the street is necessary at times when the psychiatrist's time cannot be made available for a few days. Tentative acceptance is based on a written case history and in the case of the public schools and the court, also on a psychological test. In a few cases of ubiquitous anger the child must be left alone, as it were, to exist in day-care until he finds in the adult an element of support that he increasingly seeks. He may be ready for therapy. When he has shown whether he tends to look for comfort with a male or female figure, we shall decide to whom to assign him. This decision may or may not be in terms of what he has asked for. But considering the relevance of his day-care (teacher) attachment, a complementary parent figure may be offered in therapy. Obviously we shall evaluate whether the child's immediate need for being mothered or, on the contrary, for reaching more independence needs to be gratified and by what form of staff interaction, and whether the child longs for or tolerates a twosomeness or whether he feels protected from too much attention in a small group.

## *"Talent is Shaped in Silence; character in the Gushing World"*

We could observe, through the months, the progress in psychotherapy of a mixed open group consisting of an average of four verbally communicative and socially inviting adolescents. These young girls and boys attended high school or junior high school and were not enrolled in day-care. Three of the five original members had been exposed to individual psychotherapy. For the sake of condensation we refrain here from giving the individual members' background and their earlier therapeutic development at length and the group dynamics in detail. We should like to mention only the main protagonists of this phase in therapy, a boy and a girl of the struggling classes. To quote the intelligent girl herself, the parents were the people who do the menial jobs to get their children through college. The parents of both of the young people were working: the fathers eighty hours a week, holding two jobs and "picking up" small jobs on the side. Both mothers were working full time, the boy's mother as a high-class secretary, the girl's mother at a job far below her mental capacity and social ability. The girl's mother indulged in drinking sprees with her sisters. She disappeared off and on for a few days. The girl, Corine Landis, was very ambivalent in her relationship to the mother and swayed between incestuous love for her which was imbued with a profound oral dependency, and a rejection of the mother with concomitant sympathetic identification with the father. The attitude alternated with rare and short periods of hostility and more frequent stages of apparent neutrality in her relationship with him. When "the father" or a special "father" was attacked in the group she went always to his rescue. Intelligent and intellectual in mental structure, she used these capacities as her defenses in the group. At the time of intake she functioned far below her mental abilities, but when she joined the group she was her best self in respect to studying and had been offered a science scholarship. The boy, Carol Pettis, was the contended son of a tense and suspicious man, compulsive and constantly on the verge of exploding. His wife had as little time for him as he for her. In addition to working full time, she had returned to study at a college, in the evening. She had influenced all of her children against her husband. Our patient was extremely involved with the mother when treatment started. He had liberated himself to some extent from the excess of his involvement with her but not yet from his hostility against the father. He was tired and suffered from revealing psychosomatic symptoms. The father scared him. Carol said he was taller than the father, but the father was broader and stronger and Carol was no match for him. If they could talk on even terms they would not have to fuss all the time. The more "fat" his father loses, the more Carol would get used to him and one day they may get together. The father on the other hand could not conceal the rejection of the boy. He doubted that he was his son. Carol still retorted by catering to his mother exclusively and fleeing the house as long and as often as possible. He, too, assuaged his disquietude by escaping into excessive work. At the time of referral Carol seemed on the verge of a psychotic disintegration. He related with excessive ease, was seen dependent and spoke incoherently without restraint. He talked constantly in a nagging aggressiveness. Without being aware of it, he told of his own experiences as though he had seen them in the movies and failed to recall or recognize them as his own. He brought me his short stories to read which, though extremely revealing, were loosely put together. His work in school was far below his standards, but in school and in therapy he displayed excellent artistic ability. Whatever he touched, even a few broken remnants of toys, he shaped into an abstract but aesthetically valid whole. This he did while talking, whether in individual or later in group therapy. He was always emotionally high-keyed. He considered himself a great hit with the girls and raved about all of them. Only when the group was formed did we become aware of the fact that the two, Carol and Corine, had been friends for years. They were apparently extremely fond of each other and very affectionate. They used each other for protection from real involvements of whom both were intensely afraid. In the early days of the group treatment Carol attempted to out-talk everybody else.

One of the two new members introduced to the group was these two young people's own concern. They considered the group their own, their club for helping each other. This was their own spontaneous attitude. They started out with violent aggression against their parents, considering that the parents' failure to protect and instruct them had promoted their own problems, that they would have liked to do better and could have succeeded with proper parental guidance, attention, and companionship. They resented the parents' ambitions and value system. But they were obviously proud of the parents' home ownership, though they also complained of their enslavement by debts and bills. They soon brought the school and the society structure into their discussions and at one time wanted to have a similar club in their public school. This was the reaching out for parental guidance from this symbol of society and their desire to display their adequacy on a wider forum than the Clinic. They spoke with considerable intelligence and knowledge. But soon they were concerned about themselves though not yet ready to face the problems within themselves. They needed the medium of representative figures. They began to talk about a friend of theirs, Susan Cherry, whom they considered in serious need of therapy. Her total downfall or breakdown had to be prevented, they said. Why she needed help was explained in an excited manner which amounted to an indulgence in fantasy about all the dangers from which Susan had to be saved. The young people became contrite about it and decided that help, not slander, was indicated. They became aware of the fact that they had lost their goal of helping themselves. Corine Landis had talked to Susan's mother whom she knew. A few years earlier, this lady had made an ambivalent attempt to bring us her eldest daughter but never followed through. The eldest daughter was still a problem. Therefore, she decided to bring us Susan, being aware of the great progress made by Corine. Susan's mother was her elderly husband's "baby." The same role was ascribed to Susan. Competition between mother and daughter was extreme, and, by her own behavior, Susan exaggerated the mother's characteristics to the point of being a delightful caricature of her. Susan was utterly regressed and unpredictable; she acted silly and irrational. She had unusual charm, a sense for the grotesque and seemed to capitalize on these attributes to the extreme. Contrary to the expectation that she would be unmanageable, Susan soon became a contributing member of the group, affectionate with the therapist, and a most fair-minded young girl. She verbalized her problems with the home with more obvious reluctance than Carol but, though her family problems were as involved as Corine's, her reactions to them were not as profound as Corine's. By regression, she protected herself from suffering.

A new emergency case was shortly brought to our attention. Minnie Jennings, a young orphan and a long-standing concern of the city welfare, had at one time been committed to the state for her uncontrollable behavior. The same attitude had prevailed upon her return and, to express her despair about what she considered undue rigidity of the foster home, she had made a pseudo-suicidal attempt. Minnie was found not to be in a serious emotional condition but simply in need of overcoming some adolescent adjustment difficulties. She was intelligent and serious. She had undergone individual psychotherapy in the industrial school. Change of environment was recommended by us and most successfully carried out by the city welfare. Minnie was taken into the group of Carol, Corine, and Susan, pending discussion with its existing members. Although nothing about the girl's background was revealed, the young people had found out everything about her "through the grapevine" in school with the result that Corine and Carol became disturbed by fantasies about her assumed bisexual promiscuity and both approached her by phone or at school. (We do not forbid outside contacts. Many of our patients could not be expected to comply, either because of hostility and resistance to rules or because such interdiction would represent only one more inhibition to living and to the right of being. Moreover, since the Negro group in Richmond consisting of a population of 100,000 souls, has only two high schools and until recently only two junior high schools, many of our patients know each other.)

We deal with the problem from within the group and the child-therapist relationship. This is what brought to the group's and my attention what was going on. The three main actors of the psychological involvement went through a very complex upheaval and a crisis of distrust among them. Susan, the silly infant, was of great ego support to all three of them, as will be seen. Minnie spoke in a firm and dignified way about past errors which she did not qualify in detail. She felt that she was entitled to change and to make an adjustment because she was determined to do so. She mentioned how she was being helped and how she was trying to help herself. She considered it unfair to gain information about a person without the person's knowledge and consent and not to give that person an opportunity to defend herself. Susan supported her, probably having been exposed to the same treatment. She spoke to Carol, saying that she was sorry for him, since he was bound to be totally confused. When you ask many people you get many contradictory answers. Carol and Corine suffered seriously from their social cruelty and presumption. Corine had laid herself wide open to slander because of her narcissistic, as well as masochistic needs. She exhibited her "different" behavior at one time because she longed to succumb to it by outside pressure. Minnie in the group was a catalyst for a re-exposure of Corine's problem which she had beclouded for a time by her intellectual leadership. She revealed her problem indirectly, in a new specific light. Suddenly she announced that finally she had met the great love she had always been longing for. Most unexpectedly that alleged love was an aunt of hers; but losing track she continued to speak about her mother. In her previous discussion, in individual therapy, she had aired only her frustrating dependency needs. Now the incestuous element became evident. She asked for an individual session in which her narcissistic tendencies and the implied negative aspects of the transference could be clarified.

One problem at the time of Corine's referral was her persisting intrusion upon a female teacher who was of exactly her and the mother's very tall and slender stature. She had used this adoration of the tall and slender woman in the early stages of treatment to try to cause her therapist, who was short and not slender, to be hurt and jealous and to involve her in a sado-masochistic interaction. From time to time she fell back on discussing her urgent need to see the adored teacher or to convince her of her fine adjustment. The negative aspects of the transference also were revealed as her means of keeping the therapist out of her impulsive involvement and in harmony with her censuring conscience, in other terms, as the ideal ego she had not found so far. Her relationship had long been ambivalent and the glow of her feeling was kept under the ashes of negativistic manifestations. But Corine steadily grew in depth and resisted any test of their reliability.

Only after her intermittent individual sessions was Corine able to face her share of responsibility in the group and relieve Carol from being the scapegoat in the situation to which he had been subjected. She had been the *spiritus rector* of his spying on Minnie. He was deeply disturbed to have been a dupe of Corine, the girl whom he had trusted for so long. It affected him so profoundly that, in the group session, he held onto his therapist's hands and, laying his head on them, he confessed that he had tried so hard to straighten himself out through the seven months of his treatment that his "breakdown" would mean loss of life itself. Corine was intensely impressed. Carol seemed very much afraid of losing the therapist's love and faith in him. Both he and Corine were deeply ashamed of their social prejudices and stressed the humility of their condition rather than their "upper class" status. They were painfully aware of the betrayal not only of Minnie but of themselves and of their group purpose of mutual assistance and "rehabilitation." Minnie's absence through two sessions distressed Corine and Carol. They both had gone to her home to apologize, a fact they reported in the group. Minnie consented to come for an individual session with the therapist.

To the extent that it could be revealed in fairness, she was helped to understand the underlying self-centered meaning of the young people's vexatious behavior. She understood and admitted that all of us are in need of forgiveness and that she was going to help them by forgiving. This she did.

Carol and Corine benefited from the awareness that they had competed for the same love object and indulged in voyeuristic fantasies, being confused in their sexual identification. They discovered the meaning of their enamored friendship in reference to their problem of erotic maturation, a problem Carol sensed keenly. He told the therapist, for instance, about his relationship with a girl thirteen years old, i.e., four years younger than he. He reported self-importantly the intended stages of getting closer to her, the protection he saw in the relationship with so young and "quiet" a girl and his plans to marry her eight years later.

Having thus traversed a long road of self-recognition, having suffered from their shortcomings and their honest avowal of failure, having rejoiced in being genuinely forgiven by those who knew how much in need of forgiveness one can be, having worked to deserve forgiveness and to feel free to go on struggling, these children returned to the concern about their parents. Minnie, the only one who had none, was presently privileged by the possession of ideal foster parents. She suggested that we have family sessions. She admitted that she had nothing to fear from her parents. The others were ambivalent. They had remarked lately that their parents were not as faithful as were their children in keeping appointments with their therapists (all of them had to be seen individually, if for no other reason, than their heavy working schedule). They regretted that the parents had not struggled for improvement as they had. They agreed to a monthly session in the "family group." The three real parents knew each other well and the foster family was considered supportive of the group spirit. The children's hesitancy was caused by their conviction that the parents would be "two-faced." They would be co-operative on the surface and let the children get it at home. But they were ready to challenge their parents in an orderly discussion and to brave the consequences. The goal was a final meeting of minds between the generations.

## The Oedipal Problem

The Oedipal problem as it unfolds itself in the Educational Therapy Center is based on the vicious circle established between reality factors and emotional problems. Troubled feelings and disordered facts have prevailed throughout the children's lives. The Oedipal problem therefore is almost invariably implanted on and complicated by previous levels of disharmonious or generally interfered with libidinal development.

The problem of adolescent growth toward and strivings for self-identification and independence presumes a sufficient sense of adequacy of which these children are deprived. They face inadequacy with an empty bravado or with the various fugues of regression and stubborn adherence to helplessness or insufficiency. They are not equipped to meet the challenges or implement resourcefully, imaginatively and fruitfully those positive tendencies which are still preserved. The early or late stages of erotic maturation are not refined and made wholesome by the intangible enchantment inherent in a more inspired relationship between parent and child of the other sex.

It is in the child's cradle that the beauty of such an enchantment can begin and with it a generous and all-embracing love that includes the other parent who is reborn in the child and emulated by the younger person as the image of lovableness. Such a gracious and enchanting love begets trust rather than jealousy. It inspires mutually pleasurable relationships inside and outside the family group. It redeems crude impulses and channels libidinal enjoyment. Such consummate delight is liberating. Because of the quality and the exhilarating mood of the experience the child is free to move on to the joys of comparable quality elsewhere. Guilt feelings are not annihilating in such circumstances. Where they are sensed, they do not stand in the way of the relationship between the child and the parent of the same sex but stimulate generosity in sharing and the striving to emulate the parents' model as well as to deserve their love.

Much tending is needed. Unless the child is set in the family garden, that is, in an atmosphere where sensibility can unfold, "the earth and every common sight" will not be animated by the "freshness of a dream." The child's world will not be brightened by a glowing inner abundance that defies the will-o'-the-wisp flares of ephemeral Oedipal lures. Sensibility is not only a protection because it redeems the crude reality, but it is a guide in discerning and selecting.

In taking this view we have to realize that mere skill and a methodical approach are insufficient aids for a youngster under the impact of an Oedipal involvement raised in barren and undifferentiated surroundings.

In reviewing and reliving his life under the assistance of psycho-therapy, he needs help in the unfolding of his sensibility, the source of his power to sublimate. Obviously such an opportunity is given by any therapist who can follow his patient wherever needed without losing his own sense of direction. Such a security of the therapist rests on the pillars of basic convictions, of insight and empathy and his own strong capacity for sublimation.

But how could a psychotherapist hope to relieve a child who has been submerged by crude realities all of his life, in particular the one still grounded in the sunken caravel which is his natural home? To be sure that the therapeutic impact may have sufficient resonance to carry from session to session and hold the child in its ban, he must rely on an atmosphere, a surrounding attuned to the therapeutic relationship. The therapeutic relationship must have its own world and its own landscape to be true and more than an evanescent dream or a fairy island. To fulfil its function of inciting sublimation, the therapeutic surrounding or the milieu must be populated by a variety of grown individuals who are by education and spirit the quickening founts of the child's own resourcefulness. To be animative, each of those pa-rental images need to feel approved in his or her individuality and to be in a position to consummate joyfully the privilege of being his or her true self. Such a status implies the awareness that they can be sources of uplifting gratification and answers to real promises to the young members of the therapeutic family, or important organs in an organic whole kept alive and in harmony by the community of pur-pose. Slowly the child will grow into the organism as its homogene-ous part.

One of the most obvious symptoms of the children struggling with their Oedipal involvement is suspiciousness which is transferred to the Clinic milieu. They interpret behavior and relationships in light of their jealousy and competitiveness, and see forbidden sex relationships everywhere. They spy on every newcomer in particular and attack him as a potential rival either overtly or on the sly or both.

When he begins to trust his therapist and the milieu, the child will tend to manipulate both for gain of support. The loyal coherence of the total staff and their impartial loyalty to the child will help him raise his standards of expectancy in reference to assistance and the idea of trustworthiness. These standards for the sake of love and admiration, for the sake of filiation and self-respect, the children will try to emulate.

The milieu will demonstrate by a living experience that one can hold a gratifying position with attuned parental figures; and in psychotherapy the child will be enlightened specifically about what he is trying to do. Against the uplifting elements of the therapeutic background in day-care the undesirable elements of his defenses will be more apparent and clarification will be facilitated. It is more likely that he will bring up the discussion himself at some time or another. He will be supported in his new tendency to search for more realistic issues than concentrating all of his efforts on being the parents' sole owner against his or her will. Most children learn in the milieu and the intensely gratifying psychotherapeutic relationship to consider other people's needs and enjoy the gain in one's humanity which it presumes.

A special effort by the total milieu is needed to help the child with the dissonance between his hurry to grow and its refusal. The boy wants to be the mother's provider but is too anxious and weary to implement his ambitions by the slow, stepwise process of becoming academically or technically competent. Under the impact of anxiousness and incompetence, he resorts to stealing. Or, another may hate his parents and obstruct their supportive unity. Since their delinquent acts have multiple determinations from all levels of libidinal deprivation and being substitutes for them, a review in depth of such children's lives is necessary and symbolic realization[8] in psychotherapy may benefit from support of their immediate and concrete needs in day-care. In certain instances intense therapeutic or organizational endeavors are needed to prevent parental interference with the process of recovery.

Slowly the child will have risen through self-scrutiny and exploration of relationships and mutual obligations, to a state where failure causes first qualms of conscience and where the alternative is recognized of either indulging in the anxieties inherent to temptation or accepting the cure of braving the assuming of responsibilities.

At this stage psychotherapy must be ego-supporting, though understanding. At the time a person has discovered his conscience, he is at the crossroad and the decision to move into the open and away from a dead-end road requires valor. The child's first expression of independence, however, will be his will to indulge temptation and the gratification of his "sinful" interaction with his mother. He challenges the therapist by his refusal of him or her as a parental image, and the responsibilities inherent to such an acceptance. He may express simultaneously the fear of being devoid of an anchorage which would point beyond his present and past condition and he may voice the assurance that to revolutionize his nature would be futile. But in revealing how he feels, how he doubts and how he revolts, he also learns to see in himself the struggling human being that he is and learns to believe in it.

We attempt to strew the child's path with opportunity for self-fulfilment through an intense and uplifting joy which will supercede the need of grabbing for crude matter outside, matter that resists fulfilling its function of substituting for a mother's love throughout the years.

When the child climbs on the ladder of joyful self-fulfilment to achievement and adequacy, the way itself and progressing will have become enchanting. The enchantment calls for full consummation. Rushing has ceased. The child picks the day, his very own day. School no longer is an obstacle to providing for and possessing the mother. He may be heard to say optimistically to another child, "I have only three more years and I'll be out of school."

## The Asocial and the Antisocial Child in Therapy

Individual psychotherapy at the Educational Therapy Center is by intention not different from the usual practice. Therefore, we avail ourselves of the usual procedure where possible. Deviation from it is necessary with the whole variety of uncommunicative children, the asocial as well as the antisocial ones. In reference to the latter, Aichhorn[9] led the way when he indicated and let the child in therapy know that verbal communication was not compulsory. Insistence on releasing "secrets" by verbal communication would only give the child the awareness that he is empowered to deny it. What he retains thus gains in importance as does the need to conceal and withhold. Rather than being loosened, his verbal costiveness is tightened. His resistance and his angry responses in terms of experienced denial of gratification and rigid enforcement of co-operation are encouraged.

Therefore, therapy in the milieu as well as in individual therapy consists at first in helping the child feel he is in his own room where he may tend to have his own peculiar revelatory or concealing order.

We have no experience with a child who was what might be called antisocial in reference to himself, that is, so self-defiant and self-punitive or self-deprecating that he would want only to disorganize his *own* symbolic room to the point of causing his own disorganization or disorientation, nor to the point of producing unbearable filth. We have had no child who would wantonly ransack the room for fear of loss of ownership of the toys, promise and source of joy, life and growth which also is a promise of power, or wantonly annihilate his compartment in the world for fear of losing the parent who protects him and whom he can fight as the source of all discomfort. Tantrums, which are relatively rare occurrences, are instances of such utter distress that they have a suicidal connotation and the target is everywhere and nowhere, the hitting everywhere being exhausted before the child wakes up to the futility of hitting nowhere.

To make the "room" his own and not the therapist's, the child may stress how your order of things in it differs from his. Objects, therefore, should have no assigned place; they must be allowed to be discarded, pushed around, destroyed or preserved at the child's whim in support of his defiant self-image. Objects that represent the other person, child or adult, may be allowed to be slightly damaged. But if the child is allowed to be himself, to be at war or at peace with himself, in the presence of adult equanimity, the need for self-assertion by antagonism is lost. He can live for the sake of living and in living he is bound to find in time solutions that fit the purpose of self-fulfilment by the same methods that helped to bring self-fulfilment to the adult, the one whom he could observe as well as adults in general, the ones with whose requirements he is familiar. Order no longer is synonymous with command. It becomes the helper called in by the child to liberate him from the interference by unruly matter with his important pursuits. Increasingly tolerant and aware of the benevolently impartial eye of the adult observer, the child will notice that in a disorderly place he cannot find what he needs for play. Formerly his needs were unspecific and, an emotional and mental nomad, he let himself be solicited by any excitation, at best absorbing it and by mere absorption, exhaust and annihilate its unseen potentials for stimulation. Where there is no purpose, order is not conceivable and has no function unless for the sake of self-assertion against adult coercive orders. It therefore obtains a purely negative connotation. Not listening and refusing to speak, therefore, is the safest means to resist.

The proper kind of a community between the child and parental figures has "regulating" function. The child sees his actions reflected by adult observation and by sensed or actual interpretation. He becomes naturally aware of his purposelessness. The child who has not yet discovered his need for order because he can be easily distracted from his purpose or who evades the burden of being purposeful by allowing himself to be distracted when the pursuit of a goal becomes onerous can be guided by a simple question: "Weren't we looking for the other Indians? They are waiting for a good fight." "Are the dollies not going to be hungry if we give up cooking for them?"

The child may look up to you in a friendly convinced attitude or displaying no emotions, he still may show a tendency to proceed. The therapist may comment "Let's look for the pan. Next time we won't have to look for it if we remember where we put it." When the meal is over, washing the dishes and putting them away is part of the fun in common. The therapist might be wondering where objects like dishes, cups, and saucers would look most attractive or mention the child's appealing arrangement of things in the cupboard if she can take praise. To do things in common means to be with the child or watch the child while he does it, make a token supportive gesture or a helpful comment. Exceptionally the adult may play actively with a child in view of a common purpose and the child's ego support.

A child's harmonious development in education or treatment is not invariably progressive and a step-by-step procedure. While progress is indeed built up on established foundations,[10] in the miraculous ways of moving life these steps must not be conceived in terms of mechanics and rigid architecture. Progress in one area may hang in mid-air unbuttressed until, solicited by its need to be buttressed, another mental or emotional "organ" grows to its support. The overgrowth of the first area of development may become unnecessary and recede due to the reciprocity of the "parts" in a living organism.

The antisocial, the rejected child or the one abused by self-centered parental interaction has been exposed to interference with his harmonious growth. Therefore, he has to rely for his existence on continued support which however continues to be supportive of distorted growth and adverse to wholeness and liberation. The child therefore revolts violently against discomfort. When sufficient health tendencies are preserved or can be promoted in the child, the therapist may enter in a complementary interaction with the child which promotes the inherent tendency of every organism to restore its entity at every stage of development.[11]

By the therapist's subtle and alert responsiveness, the child feels encouraged to yield to a new symbiosis, as it were, that tends to be homogeneous to the child's integrative tendencies. Feeling necessarily the comfort of becoming whole or of being "healed," the child is alerted to his state of existence, and well-being will be associated with the one who is connected with it. But in the process of developing, he becomes also slowly aware that "the one" is also "the other one." Discomfort arises again, manifested by a state of restlessness, wariness or even suspiciousness. Sensitized to and afraid of renewed heterogeneous interference, he offers as a defense or as a test a rejecting and obstructing behavior. Appropriate help will be based on the insight of the child's reasons for the apparent relapse and on sensibility to the specific areas of growth which need to come to the rescue of overgrown ones. Their growth, therefore, needs to be stimulated toward the end of restoring the harmony of the parts and the attuning of their function. Success will be achieved when the child has gained comfort and trust for positive action and aggression, and when he has no further need to defend himself by obstructionism, secretiveness, and defensive aggression.

Thus, as it were, for being recognized, the child learns to acknowledge his own existence, in time following the model of his genuinely benevolent beholders. Recreated as it were in the image of man who is penetrated by the conviction of man's dignity and respect, a respect shown to him by a convinced acknowledgment of his existence, the child learns not to waste such an austere privilege. He will fight a losing battle goodnaturedly, uncomfortable, disquieted, and deeply confounded when he fails. He will talk about his struggle. Candidly he will tell you as a big conquest of his undesirable tendencies that he has "not stolen a thing since. . . ." He thus stresses his effort and optimistically sees the gain rather than the renewed failure. He reaches out for acknowledgment of success. Such an acknowledgment is sought also for relief from the pressures of his conscience and for the support of further resistance to temptation. Struggling against his resistance or opening the floodgates of communication, he tells his helper how he feels before, when, and after he fails. At this time the stage of the usual psychotherapy is reached, though some of the children may be slow in becoming demonstrative of warmth. Their attitude is still more one of a sore, bed-ridden child though not demanding of pity. He simply feels uncomfortable and helpless but secure with you. On the other hand he may go so far as to tell his helper how much he resents him or her for interfering with the profound gratification inherent to his interaction with his mother, which is symbolized by his stealing at her silent behest. On the way to such struggle by the child, with and in view of higher issues, one may be confronted with their concrete needs or desires, the predominantly symbolic connotation of which, however, must never be overlooked. It is of major importance to the child whether he knows it or not. It determines whether the child is ready for an answer to his symbolic needs alone. When he is not ready yet, it is an indication in what intangibles to wrap the realistic gratification in order to help the child become aware of the fact that things have also imponderable values. The mere presence of the supportive adult, the slight nuances in his poised warmly approving attitude and the child's growing need motivate self-expectation and make the child vulnerable to failure. The therapist must know when and how to exploit the voice of the child's growing conscience or his sense for quality and where to prevent or temper despair about failure or inadequacy lest they nurture discouragement and new regression. An early display of expectation would further regression to a punitive and demanding attitude.

It is generally recognized that relating is the first step in therapy but to relate a child must already belong to himself and be basically himself. The antisocial child is already capable of relating, a factor which is expressed by his fear and obstruction to injurious ways of relating or in other terms by his inappropriate self-help. His deepest motives for fear and obstruction are the sensed threat to his being the one he is or believes he is, must, and wants to be. Therefore, a successful prerequisite to relating is the opportunity to find the basic comfort that he will be allowed, and is allowed, to be himself as outlined.

In relating, the child overcomes both the need for obstruction and the wariness to change. In relating with delight, he gives in to and submerges himself in an ocean of love which his overflowing feelings have helped in deepening. In producing the love that he gives and receives, he is identified with those who in their poised and reliable way taught him about dedication. Like any growing child he will learn by emulation, ways of being and behaving, of discerning in the realm of facts and of decent action and to foster aspirations implemented by endeavor. Insight and realism are parallel developments where children have opportunity as in day-care to be exposed to testing insight gained in the privacy of individual or small group treatment on the forum of real life in miniature.

The asocial child is not exposed as easily as is the antisocial child to the expectation that he respond and speak. The drawbridge is up between him and the observer and a wide moat of hopelessness spreads out between them. Even on the wings of kindness you cannot reach him. You have but one hope, to wait and let the child sense you are there with no ill intent. Then your chance may come that the iron-clad little creature starved out for and allured by the tokens of attention will move over the lowered drawbridge and accept urgent gratification. If the therapist's response fits delicately the child's needs and respects sensitive areas he may slowly be admitted and sensed as being part of the child's own life. The perceptive interaction of therapist and child unfolds growth tendencies inherent to all life when tended. The child's own perceptiveness for exquisite gratifications that may lend intangible charm to minor events can be supported at a phase of treatment when the child begins to respond and is amenable to joy but is still extremely resourceless.

We have in mind an approach first used with an unusually attractive narcissistic girl, withdrawn, unresponsive, and mute. She was referred to us by the superintendent of an industrial school because of an unsusceptible muteness and seclusiveness. She had been raised by an emotionally bland and unresponsive mother and had been committed to the state welfare department because of shoplifting and the attempt (twice) to leave the home community with a stolen suitcase. Aware of her need for the comforts of infancy we would discuss her everyday experience in the light of these needs. Waking up was made the object of interest. Did she wake up spontaneously? "No!" "What woke you up, a bell, a knock?" "The housemother." A happy surprise was shown and the attention drawn to the fact that the housemother called personally. The girl was asked, "What did she say? 'Get up girls'?" Again we were pleasantly surprised and touched that not just a thing had aroused her but the housemother. We were delighted that she was so personal and said "girls." We asked how the housemother's voice sounded, sweet, warm, or harsh, and the young girl said "sweet." By questioning and using the primeaval terms of poetry residing in all mankind she was helped to notice the weather and the mood that it promoted and therefore how she felt when she had awakened. In similar terms we helped her become aware of the warm caress of the bath and she nodded relaxing her unmoved seriousness slightly. Then we enjoyed the fond gift a bath can represent and how much recognition of her needs as a person such a gift implied. Breakfast was mentioned and in speaking about food she revealed her dislike of liquid food, in particular milk.

The length of the process of expanding necessarily depends on the intensity of the withdrawal and the nature, duration, intensity, and depth of previous traumatizations as well as the adequacy of the child's present home and the security offered. When the child begins to live, he necessarily asserts himself and having to overcome the provoked and assimilated hostility, self-assertion is likely to be imbued with hostile aggressiveness usually of a silent and sly nature first. Insight, sensibility, and empathy of the therapeutic staff make the child feel safe from interference with his growing self and protected from excessive and unfriendly challenges which in requiring incessant vigilance and reactive sallies have an adverse effect on the child's growth. Motives offered for sound self-expression and self-assertion promote a sense of increasing fitness, adequacy, and strength.

An early display of expectation would arouse guardedness in an asocial child and cause him to recoil further upon himself. Thus he will be deprived of the balance of his already stunted extratensive propensities. The greatest discretion is needed, since all interference is threatening and his discriminative potentials may lay dormant. Nor will the child necessarily appear menaced where you would expect him to be. Threatened from everywhere, he has learned to close all gateways of impressionability. A small world of potential pleasurable temptations is laid out before him in the presence of a therapist sensitive to his changing needs, which include his need of the therapist's staying out of or partaking in his first approaches to life and his appraising by what gestures partaking would be permissible.

When the child meets adversaries who are attracted to him by his weakness and residual fear or if he meets them because the world is replete with defensive aggressiveness, he will for some time to come return to his helpers and rediscover his dependency on them. But he will gain not only comfort for remaining dependent but support of awakening realism and a sense of values. Even the formerly withdrawn child whose only utterances were "throwing rocks" or the one who iterated beating two toy Indians or soldiers against each other will have learned to discern between friendly and trustworthy people and those whom it would be sensible to avoid. Later he will return for visits whether in need of help or just for the pleasure of relating, for remembering or for a return to an uplifting experience. He will find a small place where he fits for work even when his innate ability is reduced.

An example of the treatment of an asocial child, Rud Martin, is given in the Appendix.

# APPENDIX

*Dynamics of Representative Case Histories*

Case illustrating the subtle grinding down of a
child's emotional soundness by the child's
parents

# Case Summary of Nancy McLead

Nancy McLead was brought to the Educational Therapy Center at the
age of eleven by a distraught stepmother. She was extremely concerned
that Nancy was stealing petty cash from her around the house or using
her milk allowance on candy, of which she seemed to have an excessive
need.

After two years of common-law marriage Nancy's stepmother had
been legally joined to Mr. McLead, an interstate truck driver and Nancy's
father. A miscarriage suffered by the present Mrs. McLead, his second
wife, and the couple's awareness that there was no hope for a child of
their own, was a profound blow to Mr. McLead's perfectionism, of which
his second wife was well aware and which caused deep anxiety in her.
His second marriage was motivated partly by the failure of his first one
and by the self-righteous resentment it had left in its wake. According
to Mr. McLead and his second wife, his first wife (Nancy's mother)
had been unfaithful to him and had lavished on her lovers the savings
he sent home during his military service. He gave her alleged behavior
as a reason for not recognizing another daughter, born during his first
marriage, despite his first wife's contention that the child was his.

As we became more thoroughly acquainted with the case, we had every
reason to doubt that his first wife had been solely responsible for the
failure of his first marriage. We also questioned at least part of the facts,
as reported by him. In fact, using the analogy of his relationship with
his second wife, as well as with Nancy, we had every reason to assume
that he was under compulsion to promote failure in his marriages in order
to prove his superiority in virtue and power. He needed submissive and
guilty females around him and he lorded it over them, though he was not
free from guilt-feelings, which, however, he projected. His second marriage was supposed to vindicate him. Since its childlessness failed to confirm its perfection and thus the anticipation that the second wife would
reward him with everything that the first one had allegedly denied him,
he tried to shift the "assets" from his first to his second marriage. He
managed to obtain custody of Nancy—a maneuver which tended to

downgrade the first marriage and lend status to the present one. Not having compensated his resentment toward his first wife by a successful second marriage, he had to deprive her of his child, the only positive result of their life in common. Since Nancy was his one gift to her, she was the only "treasure" he could take back in lieu of the money supposedly wasted.

Actually, the first wife's alleged infidelity and her carrying another man's child while they were still married was a blow to his masculinity. Therefore, he also felt profound bitterness toward his second wife because she was incapable of providing him with a demonstrable token of his virility. He penalized her by callous infidelity at a time when she was desperate, depriving both himself and her of the desired token of their community. In this present situation, Nancy, who was still living with her mother, became an invaluable jewel. The present wife lost most of her value in relation to the husband's inner scheming and the loss of the first wife became retrospectively more painful to his ego. Hating the latter for what he saw in her and wanting her for what she had to give, i.e., Nancy, he worked coldly to inflict the hardest blow he could imagine. He wooed their child by showering her with all the gifts the little girl could dream of. He became her fairy prince, as she herself put it.

Involved with a glamorous and apparently loving father, Nancy could be prevailed upon to connive with him for a night elopement by car to Richmond, secretly leaving her mother's home.

Nancy felt extremely guilty about her betrayal of the mother, whom she described as a gentle, maternal woman. The latter lived in a common-law marriage with a man, pretending without convincing Nancy, that she was legally married to him. The man, too, was described as kind, unlike her stepmother, he did not refuse to assume educational responsibilities with the children. He worked in the daytime and went to college at night. Her mother worked also and Nancy had to take care of the mother's three younger children when she returned from school. Mr. McLead's tempting gifts made her feel like Cinderella and the prince was the father whose love she ardently desired. In the mother's home she felt confined to an humble hut while her father seemed to live in a luxurious castle from which he sent his gifts and from time to time came to visit her. The privileges bestowed upon her isolated her from her siblings, in particular from the sister whom the mother claimed was Nancy's father's also but who was denied and rejected by him.

Nancy was actually kidnapped by her father. The story she told us was never denied. He obtained a warrant against his first wife, and the child was given into his custody because of the mother's alleged immorality. Nancy told how she connived with the father and the police. The latter were supposed to knock at the mother's door at a certain hour of the evening and, pretending not to know who it was, Nancy was supposed to open it; she was then led by the police to the father's car across the street and left with him for Richmond.

Nancy reached her new home full of illusions, unaware that, like mother and stepmother, she had to play a prescribed role in the father's life. In bringing her home, he wanted her, like the mother, for what she had to give yet hated her for what he saw and feared in her: the mother's child, with a strong potential for immorality. This "immorality" was to reveal itself on short notice—he saw to that.

Nor was Nancy aware of the fact that she was wanted only ambivalently by the stepmother, unacceptable as she was as a substitute for an infant of her own, and though an artificial link between her barren self and her husband, she was as well a revival of a natural tie between him and his first wife.

In order to invalidate the first marriage, the child had to demonstrate irrevocably her mother's inherent immorality. In this respect a complete unity of interest prevailed between father and stepmother. But in spite of it and though intensely identified with her husband's righteousness, the second Mrs. McLead longed also to experience motherhood and, as we shall see, treated Nancy with similar ambivalence, lavishing upon her not only tokens of hostile aggressiveness, but of a love which, even in the process of granting, she deprived of fruitfulness. She likewise accused Nancy of unresponsiveness when actually the child's response was prevented or not accepted.

The underlying motive for enrolling the services of our Clinic was to obtain official "proof" of the child's inherited immorality and the justification of the parents' view that the child was doomed. We were chosen to support the rationalizations for the rejection of Nancy and the subjective invalidation of Mr. McLead's first marriage. The parents deeply resented the fact that the beatings of the little girl, in which both parents indulged, were considered strictly inadvisable by the Clinic.

When we met Nancy, an attractive and intelligent girl, a few months after her father had brought her to Richmond, she was in a great need of communicating her problem and most keenly aware of the realities underlying her difficulties. At first her discussion centered around the symptoms for which she had been brought to us.

Ten days after arrival in her father's home she had developed an allergy to candy and pork. Originally it was manifested by a general rash, but shortly thereafter it became localized, reduced to the formation of sores on the legs where the father was in the habit of beating her mercilessly with a strap. She soon accused herself of having deceived her mother, following the false fairy prince whom she found to be "cold, ambitious, not loving, not a father but a policeman." She felt so guilty that she thought she could never again face the mother, but longing for her, she made plans to write to her. After weeks of hesitancy she started a number of letters but never could finish them. One letter which she attempted to write in her therapist's office had to undergo the same fate: she left it unfinished and unsigned.

Nancy explained that her craving for candy had started in Richmond as a longing for pleasure, "something sweet," when everything had become strange, hard, and unrewarding. The doctor had diagnosed her rash as an allergy to candy and pork. Her parents nevertheless continued feeding her pork *daily* but were strict in carrying out the doctor's orders in reference to candy. Totally deprived of sweets, her craving increased. While her father used to beat her on the legs, the stepmother made her undress, laid her on the bed and beat her mercilessly on the lower dorsum with electric cords, the wires of which had been removed only lately. Her immorality was giving in to the temptation of candy.

Early in treatment, following the advice of the Clinic, the tabu on candy was lifted, the corporal punishment stopped, and the child lost the need to stigmatize herself for guilt feelings. The possibility of being returned to the mother was explored but found inadvisable by the authorities because the mother lived with a man married to another woman. Nancy at least had the gratification of finding out that her mother loved and wanted her without reservations.

While the cruel corporal punishment had stopped, the subtle persecution went on and Nancy was involved in the hostile interaction between her parents. The child expressed deep hurt over the father's insistence on voicing fear that she might be given to vice and immorality like her mother. He was extremely suspicious of her.

She manifested an intense eagerness to make friends and to be accepted by respectable people. In school she was successful and extremely well liked.

The little girl brought profuse evidence of the stepmother's determination to isolate her by incessant humiliation. talking for hours over the phone about her. The child sensed in this behavior the tendency of the stepmother to isolate herself from the child while Nancy regretted the waste of these long hours which could have been used to "have a good time together." Nancy also felt that the stratagem of denigrating her for hours on the telephone served the purpose of isolating her from everybody, or else enrolled everybody in the mother's rejection of her. Nancy asserted that she did not know anymore who she actually was; she began to talk in a whisper, to look around to see whether anybody heard her talk; she began to communicate in sessions by writing, rather than speaking, searching for paper and pencil as soon as she entered the room. She tiptoed instead of walking.

Nancy stated that while her parents welcomed the visit of a number of tots, their own friends' children, expecting her to tend to them while they entertained the parents, her own friends were unwelcome and were undeservingly accused of dirtying the slipcovers in the living room.

Nancy thereupon invited her friends to her own room. To this the father reacted by disapproving the use of electricity in a second room. The stepmother would listen to the conversation from across the hall, then she would enter Nancy's room and humiliate Nancy in the presence of her friends, calling her a liar because she had been indulging in happy reminiscences concerning her real mother's love and peaceful home life, in particular the table games played in the family circle. As she reported these experiences, it became evident that she boasted to herself of having a real mother which was proof that she felt she was better than just a Cinderella. Similarly Nancy's friends, who came by in the morning in order to walk to school with her, were discouraged by the stepmother's unfriendly, at times haughty ways. One such instance concerned four poorly clad motherless children whose appearance the stepmother ridiculed without compassion for their plight. Nancy commented: "My Daddy must have thought inside of himself, here she talks about others and her child is badly off herself." Invitations from "nice children" to join their clubs were totally disapproved. She did not deserve such privileges, her parents said with the obvious intent of sapping the encouragement to Nancy's self-confidence and self-respect which the invitations entailed and which joining would have maintained. As a stepmother, Mrs. McLead refused to make even minor decisions, referring the child to her father who, however, would be absent until after the event. The child's schedule of chores was planned to prevent her from reaching deadlines for invitations or favored programs. Mrs. McLead misinformed us about this, pretending, contrary to fact, that Nancy had joined the Brownies as we recommended. A radio given to her was but a false lure, a means for deprivation and punishment; finally its use was forbidden altogether under the pretext she might damage it.

Nancy tried to endear herself to the stepmother, surprising her with nice meals, ready to serve when she returned from work; but the stepmother criticized them, fearing that the child would take a place close to the hearth and therefore play a predominant and positive part in the father's heart.

On the other hand, she left father and daughter alone for hours in the evening, not saying where she was going, thus causing them to draw close together in their common experience of rejection and fear of loss. The eleven-year-old Nancy then would sit on the father's lap, her head on his shoulder, looking at television with him. She would indulge in fantasies of her deep communion with the father who loved her to the point of giving her his last nickel and who suffered silently from the stepmother's rejection of his beloved child. This aspect of her relationship to the father also promoted conflict and she expressed the fear of being a bone of contention between the parents. Rather than bring upon him the shame of a second divorce, she would like to leave the house.

In the Clinic she could be observed in a state of anxious excitement when the father was supposed to pick her up. She was requested to call him at the end of the session but could neither remember the telephone number nor dial it when it was finally found. One day she insisted that the father enter the psychiatrist's office, their relationship to him thus could be observed. She displayed an attitude of adoring submissiveness; the father, however, was cold, self-righteous, impassive, and ungratifying, but he enjoyed with obvious vanity the admiration shown to him. He actually stimulated it, and she reacted as desired. It had become her own need, the need of the loving subject to have a father as glorious and remote as a king, as well as to gratify his needs by service to him as to a prince for his love and gracious attention. He remained, however, unpredictable. He needed to bolster himself at the expense of the three main women in his life and to defend himself against giving in to Nancy's appeal and winsomeness. She could not be allowed to play a predominant part in his life lest she weaken him, deprive him of his means, like her mother, and interfere with the role he had assigned to her as a tool for punishing and disparaging her mother.

The fear of being deprived by her of his means was a very real one. It was emphasized by him in the account of her mother given at the beginning of treatment, and in the symptoms reported in reference to Nancy herself both then and during treatment; one example given was that she wasted writing paper. Therefore she was kept so short of writing paper that she had to borrow it from other children if she wanted to carry out her school work. When she was finally given funds with which to buy paper, she was so indebted to her schoolmates that she rapidly ran out of it and actually appeared to be wasteful. Nancy was extremely anxious to return the paper to maintain the sources which produced it in time of emergency.

Contrary to the father's expressed wishes, the stepmother would keep Nancy away from school and in bed with her, thus making Nancy not her father's big girl but her own infant, the one she could love and accept. Nancy then would express surprise that the stepmother appeared to love her after all, even better than her father, as it seemed, and she expressed the desire to do everything to please her. But she soon would be disappointed. Pain and uncertainty became with increasing intensity part and parcel of her life. Her parents would have violent dissensions about real or alleged infidelity and she would be torn between them, enlisted as the comforter of the injured and identifying with the misery of one or the other.

The Clinic made an intense effort to engage the parents' interest in their own treatment, but to no avail. In view of the obvious danger to the child's mental health—she became more and more confused and not knowing where to turn, became first cynical, then listless and inactive—the case was brought to the attention of the protective services. After several months of study and endeavor to improve the family interaction, during which time the parents attempted to enrol the two agencies into their own pathology, the parents finally exhausted their hope of prevailing in their unilateral incrimination of the child. Nancy was removed from the home with the parents' consent and is improving satisfactorily in a foster home.

Case illustrating traumatization of a child due to
emotional interaction with the father who
deserted the family

# Case Summary of Dayton Peterson:
# Mirage in a Fatherless Desert

Dayton was referred to the Educational Therapy Center by his mother,
Mrs. Peterson, on the advice of a probation officer at the juvenile court.
He was nine years old. Her reason for bringing the boy to court was his
tendency to steal apples and oranges from markets. Quite apparently she
needed this action against the child as an alibi for her own behavior.

Dayton had been a behavior problem for years; he was a poor learner,
did not get along with other children, and was an extreme "nuisance" in
his section of town. The child had been a patient in two other child
guidance clinics for an extended period prior to referral. Since his nervous
condition was quite obvious, an intake interview was not made in court
and he was referred to our Clinic.

Dayton came from a seriously pathological family on his father's side.
His father married the mother under an assumed name; he pretended that
his parents were dead, whereas his mother, whose maiden name he had
assumed, was actually still living. Mr. Peterson had left home at the age
of fourteen and had gone to live with a cousin in the country. He joined
the CCC at the age of sixteen, and renounced his parents when he went
into the army. Dayton's paternal grandfather was psychotic and was
hospitalized. His paternal grandmother was described as the "nervous
type." She kept a great number of neighborhood children but denied her
own descendants and asserted she would not know any of them. Her
memory for family events was very defective; however, she was sixty-
nine years old.

Dayton's beloved maternal grandmother was known to indulge in telling gruesome stories. She never left home, was submissive to Dayton's
whims, being ready to serve him hot food at any hour he chose. She always sided with him against her daughter, his mother, whose attitudes
she criticized sharply in his presence (and her daughter's absence), accusing her daughter of rejecting Dayton.

Dayton's father, although a cement finisher by trade, worked in a
bakery. He was represented by the mother as a man who could never be
satisfied, and who was unappreciative in the extreme, as well as promiscu-

ous. He had "plenty of children strewn all around one of the city streets." He had left the family once to go to a northern city but had returned. When Dayton was five years old, the father left again, and this time did not return. According to Mrs. Peterson, her husband proceeded with great cunning. While, following his wishes, she spent two hours visiting her mother who had just come back from the hospital, he removed the furniture from their home. Subsequently it was lost. This was a great shock to the family. Mrs. Peterson assumed he ran away because of his overwhelming obligations to his many illegitimate children. His mother, however, accused her daughter-in-law of being promiscuous.

After an interval of seven years, the father re-established contact with Dayton's eldest sister and sent her money for clothes. He had in the meantime become a preacher and had married again. Finally he made a short visit to his former family. Through the years Dayton ardently tried to attract the rediscovered father's attention but to no avail.

Mrs. Peterson, whom we were able to observe at intervals for a number of years, was a plump, attractive, healthy, and neat-looking woman, said to be of an irritable temperament. However, in all of her contacts with the Center this bewildered woman showed remarkable patience, endurance, and self-denial in her attitude toward Dayton. One day, he was brought into court for some delinquency. Upon her return from court, she wished to see the child's psychotherapist. Having no appointment, she necessarily had to wait, profoundly worried, frustrated, remarkably patient, and without food for the whole day, until it was possible to arrange for the last interview period to be given to her. She showed forbearance with her mother, grateful for the good education given to her large family in spite of almost insuperable difficulties which developed after her father's death.

But in reference to Dayton she was locked in an interminable battle with her mother, who appeared acceptant of the boy. Mrs. Peterson, however, was profoundly ambivalent, incapable of insight, and expectant of an absolute virtue from Dayton, which she herself was not able to achieve. She was a perfectionist who was frustrated in her eagerness to have an ideal household and to feed her children in a way she considered adequate. She felt cornered and trapped between conflicting choices. Dependent upon public assistance, she said she had to endure humiliations, interferences, and limitations; however, she admitted appreciatively that two former welfare workers had helped her considerably. Yet, if she had tried to improve her economic condition by working at a regular job, she would have had to leave her quarters, and her children would have been deprived of her care and attention. She did undertake sporadic gainful occupations, which she kept secret and which caused her and Dayton great anxiety. But honest avowal cost her a considerable part of her income and thus no improvement of her condition was brought about.

Mrs. Peterson subsequently found what seemed to her a clever solution to her emotional problem as a deserted woman and mother of five, later six, children: She gave dinner parties in her neat home, offering excellent food which her guests washed down with adequate amounts of strong liquor. This was her way of staying with her children without being deprived of an opportunity to have male companions and suitors. The men were made to pay and thus provided for an increase of her income from public assistance without working or leaving home. She was consequently very cagey when questioned by her social worker.

She was usually warm and matter-of-fact. She had organized her family on a co-operative basis that functioned well, though not without some covert opposition from her children. However, she did not seem to have appreciable difficulties with them except for Dayton.

Dayton was more readily associated by his sex and age with the image of the father, whom she rejected. She would complain worriedly how, like his father, he failed to appreciate her (undoubtedly honest and genuinely moving) attempts to satisfy both father and son.

This woman was said to have a way of life which was not desirable in all of its aspects. In her contacts with me, I found her to be straightforward and without cunning, revealing her problems as she saw them; but burdened as she was with her children, she had not succeeded in achieving her goal acceptably, which caused her great anxiety.

Dayton had adjusted poorly to the difficulties of her condition, and by making her attempts to escape these difficulties more complicated, he had made her even more vulnerable. Accordingly, the child was exposed to her irritable temperament, which further undermined his situation, and thus a vicious circle resulted. Since he cruelly exposed her shortcomings, she developed a number of mechanisms to ward off his threat, such as siding against him with unfriendly neighbors and diminishing her responsibility by temporarily disavowing him, or discouraging the child from continuing treatment in the Center because of her own insecurity and fear of our criticism.

In self-defense, Mrs. Peterson projected her own shortcomings upon others, which at times led to manifestations of overprotection of the child. A fight Dayton had on the way to the Center was made out to be the overt reason for having to protect him from any further experiences of that nature and to prevent his coming for treatment. But her motivation was of multiple determination, partly because of the insecurity she felt as a result of the child's intense positive transference to the psychotherapist and to the Center, as opposed to his ungratifying mother and home. Mrs. Peterson projected on the psychotherapist and acted out her competitive problem with her own mother, in reference to whom, personally, she had always been able to control her covert hostility and frustration.

Mrs. Peterson told us that during pregnancy with Dayton, her first son and the third of her six children, she had had a great deal of marital trouble, but physically she was well. She asserted that the child was wanted. Birth was normal and the child was well. He was breast-fed for seven or eight months and hard to wean, as he did not like the bottle. He sucked his thumb until the age of six and wetted the bed until a short time before referral. The history of early childhood was otherwise negative.

Dayton's sleep had been greatly disturbed for some time; he was restless all night long and talked in his sleep. At a later stage he kept himself awake in order to take money out of his mother's pocketbook or, conversely, to prevent her from allegedly stealing his money, which he earned by running errands and rendering services.

At the time of referral, Dayton was a neat and attractive nine-year-old. He was subject to excessive mood swings, elation, extreme anger, anxiety, and agitated despair. He loved to render services, thus trying to be good and alleviating insecurity about his acceptability, and above all getting money for these services which would compensate for his impotence in face of an overwhelming reality.

Dayton's relation to the psychotherapist was of a tempestuous nature, but he was rather a generous type, thus trying as in reference to his own mother, to achieve a status of adequacy and human dignity. He was always eager not to be too great an economic burden, and except for gifts such as shoes provided by a church needle guild, a watch (to which he contributed his honest share), and a minimum rather than a maximum of school materials, he would not ask for material objects or beg. In this respect he also emulated his mother. Though she became emotionally dependent on the child's psychotherapist, she would feel inadequate if she were not the sole provider of all of her son's needs. However, she was able to accept the fact that it was due to his pathology that the child had to refuse taking shoes from her. Dayton took pride in returning money he had borrowed. He would dream up thoughtful gifts he wished to make and find means of actually giving them at Christmas, buying these things with his own money.

Dayton was extremely hyperactive, one of the prominent aspects of this being his excessive verbalism. He spoke incessantly, and so rapidly that it was at all times difficult to follow him; his articulation, though not exactly faulty, was somewhat slovenly because he was too haunted to take pains to enunciate clearly. Though sufficiently extroverted and intensely communicative, he was too preoccupied to wonder whether his partner in conversation had difficulties in understanding him.

Dayton's verbalism proved to be a manifestation and a constant reminder of his weakness—a symptom as well as a cause of anxiety. He thought aloud. His loquaciousness was a kind of incontinence which permitted him "artlessly" to divulge information "to the whole city," a weakness of which he accused the mother whom he saw as "the horse lady who kills and throws dirt." He was not able to perceive and comprehend her anxiety. Dayton's verbalism was not under control. He would decide "I am going to talk no more," but then go on immediately and unalterably. He talked to punish the mother, thereby gaining support and relief. And yet he did not want the psychotherapist to take actions that would relieve him from insuperable traumatic conditions of an objective nature.

He would accompany his words with excessive motor expression, performing as though on stage the things he was trying to convey in his permanent disquietude. His mind was peopled with a terrifying imagery. In his Rorschach he was almost pleasantly surprised to encounter the horse lady; she had gained objective reality and was less frightening. The content of his mind at that time was not only revealing but impressive because of the profuse symbolism produced and the subtle dovetailing of his defenses. Without treatment, the early development into a paranoid condition would have been, as we see it, a certainty.

The "horse lady" was once described as having teeth like a horse; "she digs holes, kills children and puts dirt on them"; "I am scared, I am scared to death"; "I see things I dream." His avowal of fear was almost a refrain with Dayton. He did not dare go to the toilet "because it looks like a black man who is in the hall." This is a most interesting symbolism of becoming unclean, the more so as there exists no evidence whatsoever that it might have been suggested by any knowledge of the Old Testament or any other source.

"Nobody can shoot across the ocean"; thus he expressed in various ways the fear of inescapable danger and his inadequacy to cope with it. He wanted to have a stick to measure the depths of the ocean, which he thought was as deep as a house. He was afraid of rats coming into the house, and for a time was preoccupied by men breaking in, himself playing the part of the absent father and helping to defend the whole family. At a later stage he asked the psychotherapist how old the house was in which the Educational Therapy Center was located, how long she had been in it and how long he had been treated. Pretending he had known the psychotherapist as a baby, he then proceeded to make a cube out of his two hands to show how small she was. She had to be fed with an injection needle so as not to die but to grow and become fat.

He also thought of defending his mother from members of the Ku Klux Klan, which frightened him extremely and aroused loving pity for his mother. The contrast between his thin, worn little body and his dream of being a hero was pathetic. Everything had to be monstrous, in view of the intensity of his pent-up emotions and their incongruence with the resisting forces in reality. If he wanted to fish, for example, he would "dive and catch a whole gang of fish."

Dayton had been feeling very "nervous" and requested vitamins to alleviate these feelings, but he admitted taking "seventeen" at a time, "almost all at a time." He may have discarded the rest of the pills, though he pretended someone had stolen them overnight. The overdosage and the discarding of the pills showed him to be ambivalent about life and death—a desire to get well one way or the other. But at that time we could not determine whether it was only fear of himself or of others that caused the disappearance of the pills, or whether it had a symbolic meaning of deprivation.

All of his abundant fantasies of death and immolation were intertwined with his despair at being inadequate, as evident particularly in a fantasy about a rope needed to bring up money from the river. On the other hand, they were fancied or acted out as substitute satisfactions with voluptuously anticipated self-punishment, for instance his actually boring a deep, profusely bleeding hole into his wrist. At that period he seemed to have been precariously undecided between life and death; death meant escape, yielding to temptation and forfeiting life rather than struggling; it meant putting to sleep his conscience which plagued him; it meant self-punishment, punishment of the mother and the psychiatrist.

At one stage of treatment, when the mother clung to her dependency on the man who had involved her in the illicit liquor trade, Dayton continually toyed with the idea of suicide, verbalizing a variety of ideas of jumping in the river, where there were mostly rocks and where he would be smashed and could not be saved; or wading in the water where there was mud and loose ground; or jumping from the highest skyscraper in town. By magic, he would "vanish in thin air" by tearing up a railroad ticket. He imagined, at an earlier period of treatment, that he would run and run until he would disappear, and no one could find him. At one time he complained that he had run away from the city home and no one had noticed it, identifying with the father who had "run away" and the "cop had not even taken the trouble to find him." This aroused great resentment and the feeling that the father's value, as well as that of the family, was slighted.

Dayton would scratch his wrist until the blood poured profusely from the deep wound, which he did not allow to heal. He would let the psychotherapist bind it, punishing her when he saw fit by reopening the wound. He would try to keep the psychotherapist worried by riding on the window sill in a dangerous position, certainly believing himself that he was serious and would jump.

He had various fantasies of immolation, such as diving in the river for money, tying a rope to a piece of iron anchored on the bank in order not to be killed, and successfully bringing the money up for his mother, thus symbolizing his desire to be adequate and to give. Only by artificial means, only by a rope and because of dedication and the need to atone could he hold on to life and not be submerged. One day he asked whether his mother would receive insurance money if he died. But as much as he may have wished to give it, he might have begrudged her the money. He had to redeem—as well as rid—himself of unacceptable fantasies by imagined noble deeds. He told about a boy who tried to stab a girl in the stomach; Dayton took the knife away and brought it to the principal. Many months later, at the climax of his anxiety reactions, he actually threw a knife which slightly hurt a girl's leg, and he was again brought into court.

In addition to his pan-sexualistic fantasies, he was obsessed with visions of a more concrete nature about his mother's relations with men. He peeped through keyholes, as he himself reported, in order to testify to her alleged misconduct, and at the Center he eavesdropped and tried by sudden intrusion to surprise the psychotherapist with other children. He admitted that the mother was his greatest trouble and was constantly on his mind. Dayton imagined illicit relations among younger staff members, which preoccupied him intensely. The fact that they rode in a car together was for him sufficient evidence. Everything became a symbol of intercourse and was declared to be so.

Although he did not smoke, he carried books of matches, sometimes lighting a whole book at a time or a few in a row. He did this once to light up the keyhole of a car in the dark. The meaning of this behavior became quite clear when shortly after this event he made frank sexual allusion about key and keyhole to another staff member. While in the city home he threw a burning match into a middle-aged patient's bed, an act of displaced hostility against the mother's middle-aged lover.

He was always in need of new shoes, not resting until he had them, and mistreating and discarding them after short use. He insisted that only the psychiatrist should give them to him.

For months he would perform an iterative movement: Beating both his thighs back and forth with the palm and back of both hands as if in substitutional sex gratification and simultaneous punishment. He did not seem totally unaware of what he was doing, because there appeared to exist an understanding between him and another boy with masochistic tendencies who used to exhibit a similar dance before the Center audience —an understanding which the boys thought was not perceived by the psychotherapist. At a later date, when he had improved and no longer displayed this symptom, he once called his mother on the telephone (he did not live with her at the time), smiling in happy anticipation. When she came to the phone he started the movement again, but awakening to the awareness of the psychotherapist's presence, he stopped. The symptom had not been discussed between them at that time.

Dayton would slip out daily to avail himself of quantities of discarded ice cream in the nearby dairy, regardless of all warnings against possible infection, the ice cream being unsafe and unsalable. He thus satisfied forbidden needs and exposed himself to disastrous consequences. A similar substitutional procedure was the pseudo-masturbatory activity, when he gratified and punished himself almost incessantly.

However, he was very choosy about the lunch brought from home and extremely wasteful of it, though he did accept lunches from other children, and at that time still took fruit from stores. He feared that the food at home was poisoned by his mother. The mother wondered why he threw away so much food when she had such a hard time providing it. Then he would go over to the ice-box and eat ravenously. When food did not come directly from his mother, his anxiety was lessened so that gratification of hunger could prevail.

When Dayton lived in the foster home, he would complain about what seemed to be luscious breakfasts and lunches, as though they were a means of ill-treating him. He would remark that he would be forced to eat or else be punished; "would you want to eat chicken for breakfast and white potatoes, bread and chocolate milk-shakes all the time?" He thus depreciated what he felt he did not deserve, believing that he had betrayed and deserted his mother. But if the food was considered worthless and forced upon him, he could permit himself to eat it. At home, he would always be late for dinner and complain that his siblings were better fed than he.

He was unable to accept any of the mother's gifts without anxiety. He expressly did not want to accept shoes from her. She did not understand why he complained angrily that she was depriving him of the privilege of "bought clothes," when she lived in happy anticipation and told him that at certain times, like Christmas or Easter, she would have finished paying for them and could "take them out."

Dayton was extremely jealous of his siblings. The mother reported that he begrudged them everything. In the Center, other children would call him a bad boy because he tried to rob them of all of the psychotherapist's time. Indeed, there were periods when a vicious cycle arose between his anxiety and his excessive needs, the latter causing him to increase the display of anxiety so as to gain more attention, at the expense of the other children. His jealousy problem was manifested in every area of competition with his siblings, particularly with reference to food which he tried to assimilate greedily, denying the others imagined privileges. It was also a means of gaining strength, a concern expressed in bodily preoccupation. It is interesting to note his complaints about the mother's and the foster mother's habit of stealing his money.

He was greatly upset and preoccupied about the drinking habits in his family. He spoke repeatedly about people "vomiting" and about his beloved grandmother's leniency with an older cousin who had brought such a condition upon himself. At that time, he said that "vinegar" came out of his own stomach and he had to vomit. In his mind, food tasted "like dishwater because they stir it with their soapy fingers."

He also had a great many fantasies about good food, one equally concerned and confused with sex as well as his learning problem. "A boy forgot all his numbers and was sent to the hospital," where he would drink orange juice, buttermilk and sweet milk, and something prepared with sugar.

He tried intensely to inhibit himself and "to make good and be the best child that walks this earth." If he had desires, they had to be motivated by their altruistic usefulness. "If I had a wheel I would get to the woods and get berries or fruit for my mother." His imagination abounded in ideas for helping his mother or the Center by sacrificing a dime or a nickel toward their budget. He denied himself wishes for Christmas gifts so that "the whole family will have a turkey and at least food in the house." But he drew "a whole gang of chimneys for Santa Claus."

Dayton's father, an emotionally disturbed man, was the son of a psychotic father and a mother described as peculiar and rejecting. He left home when Dayton was five years old, when in all likelihood he was still in the Oedipus phase, considering his state of development. Thus the person for whom the little boy would have given up his claim on the mother disappeared from the horizon. It is not surprising that Dayton repeatedly spoke longingly of him and wanted to join him. He identified with the father and disapproved of substitute figures in the home, whom he resented explicitly.

Though the economic standards of the family changed with the father's departure, he never referred to the father as a provider, but as a protector and friend, a man of worth, thinking of him as an ideal image endowed with qualities, the respect for which would make it possible for him to rid himself of his Oedipal dependency on the mother. In his case, the father being an ideal image implied that the mother was the one at fault, or undesirable. This was a secondary gain from his fantasies about the father, who was his unknown protection from the mother's lure. He imagined that the father lived in California, was a "hotel captain" there, and had wanted to take the son along, and that the father had had two railroad tickets, one for Dayton and one for himself. He also imagined that the mother had prevented Dayton from going. The father had been his opportunity to escape and preserve his integrity; the mother had been the one who had retained and weakened him. She also had prevented his positive identification with the father.

He also tried to escape the danger that beset him by identifying with the mother. The result was sex confusion, as is evident in some of his fantasies and homosexual behavior with his younger brother, reported once by the mother. This behavior was not overt and active, as far as could be observed. But the mother was the one who allegedly went through his pockets at night and deprived him of his money, a definite symbol of strength and potency for him.

Sex confusion is evident in his attempt to injure a girl's leg. At the time he used the term leg repeatedly as the symbol for penis. It was a period of intense exhibitionism by word and act. This was a symbolic acting-out on a less threatening person of his tendency to hurt the mother and mutilate himself. After this incident he was remarkably unconcerned, especially in view of his sexual anxiety or alternatively, his extreme elation.

The mother's emotional life after the father's departure was intensely resented, as evidenced by Dayton's fantasy of the stabbed girl. Another such fantasied report had it that the father had written a letter to his mother, which she allowed "a stranger" to read.

He never seemed more frustrated by his inability to read adequately then he did in regard to the father's imagined communication, which was read by another man and which, he said, he would have liked to be able to read himself. He claimed that his mother withheld the contents from him. His resentment was expressed by his disseminating information about his mother's real or presumed way of living, in a vain attempt to take revenge and to hinder behavior he could not endure.

His habit of intriguing, stated in a school report, should be understood as a defense mechanism detached from its original source where he had to defend himself by hindering his mother's relationships through hostile interference, or by reporting her behavior. His fear of house breakers was a confusion of himself with the intruders whom he hated and feared, and whom he, son of his father, would like to supplant. The fantasy of the stabbed girl also revealed his identification with the intruder and his obedience to his conscience represented by the principal. He "dreams" of being his mother's knight and defender, of "saving" her from Ku Klux Klan intruders, the image of his worst enemies. He felt accused of crawling into her bedroom. His stealing was a symbolic substitution, and shows how hard pressed he was by his instinctive drives which broke out here and there in spite of the self-inhibiting dams he had erected in so many places. It is interesting, in this respect, to note that he liked to go to his grandmother's because "it is the best way to keep out of trouble."

At the time the mother moved away from the section of town where his grandmother lived, he became frantic. He was also unusually concerned about leaving an apple tree that grew near her house. His fantasy of the child who has forgotten his numbers, is transported to the hospital and given milk—something agreeing with an infant—expressed his longing for the paradise of innocent babyhood.

Dayton displayed at all times a desire to "have himself." "I don't know why my mother has always to accuse me of something when I try to be the nicest boy who walks the earth." This expression occurred repeatedly. He had a remarkable way of "memorizing" what he considered acceptable behavior. We may consider this a means of auto-suggestion and a way of soliciting confirmation and support from the people upon whom he leaned in his anxiety and distress. His fantasies about the father and his lionizing him to satisfy his own ideals represent another mechanism of defense against temptation.

Wrong was projected on others, over whom he established himself as censor; his mother, and later his foster mother, were accused of stealing his money as soon as it was in his pockets or piggy bank. The substitutional role of stealing because of deprivation and depletion of strength is particularly evident from these projected accusations.

He reported that his brother was supposed to have taken money from the grandmother, but "he put it all back, because to take money from your grandmother is not the thing to do." While talking he forgot about his brother and the story went on with Dayton changing his mind, and renouncing candy. His permanent fears of rats or burglars had to be considered as a symbolized projection as well as a means of disapproving of the presence of men other than his father in the house. Inasmuch as it was a projection, it shows under what stress he operated and allows us to assess what inhibitions he had to impose upon himself.

We interpret the persistent response on the Rorschach test as "guts," in particular the remarkable response "guts of an ole skunk," in relation to his fantasy of the still gory cadavers of cows and horses which he finds in the water into which he plunges, as a sign of his simultaneous temptation and revulsion. To make what he covets impalatable was one of his generalized mechanisms.

The question of whether the disgust is primary and inhibitions help him in his striving for "being the best boy that walks the earth"; or secondary, with all the fantasies being merely productions to serve a basic need for decency, is not easily decided. Both conditions probably overlap. Without the aid of natural inhibitions, moral tendencies could not easily prevail and such a profusely stocked arsenal of defenses could barely be mustered. The very fact of anxiety is an acknowledgment of standards that one is not able to live up to, and an incomplete form of humility, the anxious person being unable to confront himself with shortcomings and inadequacies which are pressing to break out to full and permanent awareness.

In Dayton the struggle was so overwhelming that it did not remain localized on the original traumatic area, but became generalized and flowed over to any area of "knowing," in particular to the field of his education and learning. "The food in school tasted like dishwater, they stir it with their soapy hands."

Insofar as the "breaking in" is a sign of disapproval, it is again directed against outsiders. This displays how much the outside at all times excited him in an area where he was already threatened from within. These factors are elucidated in two ways: first that he had to deny the threatening world outside in fairly general terms and resort to fantasy, which is autistic life; and then that he unconsciously had to reject knowledge which is dangerous. This included school learning that comes from the outside world, considered to be foul. However, lack of knowledge, as we could observe in reference to the incidents of the letters, represented exclusion and incompetence. It was an additional source or anxiety and proof of his inadequacy. He was caught between the necessity of protecting himself by inadequacy and the distress experienced by its crippling effects.

Because of the same threats inside and outside, he sometimes lost a clear awareness of his identity versus the world and confused his acts with other people's, or became confused about the origin and direction of his tendencies.

To liberate the mother and himself, Dayton began to earn money at an early age, one of his motivations for stealing being his desire to provide for the family. Now he wanted to be honest. His great efficiency, his ardor at work, and his need to brag of his success in order to bring home to himself and others his efficiency brought on him street fights and often unjustified accusations of theft. Money was stolen from him by the children who fought him. The mother's own insecurity and defensiveness caused her to believe the false accusations and to overprotect him when he should have had the support of being corrected. The boy was swayed between despair about undeserved distrust, when he struggled so ardently, and impish pleasure at being so smart that nobody could catch him—like his father, whose whereabouts were still unknown.

At that time the mother seemed involved with a man and his bootlegging activities, and the boy tried to divulge everything. He said the sisters were too scared to talk, but he wanted to save the family. At one time his lack of success brought him close to suicide. Placement in a city foster home was successful but was interfered with. The foster mother and a number of reliable observers reported that he behaved like any other child. When he had returned home, he again began to work, selling papers in the afternoon and shining shoes before school; nothing and no one could hold him. He barely allowed himself to sleep. An accusation of having sold stolen papers led to a commitment to the state, a commitment not unwelcome to the mother and her friends because of her precarious situation.

Dayton's behavior in the study unit was so exemplary that he was referred to a foster home, and day-care treatment in the Educational Therapy Center could be continued. The foster mother seemed intensely interested in the boy, but she too was on the defensive because she too was known to have drinking habits and to have her kind of parties. This kept the boy in an emotional upheaval and intensified his sexual fantasies in reference to her as a mother figure, but he struggled for control and slowly achieved a greater sense of realism than ever before. When he felt he had conquered his Oedipus involvement, he insisted on being returned home. He believed he could now take his mother as she was, and hoped to achieve a more genuine and non-ambivalent affection. When she re-

548

APPENDIX

mained unchanged, he liberated himself one day by reporting artlessly to his psychotherapist, "you wouldn't believe me, but my mother doesn't love me." The insight was gained by a diminished involvement and the awareness that also his purified love remained unacceptable. He achieved a measure of economic independence and tried to find acceptable pleasures in the city's recreational centers, and attempted to learn a trade in the Educational Therapy Center.

Case illustrating the salutary effects of good
foster home placement

# Case Summary of Daniela and Vicky Middleburg

Daniela and her sister Vicky were referred to us at the same time for diagnosis and recommendation, the one by a diagnostic clinic, the other by the City Welfare Department. Daniela, the oldest of her mother's five surviving fatherless children was considered incorrigible and unmanageable. She was a chronic absentee from school and was suspected of promiscuity. Vicky, the younger one, was also a truant, a bedwetter and our evaluation was particularly requested in reference to the nature of her sleeping spells. A few years previous to this referral she had been given a complete neurological examination in a good hospital, including a skull x-ray, electroencephalogram, the study of her blood, and spinal fluid serology. The results were negative.

The children's mother, her four daughters and her infant son lived in one single room that served also as a kitchen. For the six people there was only one large bed, which was used by the mother and three of her children. Our two patients slept together on a narrow cot which was wetted nightly by one of them. The mother was herself the dependent daughter of a domineering single woman engaged in prostitution. However, due to her attitude, the grandmother never lost status completely. Her part of their house, in a run-down section of town, was at least fairly well kept and its furnishings were objects of her anxious protection. In contrast, her daughter's room was in a state of total disorganization. The grandmother viewed her daughter's status with utter bitterness and locked her as well as her children out of her personal quarters. The children's mother suffered from several venereal diseases. Contrary to fact, she pretended having been married to a college graduate, a military man who was the father of her children. He allegedly deserted her. Actually she had lived under the assumption that to gain a husband you had to please a man sexually and tie him to yourself by having a child by him. If you were unsuccessful you just were unfortunate and should try again.

The mother being outside the home most of the time, Daniela was its acting head and could be seen, surrounded by her siblings cutting cabbage and cooking it in water on those days when food was at hand. Daniela's psychological test indicated in summary that she was functioning in the borderline range of intelligence, with slight indications of greater intellectual potential. The test was considered indicative of schizophrenia. Strong withdrawal tendencies and an infantile dependency on others were in evidence, but in a controlled manner of awareness and acceptance of her affectional needs. Her inhibitions were said to prevent her from strong emotional interaction and from being effectual in handling situations. There was denial of, and frustration over, sexual impulses with a lack of insight in coping with these problems. The need of psychotherapy was stated, but the probable results were considered unpromising.

The initial interview showed a very slender young adolescent with a whip-like body, pale and hollow faced. All of her front teeth were badly decayed. Daniela complained that she could not fall asleep until 12 and 1 A.M. It seemed as though "sleep doesn't come." She was "real sleepy in the morning"; that's when she had her best sleep she said. Assuming that this sleeplessness might be due to undernourishment, I inquired about her meals. She pretended having her main meal at 12 or 1 o'clock in the daytime: "White potatoes, green peas, and fried chicken." She asserted that she always ate that well, a contention not borne out by the observation of her social worker who saw that the best these children had to eat was a diet of watery cabbage. Actually she ate one meal a day which was, as we found out later, a free lunch at school. She pretended that she ate when she felt like it and did not have any appetite at night. She was as fantasied in indulging in dreams about the fine food she ate as her mother was about her marriage. Such dreams of "fine" food in a "fine" environment with a "fine" fatherly man open the door, as we know, to prostitution in girls who have dreams and potentials for what is "fine" and artlessly display their longing for it.

Daniela said that in their narrow cot the two sisters got in each other's way. It disturbed her sleep but Vicky slept soundly and *her* daytime sleeping had nothing to do with the bed. She used to sleep so much even as a little child. It was just "built in" her, their mother said, according to Daniela.

Her leisure activities were reading from stories which describe girls who do wrong and then get caught and sent to Peaks (the location of the Virginia Industrial School for Colored Girls) or another industrial school. Daniela said she was very curious as to how these stories ended— whether the girl got away with it or not. She wanted them to be punished. Vicarious gratification and the identification with the punitive society were Daniela's spontaneous means of experiencing temptation as well as overcoming it. She called herself a "mean girl" but wanted to be good. She reported further her ambition to become a singer and consented to sing for her interviewer. She had a tiny sweet bird-like voice but revealed no talent.

In this interview no evidence of schizophrenia was detected. The child communicated artlessly and honestly. She explained that she was irregular in school because her teacher shamed her when she came late and asked her whether she had any plans for returning home soon. Daniela was ashamed of her destitute condition and actual starvation. Considering the child's background, the preservation of so much humanity and girlish charm was more than surprising. The interviewer felt that this girl could and would make use, even at this late stage, of a better opportunity for growing up.

In her initial interview Vicky, her sister was most impressive in her own way. Her revelations made apparent the emotional nature of her narcoleptic spells as well as the tendency to sublimate her emotions and escape the haunting turmoil of her condition. She reported her delight in listening to the pastor in church. When she was irresistibly succumbing to her sleeping spells she felt she was raised in heavenly glory close to God himself. Although she had felt like dying, she would awake refreshed.

In a common conference of the two referring agencies with a representative of our Clinic, it was decided that to redeem the children's home, if at all possible, a long period of time would be required. The children's condition, however, required urgent attention. Foster home placement therefore was decided as the inevitable solution, and psychotherapy was recommended for the two girls. However, the follow-up on both these recommendations was deferred greatly and the mother's resentment promoted an intense hostility in both girls. We were never in a position to see the mother, whom the court committed for observation to the mental hospital.

When the two girls finally were sent in for treatment, their hostility was intense and their desire to be helped had ebbed down to zero. The two sisters were enrolled with another pair of intensely hostile sisters and later in a mixed group of eight children. To observe these four girls, one would think them devoid of any other experience in relating except violent verbal aggression, or withdrawal. We shall not dwell further on the composition of this therapy group and on what led to a resolution of the excessive and exclusive display of aggression at the beginning of treatment. What we noted when the two Middleburg sisters began to talk, to sing, and to enjoy the sessions was the apparent benefit incurred through foster home placement. The children obviously felt included in the human society. While her sister could make slips into lack of refinement and rough expressions of hostility and while she would verbally express the tendency to become sleepy and bring the conversation to the subject of church whenever she felt menaced, Daniela was gentle and serene, the boys flocked to her and strove by society's acceptable ways to gain her attention. The joyful relaxation was exhilarating to observe. The narcoleptic Vicky of former times, who had felt excluded from what was worth desiring, the one who had to escape into the dream of being in heaven, stood up before the group spontaneously and gave her opinion about music. She classified composers and established a hierarchy in reference to the quality of their work. She knew which she liked best. She talked to the group as though she took for granted that they were versed in the matter as well as she was. There had not been any school attendance problem ever since they were enrolled in the foster home and at the time of this writing the children were looking forward with joyful pride to a school trip to Washington. They had made definite plans and fostered definite expectations.

They were in contact with their mother who as a court commitment was in the safety building of the mental hospital. Daniela was writing for all of the siblings. She visited the younger ones and reported about their well-being. The children consented not to visit the mother as long as she could be seen only under special confinement. (Prior to the mother's commitment to the hospital and prior to the children's return to us, the mother caused grievous embarrassment to the girls and the foster parents when she visited. But with the help of their social worker the children and their foster mother agreed to let the mother continue her visits to the foster home rather than to humiliate her by meeting her at the welfare department.)

Thus the human status acknowledged in the foster home and the sense of being included in the human society despite their bondage, enabled the children to assert themselves in treatment. Feeling less isolated and exposed, they did not have to exhaust their mental and emotional resources for a defense of their status against a world from which it differed. (We omit here the mere struggle for physical survival which was now overcome.) They could use their "raised platform" as an experimental theater for testing the social graces, inviting and involving the other children of the therapeutic group. They were thus acquiring a new self, acceptable to themselves and others; they were leaving behind the "mean" self or the one that made them try to escape into temporary death and the protecting arms of God himself because the menace was so great. Vicky learned to face this menace only gradually. She went through a phase of loud behavior and a tendency to denigrate others. But Daniela showed gentility and tact from the outset. She showed her sister how to lay the cloak of love over other people's shortcomings. Finally, both girls were joyfully impressed by their own rebirth. They were exploring the possibility of even greater surprises coming from life outside as well as the wellspring pouring from within. At this time, rather than resist treatment, the children wanted it and used it to the best of their ability. However, the need for it was considerably shortened due to the merits of their foster home and their dedicated social workers, both before and after placement. This case is presented as one example among many which demonstrates the contribution of the community to the treatment of children enrolled in our Clinic.

Case illustrating a child's involvement in pervasive maternal hostility

# Case Summary of Linwood Fanhurst

Linwood Fanhurst is a representative example of a victim of ubiquitous maternal hostility. The child in such cases is used as an anvil, but also as a hammer. Hostility, being inexhaustible, has become an obsession. Nearly everything and everybody is made to serve it, and the creation of general disquietude is the means for obtaining "results." The dynamics which lead to a sado-masochistic pattern of behavior are illustrated by the following case.

Linwood Fanhurst was referred to us at the age of thirteen, by the juvenile court, after his return from the industrial school. He had a story of gradual decline in school achievement and behavioral adjustment. He had incurred his neighbor's wrath for persistent trespassing, carrying guns, causing damage by shooting, and annoying the younger children in his neighborhood.

The mother, as all three members of this family group, was a woman of at least average mental endowment, the seventh of the eight children of a poor farmer. The domineering father died when Mrs. Fanhurst was thirteen years of age. The mother allegedly was "a sweet woman," an assertion made after a number of sessions where any communication in this direction was resisted. Mrs. Fanhurst evaded the subject of her childhood which was unknown even to her husband and son. Her interaction with her present family and her inordinate resentment of authority suggested that the Oedipal involvement and the revolt against parental authority remained unresolved. Mrs. Fanhurst's first marriage was of very short duration, apparently made to legalize her unborn child, a daughter, much older than Linwood, an able young woman who, however, was divorcing her husband at the time of this writing. This daughter had been raised in Mrs. Fanhurst's second marriage. Indulged by both parents, she was unable to share with Linwood, when his turn had come, parental attention.

When Linwood was born, Mrs. Fanhurst was in the second half of her thirties and her husband ten years older. It was at this time that her psychosis broke out. She was subjected to a maximum of electroshock treatments and finally hospitalized when Linwood was eleven years old.

Mr. Fanhurst was the child of poor parents, but in his leisurely elegance and dignified appearance, he showed no trace of it. Mrs. Fanhurst maintains that his mother keeps a brothel and that her husband wants her "cheap." His father, according to her, had died of the excesses of alcoholism. During their courtship and early marriage, Mr. and Mrs. Fanhurst drank together socially. But during Mrs. Fanhurst's illness Mr. Fanhurst began to drink excessively. After thirty-six years of successful employment in a respectable position, he was placed on retirement, at half of his maximum salary. Mrs. Fanhurst's commitment to the mental hospital was considered necessary for the improvement of both marital partners' emotional problem. At the time of Linwood's referral to the Educational Therapy Center, Mr. Fanhurst had given up drinking for two years but his wife retained her delusions which she fostered also in reference to the sons of his first marriage. His first wife was also mentally ill.

The final reason for referring Linwood to us was his refusal to go to school. He was a depressed and withdrawn boy, lacking in spontaneity and taciturn. He was also extremely suspicious, projective, and irrational, like his mother. His attitudes coincided with hers, but while she had a bitter-sweet way of pursuing her goals, Linwood could be very defiant. This quality he used in a self-destructive way, provoking to the extreme the judge and the welfare workers who had been most sympathetic with him. His early neglect is said to have been appalling, the neighbors pooled resources to place him in and drive him to a day nursery. To these people he transferred much of his resentment felt for the parents and withheld from the mother. He was a very poor eater, his nails were bitten, he had a tic and a jerking of the shoulders, that seemed to express disarmament and indifference. He had an asthenic body constitution, like his mother.

His early delinquencies began with setting fires in the house, and selling his parents' silverware. He drove a car with the mother's permission but without a license. She condoned the boy's driving stolen cars and went to extremes in preventing his learning to bear the consequences and assume responsibilities for his behavior. One of Linwood's friends was in court for a physical attack on his widowed mother. Linwood's mother was interested in his friends only to "prove" her contention that they were treated leniently by the authorities while her Linwood was treated roughly.

The beginning of Linwood's treatment had to be delayed for three months because of a car accident in which he and his friends were injured. A month after recovery he was again in detention for having ridden in a stolen car. While the mother was working, the father had stayed at home, refusing to look for employment, in order to keep Linwood out of mischief.

When, after this latest incident, Linwood was seen for the first time by his psychiatrist, he projected the responsibility for the taking of the car on the one who had "no business leaving the key in the car." He was indignant about being confined in the detention home, the place being "no good" for him. The mother tried to bail him out by every means and by engaging a lawyer. Linwood made his release from detention the prerequisite for his co-operation in treatment. But some insight could be gained although no "conditions" were fulfilled to obtain his co-operation. In isolation from his mother, he was still capable of forming self-centered dependency relationships of his own. But the mother persevered in her fear that the detention home would hurt her child and in her sensitivity to the "unequal treatment of her son" as compared to other children.

The key figure in the family tragedy was the mother. Behind a righteous and puritanical attitude, she harbored fantasies inadmissible to her conscience. She projected her fantasies on her husband thus denying responsibility for their inadmissible implications and making him an object of repudiation. He was assigned a position to fit her ambivalence, that is, he was committed to fail her either by frustrating her needs or allegedly degrading her. This attitude was representative of her non-satisfiable nature and hence her incapacity to be gratified. Contacts with her necessarily carried in their wake frustration and a sense of failure. Harping relentlessly on her unfulfilled wishes she would grind down her victim without mercy, but in doing so she depleted herself to the point of becoming incapable of watering her own desert.

Lost in a world of delusions which she concealed from herself, Mrs. Fanhurst made herself impervious to outside influence. In the last resort she trusted only her inner world and those relationships which she had included in it.

The person who fitted this description was Linwood. She "needed him so bad" and therefore condoned his antisocial acts. He was her crutch in performing them, a crutch which, in a gruesome way, she used also as a stick. In order to be tolerable Linwood had to be she, otherwise, like all "outside" people he immediately became a threat to her very existence. Not to release him to an independent and mature status of his own was to protect him from becoming part of the alienated world, and thus subject to her repudiation. But the hate withdrawn from him as an object outside of her, inevitably and automatically, was instilled in him and, projected as an organ of hers, became her projectile. Having lost his identity and self-determination, and being recruited to fight an allegedly hostile world, Linwood was deprived of the mutuality of love and community with the world, and doomed, like and with his mother, to mistrust and isolation. Obviously no responsibility for his actions could be felt. But his relationship to the outside having become increasingly envenomed, he had to, for the sake of "belonging" at least to the mother, go on acting out her will. Because of this involvement of mother and son in one another, her bidding did not have to be articulated. Preverbal communication was highly effective in moving Linwood in the direction of her thinking. But as a tool of contact with the outside world Linwood inevitably carried obstacles into the mother-child relationship. The mother's satisfaction could never be real. It was reduced to dreaming, scheming, anticipating seeing—Linwood, on the other hand, though deprived of his own shadow, was nevertheless exposed to failing the mother like everybody else. Because of her predominant role in his existence, failure was annihilating. To brace himself against annihilation, he blunted his emotions. Despair and revolt, his only active defenses, were denied. They isolated him each time he was confined and exposed him to the world he was made to fear even before it had to assert itself against the "defenses" of the deluded boy.

The fear of his own impulses reflected Linwood's ambivalence between failing the mother and losing her love and offending the world which, in its turn interfered with what an "inner voice" told him to do. Since Linwood showed first a good development and had regressed in accordance with increasing deterioration of the mother's condition, some individuality was still preserved. Therefore, Linwood had two inner voices, the mother's insinuating voice and his autonomous one—hence his ambivalence and his being easily swayed. Whoever put his weight into the balance helped Linwood to be relieved from an insoluble dilemma.

In the self-contained mother-son relationship the father has no place except as an obstacle, a target of hostility and projection. But since part of Linwood's pathology, rather than an arrested development was due to a regression which occurred concomitantly with the mother's mental deterioration, he regressed to a stage where the father's existence had also been recognized. In such situations this recognition is ambivalent. Acceptance of the father is self-centered. The father senses this and tends to be subservient to the son's demands. Actually, to justify his existence, the father is drawn into a maternal role, since Linwood fostered demands and expressed them in terms of his regressed relationship with the mother. The generally noted competition between the parents for Linwood's affection was, at least in reference to this aspect of the family interaction, secondary to the father's adaptation to Linwood's pathological needs. We must, however, not forget that the father's behavior was not totally devoid of realism. When he stayed at home and forewent working to mother the boy, he hoped to make sure Linwood was not forfeiting his chances of living at home. Linwood felt handicapped in carrying out the mother's commitments. She wanted him to act out without accepting the consequence, the loss of the privilege to stay home. That the "father did not understand" lead to Linwood's expressed contempt of the father. Although the father hatched the mother's egg, as he thought, for her benefit, since she wanted the son at home, the son revolted against him, not her. Like the mother, Linwood placed the father in a position where he has no choice but to fail. The father's protecting him was unwanted, but Linwood refused to give any guarantees which made it unnecessary. The father had to be kept in his place as an obstacle and a target of hostility and projection. One of his roles was to be representative of authority, a role the father was coerced into assuming. Thus, he was drawn into the ambivalence of the mother's desire to have Linwood act up and still be at home, and into being her serf, punished for whatever service he renders.

But in addition to subservience to the mother and to competition with her for the love of the son, the father competed with Linwood on the Oedipal level. The father had an interest in letting himself be used as a baby sitter, thus promoting Linwood's regression and dependency. For once the son had no use for regression. Exposure of his dependency on the father's care embarrassed him and nurtured revolt. Revolt was nurtured also in reference to the father's role as the mother's husband. Linwood told the psychiatrist with indignation that his parents came together to see him in the detention home. In view of the self-contained mother-son relationship the father was accessory and an outsider and his being with the mother was "illegitimate." We may be at the roots of the mother's idea of reference. Due to his own interest at the Oedipal level, Linwood became involved with these ideas. The father not belonging to the family was degrading her into a "cheap" woman, if he expected her to fulfil the sexual role in their marriage. Linwood was irrational about returning home; it was not only his mother's bidding but also his jealousy which drove him home and it was this jealousy which kept him tied to the TV until late, longing for the mother, as he admitted, to come down from her bedroom shared with the father and coaxing him, lead him to bed. Since the father had brought Linwood to their common therapy sessions, Linwood had been less irrational about going home. Mrs. Fanhurst stimulated most unsoundly the boy's competition with his father. The father's positive contribution, the attractive home with its ample furnishings were taken for granted. Instead, the mother harped on his loss of income when he reached the age of retirement and encouraged Linwood's dissatisfaction with its material and social consequences. The boy's habit of staying out late and sleeping into the day was his expressed retaliation of the father's past failures, long since amended. Linwood took pride in being more reliable at work than the father. He was punctual on his paper route even though he stayed out late. The father, on the contrary, could not be relied upon, Linwood said, to go to work regularly, at the time he drank heavily. But Linwood overlooked the fact that he failed to go to school. Linwood used to echo with indignation the mother's anger over the father's past shortcomings. In order to make up for the loss in the family's income she opined that Linwood should work and not go to school. She did not favor the father's return to work because it would not help her anyway. He would keep the money for himself—an assertion that was never wholly true and certainly not at that time. The father was placed in a minor, an effeminate, or senile role. She had even tempted him at Christmas, though vainly, by buying him a quart of whiskey. It is interesting to note that the son made the following unrealistic interpretation of the father's persistence in depriving him of his guns. With an expression of contempt, he pretended the father sold them and bought himself a whole "fence" of cigars. There is nothing in the home to stimulate forming of ideals and the inspiration needed to sustain them. The influence of the home is carried over to all fathers or authority figures. She deprived the son of ideals to emulate.

Mr. Fanhurst's interest in his son was genuine. It was for his sake that he gave up drinking. Interest was expressed with warmth, patience, and tact. But Mrs. Fanhurst had obviously succeeded in alienating also her husband from himself. He was a man of above average intelligence and good insight. But when he was confronted with his return home from his therapy session with Linwood, he felt disarmed and incapable of assuming his paternal role. At the moment of leaving he sapped spontaneous and manly decisions made by Linwood and asked whether he really meant what he said or whether he wanted to reconsider his decision. Weakened himself he needed to weaken his son who could not be trusted when exposed to the mother. Thus Mr. Fanhurst indulged in exactly the same behavior displayed by his wife and noted by previous observers, that is, her habit of ignoring in the last minute a therapeutic decision painstakingly reached and of introducing her refrain of wanting Linwood back home against his best, well-explained interests. Mr. Fanhurst was aware of and admitted his motives for retreating from reason and the courage of making a decision. He understood that by induced ambivalence, he was acting out his wife's schizophrenic symptoms. Her nagging and grinding kept him preoccupied with her way of thinking. He must anticipate it at all times to prevent being influenced.

That in the past Mr. Fanhurst should have been cornered into retreating from the coercions of his family's interaction by some means or another was, as contradictory as it may sound, almost a matter of holding on to his mental and emotional composure. Retreat was his means of not becoming absorbed and totally subjugated by his wife. Although it was a means of escaping the pressures of his chains and the awareness of having sold out without ability to pay the expected toll, retreat was an ineffective attempt at escaping his loss of self-respect, a loss which made him incapable of facing other men on the level of professional dignity. It provided his wife and son with additional reasons for depreciating and isolating him. Further, it seemed that Mr. Fanhurst had a tendency to disarm himself in order to withhold giving—probably a consequence of not receiving. A vicious circle of mutual resentment and mutual deprivation resulted.

Unless Linwood can be helped to overcome dependency, the mother's articulate or inarticulate promptings will prevail and he will enrol outside supports (his "friends") for swinging the balance in her emasculating direction. Increasingly the mother's promptings will become the irrational voice from within that will prompt his acts. He will not know why. Weariness will increase and he will be more and more reluctant to question why. This is the pattern in evidence already as well as the tendency to incriminate, as responsible, those he engaged outside, for a decision. Linwood is not yet rigid and congealed like his mother. When alone, or under proper influence, he accepts the balance of reason to be weighted down. He can be made to see. If strengthened by prolonged influence, he can find himself and will be able to see for shimself.

We presented this case as an instance of a profoundly traumatic family interaction, promoted by a paranoic schizophrenic mother. Treatment in day-care was not considered because of Linwood's aggressiveness, certain psychosociological considerations, the mother's nonamenability to treatment and, above all, the need to remove Linwood from the family's interaction. Other treatment plans are being worked out in an attempt to strengthen the father's position and in a long-range program to reach the mother as well.

## Case Summary of Isaac Jones

Isaac Jones, a ward of the City of Richmond, was referred to the Educational Therapy Center, where he received treatment for two years, until he left to live in the country. After a brief stay there he was committed to the state welfare and placed in an industrial school. When he returned to the city, treatment was resumed at the Center with one session a week. However, after a short stay in the community he was again sent to the industrial school to protect him from incessant persecution by his mother. Upon release from the industrial school he was readmitted to the Educational Therapy Center and received treatment until he consented voluntarily to accept further treatment in the state mental hospital.

Isaac had become aware that he was ill equipped to cope with the pressures in the community but was determined, as he said, "to make a man of himself." Plans were then carried out with the social service bureau and with his foster mother. She had been his faithful friend for as long as we knew Isaac.

When he was first referred to us, at the age of nine and a half, he had already undergone treatment in another child guidance clinic. Our services were considered more suitable because of the advantages of the day-care program. Although Isaac showed average mental ability, with an IQ of 107, he was a non-learner. He had had serious behavior difficulties in school and in his neighborhood, being extremely agitated, anxious, and stolid in his relations to children. He could not be trusted in stores. He had changed foster homes innumerable times and his marked inability to adjust to home and neighborhood persisted until he went to the state hospital.

After each new placement Isaac would muster all his controls, creating imagery incentive for himself, which soon broke down. He would exhaust the foster parents' good will, their capacity for understanding and would deceive their expectations. As a rule he involved the whole city neighborhood or rural community in his hostility. To overcome a deep sense of inadequacy fostered by failure everywhere, he would resort to extreme arrogance. What conditions led to Isaac's aggressive and self-destroying behavior?

A light colored boy of elegant build and handsome face, Isaac always looked serious and bewildered. He stemmed from a broken home. The father, an irregularly employed truck driver, was an alcoholic. He took Isaac at an early age on his alcoholic sprees, and in the weeks and months preceding Isaac's commitment to the state hospital, he made him drink and supplied him with the means to drink. He had been committed to the road camp repeatedly for alcoholism and delinquency in providing for Isaac and his two sisters: Ginette, one year his elder, and Mary, not quite two years younger than he. During his brief periods of return to the community, the father would live with his apparently well-adjusted, unmarried sister.

The Educational Therapy Center had explored the possibility of parental assistance. The father could not be reached, usually because he was in a penal institution most of the time. But one day, due to Isaac's eager assistance, contacts were established. The man then declared himself to be an improper father.

The mother was supposed to have come from a respectable family and to have deteriorated after her own mother's death, and under her husband's influence. She too began to drink heavily. One time Isaac commented: "I was thinking how much can be broken up by the departure of one person! Ever since my grandmother died, everything went wrong with me and my sisters." He also remembered his grandfather who would tell him, and read to him, bedtime stories. For years his medium for relating to people and being close to them was by listening to stories read to him.

The boy had lost track of his mother for a period of time before he was referred to us. When she reappeared, he was between the ages of eleven and twelve. She was seen drunk and unkempt in the streets, in the company of the kind of men who exploit women prostitutes. They were either slightly intoxicated or showed signs of chronic alcoholism. She lived with one of these men and had been bailed out by another man. The mother moved around constantly, probably to escape the police but she always attempted to live close to the Educational Therapy Center, wherever its location.

She wanted her son in a peculiar way which interfered with Isaac's treatment. She would visit him in an erratic way, sizing him up as a horse dealer would a horse, discussing proudly his beauty with her male companion in front of the child and the psychiatrist. She seemed to evaluate herself as well as the child by his suitability for the sex trade. Isaac would stiffen with anxiety in their presence, but then he would be swayed by the woman's seductive powers. For weeks he would come late to the Clinic. One morning our psychiatric social worker went to see the mother. She arose naked from the bed where she had been lying with a man, and opened the door, admitting that she had expected to see Isaac. Apparently he was exposed to this situation daily. The boy was extremely disturbed and hostile at that time. The mother's interference disrupted the mutual adjustment that had prevailed between Isaac and his foster mother. The foster mother expressed intense annoyance and resentment about the mother's competition. But she too was disloyal. A new foster child was placed in the home at the foster mother's request and against our advice. She soon became quite involved with the new child, who was not a behavior problem. Having become *persona non grata* in this family, Isaac gave up.

His mother was jailed repeatedly, was committed to the state farm, and one time was convicted for forgery. Isaac's two sisters were to him the ideal figures in his own family, especially the elder one. We would invite them at intervals for a little family party. The elder sister nagged him slightly and the younger one was seductive. He overlooked both attitudes, thus able to believe them to be the accepting and ideal sisters he needed for his self-esteem.

An elderly, unmarried, motherly woman had taken an interest in Isaac ever since we had been in contact with him. Seeing that he was cruelly ostracized everywhere, she supported him for years by a naïve faith in him and at times inspired him to strive for acceptable goals. She was always there to take care of his concrete needs, one time buying him a bicycle when he longed for it most. She represented, aside from the Educational Therapy Center, the only steady element in his life; but for a long time she still remained an unrealized lure since she was, understandably, afraid of taking him into her home. Finally, she made the sacrifice generously, and was brave to the end, despite the fact that Isaac was unruly, arrogant, acted out in the community, was drunk on several occasions, and associated with most undesirable and unsound companions. One of them was the assassin of two young children unknown to him, whom he drowned in a bathtub. Isaac was most disquieted and wondered what attitude of his own could cause a real fascination for a boy as disturbed as his companion. Isaac always carried knives and guns. His benefactor, although frightened, at a loss, and without influence over him, tried to carry on until the Educational Therapy Center, becoming aware of these new developments, successfully helped Isaac find his own way to the state hospital.

However, she felt guilty and insecure; she visited him weekly in the hospital and took him home on weekends without the knowledge of his psychotherapist and without consulting our Clinic. She interfered with his treatment and finally contributed, to her own surprise, to his elopement from her home with a woman ten years his senior. She did not understand Isaac's ambivalent fondness for her. Now he sought to overcome his unresolved longing for the mother and his ambivalence between conventional and unconventional standards by the love of an unconventional woman, who probably sought to relieve herself through her affair with him, of an unsolved obsession. Isaac soon returned voluntarily to the hospital and resumed his struggle for conformity and acceptable standards.

What made Isaac desire to go to the state hospital although he knew what he was giving up for the sake of getting well? He had long felt discomfort about his inability to cope with his world although he wished ardently to do so. He had experienced in the industrial school the support of a structured milieu, isolated from the community. That school had taught him to conform outwardly but not deeply and from within when no longer under the protection represented by the institution. On the other hand, he became increasingly aware of the inner resources that psychiatric treatment might assist him in mustering. However, he still felt too weak to cope with the menace represented by the community and the tendency to project failure on outside provocation. He began to deal realistically and successfully with this problem, in treatment, when he became deeply concerned about following in his father's track and being drawn to the company of a boy who soon afterwards became the assassin of two innocent children. Therefore he was ready to reach out for treatment in a state hospital, a milieu which would offer the protection of an institution as well as psychiatric treatment.

In the early days of treatment at the Clinic, Isaac continued to roam the streets incessantly in an avowed search for his father, pretending daily he had seen or talked to him. When he finally stopped running, he incessantly talked about his father at the Clinic, or else he assumed embryonic or infant-like postures, or played the little boy who listened ecstatically to story-reading, trying to reanimate the past when he was surrounded in his grandparents' home by an apparently united family. Searching for the father was his way to the mother, as he later revealed. Isaac also dreamed of becoming a saving link between them and of causing the father to be his mother's redeemer as well as his own. He sensed, but never stated it explicitly, that the father had caused the mother's downfall. He looked to the father as the force that would repair damage to the whole family. The boy pretended that his family was Catholic and that he could not therefore allow the parents' separation to continue. The problem worried him intensely for a long time. He yearned for his mother, but he could not solve his ambivalence between acceptable and unacceptable tendencies as long as the person most ardently longed for lured him in a direction which impeded the improvement of his troubled condition.

He tried vainly to find acceptable substitutes for his mother, clinging indiscriminately to maternal women without capacity to give of himself. He usually drained the potential source of gratification.

The deep reason why Isaac was unable to solve this ambivalence was that from the onset of his illness he was obsessed by the need to restore within his own natural family conditions conducive to his proper guidance. In the early years of treatment he was bent on redeeming the parents for their and his sake, searching for guidance and love for them in a church that most obviously to him laid stress on the permanence of mutual dedication. Sensing his confusion in reference to direction and the weakness of his commitment to recommended ways, he needed the Shepherd who would come for him and make him return to the fold. The power of the church to bind what has no cohesion of its own fascinated him. The mother was helpless without the father and both needed the grandparents. Their mortality had been their weakness and the ultimate source of the family disaster. Church alone represented strong guidance and an enforcing as well as protecting shelter.

But things supposed to be good were to him but an evanescent promise because he lacked conviction and strength by action of his own to espouse them. He once compared himself to a pet turtle that would forever tend to return to its natural pool. A woman with acceptable standards was, whatever her own attitude toward his mother, by her very existence, a censure of the mother. To remain loyal to the mother, gratification from a source that would downgrade her had to be resisted. In pre-adolescence, running to the mother when he knew she was going to be unclad was not simply his yielding to temptation but making use of temptation to solve the ambivalence to be or not to be hers, to have or to forsake her. But we helped him to struggle for a less troubled condition.

In therapy he lost, through the years, much of the resentment against the therapist for her inability to resolve from without and *for* him the alternatives which so cruelly exposed him. He no longer used her merely as a shelter or a purifying brook. He no longer withdrew into mute resentment against her as a symbol of an eternally strange and unattainable world. He now was able to invest the therapeutic community with a self-redeeming ardor. In his efforts to make a decision that would help him resolve the whirl of alternative directions and deal with them without destructive effects to himself or others, he still swung back and forth between indulging a drive down to the mother's level, on the one hand, and his ideal images on the other. His problem remained for some time this: that he strove for the absolute as a panacea against the lure from the "inferno." But he also used the abyss between the two extremes as the deadly fascination and crossed it back and forth. Moreover, not to remain strange and unattainable the good had to be detectable in his own family. He venerated in his mind his elder sister, who then could redeem the whole family, substituting for the mother's defection. He visited her regularly for ever renewed evidence of the truth of her existence and as his guiding light. He had a girl friend, significantly in the country, who played a role similar to the sister's. His last step before going to the state hospital was to visit both of these young women whose inspiration he felt would guide him toward recovery. Before he left he wanted to record, in the presence of his therapist, some spirituals which he sang with religious ardor and a fine sensibility for phrasing and musical expression.

In the light of his extreme distress and in terms of his deprived social environment, Isaac was a lacerated person who could not resolve his duality.

Case illustrating severe traumatization of a child
in the sexual area, in the home

# Case Summary of John Martin McGregor

"All nobler thoughts and the longing for better things are crowded out
of my mind" was John Martin's complaint. Therapy had to be interrupted
twice because no solution could be found for the problem of creating an
adequate background for treatment.

John Martin McGregor, a physically overgrown fourteen-year-old boy,
classified as of dull-normal intelligence, lived in the crowded conditions of
a home situated in a downtown section of poor repute. He had one older
brother and four older and four younger sisters.

At the time when his initial social history was first studied by the Clinic,
three of the older sisters had five illegitimate children, and two of them
lived in the home with the young men considered, correctly or incor-
rectly, their future husbands. John Martin had no other place to sleep
than in the parents' bedroom. He never mentioned this fact, though he
spoke much about the father and expressed constant dependency needs
toward the mother. He complained again and again of his sisters' immod-
esty, constant disputes and rows, as well as their loud and inconsiderate
sex behavior in his presence. He said he hated them, and it became evident as treatment proceeded that he was also greatly disturbed by nearly
all of his older sisters; they represented help as well as impediment in
his struggle to free himself from his mother.

The sisters had a very poor reputation, and their lack of sexual reserve
when talking over the phone caused the telephone company to discon-
tinue service. One sister, a most hostile young person, was seen personally in the Center. These young women were all over twenty. Since the
economic situation did not permit the family to move into larger quarters,
it was suggested that they room out and give the young brother an opportunity to grow up under less traumatizing conditions; none of them
co-operated.

The father was a regular provider on a relatively high scale, considering his social and educational status. He had held a steady job for
many years and was regular and punctual at work. However, he could be
counted on to get drunk on weekends and retire into sleepful oblivion
from his family's life. His role was not devoid of tragic traits: Apparently he did not lack the capacity to display some of the educational guid-

ance which the boy desired and which he spoke of in explicit and ardent terms. But the boy was too involved and too young to understand the complexities of the father's situation; he held him responsible for the family's condition; in fact this was the sole power and prerogative that he did not deny the father.

Such a fate would have been spared the father, if circumstances had permitted him to remain an associate and guide to the son in those areas of living where a community of definite, shared pursuits and education by demonstration is desirable. But the father should have remained an anonymous figure in a field where the son, like every man, should do his own exploring, convinced of the uniqueness of his individual experience and of his final triumph. Parental guidance in matters sexual can be theoretical only unless in the area of finer emotional attitudes and relations or assistance in times of conflict or distress.

As a Negro in a relatively menial job, John Martin's father had to deny his personality the better part of the week. When circumstances are wholesome in the home, the spell is lifted upon return at night to his castle and on week ends he can recover his dignity. Not so with this father. New threats to his pride and dignity and new frustrations confronted him. At a time when we were successful in arousing his genuine co-operation, he visited his son in company of his wife and other family members at the state industrial school, a visit registered by the boy as "My mama came to see me yesterday."

The older man had to pilot his own storm-beaten craft through the straits of the family's contradictory passions. Because of his total withdrawal from any paternal function other than that of a provider, and because of the specific method of withdrawal, he could not enlist encouragement from the son, although father and son both longed for it. The father could never appear to the son in the enchanted glory which is the pride of every growing boy, and which he preserves unchanged in the back of his mind despite future alterations which demand an adjustment to reality.

The father thus missed the conviction that he had the vocation to guide his son. He therefore sealed his tragic condition by his weekly semi-suicide. Every additional child, under such circumstances, becomes a burden to a prematurely aging man, particularly when to each child is born a grandchild for whom there is no provider. Although we may be able to understand the man from an objective standpoint, he, himself, felt surprisingly uncomfortable about his inadequacy to cope with his humiliating situation. And he could not help resenting the dreary routine of his existence. Nor did he seem to allow himself much credit for his merit as a provider. This function of the father, however, impressed John Martin with great pride in spite of his mental negation of him.

Of the three "protagonists" in this family, the mother appeared to be the most resistant. A few years earlier she had passed through a crisis, consisting of asthmatic paroxysms, and recovered, for all practical purposes, after having made a vow to return to church, significantly as a choir member. Yet, behind her matter-of-fact attitude, she barely concealed her embarrassment and her anguish; her wandering eyes never seemed to rest on the therapist, who appeared as the representative of the higher order to which, try as she might, she could not ascend.

She was able, however, to struggle for the integrity of the family as she understood it, and she tried to redeem herself from guilt (incurred under the force of circumstances) by motherly devotion. Although she remained confused at the discrepancy between the actual condition of her family, with its extreme shortcomings, and its imagined potential, she humbly accepted whatever limitations there might be in the management of so difficult a situation. This kept her serene enough to struggle in each instance to the limit of her ability, and to yield where necessary, resigned and without any apparent resentment.

Although the boy's mother was reasonably protective and maternal, she was defensive in court, and on various occasions manifested an ambivalence toward the son, an ambivalence originating in the uneasiness which he could not help creating between her and her husband. She overcompensated her ambivalence by increased endeavor in co-operating with and assisting the boy. She often lacked judgment and was unable to refuse what was tantamount to abetting undesirable or unlawful behavior.

When John Martin became an inmate of the state industrial school, he came for treatment to the Educational Therapy Center. Each time upon arrival he would immediately ask to see his mother, but he was either very shy or unable to show any joy when she came. His attitude toward her could be partly explained by her own ambivalent attitude. She was cordial enough to arouse his desire for her warmth but so evasive as to remain altogether unsatisfactory. In the beginning, she would come, looking unkempt in spite of her Sunday finery, kindly, yet tired and strained, bringing him food packages. But being too busy with the youngest generation in the home (whether her own children or her grandchildren of the same age), she would be tardy and fatigued, feeling inadequate and guilty or anticipating wearily that again she would be faced with "missing the boat"; indeed sometimes she would call and say that she could not make it.

Occasionally the boy was allowed to go to her home. One day, after being seen on her back porch, he did not return but disappeared. She seemed concerned about him at first, but after a while, whether only at that time informed of his whereabouts, or what is more likely, tired of playing a false role, she "left it to God and trusted He would protect him."

John Martin had found his way to the home of one of his older sisters who lived in a northern industrial center. There he became part of a dope ring. The mother may have helped to work out his escape to the sister at her son's or her elder daughter's suggestion. The father was probably the only one not informed.

Both John Martin and his mother had a transference to the psychotherapist, which reiterated the boy's relationship to a condoning mother. Thus, one day the mother approached the psychotherapist requesting financial aid for John Martin's older brother who was in some "trouble" or other; she was confronted with the father's adamant refusal to be involved in it. Such behavior on the part of the father was accepted with resignation by the mother, but it isolated him in the family, where his attitude was not understood. He was considered pitiless.

From the time we met John Martin until his escape, he was profoundly depressed and inhibited; like his father, he would never raise his eyes. He had an unusual fondness for machines, in particular movie projectors, which he actually fondled and which he operated well. His delinquencies consisted of repeatedly stealing new bicycles, from which he retained only parts, dumping the rest. He begged to be sent away from his home and placed in a better section of town. He complained that when he tried to escape the evils in the home, he encountered them in the street: "There is evil everywhere."

The boy blamed this fact on his race, with which he identified reluctantly, his color being imposed upon him just like his inescapable fate in the family. He identified with the father's role as husband, which was intensified by his own role as witness. This identification became one of the main causes of his deep conflicts.

In loathing the father, he abhorred himself and his racial identity, believing his relationship with a father who never talked to him or shared with him common activities to be typical of parent-child relationships in his race, whereas the community between father and son in the white race was, as depicted in schoolbooks, always ideal. He was so preoccupied by this discrepancy that he would show as proof to the psychotherapist pages in elementary schoolbooks. He bitterly resented the father's alcoholism and characteristically, soon after leaving home, became involved with the dope ring.

The boy unconsciously had identified with the father's lack of forbearance in the family situation, from which he too withdrew passively for the sake of his integrity, though he withdrew for different reasons. In the Rorschach test he rejected all possible sex symbols, saying each time: "I cannot see anything."

The help John Martin had been desiring for a long time was not passive and pseudo-suicidal withdrawal but a stirring, active community in search of fine pursuits, with promises for a happy future. Though he deeply sensed the shame lingering between him and the father and the hostility entailed in their relationship, he discounted these situational impediments unrealistically and dreamed of what their relationship could be, if the father, the sole cause of disappointment, were different.

Under those compelling conditions within the home, the boy had experienced his first sexual sensations as a witness to other people's sex play or activities. The resulting pattern of voyeuristic sex gratification brought him into court and a second time into treatment at the Educational Therapy Center. Contrary to the habits of children of this background and physical as well as mental make-up, John Martin was inhibited in his normal sex tendencies; everything about his first sex awareness was forbidden and thus connected with strong feelings of guilt and shame, fear of torment counteracting desires. His drawings revealed this clearly. The tendency to indulge in passive sex gratification increased the painful awareness of his want of integrity. He withdrew from people of all ages and both sexes, except protective mother figures, as well as, to a certain though remarkably modest extent, from his own virility. He used to join the craft teacher, and he was satisfied for hours to weave and make rugs mutely at her side.

He attempted to solve his problem in reference to the mother by a predominantly concrete, regressive, and dependent relationship. Though his disquieting relationship to his sisters also provided material for emotional inhibition, in particular sexual inhibition, he elaborated more profound conflicts with the father. He really was "identical with him."

The son tried intensely, by approval or disapproval, to eliminate the father outside and inside himself, but they were inexorably joined by the very fact of their relation and by a common experience. Father and son maintained their relationship only in their own minds, without the least feeling of reciprocity. They were helplessly trapped and, whatever their hopes to the contrary, stood in each other's way. That John Martin, under these conditions, lacked the self-confidence to search for other objects for identification and ideal-formation must not surprise us. In fact, he had to prevent himself from thinking of it; and in his effort to improve his own status by denying his identification with the father, he was bound to arrive at the very opposite of the attempted goal. He further diminished his own status and his adequacy for identification with venerable models. That he dare not love and admire excluded him from life and reflected upon the scale of values for which it is esteemed. An eternal outcast, blocked by the alternative between dishonorable identification with the father and the self-diminishing attempt not to identify with him, he was ultimately destined to deny values altogether.

The outlook on life is narrowed by this fruitless and exhausting struggle and by the inexorable concreteness of a way of life, specifically the exposure to sexual experience. The exalting power of abstraction is broken by the shattering effects of concrete facts. The child, although afraid and inhibited, is deprived of the capacity and even of the motivation for postponement of gratification, which would be identical with integration of the instinctual drives into the higher purposes of life. The tendency and the expressed longing are in evidence, but they cannot be substantiated, and thus, cannot be implemented.

Such dynamism is perhaps sufficient to explain the passive solution sought by John Martin. However, the parental model necessarily contributed to his formation. Both parents had preserved a certain amount of capacity for struggling; the mother in the home, the father at work; that is, in the crucial areas of duty as well as of survival. Both parents surrendered partially, the father to a regular and temporary deathlike comfort, the mother to divine solace, thereby escaping the excessive demands of living as well as the conflicts of sexuality.

John Martin admired his mother for having risen to such proximity with the divine; he even tried to follow her. This was not without influence on his passive longing for better things, dreaming of them and pondering on his fate. It is noteworthy that once he had left the mother and her guidance, he followed the father's passive escape, without, however, emulating him in continuation of his active and honest struggle for survival.

Case illustrating a highly differentiated, elaborate,
and gravely pathological Electra fixation

# Case Summary of Virginia:
## Electra's Woe

Virginia, fifteen years old at the time of referral by the state industrial
school for Negro girls, had struggled so persistently through the years
that she had experienced a wealth of differentiated feelings of rebuke, of
shame and contrition, of sinfulness and unworthiness, of intense hatred
for her degradation, her vileness and her reverence of her parents. Against
each of these feelings she had built up defenses and counterdefenses, ab-
stracting more and more from reality to the point of becoming confused
about her identity.

Changing from conceit to submissiveness, from self-righteousness to
self-disdain, her overt behavior alternated between total withdrawal, angelic sweetness, and a hard, nagging argumentativeness. In view of maternal coldness and rejection, she was to herself the measure of all things.
Obsessed with her own completeness and perfection, she was determined
to have everything her way, to the point of ignoring people and violating
the elementary facts of experience.

Finally, she wanted to "be nowhere," an ambivalent term with a positive connotation. In order to avoid impediments to having things go her
way completely and constantly, she had to resort to being on the move
permanently and to running aimlessly to the point of exhaustion from
dusk to dawn.

Virginia was her mother's third child, preceded by an elder brother
and a half-sister who had run away at adolescence, leaving an illegitimate
child at home. There were six younger sisters and a three-year-old
brother.

The family lived in a dilapidated house in a slum area. The house was
in a shocking state of neglect and disrepair. The father was said to be a
steady worker and provider about whom no objective information could
be obtained. The mother had a reputation of being cold and rejecting.
A telephone contact established by the daughter and overheard by the
Clinic proved her to be totally unresponsive to her daughter's longing affection expressed impressively by voice and word. Although some information about the mother was available, there was little factual background
for assessing the reality factors in Virginia's pathological mechanisms, nor
was it possible to ascertain when her symptoms had become manifest.

Virginia was a neat girl, self-respecting in appearance. Her demeanor and appearance would never lead anyone to suspect that she could come from anything but an orderly middle-class home. She was a good student until she became delinquent at adolescence and remained an excellent worker as a student seamstress, tending to withdraw into her work. Virginia pretended to have been withdrawn at home and at school all her life because she felt rejected and vile.

She had been committed to the state for being unmanageable and running away repeatedly, with money stolen from the father. Appearing unexpectedly at the distant home of her aunt, who kept her half-sister's second child, a little boy, Virginia forced the aunt to repeat the assumed or real parental rejection. The aunt had to refuse to keep Virginia illegally and reported her to the authorities. Placed in a foster home, Virginia invited renewed traumata by her explicit and provocative fear of the foster father. She was then sent to a state industrial school from which she was referred to the Educational Therapy Center for treatment. She acted out her problems with the mother in a subtle form of negativism, directed against maternal figures at the industrial school and at times provoking obsessively the feared as well as wanted rejection without which her world would have lost its consistency. She made it, in the long run, impossible to keep her in the school. At the same time she showed to the psychotherapist in the Center an angelic Virginia, with a sweet, gentle, childlike voice, an identification with her mother as she imagined her, as a creation of her perfect self. To the school she offered her rejected and rejecting person. In order to play her angelic role convincingly, she subjected herself willingly to treatment.

However, when the Center assumed responsibility for her and she was again placed in a foster home, treatment had to be interrupted after a few months. Virginia was afraid of the trees around the home, of any men, particularly elderly ones, in the house. She was annoying to the women by her hostile, provocative fear of their husbands. Placed in the home of two extremely qualified single women, she displayed intense hostility, total negativism, was fault-finding and self-righteous. She wanted to be in a social group, by herself, among people, yet alone, finally nowhere.

This meant, as already mentioned, running from dusk to dawn until, exhausted, she would sit down on the steps of the police station, home of the images of the father and of the longed-for and feared male.

When committed to a mental hospital, Virginia felt at first relieved but later on resented the commitment bitterly. Actually she had forced the psychotherapist to become, for the sake of her protection, the rejecting mother, and therefore the girl went into a stage of intense resentment and negative transference. This she maintained for a long time, visiting and writing hostile and demanding letters after release from the hospital to her home. She tried by violent or gentle means to provoke denial of wishes which could not possibly be fulfilled and which would result in a satisfaction of her need for rejection. Later on she developed a dependency less imbued with the need to prove the mother figure ungratifying. She would come from other cities to see the psychiatrist and to be in her neighborhood, although treatment was not resumed.

Virginia's ambivalence to the rejecting mother was characteristic of all her emotions. Negative feelings were transferred onto maternal substitute figures; they expressed themselves in hostility and negativism regardless of all therapeutic efforts.

The mother, however, was depicted, contrary to all available information from other sources, as a sweet and loving image. This illusion, an ambivalent hence abstract gratification of dependency, was needed for the preservation of the girl's self-respect, her struggle for feminine identification as well as for the protection from her feeling for the father.

Virginia was equally ambivalent toward her father. Her rejection of him at the beginning of treatment was described as of indefinite origin "as long as I can think." Later this rejection was motivated by her as due to many resemblances; she emphasized particularly that she had an ugly broad face like her father, while the older sister was pretty like her mother. But Virginia also admitted her intense hatred was motivated by her loving him too much, a love which brought her in inner conflict with the mother.

Loving him, Virginia felt, she trespassed upon the domain of the mother's affection; hating him she offended the mother who cherished him. To overcome this ambivalence, she stated one day that both she and her mother hated him, intensifying thus the identification with the latter. However, she said her mother actually did not know what kind of person she was "tied up with." Implied was that the father's erotic attitude or his sex behavior was frightening to all his daughters; but Virginia's ambivalence went so far as to deny categorically the very assertions made repeatedly. When she was seven years old, her father was for Virginia the image of the male. In her dreams the father played many parts. He was the chief of police who committed her to the highest court, where she was never tried.

The intensity of her obsession involved all her sisters in incestuous fantasies with the father and increased the anguish which had become a need. She had to feel sexually threatened in order to live. At the same time, the threat was an excuse to run away from life and love. As could be expected, she was as ambivalent to homosexual as to heterosexual feelings and ran toward as well as away from them, thus being "nowhere" and unable to achieve much more than the most casual personal contacts.

Children played an important role in Virginia's dream life as objects of complementation as well as means of identifying with the sweet and kind motherhood to which she dedicated herself. Motherhood and childhood were both means for postponing womanhood. Longing for motherhood simultaneously with repression of the consummation of womanhood is representative of the ambivalence of the adolescent situation.

Motherhood is a veil for womanhood but also a path to it. An alternative is seen between sinful sexuality and divine maternity. With Virginia this subterfuge did not succeed. Her dreams revealed that she wished to take full possession of her little brother as her own child. He was the object of her nightmares. She fled from him as from a part torn from both parents, but she hurried to the aunt where her little nephew could, with less danger, take the role of the brother.

Virginia reported a number of relevant dreams which revealed her involved elaborations of her problems, as well as the representative roles played by all her close relatives in this struggle for liberation, sex maturation, and personal wholeness.

In one of her dreams she told haltingly in simple evocative language how she identified with her oldest sister who sits in a car which is carried by a truck. But she realized that the sister also represented the mother. Accompanying this maternal figure were the two children of the sister who represented also the even more important youngest sister and brother. Separated from the women and children, sat a man, in her interpretation, the father; the man sat in a separate car on the truck. They were coming in these vehicles and super-vehicles from the busiest section of town, its traffic and the department stores, symbols for this girl of many temptations. The street vanished while they crossed a bridge in the shadow and arrived in a pastoral landscape with a river crossed by a second bridge. The truck fell into the water and Virginia could see nobody after that except the little boy and the face of the little girl.

She turned around and it looked as if the little boy and the little girl were going to the theater with her. She did not know what happened in the theater, but the police came in. She repeated that she didn't know what trouble started, except that the police were calling everyone outside for questioning when she awoke.

Direct interpretation by the girl, and further interpretation by the therapist suggested, by observation of her behavior and the reading of her notes and letters, in particular those to the girls in the industrial school, that the children played a dual role, one pertaining to the father and the other taken away from the mother and sister, with Virginia thus assuming the total role of mother to the children. The conflict that arose was evaded by death and immolation of everybody but the two children. The little girl of the dream was also Virginia herself who rose from the water, which represented death as well as birth, bodiless and purified.

She could not guiltlessly enjoy her illegitimate prize that stood for so many inadmissible wishes which were gained at the expense of those who were drowned. The police appearing at the spectacle questioned everybody. She could not face the interrogation. The trouble was not only projected on "everybody" at least potentially, but the dream was inter-rupted and she awoke.

Virginia's second dream clearly showed the incipient detachment from her Oedipal dependency upon the father and the identification with her own and her sisters' femininity.

At a later stage of Virginia's sex maturation, she deprived the father and the little brother of the symbols of sex maturation, leaving them only to her older brother. The dream occurred at a time when Virginia had engaged in a correspondence, initiated by the brother who was in the service, and when both made a concerted effort to see each other at Christmas time.

I don't know what I was dreaming at first. I woke up and fell asleep again. It was raining hard. I was at home and I went upstairs to my daddy's room, and his bed was torn up, and my sister next to me, down in age, had put all the shoes of the family except my oldest brother's, on his bed. She had taken the heels off all of them, and I asked her why did she take them off, and she said there is a girl in our school called Daisy Harris who told me to take them off. I happened to look out the window and it was still raining hard [she told this in a troubled way] and there was someone knocking at the window, and I went to see who it was, and it was my little sister [the one next to the young-est], and I opened the window so she would come in and she wouldn't come in [repeats it], and all at once, she'd faded away, and I looked out in the street and all my sisters were on bicycles riding in the rain. In time they got to the corner; I heard a car sound and the wheels were rolling around the corner and they were not on the bicycles and after that I woke up.

In this second dream, Virginia acknowledged the femininity of her youngest sisters who were no longer menaced by the father. Both he and the little brother, who in the first dream emerged from the water, are de-prived of their masculinity. This is accomplished by maintaining their similarity to her. Their shoes lay with those of the rest of the family "with heels taken off," and just "flat looking," on the father's torn-up bed. The torn-up bed with the heedless shoes resting on it is a reminis-cence of the father's past role and of the desolate condition of the dis-orderly house. Explicitly excluded from placement on the father's bed was her eldest brother only. He represented the accepted symbol of young manhood outside the home at a time when Virginia tended to-ward liberation from her sex confusion. She ascended to the father's room, unafraid of him, for he had become inoffensive. Formerly he was depicted as repugnant and hateful, now she surprised us, in telling this dream, by calling him "daddy" for the first time. Home and security were symbolized by the father's room, while her former self, riding bicycles outside in the rain, is identified with her younger sisters.

In a move, parallel to the retouching of a man's portrait from fatherly to brotherly features, Virginia modified the symbolization of self in terms of the younger sisters rather than of the mother or the older sister, as previously. This movement not only corresponded to the change of her inner reality, but it is an acknowledgment of an evolution of events. As Virginia matures, history also takes its course. The father's attractive manhood has passed its prime and a new generation is asserting itself.

Those traits in the mother's image which betray her status as a grandmother are taken into account and cannot forever be glossed over, even by Virginia, though there will be reverses and renewed doubts. Indeed while she was concerned whether awake or dreaming with danger to her sisters from the father inside the home, in this dream she now sensed danger as existing outside the home. Thus she called the sisters into the protecting dwelling. But they did not listen; the outside would now represent a new future. Resigned, Virginia acknowledged and obeyed the law that rules the course of events. She saw herself in the image of the younger sisters disappearing around the corner without bicycles. Thus, she consented to accomplishing her natural destiny, to freeing herself from bisexual neutrality, and growing into maturity.

Virginia's meticulousness in working through the difficult problem of sex orientation was brought out by a variety of further dreams. In one of these her father was no longer represented by himself, in a car or by his bed, his heelless shoes and his home. Another man, a mature worker in the industrial school, accompanied by the police, represented the alluring as well as the forbidding and protective male role. In the dream the mature male worker and the police were to go to the court in Washington, which was the supreme legal symbol of her superego. Nobody was tried, however, the train moved on as on an unseen bridge in the countryside and stopped. Children appeared from underneath the train and she woke up.

Additional features of Virginia's dreams should not be overlooked. One is the window which separated Virginia from her anticipated and desired future sexual identity and "through" which she became the observer of her changing attitude. The other feature was her narcissism and introversion. The narcissistic dream started in the father's room. All persons and their sex attributes were symbolized or represented by objects, except for her sisters. Only the sisters, who were identified with herself, were represented by persons, an expression of the fact that she was now intensely self-identified. This was one of Virginia's main problems. Also in other dreams she was always represented by people, females of all ages. The father was represented under human features in his character as a male. As soon as the human character of the father was an object of concern he would be deprived of his sexual role, and the dreamer would have no human imagery at her disposal. The father then was represented by something negative as to sex. A torn-up bed, heelless shoes or other objects fraught with negative reminiscence. Virginia represented him without his protective functions. She actually never had known her father as a human being and thus could not have had any human imagery of him.

## *Case Summary of Peter Pope and His Dollhouse Play*

Peter came from a white middle-class family. His negative transference to two previous therapists was due to his sensitivity to being faced directly with the family situation which the dollhouse suggested. As a result, Peter, a gracious eleven-year-old, had unsuccessfully undergone previous treatment. At one time admission to an open ward had become necessary, but he was negativistic and withdrawn and repeatedly ran away from the ward. Family placement had been recommended, but neither the parents nor the child would accept this. The boy and his family had been dismissed as unsuitable for further treatment by the last therapist.

The father and the paternal grandfather were both sturdy tradesmen of a high caliber. The father, though not without wisdom and stoicism, was simple and robust. The grandfather, a supervisor in the factory where he had been employed for over twenty years, was much more differentiated. He was a sophisticated gardner and, on a small scale, an excellent "garden architect" as he called himself. Both he and the paternal grandmother had inherited certain antiques which they treasured, added to, and integrated into a gracious form of living.

The boy's mother was of a charming impishness, but she had a serious emotional problem which she traced back to circumstances in her childhood. These had led to profound insecurity and actual self-rejection which was reflected in her relationship to Peter. He resembled her physically, being blond and delicate, and she feared sexual inversion in him. It is noteworthy that she had no problem in reference to her dainty little blonde daughter, the youngest of her three children or with the second son, who was the image of his father. Prior to Peter's referral to me, she had been subjected to electroshock therapy. When I met her, she was absolutely truthful in facing her feelings and in the beginning of our association, equally blunt in rejecting her son. She loved men of the dark-haired, sturdy type like her husband. She was devoted to her father-in-law. Her fear that Peter might not escape becoming homosexual was based on the fact that, unlike the second son, he did not like to play boyish games. He preferred to sit by himself, drawing, which he did very well. Contrary to his brother, Peter was not successful in school, nor did he associate with others. He was teased about his daintiness and his effeminate gait.

Peter shunned the home and, whenever possible, associated with the grandfather, joining him enthusiastically in his pursuits. He had a less important relationship to the grandmother whom, nevertheless, he helped in her preparations for parties for which she used her fine old china and silverware. These antiques fascinated Peter. At a later phase of his treatment he talked about them enthusiastically. He also showed an unusual interest in the British royal family, admitting later in therapy the desire to be like them. Similarly, he pretended to have a blood kinship with the poet Pope—a conviction probably conveyed to him. The boy's name was not actually "Pope" but that of another famous English poet. The grandparents' interest in cultured living and their genuine love of antiques and historical objects had increased this child's awareness of beauty. Although his dreams carried him away from reality and were indeed an evasion of reality, the grandfather, by instinct an unusual educator, took them for granted and satisfied them, thus introducing a bridge to life and making it acceptable. Other family members joined in. An aunt, who also had artistic talent, made a portrait of Queen Elizabeth to the infinite delight of her nephew. The grandfather framed it with a crown on the frame.

When the boy was told he was going to a new psychiatrist, he immediately blocked. He announced that he was not going to talk, or reveal family relationships in play or by interpreting drawings. In his first session, however, he responded emotionally, though he tried to conceal it and though he carried out his decision not to respond verbally. His suspiciousness and mutism lasted for some time, but he occupied himself with drawing at an early period and also acted out slightly. He had a hurt expression and pinched lips as though bitter and hopeless. His gait was awkward, revealing his uneasiness at being watched.

His early drawings concerned remote countries and remote times. In order to becloud any possible communication implied in his drawings, which he had an urge to perform and which were a convenient device for introversion and withdrawal, he pretended his topics were taken from subject matter in school. In particular he liked to depict castles, the bridge drawn up, situated on top of a mountain within a wide unpopulated, though serene landscape. He refused to comment but artlessly revealed himself anyway by the few words he granted his psychiatrist. When he began to confide in her, he expressed his sense of total rejection by the mother and his love of an aunt, whom however he had refused to accept as a foster mother. Upon questioning he revealed that if he lived with her, she would become like the mother. Actually the aunt, though loved, was but a tool to cause the mother's jealousy and thus a bait held out for her to answer his love and longing. Queen Elizabeth at a distance and as a dream was the only gratifying reality for him at that period.

Peter considered his relationship to his mother hopeless, not without reason. Making his acceptability dependent upon an impossible prerequisite, namely that he be like the father, she was not only rejecting him but enrolling the father as an artless tool to smother her son with his sturdy manhood. The mother, "too nervous to bother" helping Peter with his school work, had the father do it. The father, who admitted being as inadequate in mathematics as his son, was insecure in fulfilling his task, and impatient. He frightened his son, who could work with neither parent. The boy thus could not cope with the father, nor take refuge with the mother. Neither was it possible for him to find, by identification with her, a justification of his existence that would compensate for his inadequacy in comparison to his father. In fact, identification with the mother would have been suicidal since as a person of her kind he was odious to her. It would also have underscored the difference between his frail build and the father's stolid stature. Flight into fantasy seemed his only escape, which had to be achieved by denial of the family's existence—at times of *any* family's, even of any people's existence. It was his sensitive way of "rejecting rejection" by the person he actually loved.

The grandfather never became involved in these emotional tangles, despite the mother's tendency to include him in her love of the husband and to consider them fundamentally similar. With kind dignity and determination to hold to his neutral position but through his play with Peter and his two siblings, he developed a profound kinship with the sensitive and artistic boy that Peter actually was. That the grandfather was of sturdy build therefore did not make him necessarily a husky and crude male.

In treatment, Peter had first to overcome his anxious and prejudicial anticipation that, in front of the dollhouse or similar therapeutic devices, he was going to be led to expose his annihilating problem. The mere presence in the room of the dollhouse, to which he had been sensitized since his early treatment, made him shrink and cast hostile glances at his psychotherapist. When Peter began to give in to the therapeutic relationship, he attempted to cast the therapist in the grandfather's role. Previously, he had tried to provoke the psychiatrist by every possible means, to induce a maternal rejection.

Improvement began ambivalently. He reported in detail and with enchantment his activities with the grandfather, conveying that the therapist was unnecessary and trying to provoke jealousy. But he also wanted her to understand what kind of association and activities satisfied him. Conditional acceptance was thus granted. She was deviously told to be like the grandfather just as he had been told to be like the father in order to be acceptable. As the psychiatrist was able to understand this role assignment and yet remain herself, unmistakably a woman, she was considered by Peter an equal partner for the grandfather. Both became parental figures whom he made to co-operate on his behalf. Projects started with the one were finished with the other under the pretext of wanting to complete a job which was almost done. Finished products were carried from one to the other to be admired or for the sake of adorning the other's office or shop. He realized that he could be an accepted son without being smothered.

Increasing co-operation was shown when Peter began to build his own magnificent dollhouses with an unusual feeling for exotic architecture and landscaping. His materials were dominoes and colored blocks. He talked profusely; people of foreign nations began to populate his houses, palaces, and cities; the children, their activities, and relationships were topics of his interpretations, offered without stint and without hesitation. Thus his structures gave him freedom to escape from his home and to reject his family and convey information ambivalently.

Though generous in his production of architectural treasures, he was stingy on the other hand in retaining the materials, trying to retain the psychiatrist's attention exclusively. This behavior slowly assumed major proportions. He used all available building materials, leaving his imposing undertakings unfinished for a while, thereby retaining the final possession of the achieved masterpieces. Therapist and sibling figures could, in this way, be punished for acts of infidelity. Unfinished projects, to be resumed at his own time, were used to provoke the psychiatrist's resistance to his delaying tactics.

His projects now included historical settings, the families being followed through generations. Destruction and reconstruction of the embattled castles expressed his ambivalence between annihilation and restoration. Distant fondness and respect but also his value system were expressed in terms of beauty as for instance by adornment of castles and chapels with stained glass windows. Foreigners representing his unsophisticated parents came in to buy the castles and ruin their historical style. This was restored by later members of that family who bought back the family heirloom. In this manner he linked himself to the grandfather, the image of the ancestors of historical stature and of a noble tradition degraded by the mediocre kinsfolk.

The reported therapeutic observation describes a boy who initially resisted attempts to help him. The inducement, implied in the dollhouse setting, to express himself within a predetermined framework reminded him of the strait-jacket in which the mother expected him to grow up, a factor of her own emotional disturbance. What Peter could not express within that pre-established framework he felt free to reveal at a fairly early stage of his treatment in his very own creative terms, as the creative person he was.

An example of the therapist's tolerance of child's provocations, and the gains therefrom in treatment.

# Case Summary of Nathaniel Thomas

Nathaniel's background was paradise in comparison to those of the majority of the children described. His condition at the beginning of the treatment was also less profoundly disturbed. I chose his case, though others might have been more impressive, simply because it was the most recent and most vivid in my mind. An unexpected response to his provocation brought the child so close to the psychiatrist that he poured out the problems he had partially disclosed only deviously so far. Simultaneously it helped the psychiatrist gain a relevant insight into his most obvious communication with her.

Prior to reporting the incident, we shall introduce Nathaniel to the reader to permit him an evaluation of the contents of the child's remarks and the memorable meeting between child and psychiatrist. We shall go into detail, for instance, in reporting the initial interview. It highlights the scenes upon which proceeds the child's mournful story despite the mother's efforts which are described in his report. On its fringes we see the silhouettes of other deprived children whose bereaved condition, like Nathaniel's, spoils his enjoyment of the only privilege he has, objects with which to occupy himself.

Nathaniel was referred to the Educational Therapy Center by the public school psychologist. With a low average mentality, he was a slow learner. At eleven years of age he had reached a second grade reading ability. Comparing the results of the Wechsler Intelligence scale at the age of six and at the present, no mental growth was evident during that period. He was said not to do any homework, to leave the school without permission, and to be disobedient. He was characterized as being irritable, to have a tendency to pout and withdraw from the children at play. Both mother and school reported that Nathaniel tired easily and had a great many physical complaints such as headaches and pains in the stomach; his sleep was said to be disturbed, he was restless and tossed during the night. The mother depicted him as nervous all of his life. At the period of intake he had been moved to his mother's bedroom. His mother reported that he was timid and poorly equipped to defend himself.

The mother was one of seventeen children; she was sickly in childhood and greatly attached to her father. She had one brother in this city. He took an interest in Nathaniel, who played with his three children. Nathaniel had adopted him for a father but was denied the privilege to call him so until the mother explained to her brother what the refusal meant to the child. As an eighth grade student she came to this city from a southern rural area and went to work in a factory. She remained a factory worker until new machines made many of the workers superfluous four years ago. She then took work as a maid. When we met her, she was employed in the family of an industrial executive for what seemed a pittance. She had been taking care of his three motherless children for a year and a half. She identified herself with this family and their standards. Nathaniel was raised by these new standards and was given, within the compelling limits of her condition, the same kind of toys as seen in her employer's home. What she could not afford was an electric train. At the time of this writing she had given up her work for reasons of ill health and was looking for a job that would not take her away from home from seven in the morning to seven o'clock in the evening. At this time only did she begin to co-operate with the Clinic on behalf of her child.

Nathaniel was conceived nine years after his mother arrived in Richmond. She was extremely upset when she became pregnant and for two years she needed the assistance of a case work agency to cope with her emotional condition. When she discussed pregnancy and the child's infancy in the intake interview, she still was agonized. In great hostility against the child's father she said that as far as she was concerned Nathaniel's father was dead. She bluntly stated that the child was not wanted. The reasons given were her interest in working and her desire for economic independence. We shall not stress any further her revolt against the maternal status, her revolt against the father as a progenitor, and her identification with his role as a provider.

Despite her marginal income she was able to buy a modest home in a deteriorated city area. She rented out two of her four rooms which included the kitchen. Therefore, Nathaniel had to be moved to her bedroom. She saw fulfilment of her duties in providing for his material well-being.

Nathaniel was breast fed for one month. He was nursed from the bottle at times in bed and at times in the mother's lap. The mother did not remember when he was weaned and how well he accepted the weaning. According to the mother, Nathaniel walked and talked at the age of nine months and was toilet trained before that time. At the age of five, he was sent to school and never made a successful adjustment.

When first seen, Nathaniel was an attractive full-faced boy with expressive large eyes. He was slightly plump and made an infant-like impression. He seemed depressed and timid. His head was sunken into his trunk and his shrunken posture bespoke introjected hostility. He cracked his fingers throughout the major part of the session and at its beginning stroked a rabbit's tail, caressed his cheek with it or leaned the cheek against it. Finally he laid the rabbit's tail around his neck. He seemed to indulge in some magic ritual to judge by the way he proceeded. He repeatedly mentioned that he liked the rabbit's tail. It sometimes brings you luck. Asked what gave him this idea, he answered, "Me believes it by myself." While he talked his eyes wandered around to the toys, but he did not move toward them. When given leisure to play, he made me guess what he wanted to play with. This was his way of finding out whether his choice of bow and arrow was permissible. With a tense contracted mimicry he made the first shots but soon relaxed and expanded joyfully. He was adequate at shooting. An ambulance passing in the street startled him; he tried to ignore it but could not. He laid the back of his hand on his forehead and said, "I don't like the ambulance" and upon inquiry reported that one day he fell down the steps while playing with a car "my daddy gave me." He commented, "I usually call him uncle. I was on the steps and the car rolled on and I fell." Hearing the ambulance still makes him feel "giddy," he said.

When at leisure to leave the room Nathaniel seemed hesitant. When allowed to do as he pleased, he played a war game by himself using helicopter, tanks, and sailors. A great deal of shooting was in process and he constantly talked inaudibly to himself. He also made noises with which children usually accompany the movements of vehicles and engines. He could be heard to repeat, "that is what I wish." Off and on he smiled at me, but he looked worried about his play and placed his head on his hand. He seemed to feel uncomfortable, when he became aware of being watched in his worried condition, as well as in some of his manneristic attitudes which he could not help assuming. Otherwise he enjoyed the therapist's presence and seemed in a rapport with her. This, however, he did not express verbally. His game was structured. He was obviously expert at playing alone.

During the session, a review was made of how Nathaniel spent his lonely days. When he woke up, mother was gone, but he was not alone. There was a man that stayed with them. Nathaniel liked him, but "he never brought me nothing." This man had lived with them ever since Nathaniel was a baby. He was like a daddy. He cleaned up a state building, went to work at 3 P.M. and returned at midnight. The man fixed the breakfast for Nathaniel and himself. They ate together but Nathaniel wished mother were at home. The man and he talked about school, toys, and soldiers. Nathaniel thought he had "some" friends. The uncle he hoped was a friend. The rabbit's tail was given him by a lady in the stores. He hoped it would bring him toys, bow and arrow, a target and an electric train.

After breakfast Nathaniel went to school. He expressed a dislike for his section of town and a liking for his former school. He had been in the fourth grade for three or four weeks. After school, he said, contrary to facts, he went home directly and played by himself. He did not like the children. They fought him "because my mother brings me more things and I have more things than they have. When Christmas comes, I get most every kind of toys and they don't get any kind; I get wagons, guns, some of the things like these here too." He pointed to the toys in the room, "Mother gives it to me. The children know about it because sometimes they stand in front of my door, when I bring them out to play with." He further revealed that he stayed alone until night. He did not like it. But he was not sad. He did not think of mama all the time, "I forget about her when I plays. Mama also got me a dog and I got a bicycle. I liked the dog even better." Sometimes he rode around in the street. He ate dinner when he returned home. "My uncle who stays with us had prepared the dinner, I eat alone, fried chicken sometimes. When mother comes home she does homework, we look at TV and sometimes we have cake and sweet candy. Uncle does some of the housework before she comes home."

Together with another new child, Nathaniel was enrolled in an existing group of five boys age ten to thirteen. (In order not to overburden this report we refrain here from a more complete description of the individual children assembled in this group, and give only a sketchy indication of the background to the reported session.) The oldest, Daniel Miller, was the most dependent, sensitive, and fearful child. Two of the younger children, Johnnie Richard and Johnnie Samuels, were city wards with a history of early and extreme neglect. John Richard was absent that day. They were timid and withdrawn and verbally uncommunicative, contrary to the four others. Two of the boys were deeply hurt and aggressive. One was Marvin who had been regrouped, the other Timothy Laury, the inconsolable son of an institutionalized delinquent father. Two of the children had similar problems to those of Nathaniel. Charles Lofton had, like him, to fulfil precociously the ambitions of a striving family in order to compensate for paternal failure and parental frustration. This boy had been on the verge of a schizophrenic break at the time of referral. He suffered from severe asthma and dissociated from himself a powerful bumblebee, his potent self, capable of doing everything he wanted. Charles was usually greatly elated. He made a show of his importance, but was incapable of any pursued and concentrated endeavor. With a good average ability, he was a non-learner. Daniel Miller was, like Nathaniel, a lonely child who had to wake up every morning in an empty house, for the mother was at work. This child had not even a roomer with whom to share his solitude. He had to prepare his own meals. He was constantly whining and in tears.

In the first session Nathaniel isolated himself from the children. Sitting with his back toward the room, he did clay work, commenting on what he was doing. He tried to attract the psychiatrist's attention and approval. He shaped Lincoln and George Washington and later a few anonymous figures and passed his work on to her. This resulted in the surreptitious decapitation of one of his busts by one of the city wards, who molded one of the kneaded figures into a sculpture of his own. During the following week, Nathaniel tried to impress the children with his dreamed-up status of a child raised in a home where there is a father and a mother and where the social and the educational standards are high. He played the role of a child who is successful in school and talking to the children proffered a few French phrases. Wrestling doggedly in two consecutive sessions, he fought his way into the group. Simultaneously the two withdrawn children became more outgoing and the sensitive and tearful boy more self-assured. Charles artlessly enjoyed looking at the fight. Progress was seen when the children began quite spontaneously to stage their hostility imaginatively in a court session.

In his relationship to the psychiatrist Nathaniel was extremely verbal in expressing in front of the group his appreciation for models used on two occasions. This appeared to be quite natural and artless at first. It seemed likely that he never had models to build and that he was surprised that he got them for nothing, as he said that "we did not even have to pay for them." He made the impression of a child that had to deserve acceptance. Soon the loudly voiced appreciation seemed too obvious to be accepted as spontaneous and artless. I wondered whether such manifestations were expected of him at home. His initial interview was remembered and the toys he treasured as an enviable privilege conveyed upon him by the mother's love and strivings.

From the mother's intake interview and information received from school it seemed that due to the isolation of the mother from the son through all of their days, an isolation resulting from the mother's inclinations and the economic needs of both, a language between them had been established by the medium of material things. The mother's substitutional offerings were avidly snapped up by the boy. To him the generosity with material things became a bait which hooked him. As we know, he tried to shake himself loose. But he also held on to the self-deception that the gifts stood for the unstinted acceptance he longed for. For both mother and son, moreover, toys represented an elevated social status. In the presence of the mother, the educational and emotionally gratifying value of the toys might have been more successfully explored. A child-loving, sensitive mother is likely to have invited the envious little neighbors. Instead of becoming a medium for isolating the two sets of deprived children, the toys could have become a vehicle for sharing and companionship. As it was, the toys became the pacifier of the boy who feared the lonely house and needed it as a refuge, his nursery and his crib. The mother's tendency to keep him calm and content in her absence by means of these pacifiers had invited an arrest of growth, of active and outgoing tendencies and contributed to his poor showing in school. As representatives of a higher standard that artificially raised him above his human environment, these toys also isolated him in school which was his and his neighbors' school. Thus, Nathaniel was also isolated from children who might have been his living and stimulating company for the major part of the mother's daily absence. Nathaniel found an answer to all of these unmet needs in the group sessions in the Clinic.

The following incident shows Nathaniel's response, with a sense of being accepted, to the psychiatrist's serene reaction to provocation.

Upon entering the room with the group, Marvin demanded models in a commanding tone. This was meant to say, "We don't come to see you. We come only for the models." He had every reason to expect that the monthly supply was exhausted and that I would be exposed as the unrewarding mother. Love, as we know, many of these children measure for a-long time by what material things you give them, things that must be a piece of you, hard to get. They must hurt, in the child's mind, the giver from which that piece of himself is cut off. The giver must be willing to sacrifice. Marvin had been placed away from home, at his request, yielding his mother to his stepfather. He had shown lately the tendency to isolate people from each other and constantly attempted to put a wedge between the other children of the group and me. He anticipated that if there were no models, a wealth of resistive defenses would be unleashed. It so happened that a church had given us models for these children to use. Otherwise, we would have coped with the situation by channeling their interest elsewhere. The children grabbed the models like ravenous infants who can bring bottle and mouth together only by atactic attempts.

When the children rushed toward the models, Nathaniel knocked over a toy sideboard and tread to pieces a play dish. I suggested "let's get the things back where they belong before we start playing. Then we won't have to worry about walking on them again." Barely had the children settled down, working on the models, when Nathaniel praised the psychiatrist for being "the best doctor in the whole world." She always knew what the children needed, he commented. The psychiatrist wondered silently whether gratifying these children's needs concretely, she had actually helped them and not become involved with Nathaniel's relationship with his mother. For some time the children worked silently and Nathaniel commented: "Now everybody has calmed down." Daniel responded by saying: "We have our pacifiers." Marvin could not take that without denying them the pacifiers and peace-makers. He made an enormous noise, hammering the hubcaps into his wheels. He did not succeed because he wanted a reason for going on disturbing. I suggested he try to try to tap lightly. Johnnie came to his rescue and stated, "one has to do it that (noisy) way," but he was very obviously tapping on his hubcaps lightly and elegantly.

Then for a long time Nathaniel talked alone. His mother, he said, never "considered" that he might have dropped something (apparently referring to my reaction to his pushing over the doll dishes). "She always thinks I throw things. I can't correct her views, she insists." He cannot talk back because he does not want to go to the "form school." Marvin interjects, "they won't send you to the 'form school' for that." "When mother is tired," Nathaniel pursues, "she is worse. She makes me nervous. She always takes everything a bad way. But honestly I do not throw things because I am mad. It happens because I am nervous. Mother does not keep her promises and when she says something, I always asks her to give her word of honor. Father doesn't say much, but he is not more peaceful, oh no!" Then he quotes his mother as saying "enough is enough, too much will make a dog sick." He asked how many more minutes he had to finish his car. "When I do something" he comments further "I get into a rush, I cannot wait until I get home." Apparently he is eager to show his achievement. This is assumed because he starts to show us how well he can sing and defies everybody to hold the tone as long as he does. He wants to go to Hollywood. People said he had a good voice. "It makes me feel good. In Hollywood no beatings, no people yelling, no policeman any more." He asked me, "would you fight for a girl?" Marvin told him to shut up and not to trust Dr. Riese, to which Nathaniel responded: "That is my business with Dr. Riese" and went on to say, "my boyfriend and I like the same girl. When I was six years old I knocked a boy with a brick. He treated me like a dog. My boyfriend does not react to the brick." Marvin interfered: "he is 'flicted like you." Nathaniel answered "he does it on purpose," meaning to disarm his (Nathaniel's) aggressiveness. "But I have to do something." Johnnie dryly asked whether the girl liked Nathaniel or whether she liked his boyfriend. Meanwhile Marvin had displaced his wheels and instead of looking for them first, he accused someone of having taken them and only then looked and found them.

Johnnie said something to Marvin, whose aggressive hostility is gratifying to him who cannot release it. In response to my question what he said, naturally implying that he talked to all of us, he answered "I talked to him."

Nathaniel then discussed a neighbor who curses constantly and lies, swearing at the same time "it's God's truth." "She will say, 'I will go to church and sin no more as long as I live,' then turns around and do it again right away. Easier said than done," he comments, allegedly quoting his mother. Finally he begins to explore whether the psychiatrist is always the way she was today. She might be different, for instance, to her secretary. The week before, Timothy, who was absent this day, had commented that if the secretary could afford to be without an income, she would not be my slave, possibly revealing and identifying with his father's motives for stealing rather than working.

During the rest of the session the children spoke about what the models meant to them. They liked them, they collected them, they decorated their rooms with them, exposed them on the mantelpiece in the living room; it gave them something to do. They were an escape from resource-lessness and boredom and a structuring of their activity. All of them had done a neat and complete job and had helped each other at the end of the session. Working on a model was their timid, introverted and their emotionally, as well as mentally, reduced way of relating. They thus re-vealed that the model as a pacifier had become an avenue of life, action, and liberation from dependency and the drudgery of an existence under the pressure of necessity. Some measure of spontaneously expressed ap-preciation was evident among all of them and some giving in return for receiving. For Nathaniel the benefit of this session was his coming up with meaningful revelations under the impact of an unexpected lack of irrita-tion and punitiveness from the psychiatrist when he knocked down the sideboard. This impact struck him at a propitious moment.

# Case Summary of Rud Martin

Rud had been referred to two mental hygiene clinics before becoming a patient in the Educational Therapy Center. Three years had elapsed between his first clinic referral and his joining our own Clinic. Actually, Rud did not qualify for either of the two other clinics. Only recommendations were made and not carried out. Nor did they make any provisions for assisting children as lost as Rud, lost in a no-man's land, and as devoid of any experience usually taken for granted. Rud was simply excluded from school and left to his own devices. Reasons for Rud's first clinic referral were irregular school attendance, temper tantrums, extreme shyness, hiding from the teacher, and playing marbles on the classroom floor. The psychologist noted that he was seen in new clothes too big for him and in which he felt uncomfortable.

He was unhappy, self-conscious, sad, inhibited, and rebellious. He was non-spontaneous but mentioned the absence of a father or big brother. His unfamiliarity with objects was noted, in particular with pictures and puzzles. His academic achievement at the age of ten years and four months was on the first grade level, except for arithmetic which was on the second grade level. His mental rating was considered reduced because of his very limited mental environment.

In spite of repeated requests by his mother of the public schools, Rud was left neglected, untaught, and isolated for three whole years. His mother reports that mostly he stayed in bed sleeping until his siblings returned from school. When he got into a brawl with them, the mother sent him into room confinement, thus once more isolating the little boy, deprived all day of opportunity for experience, human company, and communication—almost a Kasper Hauser. Referral to the Educational Therapy Center was made by a policewoman when neighbors had complained about Rud throwing rocks on their premises.

The mother, Mrs. Martin, was a very attractive woman but extremely rigid, lacking in warmth, and the ability to appreciate the negative factors in Rud's life, and to gain insight into his inner experiences. But she did show some ego strength and aggressiveness in following up the policewoman's recommendations immediately, as well as in having repeatedly contacted the schools in the past on his behalf. She came from a broken home and expressed indifference to her father's departure, since at all times it had been the mother who had been the mainstay of the family. She manifested the same overt indifference to her husband's departure, an indifference which, however, covered poorly repressed hostility.

One of our workers who visited the home, in a depressed section of town, noted cramped living quarters, utmost confusion, lack of material objects and of maternal supervision. Another of our workers found the home totally devoid of the bare necessities, including utilities on the coldest days of winter. The door of the unheated home had to be kept open to allow some light to pour in when the worker talked to the mother.

Since then an observation was made in the home of the family eating a chicken breakfast in a picnic-like way (there was no table), from which Rud was excluded, lying in bed alone on the upper floor. No food was offered nor any friendliness shown, nor was he conveyed to the door when he left with our worker. Had the worker failed to get Rud, he would have missed the longed-for camping trip which he enjoyed and from which he benefited, though he left without a blanket or any of the submarginal belongings required.

In respect to this observation Rud's eating habits, as observed in the Clinic, are worth noting. He ate only a few things, liked to eat alone and ate little in the group. He accepted suckers which were distributed to all children but when in need of food he was extremely shy in letting it be known. However, he has felt free to accept gifts from his therapist for gratification of his mental and social growth.

As time went on, it was observed that the mother felt menaced by the opportunities the Educational Therapy Center had to offer Rud, and which unfortunately she was not able to match. Every attempt had been made to help her improve her situation, but she was confronted with insuperable obstacles as, for instance, spending carfare to the employment office (and getting no job), when it could have been used to buy bread. In her despair, Mrs. Martin exposed Rud to renewed danger and promoted a crisis by trying to rule out the "competitor," the Clinic. "My mother does not want me to come to the Center no more, but she has nothing to offer instead," Rud said once.

Rud was born to his mother and Melvin Martin, a laborer. He was not familiar with the fact that his parents were married when he was six months old. The couple separated when Rud was six years old, but the father has been contributing $15 a week to the family's support. A sister, three years younger than Rud, and a brother, five years younger, also sprang from this union; two other children were born to Mrs. Martin and a companion who does not share quarters with the family. The family actually lives with the maternal grandmother. Rud barely ever saw his father; he was said to like his stepbrother's father but has never mentioned him in therapy. In fact Rud has avoided persistently and for a long period of time to talk of his family.

Pregnancy with Rud was normal; birth very difficult. The mother's statement that Rud was a desired baby deserves to be taken with some doubt. He was bottle fed in his crib, never being held or cuddled. It seems entirely possible that lack of attention resulted in Rud's not walking until he was eighteen months and not talking until about the same time.

When Rud entered the Center he was almost completely out of contact with reality, semi-stuporous, a glazed expression in his eyes which were focused on nothing; he was non-verbal. He did not attend regularly because of his lack of contact with reality, his inability to relate or communicate, his anxious sensitivity, and fear of human interaction. At times he must have simply lost himself in autistic play in the street. When he had been at home for several days all progress seemed lost again and he returned to mutism and isolation. In individual treatment he was nursed by sheer togetherness at first. One day he could be observed coming out of his daze suddenly when he saw his therapist approach the porch where he stood. This incipient relation motivated him to attend regularly. He began to play with marbles comfortably within the Clinic, rather than in the street, but still oblivious most of the time of the other children. For months he was perched on trees or on top of the steps of a fire escape stairway, if not totally oblivious of the world, at best only watching the children.

At first he was afraid to enter; then he was able to endure his sessions for only part of the allotted time. He seemed to sit without an awareness of self or his surroundings, suddenly he would awake and run. But the time came when he sensed the psychiatrist's presence with comfort and finally he looked up acknowledging the acceptant attention with a smile. This smile might freeze and appear silly because its spontaneity could not be maintained at first, but it became language and his fond acknowledgment of a treasured community. He began furtively to touch small toys lying on the table and let them go, not knowing what to do with them and afraid of consequences. He began to watch the psychiatrist for her reaction. Communication thus was further established and the child began to smile as though saying, "we understand each other." Gradually his activity became slightly more varied, and subsequently trust in himself and our relation emboldened him to draw houses. The designs, which he refused to color, were so elementary that he remarked about it despondently and soon gave up. However, he was discouraged only in this one area. He began to play with small toy figures hitting one against the other. Inarticulate sounds were uttered and soon he could be asked "what was going on." Since he was unaware of the fact that something could be going on, to question him was arousing him to such an awareness. In the long run he began increasingly to dramatize simple fights or other events, setting them in a world for which available toy buildings and planes were obtained. He began to be interested in the mechanism of certain toys—a wind-up vehicle that played a tune. Rud's demandingness had been huge for some time, but he had been content to absorb the psychiatrist's time as his opportunity for an approach to life. At this time, however, he began to be helped to the point of enjoying life between sessions also. He looked at store displays and asked to be given a guitar. He began to look at television and to identify with Elvis Presley. Music began to appeal to Rud. But he overrated the difficulties of performance and the instrument was soon broken. At this time its function was to reveal maternal gratification, and encouragement was derived from the gift as a token of appreciated dedication. A car with an electric motor was another of his wishes. Slowly Rud brought his own world from the community into these sessions and showed signs that he wanted his relationship with the psychiatrist to be pursued symbolically outside the session and the Clinic. He began to discuss his associations with children in his part of town, as well as the objects needed for help along these associations and joining the children on equal terms; a bicycle was wanted and finally a BB rifle.

The latter wish caused the psychiatrist a great deal of soul-searching. Neither the mother nor the police objected and the responsibility was thrust solely on the psychiatrist and her collaborators.

Rud at this time could plead with few words for trust and proved to be trustworthy. He was surprisingly tactful, considerate, spontaneously realistic, and appreciative in all of his demands as well as positive or negative responses to them. He soon rose to a stage where he wanted to contribute his share of money to the deals he made and requested that the psychiatrist make only part of the investment. He tried and often succeeded in getting his mother to co-operate and provided some money by doing odd jobs himself. When a week-end would pass without his earning his share, he might voluntarily postpone or totally give up fulfilment of his wishes. Irrational responses from him would, at times, have to be conquered. He was so appreciative that he seemed always to feel as though a miracle had occurred to him.

But turning to life exposed him to the danger of perceiving some of its overwhelming pangs from which he had previously withdrawn. This caused him to act out in the group by spitting and cursing and by teasing sibling figures, who, however, increasingly liked him and impressively understood his awkward and frankly negative bids for attention and acceptance. One youngster commented lovingly, "Rud is but a little boy. He wants to play with us and if each of us gives him a little time daily, he'll stop being a nuisance." Turning to life moreover caused him to be increasingly panicky when he had to return home. It put the inadequate mother and grandmother more and more on the defensive.

Rud began to want to be like others and approached us with added resourcefulness and versatility. When the time had passed when he wanted to have toys like others and to manipulate them like others, thus gaining a sense of self and self-esteem, he wanted to be dressed like others and go to church in his respectable attire. He was spontaneously interested in detail, paid attention to the variety of colors, from his pants to the matching of shirt and tie; he wanted a hat for church and a beret for weekdays. He loved the Clinic so dearly that he once walked there two miles protecting himself from a pouring rain by holding a pair of bathing trunks over his head. He would come the two miles on icy winter days, through the snow, wearing torn shoes, with loose soles. He thoroughly enjoyed the shoes that were provided, seeing them above all as a symbol of acceptance and recognition of his human dignity.

But finally Rud realized that further growth and gain in self-respect could not be achieved in his home as it was, nor in the neighborhood. He first worked for an improvement of his own home. He had always spared his mother. His delayed willingness to mention her in therapy was at first motivated by his covering up for himself what was unbearable. He was ashamed and most embarrassed why things should be that way, but he was also tactful and could not easily expose his mother consciously. He asked that his mother move from their section of town. He also had difficulty in overcoming prejudice that had arisen in a year-long interaction between him and the community where he was hurt and marked as a child excluded from school. Both his mother and he needed a change. His choice was a place in the city's housing project close to the Clinic, the place of his rebirth. But although the mother seemed willing to co-operate, things moved entirely too slowly, partly because of reality factors, partly because of an intense inertia of the family to attempt a new adjustment. The mother and grandmother felt uncertain about their ability to meet the requirements of a higher social standard. Finally Rud sensed it and with great emotion verbalized it. He said that both women at home were "crazy" not to desire and work for improvement of their condition.

Rud asked for a second foster home placement with repeated insistence. A previous attempt, made at his request, had failed. Not supported genuinely and wholeheartedly by mother and grandmother, he became panicky when the foster mother pulled another child's arm. In his taciturn way he explained that he felt bad to have deserted the family for the sake of his own salvation. He seemed in extreme fear of some magic punishment, which became an imminent threat when he saw the other child in trouble with the foster mother. This second time he felt he was ready for an adjustment. He needed only a kind foster mother, he said, nothing else. He said he would sacrifice his bad habits of smoking and cursing, since he knew "nobody could take that."

# NOTES

## Introduction

1. D. D. Jackson in Carl A. Whitaker (ed.), *Psychotherapy of Chronic Schizophrenic Patients* (Boston: Little, Brown, & Co., 1958).
2. Theodor Reik, *The Compulsion To Confess* (New York: Farrar, Strauss & Cudahy, 1959).
3. Sol Nichtern, *et al.*, "A Community Educational Program for the Emotionally Disturbed Child" (Paper read at American Orthopsychiatric Convention, New York, March, 1961); W. T. Vaughan and Maxwell Schleifer, *A Day Hospital Program for Certain Psychotic Children* (Waltham, Mass.: Metropolitan State Hospital, NIMH Grant No. OM–34, 1957–60).

## Chapter One

1. Mathew P. Andrews, *Virginia, the Old Dominion* (Richmond, Va.: Dietz Press, n.d.).
2. Wilfred C. Hulse, "Private Practice," in S. R. Slavson (ed.), *Fields of Group Psychotherapy* (New York: International University Press, 1956).

## Chapter Two

1. Erik H. Erikson, "Growth and Crisis of the Healthy Personality," in Clyde Kluckhohn and Henry A. Murray (eds.), *Personality: In Nature, Society, and Culture* (New York: A. A. Knopf, 1956).
2. John Rosen in Carl A. Whitaker (ed.), *Psychotherapy of Chronic Schizophrenic Patients* (Boston: Little, Brown & Co., 1958).
3. D. D. Jackson in Whitaker, *Psychotherapy of Chronic Schizophrenic Patients*.
4. Rene A. Spitz, "Hospitalization: An Inquiry into the Genesis of Psychiatric Conditions of Early Childhood," *Psychoanalytic Study of the Child*, Vol. I (New York: International University Press, 1945).
5. Jurgen Ruesch, "The Infant Personality: The Core Problem of Psychosomatic Medicine," *Psychosomatic Medicine*, X (1948), 134–44.
6. Walter G. Eliasberg, *Psychotherapy and Society* (New York: Philosophical Library, 1959).
7. L. T. Vigotsky, "Thought and Speech," *Psychiatry*, II (1939), 29–52; Walther Riese, "J. Hughlings Jackson's Doctrine of Aphasia and Its Significance Today," *Journal of Nervous and Mental Disease*, CXXII (1955), 1–13.

## Chapter Three

1. Irving Bieber, *et al.*, *Homosexuality: A Psychoanalytic Study of Male Homosexuals* (New York: Basic Books, 1962).

2. Walther Riese, *Principles of Neurology* (Baltimore: Williams & Wilkins, 1950); "An Outline of a History of Ideas in Neurology, *Bulletin of the History of Medicine* (Baltimore, 1949).

3. Relative to this act of giving as well as the stuffing of objects into the back of pants, it is interesting to consider Freud's remark that "Faeces are the child's first gift, the first sacrifice of his affection, a portion of his own body which he is ready to part with, but only for the sake of someone he loves" (Sigmund Freud, *The Problem of Anxiety* [New York: W. W. Norton, 1936]).

4. Sigmund Freud, *Interpretation of Dreams* (New York: Modern Library).

## Chapter Four

1. Erich Fromm, *Escape from Freedom*. (New York and Toronto: Farrar & Rinehart, 1941).

2. Erich Fromm, *The Art of Loving* (New York: Harper & Bros., 1956).

3. Nathan W. Ackerman, *The Psychodynamics of Family Life* (New York: Basic Books, 1958).

## Chapter Five

1. Provided by Mrs. Edythe Allen and Mr. Lawrence Parker.

2. Jack J. Burnette, *et al.*, "Characteristics and Motivations of Thirty-six Single Negro Parents Whose Emotionally Disturbed Children Have Been Seen at the Educational Therapy Center" (unpublished master's thesis, Richmond Professional Institute, 1961).

3. Carl A. Whitaker (ed.), *Psychotherapy of Chronic Schizophrenic Patients* (Boston: Little, Brown & Co., 1958).

4. Burnette, Boston, *et al.*

5. *Ibid.*

6. Benjamin O. Hendricks, *et al.*, "A Study of Characteristics and Motivations of Foster Parents of the Richmond Children's Aid Society, Inc." (unpublished master's thesis, Richmond Professional Institute, 1961.

7. Whitaker, *Psychotherapy of Chronic Schizophrenic Patients*.

## Chapter Six

1. Rene Spitz, *The Psychoanalytic Study of the Child*, Vol. I (New York: International University Press, 1945).

## Chapter Seven

1. Hertha Riese, "Suggestions for the Teaching of Geography," *Virginia Journal of Education*, XXXVII, No. 5, 182 ff.

## Chapter Eight

1. Eric Partridge, *Origins* (New York: Macmillan, 1959).

2. Gaston Bachelard, *La terre et les reveries de la volonté* (Paris: J. Corty, 1948).

## Chapter Nine

1. Sandor Ferenczi, *Contributions to Psychoanalysis* (Boston: Richard C. Badger, 1916).
2. Theodor Reik, *Listening with the Third Ear* (New York: Farrar, Strauss, & Cudahy, 1948).
3. Carl Rogers, "Two Divergent Trends" in Rollo May (ed.), *Existential Psychology* (New York: Random House, 1961).
4. Gaston Bachelard, *La terre et les reveries du repos* (Paris: J. Corty, 1948).

## Chapter Eleven

1. Irving Kaufman, "Crimes of Violence," *Journal of the American Academy of Child Psychiatry*, I, No. 2, 277.
2. August Aichhorn, *Wayward Youth* (New York: Meridian, 1955); Kate Friedlander, "Antisocial Character," *Psychoanalytic Study of the Child*, Vol. I (New York: International University Press, 1945).
3. Trigant Burrow, *The Neurosis of Man* (New York: Harcourt, Brace & Co., 1949).
4. Erik H. Erikson, *Childhood and Society* (New York: W. W. Norton, 1950).

## Chapter Twelve

1. Charlotte Buhler, quoted in Rene Spitz, *A Genetic Field Theory of Ego Formation* (New York: International University Press, 1959).
2. Hertha Riese, "Educational Therapy for Problem Children," *Virginia Journal of Education*, XXXVI, No. 6, 222–27.
3. Hertha Riese, "Suggestions for the Teaching of Geography," *Virginia Journal of Education*, XXXVII, No. 5, 182–83.
4. Hertha Riese, "Reading Difficulties Explained by Analysis of the Reading Process and Suggestions for Improvement of the Teaching Method" (paper read before the Virginia Academy of Science, May, 1948).
5. Edgar Rubin, *Visuell wahrgenommene Figuren* (Copenhagen, 1931).
6. Walther Riese, "J. Hughlings Jackson's Doctrine of Aphasia and Its Significance Today," *Journal of Nervous and Mental Disease*, CXXII (1955), 1–13.

## Chapter Thirteen

1. C. J. Kilczweski, "The Half-way House and Its Place in Rehabilitating the Mentally Handicapped," *Virginia Medical Journal*, Vol. LXXXIII, No. 11.
2. Lawrence S. Kubie, "Say You Are Sorry," *Psychoanalytic Study of the Child*, Vol. X (New York: International University Press, 1955).
3. Warren T. Vaughan and Maxwell Schleifer, *A Day Hospital Program for Certain Psychotic Children* (Waltham, Mass.: Metropolitan State Hospital,

NIMH Grant No. OM–34, 1957–60).

4. J. Ragufrey, "Les Carences psychiques du permier age," *Semaine Medicale, professionnelle, et medico-sociale*, January 14, 1956.

*Chapter Fourteen*

1. Franz Alexander and Helen Ross (eds.), *Dynamic Psychiatry* (Chicago: University of Chicago Press, 1952); Nathan Ackerman, *The Psychodynamics of Family Life* (New York: Basic Books, 1958).

2. Edward Glover, *Techniques of Psychoanalysis* (New York: International University Press, 1955).

3. *Ibid.*

4. Haim Ginott, *Group Psychotherapy with Children* (New York: McGraw-Hill Co., Inc., 1961).

5. *Ibid.*

6. Maxwell S. Jones, "The Therapeutic Community" (unpublished data).

7. Fritz Redl and David Wineman, *Children Who Hate* (Glencoe, Ill.: Free Press, 1951).

8. M. A. Sechehaye, *Symbolic Realization* (New York: International University Press, 1952).

9. August Aichhorn, *Wayward Youth* (New York: Meridian, 1955).

10. Rene Spitz, *A Genetic Field Theory of Ego Formation* (New York: International University Press, 1959).

11. Hans A. E. Driesch, *Science and Philosophy of the Organism* (Gifford Lectures, 1907–8).

# COLLATERAL READING

*Preface*

NASH, HARVEY. "Freud and Metaphor," *General Psychiatry*, VII, 25–30.

*Introduction*

AICHHORN, AUGUST. *Wayward Youth*. New York: Viking Press, 1945.

ALGER, IAN. "Therapy with Schizophrenic Patients," *American Journal of Orthopsychiatry*, XXX (July, 1960), 521–24.

ANDERSON, FOREST N., and H. C. DEAN. "Some Aspects of Child Guidance Intake Policy and Practices," *Public Health Monograph* No. 42. Washington, D.C.: Department of Health, Education and Welfare, 1956.

BETTELHEIM, BRUNO. *Love Is Not Enough*. Glencoe, Ill.: Free Press, 1950.

———. *Truant from Life*. Glencoe, Ill.: Free Press, 1955.

BOWLBY, JOHN. *Maternal Care and Mental Health*. Geneva: World Health Organization, 1952.

DEVEREUX, GEORGE. *Therapeutic Education*. New York: Harper & Bros., 1956.

GOLDFARB, W. "Report on Henry Ittleson Center for Child Research, Bronx, New York." N.d.

JONES, CHARLES H. "A Day-Care Program for Adolescents in a Private Hospital." Unpublished.

KARPMAN, BEN, *et al. Child and Juvenile Delinquency*. Washington, D.C.: University Press of Washington, D.C., 1960.

LA VIETIES, RUTH, WILFRED C. HULSE, and ABRAM BLAU. "A Psychiatric Day Care Center and School for Young Children and Their Parents," *American Journal of Orthopsychiatry*, XXX, 468–82.

NEILL, A. S. *Summerhill*. New York: Hart Publishing Co., Inc., 1960.

NEWMAN, RUTH G., CHRISTOPHER FEAGRE, and FLORENCE GLASER. *The Assessment of Progress in the Treatment of Learning Disturbances of Hyper-Aggressive Children within a School Setting*. New York: National Institute of Mental Health, Child Research Branch, 1958/59.

NICHTERN, SOL, *et al.* "Community Educational Program for the Emotionally Disturbed Child." American Orthopsychiatric Convention, New York, March, 1961.

REDL, FRITZ, and DAVID WINEMAN. *The Aggressive Child*. 2 v. Glencoe, Ill.: Free Press, 1957.

RIESE, HERTHA. "Psychiatric Approach in Educational Therapy with Emotionally Disturbed Children," *Journal of the American Women's Association*, XII, 369–76.

———. "Educational Therapy: A New Approach in Child Guidance," *Psychiatry, Journal for the Study of Interpersonal Processes*, XIII, 465–88.

———. "Educational Therapy: A Methodical Approach to the Problems of the Untreatable Child," *Group Psychotherapy*, XII, 58–66.

VAUGHAN, W. T., and MAXWELL SCHLEIFER. *A Day Hospital Program for*

*Certain Psychotic Children.* Waltham, Mass.: Metropolitan State Hospital, NIMH Grant No. OM–34, 1957–60.

WITMER, HELEN LELAND. *Psychiatric Interviews with Children.* Cambridge: Harvard University Press, 1952.

### Chapter Two

ALEXANDER, FRANZ, and W. HEALY. *Roots of Crime.* New York: Alfred A. Knopf, 1935.

PIAGET, JEAN. *Language and Thought of the Child.* New York: Humanities Press, 1955.

REDL, FRITZ, and DAVID WINEMAN. *Children Who Hate.* Glencoe. Ill.: Free Press, 1951.

SPITZ, RENE. *Genetic Field Theory of Ego Formation.* New York: International University Press, 1957.

SULLIVAN, H. S. "Language of Schizophrenics," in J. S. KASANIN (ed.), *Language and Thought in Schizophrenia.* Berkeley: University of California, 1944.

WHITAKER, CARL A., *et al. Psychotherapy of Chronic Schizophrenic Patients.* Boston: Little, Brown & Co., 1958.

### Chapter Three

BOYER, L. BRYCE. "Maternal Overstimulation and Ego Defects," *Psychoanalytic Study of the Child,* XI, 236–57.

BENNETT, IVY. *Delinquent and Neurotic Children.* New York: Basic Books, 1960.

DAVIDSON, SUSANNAH. "School Phobias as a Manifestation of Family Disturbance: Its Structure and Treatment." Unpublished.

KARPMAN, BEN, *et al. Child and Juvenile Delinquency.* Washington, D.C.: University Press of Washington, D.C., 1960.

RIESE, WALTHER. *Principles of Neurology in the Light of History; and Their Present Use.* Baltimore: Williams & Wilkins, 1950.

WILLIAMS, JESSIE M. "Children Who Break Down in Foster Homes: A Psychological Study of Personality Patterns of Grossly Deprived Children," *Journal of Child Psychology and Psychiatry,* II, 5–20.

### Chapter Four

AICHHORN, AUGUST. *Wayward Youth.* New York: Viking Press, 1945.

ANSHEN, RUTH NANDA. "The Family in Transition," in *The Family.* New York: Harper & Bros., 1959.

BOWLBY, JOHN. "Separation Anxiety: A Critical Review of the Literature," *Journal of Child Psychology and Psychiatry,* I, 251–69.

BURNETTE, JACK J., *et al.* "Characteristics and Motivations of Thirty-six Single Negro Parents Whose Emotionally Disturbed Children Have Been Seen at the Educational Therapy Center between July 1955 and September 1960." Unpublished Master's thesis, Richmond Professional Institute, 1961.

CEVON, RUTH SHAPLE. "Negro Family Disorganization and Juvenile Delinquency," *Journal of Negro Education,* XXVIII, 230–39.

DEUTSCH, HELENE. *Psychology of Women.* 2 v. New York: Grune & Stratton, 1945.

ERIKSON, ERIK H. *Childhood and Society.* New York: W. W. Norton, 1950.

FENICHEL, OTTO. *Psychoanalytic Theory of Neurosis.* New York: W. W. Norton, 1945.

FRAZIER, E. FRANKLIN. *The Negro Family in the United States.* New York: Macmillan, 1949.

FREUDENTHAL, KURT. "Problems of the One-Parent Family," *Social Work,* IV, 44–48.

FROMM, ERIC. *Escape from Freedom.* New York and Toronto: Farrar & Rinehart, 1947.

HEALY, W. *Mental Conflict and Misconduct.* Boston: Little, Brown & Co., 1921.

SILVERBERG, WILLIAM V. *Childhood Experience and Personal Destiny.* New York: Springer Publishing Co., Inc., 1952.

SPITZ, RENE. *No and Yes: On the Genesis of Human Communication.* New York: International University Press, 1957.

## Chapter Five

ACKERMAN, NATHAN W. *The Psychodynamics of Family Life.* New York: Basic Books, 1958.

ALPERT, AUGUSTA. "Reversibility of Pathological Fixations Associated with Maternal Deprivation in Infancy," *Psychoanalytic Study of the Child,* XIV, 169–85.

BASAMANIA, BETTY W. "The Family as the Unit of Study and Treatment," *American Journal of Orthopsychiatry,* XXXI (Jan., 1961), 74–85.

BELL, ANITA. "The Role of Parents," in SANDOR LORAND and HENRY SCHNEER (eds.), *Adolescents: Psychoanalytic Perspectives.* New York: Harper & Bros., 1961.

BERES, D., and S. OBERS. "The Effects of Extreme Deprivation in Infancy on Psychic Structure in Adolescence; A Study in Ego Development," *Psychoanalytic Study of the Child,* V, 212–35.

BOWEN, MURRAY. "Family Psychotherapy," *American Journal of Orthopsychiatry,* XXXI (Jan., 1961), 40–60.

BOYER, L. BRYCE. "Maternal Overstimulation and Ego Defects," *Psychoanalytic Study of the Child,* XI, 236–57.

BURLINGHAM, DOROTHY T. "Handling of Mother-Child Relationships," *Psychoanalytic Study of the Child,* VI, 31–37.

BUXBAUM, EDITH. "Transference and Group Formation," *Psychoanalytic Study of the Child,* I, 351–65.

CEVON, RUTH SHAPLE. "Negro Family Disorganization and Juvenile Delinquency," *Journal of Negro Education,* XXVIII, 230–39.

EISSLER, K. R. "Ego-Psychological Implications of the Psychoanalytic Treatment of Delinquents," *Psychoanalytic Study of the Child,* V, 97–121.

FRAZIER, E. FRANKLIN. *The Negro Family in the United States.* New York: Macmillan, 1949.

FRIEDLANDER, KATE. "Formation of the Antisocial Character," *Psychoanalytic Study of the Child,* I, 189–203.

COLLATERAL READING

FREUD, ANNA. "Child Observation and Prediction," *Psychoanalytic Study of the Child*, XIII, 92–124.

FREUDENTHAL, KURT. "Problems of the One-Parent Family," *Social Work*, IV, 44–48.

GELEERD, ELIZABETH R. "Borderline States in Childhood and Adolescence," *Psychoanalytic Study of the Child*, XIII, 279–95.

GREENACRE, PHYLLIS. *Trauma, Growth, and Personality*. New York: W. W. Norton, 1952.

GROTJAHN, MARTIN. *The Psychoanalytic Treatment of the Family*. New York: W. W. Norton, 1959.

KARPMAN, BEN, et al. *Child and Juvenile Delinquency*. Washington, D.C.: University Press of Washington, D.C., 1960.

MASSERMAN, JULES H. *Individual and Familial Dynamics*. New York: Grune & Stratton, 1959.

MEYERS, M., and W. GOLDFARB. "Studies of Perplexity in Mothers of Schizophrenic Children," *American Journal of Orthopsychiatry*, XXXI (July, 1961), 551–64.

RANK, BEATA, and DOROTHY MacNAUGHTON. "A Clinical Contribution to Early Ego Development;" *Psychoanalytic Study of the Child*, V, 53–65.

SANDLER, ANNE MARIE, ELIZABETH DAUNTON, and ANNELIESE SCHNURMANN. "Inconsistency in the Mother as a Factor in Character Development: A Comparative Study of Three Cases," *Psychoanalytic Study of the Child*, XII, 202–25.

SCHEIDLINGER, SAUL, and MARJORY PYRKE. "Group Therapy of Women with Severe Dependency Problems," *American Journal of Orthopsychiatry*, XXXI (Oct., 1961), 776–85.

SPITZ, RENE. "Anaclitic Depression," *Psychoanalytic Study of the Child*, II, 313–42.

———. "Psychogenic Diseases in Infancy," *Psychoanalytic Study of the Child*, VI, 255–75.

SPITZ, RENE, and M. WOLF. "Autoeroticism," *Psychoanalytic Study of the Child*, III/IV, 85–120.

## Chapter Six

ACKERMAN, NATHAN W. *The Psychodynamics of Family Life*. New York: Basic Books, 1958.

DAVIS, MAXINE. *Sex and the Adolescent*. New York: Dial Press, Inc., 1958.

DEUTSCH, HELENE. *Psychology of Women*. 2 v. New York: Grune & Stratton, 1945.

ERIKSON, ERIK H. "Growth and Crisis of the Healthy Personality," in CLYDE KLUCKHOHN and HENRY A. MURRAY (eds.), *Personality: In Nature, Society, and Culture*. New York: A. A. Knopf, 1953.

FROMM, ERIC. *The Art of Loving*. Ed. by RUTH NANDA ANSHEN. New York: Harper & Bros., 1956.

NEILL, A. S. *Summerhill*. New York: Hart Publishing Co., Inc., 1960.

WITTENBERG, RUDOLPH. *Adolescence and Discipline*. New York: Association Press, 1959.

## Chapter Seven

ARTHUR, HELEN. "A Comparison of the Techniques Employed in Psychotherapy and Psychoanalysis of Children," *American Journal of Orthopsychiatry*, XII, 484–98.

AXLINE, VIRGINIA MAE. *Play Therapy*. Boston: Houghton Mifflin Co., 1947.

GELEERD, ELIZABETH R. "Borderline States in Childhood and Adolescence," *Psychoanalytic Study of the Child*, XIII, 279–95.

GINOTT, HAIM. *Group Psychotherapy with Children*. New York: McGraw-Hill Book Co., 1961.

GREENACRE, PHYLLIS. "Play in Relation to Creative Imagination," *Psychoanalytic Study of the Child*, XIV, 61–80.

KRIS, ERNST. "Neutralization and Sublimation," *Psychoanalytic Study of the Child*, X, 30–46.

LEBO, DELL. "A Formula for Selecting Toys for Non-Directive Therapy," *Journal of Genetic Psychology*, XCII, 23–34.

PELLER, LILI. "Libidinal Phases, Ego Development, and Play," *Psychoanalytic Study of the Child*, IX, 178–97.

MORENO, J. L. *Psychodrama*. Boston: Beacon Press, 1946.

MOUSTAKAS, CLARK E. *Children in Play Therapy*. New York: McGraw-Hill Book Co., Inc., 1953.

RAMBERT, MADELEINE. *Children in Conflict*. New York: International University Press, 1949.

RANK, BEATA, and DOROTHY MACNAUGHTON. "A Clinical Contribution to Early Ego Development," *Psychoanalytic Study of the Child*, V, 53–65.

SLAVSON, S. R. *An Introduction to Group Therapy*. Cambridge: Harvard University Press, 1943.

SPITZ, RENE. "Anaclitic Depression," *Psychoanalytic Study of the Child*, II, 313–42.

WAELDER, R. "The Psychoanalytic Theory of Play," *Psychoanalytic Quarterly*, II, 208–24.

WILSON, GERTRUDE, and GLADYS RYLAND. *Social Group Work Practice*. Boston: Houghton Mifflin, 1949.

## Chapter Nine

CASSIRER, ERNST. *Language and Myth*. New York: Harper & Bros., 1946.

DECORDES, V. "Le Jardin d'enfants a l'Ecole Decroly." Comité d'iniative pour la renovation de l'enseignment en Belgique, 1952.

———. *Le Docteur Decroly et quelques uns de ses principes educatifs*. Uccle-Bruxelles, 1947.

ENELOW, A. J. "The Silent Patient," *Psychiatry*, XVIII, 153–58.

EISSLER, RUTH, et al. *Psychoanalytic Study of the Child*, Vol. I. New York: International University Press, 1945.

KASANIN, J. S. *Language and Thought in Schizophrenia*. Berkeley: University of California Press, 1944.

PARKER, BEULAH. *My Language Is Me*. New York: Basic Books, 1962.

PIAGET, JEAN. *Language and Thought of the Child*. New York: Humanities Press, 1955.

REUSCH, JURGEN. "Non-Verbal Language and Therapy," *Psychiatry*, XVIII, 323–30.

## Chapter Ten

BACHELARD, GASTON. *La terre et les reveries du repos*. Paris: J. Corty, 1948.
BENDER, L., and H. YARNELL. "An Observation Nursery," *American Journal of Psychiatry*, XCVII, 1158–74.
BERES, DAVID. "Ego Deviation and the Concept of Schizophrenia," *Psychoanalytic Study of the Child*, XI, 164–235.
BETTELHEIM, BRUNO, and EMMY SYLVESTER. "A Therapeutic Milieu," *American Journal of Orthopsychiatry*, XXII, 314–34.
DEUTSCH, HELENE. *Psychology of Women*. 2 v. New York: Grune & Stratton, 1945.
EISSLER, K. R. "Ego-Psychological Implications of the Psychoanalytic Treatment of Delinquents," *Psychoanalytic Study of the Child*, V, 97–121.
FREUD, ANNA. "Psychoanalysis and Education," *Psychoanalytic Study of the Child*, IX, 9–15.
———. "Child Observation and Prediction," *Psychoanalytic Study of the Child*, XIII, 92–124.
FRIEDLANDER, KATE. "The Formation of the Antisocial Character," *Psychoanalytic Study of the Child*, I, 189–203.
FROMM-REICHMANN, FREIDA. *Principles of Intensive Psycotherapy*. Chicago: University of Chicago Press, 1950.
GELEERD, ELIZABETH R. "Some Aspects of Psychoanalytic Technique in Adolescence," *Psychoanalytic Study of the Child*, XII, 263–83.
KRIS, ERNST, *et al.* "Problems of Infantile Neurosis," *Psychoanalytic Study of the Child*, IX, 16–71.
KULKA, ANNA, CAROL FRY, and FRED J. GOLDSTEIN. "Kinesthetic Needs in Infancy," *American Journal of Orthopsychiatry*, XXX (July, 1960), 562–71.
MAHLER, MARGARET SCHOENBERGER. "On Child Psychosis and Schizophrenia," *Psychoanalytic Study of the Child*, VII, 286–305.
MEERLOO, JOOST A. M. *The Two Faces of Man*. New York: International University Press, 1954.
MULLAN, H., and I. SANGUILIANO. "The Discovery of Existential Components Inherent in Contemporary Psychotherapy," *Journal of Existential Psychiatry*, III (1960), 330–45.
RANK, BEATA, and DOROTHY MacNAUGHTON. "A Clinical Contribution to Early Ego Development," *Psychoanalytic Study of the Child*, V, 53–65.
RAUSCH, H. L., and E. S. BORDIN. "Warmth in Personality Development and in Psychotherapy," *Psychiatry*, XX (1957), 351–63.
SYLVESTER, EMMY. "Discussions of Techniques Used To Prepare Young Children for Analysis," *Psychoanalytic Study of the Child*, VII, 306–21.
WEIGERT, EDITH. "The Nature of Sympathy in the Art of Psychotherapy," *Psychiatry*, XXIV (1961), 187–96.

## Chapter Eleven

BALDWIN, A. L., J. KALHORN, and F. H. BREECE. "Patterns of Parent Behavior," *Psychological Monograph* No. 58 (1945).

BETTELHEIM, BRUNO. *Love Is Not Enough.* Glencoe, Ill.: Free Press, 1950.
————. *Truants from Life.* Glencoe, Ill.: Free Press, 1955.
DEVEREUX, GEORGE. *Therapeutic Education.* New York: Harper & Bros., 1956.
EISSLER, K. R. "Ego-Psychological Implications of the Psychoanalytic Treat-
ment of Delinquents," *Psychoanalytic Study of the Child,* V, 97–121.
JACKSON, EDITH B., ETHELYN KLATSKIN, and LOUISE C. WILKIN. "Early Child
Development in Relation to Degree of Flexibility of Maternal Attitude,"
*Psychoanalytic Study of the Child,* VII, 393–428.
NEILL, A. S. *Summerhill.* New York: Hart Publishing Co., 1960.
PEARSON, GERALD H. J. *Adolescence and the Conflict of Generations.* New
York: W. W. Norton, 1958.
PIAGET, JEAN. *The Language and Thought of the Child.* New York: Humanities
Press, 1955.
POLLACK, OTTO. *Social Science and Psychotherapy for Children.* New York:
Russell Sage Foundation, 1952.
RADKE, M. J. *The Relation of Parental Authority to Children's Behavior and
Attitudes.* Minneapolis: University of Minnesota Press, 1946.
RANK, BEATA, and DOROTHY MACNAUGHTON. "A Clinical Contribution to Early
Ego Development," *Psychoanalytic Study of the Child,* V, 53–65.
REDL, FRITZ. "Strategy and Techniques of the Life Space Interview" (from the
Life Space Interview Workshop, 1957), *American Journal of Orthopsychia-
try,* XXIX, 1–18.
ROBINSON, J. FRANKLIN. "Psychotherapy of Adolescents at School Plus In-
patient Treatment," in BENJAMIN H. BALSER (ed.), *Psychotherapy of the
Adolescent.* New York: International University Press, 1957.
WATSON, R. I. *Psychology of the Child.* New York: Wiley & Sons, 1959.
WHITING, J. W. M., and I. L. CHILD. *Child Training and Personality.* New Ha-
ven: Yale University Press, 1953.
WITTENBERG, RUDOLPH. *Adolescence and Discipline.* New York: Association
Press, 1959.

*Chapter Twelve*

BLANCHARD, PHYLLIS. "Psychoanalytic Contributions to the Problems of Read-
ing Disabilities," *Psychoanalytic Study of the Child,* II, 163–87.
DEVEREUX, GEORGE. *Therapeutic Education.* New York: Harper & Bros., 1956.
COLVIN, RALPH W. "An Educational Program in Residential Treatment," *Amer-
ican Journal of Orthopsychiatry,* Vol. XXXI (July, 1961).
EISSLER, RUTH, et al. *The Psychoanalytic Study of the Child,* Vols. VII, XI.
New York: International University Press,
FREUD, ANNA, and DOROTHY T. BURLINGTON. *War and Children.* New York: In-
ternational University Press, 1943.
GALLIEN, LIBOIS-FONTEYNE, CLARET. *Initiation à la method Decroly.* Uccle-
Bruxelles, 1946.
NAMNUM, ALFREDO, and ERNST PRELINGER, "On Psychology of the Reading
Process," *American Journal of Orthopsychiatry,* Vol. XXXI (July, 1961).
PEARSON, GERALD H. J. *Psychoanalysis and the Education of the Child.* New
York: W. W. Norton, 1954.
PELLER, LILI. "The School's Role in Promoting Sublimation," *Psychoanalytic
Study of the Child,* XI, 437–49.

COLLATERAL READING

PIAGET, JEAN. *The Origins of Intelligence in Children*. New York: International University Press, 1952.

———. *The Judgment and Reasoning of the Child*. New York: Littlefield, 1959.

———. *Language and Thought of the Child*. New York: Humanities Press, 1959.

———. *The Construction of Reality in the Child*. New York: Basic Books, 1960.

———. *The Child's Conception of Number*. New York: Humanities Press, 1960.

RABINOW, BARNEY. "An Agenda of Educators in Residential Settings," *American Journal of Orthopsychiatry*, Vol. XXXI (July, 1961).

SYLVESTER, EMMY, and M. S. KUNST. "Psychodynamic Aspects of the Reading Problem," *American Journal of Orthopsychiatry*, XIII, 69–76.

WILSON, GERTRUDE, and GLADYS RYLAND. *Social Group Work Practice*. Boston: Houghton Mifflin, 1949.

WITMER, HELEN LELAND. *Psychiatric Interviews with Children*. Cambridge: Harvard University Press, 1946.

*Chapter Thirteen*

BENDA, C. E. "The Existential Approach in Psychiatry," *Journal of Existential Psychiatry*, I, 24–40.

BETTELHEIM, BRUNO. *Love Is Not Enough*. Glencoe, Ill.: Free Press, 1950.

BETTELHEIM, BRUNO, and EMMY SYLVESTER. "A Therapeutic Milieu," *American Journal of Orthopsychiatry*, XXII, 314–34.

ENELOW, A. J. "The Silent Patient," *Psychiatry*, XXIII, 153–58.

FRIEDLANDER, KATE. "Formation of the Antisocial Character," *Psychoanalytic Study of the Child*, I, 189–203.

FROMM-REICHMANN, FRIEDA. *Principles of Intensive Psychotherapy*. Chicago: University of Chicago Press, 1950.

LIDZ, T. *et al.* "The Intrafamilial Environment of the Schizophrenic Patient: I. The Father," *Psychiatry*, XX, 329–42.

LU, YI-CHUANG. "Mother-Child Relationships in Schizophrenia," *Psychiatry*, XXIV, 133–42.

LYKETOS, G. L. "On the Formation of Mother-Daughter Symbiotic Relationship Patterns in Schizophrenia," *Psychiatry*, XXII, 161–66.

MONTAGU, M. F. A. "Human Nature and Religion," *Journal of Existential Psychiatry*, IV, 441–54.

MORENO, J. L. *Group Psychotherapy: A Symposium*. Boston: Beacon Press, Inc., 1945.

MULLAN, H., and I. SANGUILIANO. "The Discovery of Existential Components Inherent in Contemporary Psychotherapy," *Journal of Existential Psychiatry*, III, 330–45.

MOUSTAKAS, C. E. "Confrontation and Encounter," *Journal of Existential Psychiatry*, VII, 263–90.

RAUSH, H. L., and E. S. BORDIN, "Warmth in Personality Development and in Psychotherapy," *Psychiatry*, XX, 351–63.

RIOCH, D. McK., and A. H. STANTON. "Milieu Therapy," *Psychiatry*, XVI, 65–72.

RUESCH, JURGEN. "Non-Verbal Language and Therapy," *Psychiatry*, XVIII, 323–30.

SCHER, J. M. "The Concept of Self in Schizophrenia," *Journal of Existential Psychiatry*, I, 64–88.

STRUPP, H. H. "Toward an Analysis of the Therapist's Contribution to the Treatment Process," *Psychiatry*, XXII, 349–62.

VARGUS, M. J. "Some Observations on Knowing," *Journal of Existential Psychiatry*, VI, 231–36.

WEIGERT, EDITH. "The Nature of Sympathy in the Art of Psychotherapy," *Psychiatry*, XXIV, 187–96.

*Chapter Fourteen*

AUBREY, J. "The Effects of Lack of Maternal Care," in GERALD CAPLAN, *Emotional Problems of Early Childhood*. New York: Basic Books, 1955.

BELL, JOHN E. *Family Group Therapy*. U.S. Public Monograph, No. 64.

BELLAK, LEOPOLD, and BERTRAM J. BLACK. "The Rehabilitation of Psychotics in the Community," *American Journal of Orthopsychiatry*, XXX, 346–55.

BERGER, M. M. "Non-Verbal Communicants in Group Therapy," *International Journal of Group Therapy*, VIII, 161.

BIDDLE, SYDNEY. "Transference in Dealing with Delinquents," *American Journal of Orthopsychiatry*, III, 14–25.

BRESS, R. B. "The Family Unit in Group Psychotherapy," *International Journal of Group Therapy*, IV, 393.

BUXBAUM, EDITH. "Technique of Child Therapy," *Psychoanalytic Study of the Child*, IX, 297–333.

EISSLER, K. R. "Ego-Psychological Implications of the Psychoanalytic Treatment of Delinquents," *Psychoanalytic Study of the Child*, V, 97–121.

FABIAN, A. A. "Group Treatment of Chronic Patients in a Child Guidance Clinic," *International Journal of Group Therapy*, IV, 243.

FRAIBERG, SELMA. "Some Considerations in the Introduction to Therapy in Puberty," *Psychoanalytic Study of the Child*, X, 264–86.

FREEDMAN, M. B., and B. S. SWEET. "Some Specific Features of Group Psychotherapy and Their Implications for Selection of Patients," *International Journal of Group Therapy*, IV, 355.

FRIED, EDRITA. "Ego Emancipation of Adolescents through Group Therapy," *International Journal of Group Therapy*, VI, 358.

FRIEDLANDER, KATE. *The Psychoanalytic Approach to Juvenile Delinquency*. London: Routledge & Kegan Paul, 1959.

GREENACRE, PHYLLIS. *Trauma, Growth, and Personality*. New York: W. W. Norton, 1952.

GRINKER, ROY, *et al. Psychiatric Social Work*. New York: Basic Books, 1961.

KUBIE, LAWRENCE, and HYMAN A. ISRAEL. "Say You Are Sorry," *Psychoanalytic Study of the Child*, X, 289–99.

MAIER, H. W., and E. A. LOOMIS, JR. "Effecting Impulse Control in Children through Group Therapy," *International Journal of Group Therapy*, IV, 312.

MARCUS, W. R. "Psychoanalytic Group Therapy with Fathers of Emotionally Disturbed Pre-School Children," *International Journal of Group Therapy*, VI, 61.

MILLER, A. A. "Diagnostic Evaluation for Determining the Use of Psychiatric

Resources or Family Casework Resources," *American Journal of Ortho-psychiatry*, Vol. XXXI (July, 1961).

MORROW, TARLTON, and EARL A. LOOMIS. "Symbiotic Aspects of a Seven-Year-Old," in GERALD CAPLAN, *Emotional Problems of Early Childhood*. New York: Basic Books, 1955.

PELLER, LILI. "Libidinal Phases, Ego Development, and Play," *Psychoanalytic Study of the Child*, IX, 178–97.

SLAVSON, S. R. "The Nature and Treatment of Acting Out in Group Psychotherapy," *International Journal of Group Therapy*, VI, 3.

STRANCHAN, H., C. SCHWASTMANN, and E. ATKINS. "Active Group Therapy with Emotionally Disturbed and Delinquent Adolescents," *International Journal of Group Therapy*, VII, 425.

*Appendix*

DEUTSCH, HELENE. *Psychology of Women*. 2 v. New York: Grune & Stratton, 1945.

FRIEDLANDER, KATE. "Formation of the Antisocial Character," *Psychoanalytic Study of the Child*, I, 189–203.

WEISMAN, AVERY D. "Silence and Psychotherapy," *Psychiatry*, XVIII, 241–60.

# INDEX